THE AIDS READER
Social, Political, Ethical Issues

The comprehensive collection of writings about the AIDS crisis encompasses a wide range of timely issues and debates—from Anthony Fauci's "The Human Immuno-deficiency virus," which offers a clear and concise examination of the latest biological facts, to June Osborn's "Prevention: Can We Mobilize What Has Been Learned?", an address to the 1988 International AIDS Conference which stresses that the rapid advances of science must be matched by increased public understanding and commitment to fight discrimination against the affected. The many facets of the social context of AIDS are explored in essays such as Larry Kramer's "The Plague Years" and Kathyrn Anastos and Carola Marte's "Women—The Missing Persons in the AIDS Epidemic." Complicated ethical issues such as the role individual privacy plays in AIDS policy are examined here, as are the special problems of populations at risk confronting an overburdened and unresponsive health care system. These are informative, thought-provoking writings that illuminate one of the most important issues of our day.

NANCY F. MCKENZIE, Ph.D., is a philosopher and human rights activist who is currently the executive director of the Health Policy Advisory Center (Health/AC), an independent national organization that focuses on health care delivery in America. McKenzie teaches philosophy at the New School for Social Research. She is the editor of *The Crisis in Health Care: Ethical Issues,* available in a Meridian edition. She lives in New York City.

THE
AIDS
READER

SOCIAL, POLITICAL,
AND
ETHICAL ISSUES

EDITED BY

NANCY F. MCKENZIE, PH.D.

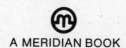

A MERIDIAN BOOK

MERIDIAN
Published by the Penguin Group
Penguin Books USA Inc., 375 Hudson Street,
New York, New York 10014, U.S.A.
Penguin Books Ltd, 27 Wrights Lane,
London W8 5TZ, England
Penguin Books Australia Ltd, Ringwood,
Victoria, Australia
Penguin Books Canada Ltd, 2801 John Street,
Markham, Ontario, Canada L3R 1B4
Penguin Books (N.Z.) Ltd, 182-190 Wairau Road,
Auckland 10, New Zealand

Penguin Books Ltd, Registered Offices:
Harmondsworth, Middlesex, England

First published by Meridian, an imprint of New American Library, a
division of Penguin Books USA Inc.

First Printing, April, 1991
10 9 8 7 6 5 4 3 2 1

REGISTERED TRADEMARK—MARCA REGISTRADA

Library of Congress Cataloging-in-Publication Data

The AIDS reader : social, political, ethical issues / edited by Nancy
  F. McKenzie.
        p.   cm.
      Includes bibliographical references.
      ISBN 0-452-01072-1
      1. AIDS (Disease)—Social aspects.   2. AIDS (Disease)—Political
  aspects.   3. AIDS (Disease)—Moral and ethical aspects.
  I. McKenzie, Nancy F.
  RC607.A26A348914   1991
  362.1′969792—dc20   90-20125
                                                   CIP

PRINTED IN THE UNITED STATES OF AMERICA
Set in Century Book
Designed by Leonard Telesca

Contents

SECTION THREE HIV AND THE RIGHT TO HEALTH CARE

SECTION FOUR HIV AND THE ISSUES OF PREVENTION

Acknowledgments

THE MATERIALS FOR THIS book grew out of a course entitled "AIDS and the Expectations of Democracy" that I taught at Vassar College in the winter of 1988. I must thank the Department of Philosophy for its support of the course(s), Professor Mitchell Miller for his strong encouragement of it, the Dean of the College for his financial support of the speakers' project that accompanied the course, the library for its genuine interest and help, and, finally, my student assistant, Ann Otto, who worked tirelessly on organizing and readying materials for the course. I must also thank my students, who suffered through disorganization and split schedules in order to attend sections of the course. I learned a great deal from teaching the course and working through for myself the issues of racism, sexism, heterosexism, and classism that form the contours of this epidemic. I especially appreciated what I learned from those who supplemented the course with their works: Lew Katoff of Gay Men's Health Crisis and his partner Phil; David Wertheimer of the New York City Gay and Lesbian Anti-Violence Project; Rebecca Rosenfeld of P.R.O.M.E.S.A.; Betsy Mayer, M.D., Dawn McGuire, M.D., and Marie Farrell, Ph.D., of the World Health Organization, and Dan Farrell. Rodney Sorge was also an ever-present worker and critic. I also thank the New School's Vera List Center, and especially Sondra Silverman, its director, for the opportunity to offer the course in a mini-version in the summer of 1988.

The materials for this book were further developed by my work at the New York City Commission on Human Rights, AIDS Discrimination Unit—a place of extreme dedication and resourcefulness and a part of my life that I will never forget. To the Unit I offer my great appreciation for their love and for what I learned from the Unit as a whole and from individuals. I owe appreciation to Azi Khalili who taught me a lot about how to think through the resource-needs of caretaking. To Otto DeMendoza who was patient and helpful with the development of a legal argument. To Katherine Franke who supplied with many articles and her own thoughts on the longer view of access to health care. To Mitchell Karp who provided much encouragement and help with the general effort at response to the HIV-affected. To Nitza Escalera for her patience, support and for her person. To Alma Torres for her genuine encouragement. To Alba Santiago for her help. To Amber Hollibaugh for her struggle with me and her insightfulness. To Celeste Davis for our long talks and her continuing political and-otherwise wisdom. To Suzanne Sangree for her collaboration and her continuing resourcefulness. And finally, to Keith O'Connor, director of the unit, who read more than his share of my ideas, edited them, and was a continuing intellectual partner in this project. And whose care of the "invisible" is beyond articulation but serves as inspiration for me.

I also wish to offer appreciation to those who gave me the gift of life by sharing with me their struggle with the disease and with the impossible odds of abandonment; with the miracle of their hope. To the PWA Coalition. To the Brooklyn AIDS Taskforce. To my complainants at the Commission, particularly Charles V., Bill L., Michael B. To Bob Tarbox at Gay Men's Health Crisis.

Much appreciation goes to Carol Levine for her offerings in this book. To Michael Seltzer for his work. Again, to Dawn McGuire, M.D., for her continuing support of my ideas and for her love. Finally, I wish to thank Edna McCown who was to be coauthor of this book. She began this project with me, talking through each step and she continues to see me through it. She is invaluable to all my efforts.

Additional thanks go to my editor, Susan Rogers, who really gave me the possibility of this work at no little trouble to herself; to my current editor, Rosemary Ahern, who worked very carefully with a difficult manuscript and improved it immensely; and to my agent, Frances Goldin.

Introduction:

The Demands of the HIV Epidemic

THIS BOOK IS DESIGNED to acquaint the reader with the major issues confronting America's experience with the HIV epidemic. *The AIDS Reader: Social, Political, Ethical Issues* is organized into six sections that examine the social, political, and ethical issues of the epidemic. The first and second sections are fact-based sections and discuss the scientific aspects of the virus and the social context of those that are affected. The remaining four sections deal with some aspects of the epidemic that require us, as a people, to make decisions: political decisions, ethical decisions, humane decisions. Each section begins with an introductory essay. My essays are designed to facilitate the understanding of salient features of the articles contained within the sections, to point out controversies, and to tie the articles together conceptually for the reader.

What is unique, terrifying, and challenging about the HIV epidemic is its position within the current institutional and economic crisis of nonprosperous America. With respect to the populations affected, we are in an economic situation unparalleled in this century of American history, with the exception of the 1930s. The disarray is primarily seen in our unfulfilled housing, education, and medical and mental health needs. Of course, all directly affect any national health crisis, for sick people need a stable environment, relevant information, and ultimately, a permanent continuum of health care resources. Sick people who are also *poor* people spend most of their waking, energy-expending hours trying to procure one or all three.

The people affected by the HIV virus are now largely poor. When they manage to secure their institutionally unmet housing, education, and medical needs they do so through a network of resources which is now acknowledged to be an alternative health care system—a community born equally of care and necessity. This network—led by the Gay Men's Health Crisis in New York City, the Shanti Project at San Francisco General Hospital and the City of San Francisco itself, as well as a host of community-based care groups in other major cities—exemplifies a decentralized way of organizing health care and, like the community health clinics of the 1960s, carries with its existence an indictment of the current organization of health care in the United States.[1]

The AIDS Reader begins by offering the reader the largely unassailable medical facts about the HIV epidemic. It moves from the biological, pathological, and clinical manifestations of the epidemic to issues of epidemiology. It is here that ambiguity blurs the scientific, biomedical portrait of AIDS; it is here that medical imperatives become unclear as they are intertwined with social and economic issues.

Scientific and medical initiatives in the first ten years of the epidemic have been largely organized around the morphology of the virus and the possibility of interventions—either through vaccine, through the direct cellular interdiction of the virus as it assaults its hosts, or through ways of shoring up the host to meet the assault. The other place energies have been almost single-mindedly directed has been in the area of transmission—the public health need for containment.

Perhaps because no one could predict the course of the HIV disease; or perhaps because the reality of suffering and death is eclipsed by our emphasis on bureaucracy and technology; or because the American media has conditioned us to expect medical bad news to have a rapid solution; or because the HIV-affected themselves have become the scapegoats of a public reluctant to take responsible action, very little attention has been paid to the fact that *the meaning of the HIV epidemic is the suffering it causes the individual.* The current medical crisis is singular in its wholesale lack of compassion for its casualties.

Understanding the HIV epidemic means understanding the significance of HIV infection in someone's life. It cannot be viewed as though its significance lay in the numbers of people affected. (Although the numbers are daunting—1.5 to 2 million Americans known to be HIV-antibody-positive; 135,000 AIDS cases; 83,000 dead. AIDS has already become the leading cause of death among people under forty in some large cities.)[2] Its significance may be how close it lies to you, or how far away from me, or from "us," but that is only a way of putting off the question of its actual significance in our lives.

The significance of the HIV epidemic is not that it now affects blacks and Hispanics at higher rates than whites but that it is unnecessary that anyone get it at all. And if they do, eight years after we have figured out how AIDS is transmitted and eliminated the infection from our blood supply, what does that say about "a country within a country"—about who counts in this country and who does not?

The significance of the HIV epidemic is not its existence in someone as the result of "high-risk behavior" but what it means for people to *blame* the affected—people they may already hate or fear—for being gravely ill.

The significance of the HIV epidemic is not how it is transmitted, as if the process were mysterious and the intentional result of cunning and deceit. (HIV is transmitted through blood injection and the sexual exchange of semen and vaginal fluid.) The significance is that the almost single-minded focus on transmission allows us to continue to internalize medical technology as The Answer and to continue to deny that our institutions are largely unable to offer comfort or care to the HIV-affected, and most other individuals suffering a debilitating chronic disease. It allows us to continue the illusion that we as a society are all educated individuals living, working, and playing within functioning institutions. It allows us to disregard the fact that our health care facilities are, for fully one-third of the population, impoverished and worn out. It allows us to ignore our predominantly two-class system of medical care; to ignore the medical triage that substitutes for sustained medical care in most urban hospitals. Wholesale, it allows us to fail to focus on the criminal inadequacies of our health, education, employment, and justice systems. Finally, more than anything else, it allows us to deny what we intuitively know is true: As people lose their communities, their social and interpersonal networks, because of sickness or through employment and housing displacement, they lose a major basis for good health. By focusing only on issues of transmission, we give ourselves license to ignore the relation between homelessness, drug abuse/mental illness, and HIV infection and to fail to understand how the three relate to the worsening economic condition of our cities.

The HIV virus may, or as it turns out, may *not* be the cause of the myriad catastrophic conditions we call AIDS. Only time will tell whether the single invasive agent theory will prevail historically.

The alternative—that the HIV virus is one factor among many undermining already immunosuppressed human organisms—has many implications, not the least of which involve the *general* state of Americans' health.

The medical exigencies of HIV infection nonetheless require that we "medicalize" the condition of those who are infected. This simply means that it is imperative that health professionals speak out about the epidemic and give those infected a hand with their uphill battle to be respected as sick people, not shunned as moral deviants. An indication that this imperative has not been met, ten years into the epidemic, is the data on physician willingness to treat the HIV-infected.[3] Another important indication that the HIV-infected are not considered first and foremost sick people, and thus deserving of the same rights as others, is the recent New York State decision to *waive* the ethical and legal requirements for providing contraception and abortion services, safer sex, and drug education in skilled nursing facilities that predominantly house people with AIDS.[4] At this late juncture in the epidemic, it remains urgent to remind ourselves to focus on the over 1.5 million HIV-positive people, as well as the over 135,000 people with AIDS as individual people in great physical and mental need.

While it is important to focus on the spread of the disease, the fear of spread is, in fact, only a direct result of the dire consequences of being infected. We must begin to affect the medical urgency of HIV infection, to redirect its focus from those who aren't infected to those who are.

The Medical Needs of People with AIDS

The needs of the HIV-infected highlight inequities in our economic and health care systems. They are needs left unmet that, when we focus upon them, appall us in their magnitude. Only the judgment that the afflicted somehow *deserve* what they get can insulate us from the person with AIDS—the PWA. Data from New York City and San Francisco provide two major profiles. The profiles are not meant to depersonalize but to draw into the medical outline features that point to structural resources not ordinarily focused upon.

Fifty to 60 percent of the over 200,000 intravenous drug users in New York City are HIV-antibody-positive. Of these, approximately 25 percent are women and 75 percent are men. Most of the women have at least one child, and that child or those children on average are under ten years old. Of the men, two-thirds have children with average ages between eleven and sixteen.

Consider the fate of the HIV-affected drug user. Naturally, intravenous drug use introduces a complex picture, one that includes unnecessary deprivation. While intravenous drug use designates a troubled individual, it also often indicates one who cannot find a treatment program and one who is primarily unemployed, and often because of addiction, unemployable. The economic outlook for this individual is now predictable. Unemployment means public assistance and drug use without treatment. No job and public assistance means housing instability—transient residences in hotels or shelters or with intolerant family members. Add children; add a public entitlement bureaucracy designed to thin out assistance rolls; add stigma; and, most important, subtract medical, emotional, or social support except through entirely overcrowded public hospitals. The total picture is beyond tragedy.

Treatment of people with AIDS is largely treatment of people bereft of family, community, or medical support. It is treatment that requires long-term care in a context that is totally devoid of *locations* for it. It is treatment that places a heavy burden on families and communities when they do exist and a crushingly impossible burden on social workers and advocates when they don't. PWAs stay in the hospital for months longer than they have to for lack of a place to live. Their attempts at parenting, at partnership, at life continuity are thwarted not only by their illness but, given a brief respite from the latest medical crisis, by their addiction. Transportation to and from public assistance agencies may, in fact, be an impossible $1.15 away. Inadequate shelter may kill a body already weakened. Looking at urban centers, we see, clearly and startlingly, how vital the physical resources of housing and home care are to wellness and, shamefully, how inaccessible these two have become, to the point that they are practically nonexistent for people who are slowly dying.

The elderly, the disabled, and the terminally ill have long tried to express the real impossibility of obtaining care for chronic conditions as middle- or low-income Americans. They have continually pleaded that we recognize the lack of home care structures; child care resources; humane policies for the difficulties of procurement in general (entitlement applications, transportation, groceries, etc.) for those who are "differently abled" but become "handicapped" by structures; for those who have the will, if not the complete stamina, to lead a meaningful life; and for those who hope and plan for a meaningful death. Continuity of medical care, hospice care, group residences, support groups, meal groups, recreational outlets, and child care are all necessities for those who have a catastrophic illness. They are crucial elements of health care for those who lack meaningful social networks. If the intravenous drug user who has AIDS cannot find a program in which he/she can be helped to get off drugs, is it likely that this individual could find these other ancillary but necessary medical services? The situation is impossible. It leads those medical professionals who work with people who have AIDS to reflect upon this system as one they no longer understand, one that frightens them and makes them regard it as a political more than a medical reality. One social worker concerned about the PWAs he works with revealed the potential seriousness of this problem when he said, "I'm hopeful that quarantine or encampment never becomes a reality in this country like it was during the Second World War for Japanese citizens."[5]

Ernest Drucker's investigation of intravenous drug users with AIDS in New York City (see article in Section 2) makes it clear that the picture of the person with AIDS in New York City is a picture of a person who is twice ill, a person whose children will probably grow up in foster care or be raised by a grandmother. The picture is contrasted by the picture of the white gay male who first made the American epidemic visible. That picture, in turn, is different from the picture of the intravenous drug user, although the gay PWA meets the same debilitated medical/social system as the nonwealthy. In the gay-identified male population, drug addiction is less frequent than in other population groups intimately tied to the epidemic. But the lack of social support because of the stigma of sexual preference is still operative. To understand the situation of gay men in the epidemic, one must recognize the violence directed against gay males and the complexities of internalized oppression. Almost invariably the PWA is at the mercy of public programs inadequately funded and stressed beyond responsiveness because the insurance industry refuses to underwrite them. A focus on the person with AIDS forces a confrontation with the unfulfilled promises of the American way of life that most Americans so studiously avoid until they are seriously ill and find (as many Americans are only now finding) that they cannot afford help. It is a focus, when trained on medical and social services, that darkens rather than illuminates. It demoralizes quicker than it informs. But this will change. As we truly confront the medical requirements of the HIV-affected, we will come to terms with the need for medical insurance for everyone and for a health care system that is truly responsive to medical needs rather than to esoteric research agenda.

The Psychological Needs
of People with AIDS

Judging by the extent to which the HIV-infected are *not* being studied or treated, psychological and psychiatric help for those with HIV disease has yet to be invented. And yet, what could be more stressful, more catastrophic, more debilitating than finding out that one is HIV-antibody-positive; that one has an almost always fatal disease; or that this almost always fatal disease causes severe neurological disorders in one-third of the afflicted? Again, most of the professional energy with respect to the psychological and neurological dysfunction that is associated with the virus has been focused upon detection—finding out who is likely to suffer the impairment so that they can be screened out of employment and insurance rolls.

There has been no national call from the American Psychological Association or from the American Medical Association's Psychiatric division for stepped-up efforts to treat the various emotional and neurological disturbances related to HIV infection. Few programs have been designed to deal with the problems of addiction that are so much a part of the American way of life and of poverty. What little help there is comes from "support groups" provided by communities meeting the needs of addiction, bereavement, depression, suicide prevention, and stress-related illnesses. Mental health experts have largely ignored the HIV-affected.

Of the 1.5 to 2 million Americans who are HIV-antibody-positive, perhaps half have knowledge either that they are at risk or that they are infected. This translates into the fact that over one million Americans are trying to negotiate their lives with the knowledge that they possibly have only a few years, even a few months, to live. They are facing these prospects with the social encouragement that they internalize a shame and an exaggerated notion of personal choice that makes them responsible for their own addiction, their own destitution, and ultimately, their own death. The HIV-affected carry not only a view of their own imminent dysfunction, deterioration, and demise but also a social guilt *undeserved and intractable*— the burden of culpability for their own illness.

The medical section of this book is truly a biomedical section. What has not been sufficiently investigated and documented and, more important, for which few interventions have been devised, is the sheer physical and mental discomfort and dis-ease of the HIV-affected. This medical and human concern requires that we begin to set up a broad range of medical responses to HIV infection that emphasizes *caretaking:* drug/alcohol rehabilitation, stress management; residential treatment centers; support networks; pain management; grief counseling; family therapy; child care and child therapy; rehabilitation therapy, suicide prevention, life-continuity counseling; recreational therapy; and psychotherapy. If HIV infection is, in the final analysis, an epidemic, it is in the *first* analysis an individual medical and psychological catastrophe. It makes little sense to be urgent about its spread, if we cannot muster urgency about its victims.

The issues of transmission *are* important. However, they are issues that we are equipped to handle. As much as we are interested in comparisons as theoreticians and scholars of epidemics and major public health events, it remains true that very little is shared between one epidemic and another. Epidemics are the same, some maintain, because they involve a contagious agent and largely affect populations that are disenfranchised and therefore either unknowledgeable about their actions and their relation to the contagious agent or distrustful enough of the medical establishment not to follow public health recommendations. Even though this view has great social currency right now, I would like to offer a different and, I believe, more complex scenario for the HIV epidemic.

It may be the case that epidemics largely affect the disenfranchised. But this really tells us very little. Poor people, by definition, are more subject to life's risks than the well-off, by any scale. And to emphasize that the nearness of epidemics takes a long time to be acknowledged within a culture, and that therefore, for a crucial period of time epidemiologically this means that populations will not only not identify with those who are sick but will treat them disparagingly as the "other," does not say much about *epidemics* per se but speaks volumes about racism, sexism, and, most important, the effects of classism on the perceptions of danger, suffering, and accountability. Epidemics are treated by epidemiologists as though their important feature were that they are *mass* events. That is the intended macroscopic understanding. But little is learned from such a gross measure of sickness, or even such a gross measure of transmission, particularly when the agent, like HIV, is so *difficult* to transmit.

The issue of transmission in the HIV epidemic is indeed similar to the issue of transmission of sexually transmitted diseases, but is also very different. HIV is transmitted through very intimate activity, but very concentrated intimate activity—the exchange of semen or blood. The word *exchange* should be emphasized. Transmission almost always involves "injection"—the mainlining of semen or vaginal fluid into the body or the mainlining of blood into the veins of the body. Cuts or wounds don't ordinarily pose a danger of HIV transmission. The body bleeds outward—cuts are openings whose flow is directed out of the body. In order for one to be exposed to HIV through blood, the infected person's blood must travel well into the body of the uninfected person. If we are speaking about infection with wounds, the infecting agent must overcome the natural outward-flowing tendency. Like the required puncture wound for infection with tetanus, HIV requires insertion deep into the body. This emphasis is not to dissuade one from taking every precaution in sexual activity; it is intended to highlight just how difficult HIV is to transmit and to show how *different* HIV is from some other sexually transmitted diseases, where mere contact can expose one to syphilis, gonorrhea, chlamydia.[6]

If HIV transmission were wholly like sexual transmission, it would still not necessitate mandatory testing or containment measures like isolation and contact tracing. These measures, as has been demonstrated over and over again, did not work with syphilis or gonorrhea because, during those epidemics, the only people who could be isolated or required to undergo drastic public health measures were people whose rights could be easily violated.[7] As surprising as it may seem, the reason we immediately go after sex workers during epidemics is because they are already doing something largely illegal. We don't restrict their clients or even attempt to find out who they are. This is because such investigations would violate the privacy of those individuals whose rights we automatically protect. Sex workers, by and large, have learned to protect themselves against infectious and contagious disease. They are the least likely to be transmitters. History shows, however, that what sex workers have not learned is how to garner the power to cry a collective "foul" when they get blamed for being "vectors" of disease. The most dangerous transmitters are those who are literally "invisible"—those people who have sexual lives unknown to their other contacts or even their life partners; or more tragically, even to themselves (those people whose cultural background prevents them from understanding their sexual identity as other than heterosexual, no matter what their actual sexual activity).[8] This is not to say that there are not sex workers who are wholly irresponsible; or that there are not many individuals who are incapacitated by drug use and other desperate factors. It is, again, just to emphasize that although epidemics look the same, the comparisons are profoundly complicated by individual, collective, and social participation, as well as by the level of individual, collective, and social denial that often accompanies controversial practices.

There have been criticisms by public health officials that different groups have refused to cooperate in the standard public health efforts necessitated by the epidemic. And it is true that public health measures in response to this epidemic *have* been influenced by political decisions. Groups have resisted standard public health measures, wishing to find measures with some promise of efficacy. It is undeniable that the homosexual community has interrupted the transmission of HIV. The rate of new infection among homosexual men is much lower than anyone thought it could be. And it is undeniable that the gay community has accomplished this without the traditional strategies of mass testing, isolation, and contact tracing. By not opting for mass testing, the communities of New York City and San Francisco took a microscopic approach to HIV. They had to define individual and collective practices that were dangerous and go about convincing each other how to avoid those dangers. The homosexual community has indeed made a difference in this epidemic. They have highlighted the extent to which only communities themselves and individuals within communities can deal with the transmission of disease. Any larger or more depersonalized measures like mass screening or contact tracing do little to stop the spread of disease and much to further demoralize and depress individuals who need every optimistic hope and incentive to believe that their behavior will make a difference to their health and the health of their partners. What is different about the HIV epidemic is that a group of people took into their own hands the job of educating themselves to the dangers of the virus. They did yell a collective "foul" when it seemed that they could be scapegoated for the epidemic.

Homosexuals not only have been effective in the area of transmission, where no one else has, they have been imaginative and resourceful in responding to the illnesses that accompany HIV infection—something that has not happened at any governmental level. Gay Men's Health Crisis in New York City, the Shanti Project in San Francisco, the Community Research Initiative, and Project Inform are at the forefront of knowledge about the epidemic and about the medical and psychological needs of the HIV-affected. As the epidemic progresses, the federal government increasingly adopts medical measures that were originated by these communities.[9]

Epidemics are highly complex phenomena. They involve not only a "germ," they involve practices that transmit it, and probably what will prove ultimately to be the most important factor, "hosts" that are vulnerable to the "germ." The host factor, besides the myriad practices that are involved in epidemics, is the individuating factor of epidemics. Populations, according to their lifestyles, nutrition, and relative ease or difficulty in maintaining continuity of health care, differ in their susceptibility to disease. But these factors are rarely emphasized by the epidemiologist. Only communities themselves have access to this information and the will to address the issues in the way that they have to be addressed if epidemics are to be halted. To say that epidemics largely affect the ignorant or the disenfranchised is to say little; it is to view the epidemic from the height of the unaffected. To say that they affect communities of differing vulnerabilities and resources is to say quite a lot and to commit oneself to allowing the differences to emerge and play their part in resolving the epidemic. It is to view the epidemic from the base of community.

Transmission of the virus has not been halted. This is not because the virus takes advantage of every opportunity to infect the unwary but because the populations that are currently being affected are ones that have no institutional affiliation. The high school dropout is also the unemployed, the medically invisible, the person confronting psychological problems alone. For instance, there is no realistic appraisal of the extent of illness among intravenous drug users, their partners, and their children, as well as the growing numbers of women and adolescents at high risk for their addictions to alcohol and cocaine, heroin and crack. Nor have there been attempts to understand the intertwining epidemics of drug use, homelessness, and HIV infection or the extent of their reflection upon poverty and its ranks. No plans for drug treatment—none at all. And short-term preventive interventions like the education about cleaning needles or exchanging old ones for clean ones meets the same resistance that condoms do with the Catholic Church, despite very effective containment programs around the globe through state-sponsored needle-exchange schemes or programs.

People with no formal affiliation with health professionals or educators will not be reached by public health information packets or posters. Certainly not when they distrust health systems that might report their immigration status; or require cash; or find out about a stigmatizing condition such as drug use, unemployment, or homosexuality. It is far too easy to avoid a health care system altogether—one that has been wholesale in its callousness. It is not easy to bring a person who may be at risk for HIV into a health care system that is largely nonexistent[10] or whose experience with that system has involved enduring long, numbing waits for less-than-compassionate caregivers. Transmission of the virus continues because the people most at risk are unreachable through "normal" institutional channels and no one has been imaginative enough or courageous enough to fund the use of the "media" that serve as a network within *communities*—radio, TV, churches, bars, and community organizations.

The transmission issue as it is defined by the American media is a red herring. The true issues of transmission relate more to *disconnectedness and concealment* than they do morality and responsibility. The greatest tool for halting transmission is the assurance of a lack of reprisals for those who are infected.

If one begins to imagine the concrete measures needed to create a climate in which people will come forward to health centers for treatment and testing, one sees first a health care system that does not rely primarily on the emergency room and that has physicians willing to treat the HIV-affected. In addition, one envisions an effective application of law and effective leadership. Amnesty proved more effective in documenting immigrants than punishment and reprisals for illegal status. HIV-affected people, or those who suspect that they may be affected, are not "illegal." They don't require amnesty. They require help against threats and abandonment. They require protection. A national effort to enforce federal antidiscrimination laws would do more to bring people forward than all the public health or police restrictions one could invent. It is that simple. Strict enforcement of antidiscrimination law at the federal level with highly visible encouragement of state enforcement would bring people closer to those centers that can help them and interrupt the spread of the HIV virus.[11]

But this is not enough. Like the issues of the medical and psychological needs of the HIV-affected, effective transmission policy cannot be formulated within structures that are moribund and cynical. Effective public health policy, like effective medical policy, cannot be developed within the usual institutional settings, settings that have been more gatekeeping and warehouses for the poor than places of responsiveness. The epidemic requires wholly new structures, not new policies installed within old structures. The issues of transmission require that people police themselves and that they do so with respect and dignity. This requirement is hard met by public health officials within medical and social service institutions designed more for efficiency and compliance than responsiveness and compassion.

All major progressive studies of the HIV epidemic contain the same sets of recommendations:[12]

1. Access to basic health care that is organized care—care that is coordinated. This is health care that is able to identify patient needs as patients move through the trajectory of sickness. It focuses on

different stages of illness that urgently require various medical, mental health, and social services. Ideally, it is community-based, accessible geographically and culturally, since "needs" depend not only on levels of morbidity and disability but also on the strengths of social, familial, and community networks, as well as on the commitment of caretakers and health institutions.

2. Housing—a network of permanent, temporary, and hospice care centers must be set up for the HIV-affected. These facilities must include extensive support services, including child care, drug addiction counseling, and social services designed to enhance, or at least preserve, continuity of life experience.

3. Drug treatment programs that work—that lead to detoxification and the learning of coping mechanisms that do not rely on drugs for problem solving. These programs must be attached to centers that also provide basic health care.

4. Family support and group support. The home care, psychological counseling, and child-care needs of the HIV-affected are currently being borne by social workers at public hospitals or immediate family members. Special assistance should be integral to the medical care of the sick. This mandates support external to the hospital setting, such as the establishment of peer support groups, community and family networks, and advocacy for the HIV-affected among their peers, families, and communities. Models exist among gay advocacy groups, the hospice movement, and community health care centers of the past twenty years; among AA and Alanon, cancer and Alzheimer groups, as well as in "poor clinics," "women's clinics," union houses, and even the settlement movements of the turn of the century. Some resources already exist in communities themselves through a history of reliance on informal networks. Many more existed prior to the federal cuts by the Republican administrations of Reagan and Bush.[13]

The suggestions and recommendations above point to the need for a large structural change in health care delivery and public health response. The greatest change, the decentralization of health care, is one that has been needed for quite a long time in America—and is demonstrated by the phenomenon of crowding and dysfunction in urban hospitals. The university health care setting has benefited research efforts but little else. There is really no sense in continuing with the centralization of health care, except for esoteric research efforts. The care of sick people demands, at the minimum, proximity and identification, attributes associated with health care based in communities. "Community-based AIDS care models must be developed both to provide services and to create a framework for the recruitment, training, and employment of additional health care providers and assistants drawn from the very communities most heavily affected by the AIDs epidemic."[14] Someone must make this demand a reality. As evidenced by the coordination of services in San Francisco, communities can do it themselves. They can "relocate" health care on the local level with extensive rehabilitation, advocacy, and treatment facilities given the financial and government resources and, above all, the political will. They cannot do it without such resources. (The lessons of San Francisco indicate that even with an alternative health care system, without federal backing, responsiveness is not sustainable. See Section VI.)

The HIV-affected are not the only ones lost to the American health care system. Minority communities and poor people have struggled for over thirty years with a system that is unresponsive to their needs. What AIDS brings to the ongoing debate about the crisis in health care is not only a greater burden on strained medical systems but a wholesale disclosure of the reality of this dysfunction.

One further set of issues concern testing for the HIV virus in order for people to get treated by drugs that might stave off those symptoms of HIV infection that result in the disease of AIDS. There are many drugs now available that offer some hope of longevity with an HIV diagnosis. Given that these drugs currently make up the American arsenal of "treatments," many are calling for larger numbers of people to be tested for the virus. Sometimes these calls are directed at certain groups that are at risk, such as those most vulnerable to infection—the newborn of HIV-affected mothers. The basic assumption here is that because there are "treatments," it is irresponsible not to somehow force people to know their serostatus or the status of their child. A word of caution should be expressed. Relative to the first five years of the epidemic, the current pharmaceutical methods of staving off infection do constitute "treatments" for, or interventions into, the progress of the HIV virus. But only *relatively* speaking. The current drugs are highly toxic, largely untested, and, equally important, available only to the affluent. They are effective only in conjunction with very close monitoring by a physician—who for a large percentage of the infected is not available. As more drugs come on the market, it is necessary to re-evaluate the national consensus against involuntary testing. But this re-evaluation should always be done with a realistic appraisal of what medical (and not just pharmaceutical) interventions are available to patients with HIV and their children. The ethical issue here is whether the knowledge of one's HIV status can bring about any change in one's condition. The issue is one of knowledge and its efficacy. If we have no treatment for newborn infants who are HIV-antibody-positive (but who have only a 30 percent chance of developing AIDS), is it necessary that they be tested, since what this may tell us is that their mothers were or are HIV-antibody-positive—jeopardizing not only her fundamental right to refuse consent to the HIV antibody test herself but also jeopardizing her standing with respect to private insurance, job security, and housing? The debate will continue as drugs and other treatments develop. We should be armed with the proper kinds of questions not merely with respect to the progress of medical technology but equally with respect to access to health care and the importance of official respect for the rights of the affected.

What the last ten years has taught us is that very little of traditional public health thinking "works" with this epidemic. The epidemic requires us to think anew—both about transmission and response. It requires that we address as indicated above what we have singularly refused to acknowledge about current inadequacies in our national systems. In an attempt to give both an overview of this book and of the epidemic so far, I've offered the above points as ways to *reorient* our thinking to more adequately respond to the epidemic as it really is.

NOTES

1. The numbers of AIDs organizations nationally must be in the thousands. It is possible in every city to find a resource directory for such organizations by contacting the department of health of the city or the state.

2. World Health Organization, June 1990.

3. See Section 5.

4. *New York Times*, July 27, 1990.

5. "IV Drug Users with AIDS in New York City: A Study of Dependent Children, Housing and Drug Addiction Treatment," Ernest Drucker, Principal Investigator, Department of Epidemiology and Social Medicine, Montefiore Medical Center. See Section 2.

6. Cf. the Duesberg article in Section 1 and the Osborn article in Section 4.

7. "Traditional Public Health Strategies," in Larry Gostin, ed., *AIDS and the Law* (New Haven: Yale University Press, 1986), pp. 47–65.

8. The New York City Department of Health changed its surveillance category of homosexual transmission of HIV to "male to male" transmission because in many communities men have sex with men but do not

reflect upon it with a sense of "identity." After tracing down risk behavior by asking if the patient who had HIV was homosexual and getting repeated answers of "no," it was discovered that this question had little meaning to the Hispanic male, for instance, who might engage in male-to-male sex but be, to his mind, definitively heterosexual.

9. For instance, ACT UP (AIDS Coalition to Unleash Power), one of the most visible AIDS activists groups, regularly confers with the National Institutes of Health about NIH's drug research protocol. At the end of the Sixth International Conference on AIDS, in June 1990, one newspaper editorial headlined its applause of ACT UP by naming its members the "The Scientists from ACT UP." This was prompted, no doubt, by an ACT UP research agenda handed out at the conference outlining new drugs to be researched, as well as by National Institute of Allergy and Infectious Diseases Director Anthony Fauci's address to the convention on the closing day. In that address Dr. Fauci applauded ACT UP's partnership in the research at the National Institutes of Health. AIDS activism has had an effect on life-preserving drugs for other diseases as well. Cancer patients are also getting drugs for opportunistic infections associated with immunosuppression years earlier than they would have had the epidemic not occurred. Of eighteen drugs approved for early release by the FDA under a new ruling in 1987 after pressure from AIDS activists, twelve are for treating non-HIV-related infections, mostly cancer.

10. According to the Community Service Society, the availability of primary care in nine of New York City's low-income communities—the kind of care that places one within a health care system through diagnosis, referral, and monitoring—is practically nonexistent. In a two-year study of clinics, emergency rooms, and private practices, the society found a total of twenty-eight full-time-equivalent primary-care physicians for 1.7 million New Yorkers. "Building Primary Care Health Services in New York's Low-Income Communities," by Christel Brellochs, Anjean Carter, Amy Golman, and Barbara Caress, 1989.

11. (Summer of 1990), Congress just passed and President Bush signed a bill that will prohibit discrimination against the disabled. People with AIDS are covered under this legislation.

12. *Confronting AIDs: 1988 Update*, the National Academy of Sciences, 1988, "Care of Persons Infected with HIV: Recommendations;" *The Invisible Emergency: Children with AIDS*, Citizens Commission for Children of New York, Inc., Report, February, 1989; "The Crisis in AIDS Care: A Call to Action," Citizens Commission on AIDS, 1989; "Recommendations."

13. The deficit for New York State in 1990 is over $1 billion. Federal contributions to New York City, which has the greatest number of HIV-affected in the country, declined by 50 percent since 1980. In 1980 the federal government cut programs to the poor in America by $57 billion.

14. Drucker, "IV Drug Users with AIDS in New York City," p. 24.

THE HIV VIRUS AND ITS EPIDEMIOLOGY

Introduction

It took Americans a while to demystify the disease of AIDS.[1] After ten years it is clear that HIV (Human Immunodeficiency Virus) is but a biological phenomenon. As a biological phenomenon, HIV is really indifferent to politics, to status, to lifestyle, to sexual preference. A pathogen is no respecter of persons. It grows where it can, when it can, and does not itself survive without a host. Its hosts, so far, have been people of various political vulnerabilities.

AIDS is thought by an overwhelming majority of scientists and clinicians to be caused by the HIV (Human Immunodeficiency Virus). But there are some truly anomalous features of the virus and of the virus's link to the disease we have come to know as AIDs. HIV has morphological, biological, and molecular similarities to viruses affecting animals, but until now not known to affect humans. These viruses are "retroviruses"—ones that are regressive—they "go backward." A retrovirus changes the original molecular structure of its host cell. Most viruses maintain themselves within a cell and the cell replicates itself from its basic genetic structure. This means that ordinary viruses produce enzymes of RNA from a reliable and fixed DNA base. Retroviruses work in the opposite direction. Through an enzyme called reverse transcriptase, they communicate from the RNA of the cell and send information to the basic DNA blocks. These messages, or this infiltration, change the DNA and, thus, the genetic structure of the cell that the virus inhabits. These cells become HIV cells forever.

Retroviruses have been found in most species. Their presence is associated with tumors or progressive illness affecting blood, respiratory function, or the central nervous system. Until 1980 no human retrovirus had been identified. In 1980 Robert Gallo and his working group at the National Cancer Institute, a part of the National Institutes of Health (NIH) identified a new retrovirus that had an affinity for human lymphocytes—a lymphoid cell that controls or mediates the immunity of the body.[2] Certain forms of cancer work the same way and are also called retroviruses. What is challenging about the Gallo finding is its insistence that a certain kind of leukemia and HIV share not only this molecular idiosyncrasy but that both are infectious agents. The conclusion that cancer may be caused by an infectious agent is not uncontroversial for cancer. Nor, as we shall see in this section, is the conclusion that AIDS is caused by an infectious agent.

"The Human Immunodeficiency Virus: Infectivity and Mechanisms of Pathogenesis," by Anthony Fauci, director of the National Institute of Allergy and Infectious Diseases at the National Institutes of Health, tells the story of HIV infection. This is the story of the affinity HIV has for certain kinds of cells in the body and the implications of that affinity. HIV has a natural inclination for the T4 helper cell of the immune system. What this essentially means is that HIV attacks the very cells that are crucial to signaling to all cells that there is an enemy present—a foreign agent afoot in the organism. Evolutionary biology will probably one day say that HIV was a great threat to the human species precisely because it disrupts the ability of the human organism to distinguish itself from its environment—it disrupts the ability of a body to welcome what nourishes it and to fight what is dangerous to it. It is not merely the T4 helper cell that is a target. HIV evidently also has an affinity for macrophages—cells also associated with the immune system which, smother, absorb, or eat up foreign agents in the blood. Once HIV infiltrates macrophages, it changes their DNA structure and cripples their ability to do battle. Recently, it has been shown that HIV can infiltrate any type of cell.[3]

The Fauci article gives vivid clinical indication of just how the immune system, now ravaged by HIV, is open to parasitic pathogens and how this pathogenesis is not merely confined to the body but is directly targeted at the brain—brain infections occurring in over 30 percent of all AIDS cases.

The Fauci article also goes into some detail on the molecular biology of the HIV and indicates that, in fact, there are now *two* identifiable viruses to contend with: HIV-1 and HIV-2. Fauci discusses the complication in the research caused by the two strains of HIV as well as the equally baffling problem of the latency of the viruses. Some patients infected with HIV develop symptoms quickly and some don't. The mean incubation period has recently been revised to 8.2 years.[4] General wisdom by the medical community is that HIV may actually live in the body for up to twenty years, although there is little data beyond the almost yearly discovery of individuals who have superceded the latest figures on incubation.

Dr. Fauci also explains the difficulty of transmission of the virus. After all, the virus is not airborne. It requires a particular kind of activity to transmit which involves the insertion of the virus into the body either through unprotected sexual activity, the sharing of contaminated needles, or exchange of bodily fluids from mother to child.

There are few researchers in America who hold that AIDS is not caused by the HIV virus. On the other hand, one learns a great deal by questioning the reigning assumption of any explanation. Particularly when the explanation of a phenomenon carries its weight descriptively. That is, when its evidence is derived from the repeated coincidence of two events. The weight of evidence for HIV as the cause of AIDS has largely been established by epidemiology rather than by etiology (causal demonstration). How valid a premise, then, is it that HIV is an infectious *cause* of AIDS and AIDS Related Complex (ARC) rather than an *effect* or only *one factor* in the etiology of the disease? The controversy has broadened from the issue of cofactors that Dr. Fauci mentions in his article to an alternative interpretation of the relation between HIV and AIDS. At direct contention is whether HIV itself is an opportunistic infection that appears on the scene when the immune system is catastrophically weakened by something else. Recent research by Dr. Montagnier of the Pasteur Institute in Paris indicates that AIDS may be caused by a *partnership* between the HIV virus and a microbe—a small bacteriumlike organism cell called mycoplasma.[5]

In "Human Immunodeficiency Virus and Acquired Immunodeficiency Syndrome: Correlation, but Not Causation," Dr. Peter Duesberg, a retroviral researcher from the University of California at Berkeley, addresses the fact that the disease profile that we have come to know and name through its clinical manifestations in diverse diseases (AIDS) may be wholly caused by the pathogens that constitute these "opportunistic infections."[6] Dr. Duesberg's reasoning takes us step by step through the structure of the virus and its relation to infection. It asks us to compare the HIV virus with the medical, biological, chemical, and evolutionary characteristics of viruses in general to see whether, in the final analysis, it would be just as useful to view HIV as yet another infection in the matrix of infections associated with AIDS as to designate it as the cause of AIDS. Dr. Duesberg's article is explosive and provides a fascinating look at the role of logic in the development of disease investigation.

Both theories of the etiology of AIDS are coherent and exhaustive ones, epidemiologically speaking. That is, given the clinical and biological data on AIDS, it is possible to use either the virus explanation or the diverse-infection explanation to account for this data. Since indications of HIV's presence exists only through antibodies and depleted T4 cells and not through direct evidence of cell infiltration, it is open to question what is the direct pathogen in the disease called AIDS.

The debate about the HIV virus is important for its implications for public health policy on venereal diseases, drug use, and malnutrition. The Duesberg challenge is also helpful for highlighting the debate between "disease-as-powerful-foreigner-invader," or "disease-as-weakened-host": a medical debate that prompts us to rethink both our expectations of medical science and our fundamental understanding of basic health.

"HIV Infection and Its Epidemiology," by the National Academy of Sciences, outlines the basic epidemiology of the virus and should be read closely. This article offers an extensive look at the magnitude of the HIV epidemic in America, as well as a short comparison with the pattern of HIV infection in Africa, the other region of the world experiencing a high incidence of infection.

In strong disagreement with Dr. Duesberg, the National Academy of Sciences stresses that HIV is the etiologic cause of AIDS and supports its position with the most widely accepted data on the subject. Although the pathogenesis of HIV infection is not wholly understood, such complete understanding is not entirely requisite to stipulate that HIV is the cause of what we know as Acquired Immunodeficiency Syndrome.

Over the ten-year history of the AIDS epidemic in America there have been changes in the pattern of HIV infection. The National Academy of Sciences gives precise indications of the spectrum of infection, the Centers for Disease Control's definition of AIDS (and the need for a broader definition to include asymptomatic infection), the modes of transmission, the HIV prevalence in groups [sic][7] understood to be at risk for infection. Current data indicate a lower incidence of HIV infection as a result of male-to-male transmission (due to changes in sexual practices) and a lower incidence of infection among transfusion recipients due to serologic screening of blood and plasma products. In contrast, data also suggests an increase in HIV infection among intravenous drug users in New York

City and San Francisco, as well as an alarming rise in HIV infection related to drug use among women and youth. As of this writing (July 1990), the number of AIDS cases reported by the Centers for Disease Control is over 130,000, with more than 85,000 persons dead. The largest increases in new cases have been in heterosexual partners of HIV-infected individuals and the children of mothers who are HIV-infected. Blacks and Hispanics are disproportionately represented in both groups. The incidence of infection in black and Hispanic populations in San Francisco is three times that of whites; it is twelve times that of whites in New York City.

All of the articles in this first section indicate just how much progress has been made on the biology and epidemiology of AIDS and just how much speculation and controversy still remain after ten years of concentrated effort. The last article shows us that there has been great achievement on the political front, as well. "The Terrifying Normalcy of AIDS," by one of America's most renowned biologists, shows that, even in 1987, it was still necessary to tell Americans that AIDS is caused by a biological agent and not by sexual preference. As progressive as Dr. Gould's article seemed at the time, it left out the "faces" of AIDS and the political realities at the heart of the epidemic—realities we have now come to regard as essential parts of our medical understanding of the epidemic.

NOTES

1. There is really a spectrum of HIV disease, which includes asymptomatic infection with the virus, generalized infection, AIDS Related Complex—a constellation of symptoms which are less severe than full-blown AIDS. AIDS, or Acquired Immunodeficiency Disease, is an end-stage syndrome of HIV infection. It is therefore somewhat inaccurate to term the epidemic an epidemic of AIDS, since this leaves out the progressive nature of HIV-related illnesses and the crisis that each level has for the individual. Asymptomatic HIV infection is itself debilitating given its relation to the medical emergency we have come to know as AIDS.

2. Robert Gallo, "The First Human Retrovirus," *Scientific American* 255 (1986). See also Robert Gallo, "The AIDS Virus," *Scientific American* 256 (1986). Dr. Gallo is no longer considered the sole identifier of the HIV virus. Dr. Gallo identified his virus after his lab received samples of a French virus. A Pasteur Institute researcher, Dr. Luc Montagnier, had forwarded the sample discovered by his Paris team to Dr. Gallo six months prior to Dr. Gallo's announcement. Dr. Montagnier sued Dr. Gallo and an international compromise was reached. The universal name of the virus would be

"HIV" and both researchers would share the title of "discoverer." Recently, the controversy over Dr. Gallo's behavior has reemerged, not only because of the ethical questions of research collaboration but because of indications that Dr. Gallo forged some research documents. A long NIH investigation of Dr. Gallo, concluded in June 1990, exonerated him of criminal charges.

3. Jay Levy, professor of medicine and research, University of California, San Francisco, "Changing Concepts in HIV Infections" (Paper presented at VI International AIDS Conference, San Francisco, California, June 1990).

4. Cf. A. R. Moss, P. Bacchetti, D. Osmond, W. Krampf, R. E. Chaisson, D. Stites, and J. Wilber, J. F. Allain, and J. Carlson, "Seropositivity for HIV and the Development of AIDS or AIDS Related Condition: Three year follow-up of the San Francisco General Hospital Cohort," *British Medical Journal* 296 (1988): 745–750.

5. Dr. Luc Montagnier, Louis Pasteur Institute, Paris, France, "HIV Pathogenesis" (Paper presented at the VI International AIDS Conference, San Francisco, California, June 1990).

6. Cf. Peter Duesberg, "HIV Is Not the Cause of AIDS," and the answer from Blattner, Gallo, and Jemin that "HIV Causes AIDS," *Science* 241 (July 29, 1988).

7. Language does matter. Although the National Academy of Sciences refers to the "risk groups" associated with AIDS, the general consensus now is to refer to "risk behavior" so that the focus on transmission is not upon categories of *people* but upon categories of action that people engage in.

The Human Immunodeficiency Virus: Infectivity and Mechanisms of Pathogenesis

Anthony S. Fauci

THE HUMAN IMMUNODEFICIENCY VIRUS (HIV), the etiologic agent of the acquired immunodeficiency syndrome (AIDS), has the capability of selectively infecting and ultimately incapacitating the immune system whose function is to protect the body against such invaders.[1,2] HIV-induced immunosuppression results in a host defense defect that renders the body highly susceptible to "opportunistic" infections and neoplasms. The immune defect appears to be progressive and irreversible, with a high mortality rate that may well approach 100 percent over several years. From the time that the first cases were reported to the Centers for Disease Control (CDC) in the summer of 1981 until 1 December 1987, there have been approximately 47,000 cases of AIDS in the United States, and 58 percent of the patients have already died.[3] It is estimated that between 1 and 2 million individuals in the United States are infected with HIV and are at present without symptoms. Given the fact that approximately 20 to 30 percent of infected individuals will develop AIDS within 5 years of infection, it is projected that there will be 270,000 cumulative cases of AIDS by 1991.[4] Although the majority of reported cases have occurred in the United States, AIDS is a worldwide epidemic including thousands of cases reported in Europe. Despite the difficulties in epidemiologic surveillance, it is estimated that there are millions of infected individuals in Central Africa.[5]

Anthony Fauci, "The Human Immunodeficiency Virus," *Science* 239 (February 5, 1988) 617–622. Copyright © 1988 American Association for the Advancement of Science. Reprinted by Permission of the Author and of *Science*.

HIV infection is spread by sexual contact, by infected blood or blood products, and perinatally by mother to infant.[6] Regardless of the portal of entry of the virus, the common denominator of HIV infection is a selective tropism of the virus for certain cells of the immune system and the central nervous system (CNS), which results in immunosuppression and neuropsychiatric abnormalities.[1,2]

The Virus

Nature of HIV

In order to fully understand the pathogenic mechanisms of HIV infection, one must consider the unique nature of the causative microbe. HIV is an RNA retrovirus that was originally designated human T lymphotropic virus (HTLV)-III,[7] lymphadenopathy-associated virus (LAV),[8] or AIDS-associated retrovirus (ARV).[9] It shares many features with other members of the nontransforming and cytopathic lentivirus family of retroviruses. Of particular note are its morphological, biological, and molecular similarities to the visna virus of sheep,[10] equine infectious anemia virus,[11] and the recently described feline immunodeficiency virus.[12] These viruses, including HIV in humans, cause a slowly progressive and inevitably fatal disease in their hosts. HIV is also related to other recently isolated primate retroviruses such as simian T lymphotropic virus (STLV)-III, which causes disease in captive macaques but is apparently not pathogenic for wild African Green monkeys.[13] HTLV-IV has been isolated from healthy West Africans.[14] Others have reported that this latter virus may be indistinguishable from STLV-III.[15] HIV is increasingly referred to as HIV-1 to differentiate it from HIV-2 (or LAV-2), which shares serologic reactivity and polynucleotide sequence homology with STLV-III and has been isolated from West African patients with a clinical syndrome indistinguishable from HIV-induced AIDS and AIDS-related condition (ARC).[16]

The HIV Genome

As visualized by electron microscopy, HIV has a dense cylindrical core whose structural elements are coded for by the viral *gag* gene and encase two molecules of the viral RNA genome.[17,18] The central core is surrounded by a lipid envelope acquired as the virion buds from the surface of an infected cell. Virus-encoded enzymes required for efficient replication, such as the reverse transcriptase and integrase, are also incorporated into the virus particle. The HIV proviral genome has been well characterized. It is approximately 10 kb in length and comprises the flanking long terminal repeat (LTR) sequences that contain regulatory segments for HIV replication as well as the *gag*, *pol*, and *env* genes coding for the core proteins, the reverse transcriptase-protease-endonuclease, and the internal and external envelope glycoproteins, respectively.[17,18] HIV also has at least five additional genes, three of which have known regulatory functions, and the expression of these genes almost certainly has an impact on the pathogenic mechanisms exerted by the virus. The *tat* gene plays an important role in the amplification of virus replication by encoding a protein that functions as a potent trans-activator of HIV gene expression.[19] The *trs/art* gene also upregulates HIV synthesis by a trans-acting antirepression mechanism.[20] In contrast, the *3' orf* gene may downregulate virus expression, as one group has reported that deletion of the gene results in an approximately fivefold increase in viral DNA synthesis and viral replication;[21] however, others have not seen such an effect.[22] Although the *sor* gene is not absolutely required for HIV virion formation, it clearly influences virus transmission in vitro and is critical to the efficient generation of infectious virions.[23] Finally, the *R* gene codes for an immunogenic protein whose function is currently unknown.[24]

Immunopathogenic Mechanisms of HIV Infection

Scope of the Immunologic Defect

The critical basis for the immunopathogenesis of HIV infection is the depletion of the helper/inducer subset of T lymphocytes, which express the CD4 phenotypic marker (the T4 cell), resulting in profound immunosuppression. Although a large number of immunologic abnormalities that accompany HIV infection have been described, all but a few can be attributed to the selective defect in the T4 subset of lymphocytes. The T4 lymphocyte is the focal and critical cell involved directly or indirectly in the induction of most immunologic functions.[25] Hence, a functional defect of T4 cells would result in a decrease in inductive signals to multiple limbs of the immune response, and this would explain the apparent paradox of a selective defect in a single subset of cells causing a global immune defect.

HIV Infection

HIV has a selective tropism for the T4 cell, and a convincing body of evidence has suggested that the CD4 molecule is, in fact, the high-affinity receptor for the virus.[26] After HIV binds to the CD4 molecule, the virus is internalized and uncoated. The precise mechanism of virus entry into the target cell is unclear. It has been suggested that receptor-mediated endocytosis plays a role in this process.[27] However, it has recently been demonstrated that pH-independent fusion of the transmembrane portion (gp41) of the virus envelope with the cell membrane is required for virus entry.[28] In addition, the inability of mouse cells transfected with the CD4 gene and expressing the human CD4 protein to be productively infected with HIV in the face of viral binding suggests that other proteins expressed on the human T4 cell may be required for virus internalization.

Once internalized, the genomic RNA is transcribed to DNA by the enzyme reverse transcriptase. The proviral DNA, which can exist in a linear or circularized form, is integrated into the host chromosomal DNA in a process dependent on an endonuclease encoded by the viral *pol* gene. An unusual feature of HIV infection compared to most other retroviruses is the accumulation of large amounts of unintegrated viral DNA in the infected cells.[29] When this phenomenon does occur in other retroviral systems, it is usually associated with a significant cytopathic effect and has been suggested as an important factor in the cytopathicity of HIV.[29]

After integration of provirus, the infection may assume a latent phase with restriction of the cycle until the infected cell is activated. Once cell activation occurs, the proviral DNA transcribes viral genomic RNA and messenger RNA (mRNA). Protein synthesis, processing, and virus assembly occur with budding of the mature virion from the cell surface.

Mechanisms of Cytopathic Effect

When active replication of virus occurs, the host cell is usually killed. However, one of the critical unknowns in the immunopathogenesis of HIV infection is the precise mechanisms of the cytopathic effect in T4 cells. The potential role of accumulation of unintegrated viral DNA has been discussed above. Another mechanism that has been proposed is a massive increase in permeability of the cell membrane when large amounts of virus are produced and bud off the cell surface.[30] Others have speculated that HIV may induce terminal differentiation of the infected T4 cell, leading to a shortened life span;[31] however, the evidence for this is meager.

There is mounting evidence that both the CD4 molecule and the virus envelope play a role in the cytopathic effect in infected T4 cells. Certain subsets of monocytes and macrophages express the CD4 molecule,[32] and these cells can bind to and be infected with HIV (see below); however, HIV does not induce a significant cytopathic effect in monocytes. Since the level of expression of CD4 on the monocyte is considerably less than that of the T4 cell,[33] it is possible that the density of this receptor is important in determining the presence or degree of cytopathic effect of the bound and internalized virus. Furthermore, superinfection of HTLV I-infected T cell clones of either the T4 or T8 phenotype with HIV resulted in a productive infection and accumulation of unintegrated HIV DNA. However, a cytopathic effect was seen only in the T4 clones; the T8 clone was resistant to the cytopathic effect.[34]

A potentially important mechanism of cell death in HIV infection involving CD4-envelope protein interaction is cell fusion. The high level of HIV *env* gene expression in infected T4 cells, as manifested by the budding of viral particles from the plasma membrane, results in cell fusion with neighboring uninfected T4 cells and leads to the formation of multinucleated giant cells (syncytia) that comprise both infected and uninfected cells.[35] Depending on the virus isolate in question, cytolysis and death of the fused cells occurs, usually within forty-eight hours. It is also possible that intracellular complexing of CD4 and envelope proteins may play a role in the cytopathic effect of HIV.[36]

It has been proposed that autoimmune phenomena play a role in the cytopathicity associated with HIV infection. Some examples are the immune clearance of infected T4 cells expressing envelope proteins on their surface that are recognized as non-self, or, alternatively, the binding of free envelope protein (gp120) to the CD4 molecule of uninfected T4 cells, resulting in similar immune clearance[37] or the elimination of such cells by antibody-dependent cellular cytotoxicity.[38] Others have reported an AIDS-related cytotoxic antibody reacting with a specific antigen on stimulated T4 cells.[39] Another hypothesis is autoimmunization with class II-like antigens.[40] This theory is based on the fact that the CD4 molecule on the T4 cell recognizes a portion of the class II major histocompatibility complex (MHC) molecule. Since the HIV envelope binds to the CD4 molecule, it can mimic the configuration of a portion of the class II MHC antigen. Hence, antibodies and cytotoxic lymphocytes directed against the HIV envelope can potentially cross-react with class II

MHC antigens. The extent if any to which these autoimmune phenomena are involved in cytopathicity of HIV infection is unclear at present.

Quantitative Deficiency of T4 Lymphocytes

The most conspicuous immunologic abnormality resulting from HIV infection is a quantitative deficiency of T4 lymphocytes. The question arises whether the depletion of T4 cells can be explained totally by the direct cytopathic effects discussed above or whether other indirect mechanisms contribute. The use of fluoresceinated antibodies against viral encoded proteins[41] and in situ hybridization techniques[42] to detect cells expressing viral proteins or mRNA, respectively, has shown that only an extremely small percentage of cells (in the range of 1 in 10^5) in the peripheral blood of HIV-infected individuals are expressing virus at any given time. It should be pointed out, however, that somewhat larger proportions of cells might be latently infected (see below). These cells are not expressing virus and therefore are not readily detractable by currently available techniques. Nonetheless, although the precise half-life of T4 cells is not known, in view of the normal turnover of T lymphocytes in the body[43] it would seem that the T cell pool would be able to compensate for such a seemingly low rate of T4 cell destruction. Thus, it has been hypothesized that in addition to a direct HIV-induced cytopathic effect on a given T4 cell, other potential mechanisms of T4 depletion may be operable.[44] For example, it is possible that HIV infects a T4 cell precursor or stem cell and that this leads to lack of production of mature cells. In addition, HIV might infect and selectively deplete a subset of T4 cells or even CD4$^+$ nonlymphoid cells that are critical to the propagation of the entire T4 cell pool. In this regard, it is known that T4 lymphocytes elaborate factors, including interleukin-2 (IL-2), that are trophic for lymphocytes[45] as well as for cells of the myeloid series.[46] Finally, another potential mechanism of T4 cell depletion is the induction by HIV or the secretion by HIV-infected cells of soluble factors that are toxic to T4 lymphocytes.[47]

Functional Abnormalities of T4 Lymphocytes

Although quantitative depletion of T4 lymphocytes is the most obvious immunologic abnormality in HIV-infected individuals, a qualitative or functional defect of a selective subset of T4 cells is also a consistent finding. It has been clearly demonstrated that the subset of T4 cells that recognizes and responds to soluble antigen is selectively deficient in patients with AIDS and that this deficiency occurs early in the course of the disease.[48] This defect is not due to an abnormality of antigen-presenting cells required for such responses. In a series of studies of identical twins, one of whom had AIDS and the other of whom was seronegative and healthy, monocytes from the seronegative twin, when cocultured with his autologous T cells, supported good proliferative responses to tetanus toxoid (TT) in vitro. However, monocytes from the seronegative twin failed to reconstitute the defective TT response when cocultured with T4 cells from the twin with AIDS.[49] Furthermore, we recently studied a large cohort of asymptomatic, seropositive homosexual men and noted the absence of an in vitro proliferative response to TT even after booster immunization in a substantial proportion of the subjects, many of whom had normal numbers of circulating T4 lymphocytes.[49] This observation could be explained by a selective depletion of this functional subset of T4 cells, a functional abnormality of the subset, or both. Since this defect has also been seen with other test antigens,[50] it is likely that it reflects abnormalities across the scope of the antigen-specific T cell repertoire. If this were explained completely by a depletion of this repertoire, one would have expected a significant quantitative deficiency in the total T4 cell pool, as was not noted in the above study. Hence, it is highly likely that a functional defect of T4 lymphocytes contributes to the observed abnormalities.

Functional abnormalities of T4 cells directly related to HIV can be explained by a noninfectious exposure of the T4 cell to HIV or by a noncytopathic infection of the T4 cell. We demonstrated earlier that exposure to HIV without infection of T4 cells results in a negative or tolerance-inducing signal, with the result that these cells are markedly defective in their responses to the subsequent exposure to soluble antigen and, to a lesser extent, mitogen.[51] Other studies have also shown that subunits of HIV, particularly the envelope, which certainly cannot induce infection, are capable of inhibiting cell function.[52]

There are a number of potential mechanisms of direct inhibition of T4 cell function by HIV in the absence of infection of the cell. Antigen-specific responses of T4 cells require the interaction of the CD4 molecule of the T4 cell with the class II major histocompatibility complex (MHC) molecule of the antigen-presenting cell during presentation of processed antigen to the CD3-Ti antigen receptor complex on the T4 cell.[53] Since the envelope of HIV binds avidly to the CD4 molecule of the T4 cell, this could readily block the critical interaction with the class II MHC molecule. Responses of T4 cells to mitogens are not critically dependent on this CD4–class II MHC molecule interaction, and therefore mitogens might override the block seen with antigen responses. This hypothesis is consistent with the observation that mitogen responses are normal in certain circumstances in which a selective defect in antigen responses is seen.

Another hypothesis is that noninfectious interaction of HIV with the T4 cell results in a defect in postreceptor signal transduction, either after ligand binding at the level of the CD4 molecule or at the level of antigen receptor (CD3-Ti complex) itself. Since triggering of cells by certain mitogens occurs through a different activation pathway than that of the cell's antigen receptor pathway,[54] this again might explain in part the discrepancy between suppression of antigen responses as opposed to mitogen responses.

Functional impairment of T4 cells may also occur after noncytopathic infection with HIV. After infection with HIV, T4 cells no longer express CD4 molecules on their cell surfaces. The lack of expression of CD4 on these infected antigen-responsive T4 cells could interfere with the required interaction of CD4 molecules and class II MHC molecules described above. Finally, infected Jurkat T cells surviving cyptopathic infection with HIV not only fail to express CD4 molecules on their surfaces, but also have decreased expression of the IL-2 gene in the face of normal expression of the IL-2 receptor gene.[55] A functional defect in IL-2 gene expression may well contribute to the antigen-specific defect that requires IL-2 for amplification of response.

B Cell Abnormalities

Persons with AIDS also have significant abnormalities of B cell function as manifested by polyclonal activation, hypergammaglobulinemia, circulating immune complexes, and autoantibodies. Despite the heightened spontaneous responsiveness of the B cell repertoire of these individuals, there is a deficient antibody response to new antigens such as keyhole limpet hemocyanin (KLH).[56] Although certain T cell-dependent B cell responses may be abnormal as a result of defects in helper function of the T4 cell, as described above, it is clear that other defective responses result from abnormalities at the B cell level. The humoral defect is manifested most obviously in an inability to mount an adequate immunoglobulin M (IgM) response to antigenic challenge. This has most severe consequences in infants and children infected with HIV who have not had previous exposure to a variety of pathogenic bacterial organisms and who must rely on an initial IgM response for adequate host defenses.[57] However, certain adult patients also manifest an increased susceptibility to various pyogenic bacteria, and this may also be related to the defect in humoral immune responses.[58] In addition, the defective humoral response may render the serologic diagnosis of certain infections unreliable.

The polyclonal hyperactivity of the B cell limb of the immune response is likely due to multiple factors. The high incidence of infection with Epstein-Barr virus (EBV) and cytomegalovirus (CMV), both of which are polyclonal B cell activators, certainly contributes to this phenomenon. Of importance is the fact that the HIV itself or subunits of the virus can polyclonally activate B cells in vitro.[59] In this regard, it has been demonstrated that a stretch of amino acids from a conserved region of the HIV envelope is partially homologous to neuroleukin, a factor that enhances B cell growth and differentiation.[60] However, it is unclear at present whether this is related to the HIV-induced polyclonal B cell activation.

Natural Killer Cells

The number of circulating natural killer (NK) cells is not significantly diminished in HIV-infected individuals, including patients who have developed AIDS, and these cells bind normally to their target cells.[61] However, their cytotoxic capability is diminished compared to that of normal individuals[62,63] but can be normalized when activated in vitro with a variety of inductive signals such as IL-2, concanavalin A, or phorbol ester and calcium ionophore.[63,64] These findings are in accord with the model of relative selectivity of defect at the level of the inductive T cell population, with secondary effects on those cell populations that rely on these inductive signals for functional integrity.

Monocytes in HIV Infection

Evidence is accumulating to support the concept that monocytes and macrophages play a major role in the propagation and pathogenesis of HIV infection. These phagocytic cells can engulf the virus. Certain subsets of monocytes express the CD4 surface antigen and therefore can bind to the envelope of HIV. It was demonstrated recently that monocytes can be infected in vitro with HIV, and the virus can be isolated from monocytes obtained from the blood and various organs of HIV-infected individuals.[65,66] In the brain, the major cell type infected with HIV appears to be the monocyte/macrophage,[67-69] and this may have important consequences for the development of neuropsychiatric manifestations associated with HIV infection (see below). Infected pulmonary alveolar macrophages may play a role in the interstitial pneumonitis seen in certain patients with AIDS[69] although EBV is responsible for this condition in certain pediatric patients.[70]

A number of monocyte functional abnormalities have been reported in AIDS patients, including defective chemotaxis and killing of certain organisms.[71] Although these abnormalities may be due to direct infection of monocytes by HIV, this explanation seems to be incomplete in view of the low frequency of infection of circulating blood monocytes. It is likely that the deficiency of inductive signals from the T4 cell (see above) is responsible for many of the functional defects of monocytes, a hypothesis that is supported by the fact that interferon-γ produced by T4 cells is capable of reconstituting certain defective functions of monocytes.[72]

It is also possible that secretion of monokines is directly or indirectly influenced by HIV infection. Monocytes from some AIDS patients spontaneously secrete increased amounts of IL-1, even though the induction of secretion of this factor is deficient.[73] It is quite possible that certain of the fevers and the wasting syndromes seen in AIDS patients are related to increased secretion of monokines such as IL-1 and tumor necrosis factor (cachectin).[74]

Perhaps the most important implication of the infectivity of monocytes with HIV is the possibility that the monocyte serves as the major reservoir for HIV in the body. Unlike the T4 lymphocyte, the monocyte is relatively refractory to the cytopathic effects of HIV so that not only can the virus survive in this cell but it can be transported to various organs in the body such as the lung and the brain. We recently developed cloned promonocyte cell lines derived from U-937 cells chronically infected with HIV.[75] One of these clones (U1) does not constitutively express virus but is latently infected with two integrated copies of provirus per cell and can be induced to express virus by certain cytokines (see below). Thus, monocyte precursors may be noncytopathologically infected and capable of secreting virus upon appropriate induction. In addition, HIV infection of the U1 clone results in the upregulation of IL-1β expression, an indication that HIV infection may have important influences on the expression of certain cellular genes.

Of particular interest is the recent finding of Gendelman et al.[76] that not only can monocytes harbor virus, but under certain circumstances they can actually serve as a major source of virus production in vitro. If this holds true in the in vivo situation, the monocyte may not only serve as a reservoir for the virus, but may be a major contributor to the viral burden of an infected host. The noncytopathic, low-replication infection of monocytes with HIV is somewhat analogous to infection with other lentiviruses such as the visna virus of sheep[77] against which effective immune surveillance does not develop. Similarly, persistence of HIV in human monocytes may explain in part the inability of an HIV-specific immune response to completely clear the body of virus.[78]

Latency or Low-Level Chronicity of HIV Infection

It is clear that upon infection of susceptible cell cultures with HIV, certain cells survive that are either latently (integrated provirus without virus expression) or chronically (low-level virus expression) infected. This can be demonstrated with infection of human peripheral blood lymphocytes[79] or CD4[+]T cell lines.[80] It is also clear that activation signals are required for the establishment of a productive HIV infection in vitro.[81] Given the extended time frame (up to 5 years or longer) from initial infection with HIV to clinically detectable immunologic abnormalities and disease manifestations, it is highly likely that the virus exists for prolonged periods in a latent or chronic form in both lymphocytes and monocytes. Gradual attrition of the T4 cells usually occurs in a linearly progressive fashion. However, intermittent bursts of virus production may result in accelerated killing of infected T4 cells and spread of infection to other T4 cells and monocytes. The length of time for clinically relevant immunosuppression to occur will depend upon the rate of this process, which might vary greatly from individual to individual. Since activation signals are required for the establishment of a productive HIV infection in vitro, it is likely that various activation signals in vivo contribute to conversion of a latent or chronic infection to a productive one. Phytohemagglutinin (PHA) has been used to induce productive infections in vitro. For the HIV-infected individual, the wide range of in vivo antigenic stimuli would serve as more physiologically relevant cellular activators than the global stimulation observed in vitro with mitogens. In this regard, when cultures of human lymphocytes were exposed to HIV in the presence or absence of soluble antigens such as TT or KLH, virus production as measured by reverse transcriptase activity was noted in the cultures exposed to antigen, whereas no virus was expressed in the absence of antigenic stimulation.

It has been postulated that other concomitant viral infections—for example, with EBV, CMV, hepatitis B, or herpes simplex virus

(HSV)—could induce HIV expression. When HIV-susceptible cells were simultaneously cotransfected with a plasmid containing the HIV LTR linked to the chloramphenicol acetyltransferase gene along with plasmids containing the *tat-III* gene and the immediate early genes from a variety of heterologous DNA viruses, it was clear that the presence of genes of these other viruses such as HSV in the presence of *tat-III* upregulated the expression of HIV.[82]

In addition to mitogens, antigens, and heterologous viruses, physiologic cellular inductive signals that might be encountered as part of the normal immune response might play a role in the induction of virus expression. We recently showed that cytokine-containing delectinized supernatants of PHA-stimulated human mononuclear cells as well as recombinant granulocyte-macrophage colony-stimulating factor (GM-CSF) are capable of inducing expression of virus in a chronically infected cloned promonocyte cell line (U1), which did not constitutively express virus (see above).[75] Although this phenomenon was observed in a cloned promonocyte cell line and may not be generally reflective of the total mononuclear cell repertoire, it nonetheless serves as a model to delineate the normal physiologic mechanisms that might be operable in the induction of virus expression from a latent or chronically infected state, with resultant cytopathicity, immunosuppression, and disease manifestations.

Pathogenesis of Neuropsychiatric Manifestations of HIV Infection

Neurologic abnormalities are quite common in AIDS and occur to varying degrees in at least 60 percent of patients. Details of the clinical and pathologic manifestations are reviewed elsewhere[83] and in this issue.[84] At least three currently recognized potential pathogenic mechanisms can explain the neuropsychiatric manifestations of HIV infection.

Monocyte/Macrophage–induced Pathogenic effects

It appears that the predominant cell type in the brain that is infected with HIV is the monocyte/macrophage. We previously demonstrated by simultaneous in situ hybridization and immunohistochemical staining that HIV mRNA was expressed selectively in multinucleated giant cells exhibiting monocyte markers in the brains of two patients with AIDS encephalopathy. Similar results were reported when immunoperoxidase techniques were used. Others have also reported infection of mononuclear cells and multinucleated giant cells, as well as endothelial cells and, rarely, astrocytes and neurons, in the brain. It is likely that the virus enters the brain through infected monocytes and releases monokines and enzymes that are toxic to neurons, as well as chemotactic factors that lead to infiltration of brain substance with inflammatory cells.

Direct Infection of Neuronal Tissue

It has been difficult to demonstrate direct infection of neuronal cells with HIV. Nonetheless, there are scattered reports of the demonstration of virus in neurons, oligodendrocytes, and astrocytes.[85] A number of studies have demonstrated the presence of CD4 molecules or mRNA for CD4 in neurons and glial cells from various areas of the brain[86] and so the potential exists for the binding to and infection of brain cells by HIV. The precise role of direct infection of the neuronal cells of the brain with HIV remains to be determined.

Inhibition of Neuroleukin

Finally, of particular interest is a recent report that the gp120 of the HIV envelope inhibited the growth of neurons in the presence of neuroleukin, but did not inhibit their growth in the presence of nerve growth factor.[87] It was postulated that the inhibition was due to the partial sequence homology between the gp120 and neuroleukin.

In conclusion, an extraordinary amount has been learned about the pathogenic mechanisms of HIV infection, particularly with regard to its effects on the human immune system. Certainly, further delineation of the nature of HIV-induced immunopathogenesis will be critical to the study, treatment, and prevention of HIV-related conditions and will also serve as a model for further understanding of the precise mechanisms of immunoregulation of the normal immune response.[88]

NOTES

1. A. S. Fauci, *Clin. Res.* 32,491 (1985); A. S. Fauci *et al.*, *Ann. Inter. Med.* 102, 800 (1985); D. L. Bowen, H. C. Lane, A. S. Fauci, *ibid.* 103, 704 (1985).

2. D. D. Ho, R. J. Pomerantz, J. C. Kaplan, *N. Engl. J. Med.* 317, 278 (1987).

3. Centers for Disease Control, *AIDS Weekly Surveillance Report—United States*, 30 November 1987.

4. U.S. Public Health Service, *Public Health Rep.* 101, 341 (1986).

5. T. C. Quinn, J. M. Mann, J. W. Curran, P. Piot, *Science* 234, 955 (1986).

6. A. S. Fauci *et al. Ann. Intern. Med.* 100, 92 (1984); J. W. Curran *et al., Science* 229, 1352 (1985).

7. R. C. Gallo *et al., Science* 224, 500 (1984).

8. F. Barré-Sinoussi *et al., ibid.* 220, 868 (1983).

9. J. A. Levy *et al., ibid.* 225, 840 (1984).

10. N. Nathanson *et al., Rev. Infect. Dis.*7, 75 (1985).

11. W. P. Cheevers and T. C. McGuire, *ibid.*, p. 83.

12. N. C. Pedersen, E. W. Ho, M. L. Brown, J. K. Yamamoto, *Science* 235, 790 (1987).

13. P. J. Kanki *et al., ibid.* 228, 1199 (1985); P. J. Kanki, J. Alroy, M. Essex, *ibid.* 230, 951 (1985); M. D. Daniel *et al., ibid.*, 228, 1201 (1985).

14. P. J. Kanki *et al., ibid.* 232, 238 (1986).

15. H. Kornfeld, N. Riedel, G. A. Viglianti, V. Hirsch, J. I. Mullins, *Nature (London)* 326, 610 (1987).

16. F. Clavel *et al., N. Engl. J. Med.* 316, 1180 (1987).

17. A. B. Rabson and M. A. Martin, *Cell* 40, 477 (1985).

18. A. B. Rabson, in *AIDS: Pathogenesis and Treatment*, J. A. Levy, Ed. (Dekker, New York, in press).

19. S. K. Arya, C. Guo, S. F. Josephs, F. Wong-Staal, *Science* 229, 69 (1985); A. G. Fisher *et al., Nature (London)* 320, 367 (1986); A. I. Dayton, J. G. Sodroski, C. A. Rosen, W. C. Goh, W. A. Haseltine, *Cell* 44, 941 (1986).

20. J. Sodroski *et al., Nature (London)* 321, 412 (1986); M. B. Feinberg, R. F. Jarrett, A. Aldorini, R. C. Gallo, F. Wong-Staal, *Cell* 46, 807 (1986).

21. P. A. Luciw, C. Cheng-Mayer, J. A. Levy, *Proc. Natl. Acad. Sci. U.S.A.* 84, 1434 (1987).

22. E. Terwilliger, J. G. Sodroski, C. A. Rosen, W. A. Haseltine, *J. Virol.* 60, 754 (1986).

23. K. Strebel *et al., Nature (London)* 328, 728 (1987); A. G. Fisher *et al., Science* 237, 888 (1987).

24. F. Wong-Staal, P. K. Chanda, J. Ghrayeb, *AIDS Res. Human Retroviruses* 3, 33 (1987).

25. D. L. Bowen, H. C. Lane, A. S. Fauci, *Ann. Intern. Med* 103, 704 (1985); J. B. Margolick and A. S. Fauci, in *Current Topics in AIDS*, M. S. Gottlieb *et al.*, Eds. (Wiley, New York, 1987), vol. 1, pp. 119–232; J. B. Margolick, H. C. Lane, A. S. Fauci, in *Viruses and Human Cancer*, R. C. Gallo, W. Haseltine, G. Klein, H. zur Hausen, Eds. (Liss, New York, 1987), vol. 43, pp. 59–79.

26. A. G. Dalgleish *et al.*, *Nature (London)* 312, 763 (1984); D. Klatzmann *et al.*, *ibid.*, p. 767; J. S. McDougal *et al.*, *Science* 231, 382 (1986).

27. P. J. Maddon *et al.*, *Cell* 47, 333 (1986).

28. B. S. Stein *et al.*, *ibid.* 49, 659 (1987).

29. G. M. Shaw *et al.*, *Science* 226, 1165 (1984).

30. R. C. Gallo, unpublished data.

31. D. Zagury *et al.*, *Science* 231, 850 (1986).

32. M. A. Talle *et al.*, *Cell Immunol.* 78, 83 (1983).

33. S. J. Stewart, J. Fujimoto, R. Levy, *J. Immunol.* 136, 3773 (1986); B. Åsjö *et al.*, *Virology* 157, 359 (1987).

34. A. DeRossi *et al.*, *Proc. Natl. Acad. Sci. U.S.A.* 83, 4297 (1986).

35. J. Sodroski, W. C. Goh, C. Rosen, K. Campbell, W. A. Haseltine, *Nature (London)* 322, 470 (1986); J. D. Lifson, G. R. Reyes, M. S. McGrath, B. S. Stein, E. G. Engleman, *Science* 232, 1123 (1986); J. D. Lifson *et al.*, *Nature (London)* 323, 725 (1986).

36. J. A. Hoxie *et al.*, *Science* 234, 1123 (1986).

37. D. Klatzmann and J. C. Gluckman, *Immunol. Today* 7, 291 (1986).

38. H. K. Lyerly, T. J. Matthews, A. J. Langlois, D. P. Bolognesi, K. J. Weinhold, *Proc. Natl. Acad. Sci. U.S.A.* 84, 4601 (1987).

39. R. B. Stricker *et al.*, *Nature (London)* 327, 710 (1987).

40. J. L. Ziegler and D. P. Stites, *Clin. Immunol. Immunopathol.* 41, 305 (1986).

41. T. M. Folks and A. S. Fauci, unpublished data.

42. M. E. Harper, L. M. Marselle, R. C. Gallo, F. Wong-Staal, *Proc. Natl. Acad. Sci. U.S.A.* 83, 772 (1986).

43. J. Sprent, in *B and T Cells in Immune Recognition*, F. Loor and R. F. Roelants, Eds. (Wiley, New York, 1977), pp. 59–82.

44. A. S. Fauci, *Proc. Natl. Acad. Sci. U.S.A.* 83, 9278 (1986).

45. T. A. Luger *et al.*, *J. Clin. Invest.* 70, 470 (1982).

46. S. C. Clark and R. Kamen, *Science* 236, 1229 (1987).

47. J. Laurence and L. Mayer, *ibid.* 225, 66 (1984).

48. H. C. Lane *et al.*, *N. Engl. J. Med.* 313, 79 (1984).

49. A. S. Fauci, *Clin. Res.* 35, 503 (1987).

50. G. M. Shearer *et al.*, *J. Immunol.* 137, 2514 (1986).

51. J. B. Margolick, D. J. Volkman, T. M. Folks, A. S. Fauci, *ibid.* 138, 1719 (1987).

52. D. L. Mann *et al.*, *ibid.*, p. 2640; M. R. Shalaby *et al.*, *Cell. Immunol.* 110, 140 (1987).

53. D. Gay *et al.*, *Nature (London)* 328, 626 (1987).

54. A. Alcover, D. Ramarli, N. E. Richardson, H.-C. Chang, E. L. Reinherz, *Immunol. Rev.* 95, 5 (1987).

55. W. C. Greene *et al.*, unpublished data.

56. H. C. Lane *et al.*, *N. Engl. J. Med.* 309, 453 (1983).

57. G. B. Scott, B. E. Buck, J. G. Letterman, F. L. Bloom, W. P. Parks, *ibid.* 310, 76 (1984).

58. B. Polsky *et al.*, *Ann. Intern. Med.* 104, 38 (1986).

59. S. Pahwa, R. Pahwa, C. Saxinger, R. C. Gallo, R. A. Good, *Proc. Natl. Acad. Sci. U.S.A.* 82, 8198 (1985); S. Pahwa, R. Pahwa, R. A. Good, R. C. Gallo, C. Saxinger, *ibid.* 83, 9124 (1986); R. Yarchoan, R. R. Redfield, S. Broder, *J. Clin. Invest.* 78, 439 (1986); S. M. Schnittman, H. C. Lane, S. E. Higgins, T. Folks, A. S. Fauci, *Science* 233, 1084 (1986).

60. M. E. Gurney *et al.*, *Science* 234, 574 (1986).

61. M. Katzman and M. M. Lederman, *J. Clin. Invest.* 77, 1057 (1986).

62. A. H. Rook *et al.*, *ibid.* 72, 398 (1983); M. M. Reddy, P. Chinoy, M. H. Grieco, *J. Biol. Res. Mod.* 3, 379 (1984).

63. A. H. Rook *et al.*, *J. Immunol.* 134, 1503 (1985).

64. B. Bonavida, J. Katz, M. Gottlieb, *ibid.* 137, 1157 (1986).

65. J. A. Levy *et al.*, *Virology* 147, 441 (1985); D. D. Ho, T. R. Rota, M. S. Hirsch, *J. Clin. Invest.* 77, 1712 (1986); J. K. Nicholson, K. A. Cross, G. D. Callaway, S. Carey, J. S. McDougal, *J. Immunol.* 137, 323 (1986); S. Gartner *et al.*, *Science* 233, 215 (1986).

66. S. Z. Salahuddin, R. M. Rose, J. E. Groopman, P. D. Markham, R. C. Gallo, *Blood* 68, 281 (1986).

67. S. Koenig *et al.*, *Science* 233, 1089 (1986).

68. C. A. Wiley, R. D. Schrier, J. A. Nelson, P. W. Lampert, M. A. Oldstone, *Proc. Natl. Acad. Sci. U.S.A.* 83, 7089 (1986).

69. B. H. Gabuzda *et al.*, *Ann. Neurol.* 20, 289 (1986).

70. W. A. Andiman *et al.*, *Lancet* 1985-II, 1390 (1985).

71. P. D. Smith *et al.*, *J. Clin. Invest.* 74, 2121 (1984); H. E. Prince, D. J. Moody, B. I. Shubin, J. L. Fahey, *J. Clin. Immunol.* 5, 21 (1985); G. Poli *et al.*, *Clin. Exp. Immunol.* 62, 136 (1985).

72. H. W. Murray, B. Y. Rubin, H. Masur, R. B. Roberts, *N. Engl. J. Med.* 310, 883 (1984).

73. P. D. Smith, L. M. Wahl, I. M. Katonah, Y. Miyake, S. M. Wahl, in preparation.

74. C. A. Dinarello, *Rev. Infect. Dis.* 6, 51 (1984); B. Beutler and A. Cerami, *Nature (London)* 320, 584 (1986).

75. T. M. Folks *et al.*, *Science* 238, 800 (1987).

76. H. E. Gendelman *et al.*, in preparation.

77. H. E. Gendelman, O. Narayan, S. Molineaux, J. E. Clements, Z. Ghotbi, *Proc. Natl. Acad. Sci. U.S.A.* 82, 7086 (1985).

78. S. Koenig and A. S. Fauci in *Cancer: Principles and Practice of Oncology*, V. T. DeVita, Jr., S. Hellman, S. A. Rosenberg, Eds. (Lippincott, Philadelphia, in press).

79. J. A. Hoxie, B. S. Haggarty, J. L. Rackowski, N. Pillsbury, J. A. Levy, *Science* 229, 1400 (1985).

80. T. Folks *et al.*, *ibid.* 231, 600 (1986).

81. J. S. McDougal *et al.*, *J. Immunol.* 135, 3151 (1985); T. M. Folks *et al.*, *ibid.* 136, 4049 (1986).

82. H. E. Gendelman *et al.*, *Proc. Natl. Acad. Sci. U.S.A.* 83, 9759 (1986); J. D. Mosca *et al.*, *Nature (London)* 325, 67 (1987).

83. W. D. Snider *et al.*, *Ann. Neurol.* 14, 403 (1983); S. L. Nielson, C. K. Petito, C. D. Urmacher, J. B. Posner, *Am. J. Clin. Pathol.* 82, 678 (1984); B. A. Navia, B. D. Jordan, R. W. Price, *Ann. Neurol.* 19, 517 (1986); S. M. de la Monte, D. D. Ho, R. T. Schooley, M. S. Hirsch, F. P. Richardson, Jr., *Neurology* 37, 562 (1987).

84. R. Price *et al.*, *Science* 239, 586 (1988).

85. M. H. Stoler, T. A. Eskin, S. Benn, R. C. Angerer, L. M. Angerer, *J. Am. Med. Assoc.* 256, 2360 (1986); F. Gyorkey, J. L. Melnick, P. Gyorkey, *J. Infect. Dis.* 155, 870 (1987).

86. I. Funke, A. Hahn, E. P. Rieber, E. Weiss, G. Riethmüller, *J. Exp. Med.* 165, 1230 (1987).

87. M. R. Lee, D. D. Ho, M. E. Gurney, *Science* 237 1047 (1987).

88. The author thanks Z. Rosenberg, T. M. Folks, H. C. Lane, S. Koenig, S. M. Schnittman, G. Poli, M. Martin, H. E. Gendelman, and A. B. Rabson for helpful discussions and A. C. London for expert editorial assistance.

Human Immunodeficiency Virus and Acquired Immunodeficiency Syndrome: Correlation but Not Causation

Peter H. Duesberg

October 21, 1988

Abstract

AIDS is an acquired immunodeficiency syndrome defined by a severe depletion of T cells and over 20 conventional degenerative and neoplastic diseases. In the U.S. and Europe, AIDS correlates to 95 percent with risk factors, such as about 8 years of promiscuous male homosexuality, intravenous drug use, or hemophilia. Since AIDS also correlates with antibody to a retrovirus, confirmed in about 40 percent of American cases, it has been hypothesized that this virus causes AIDS by killing T cells. Consequently, the virus was termed human immunodeficiency virus (HIV), and antibody to HIV became part of the definition of AIDS. The hypothesis that HIV causes AIDS is examined in terms of Koch's postulates and epidemiological, biochemical, genetic, and evolutionary conditions of viral pathology. HIV does not fulfill Koch's postulates: (i) free virus is not detectable in most cases of AIDS; (ii) virus can only be isolated by reactivating virus in vitro *from a few latently infected lymphocytes among millions of uninfected ones; (iii) pure HIV*

Peter H. Duesberg, "Human Immunodeficiency Virus and Acquired Immunodeficiency Syndrome: Correlation but Not Causation," *National Academy of Sciences* (National Academy of Science Press, February 1989). Reprinted by Permission of the National Academy of Sciences, Washington, D.C.

Abbreviations: AIDS, acquired immunodeficiency syndrome; AZT, azidothymidine; EBV, Epstein-Barr virus; HIV, human immunodeficiency virus.

does not cause AIDS upon experimental infection of chimpanzees or accidental infection of healthy humans. Further, HIV violates classical conditions of viral pathology. (i) Epidemiological surveys indicate that the annual incidence of AIDS among antibody-positive persons varies from nearly 0 to over 10 percent, depending critically on nonviral risk factors. (ii) HIV is expressed in .2831 of every 10^4 T cells it supposedly kills in AIDS, whereas about 5 percent of all T cells are regenerated during the 2 days it takes the virus to infect a cell. (iii) If HIV were the cause of AIDS, it would be the first virus to cause a disease only after the onset of antiviral immunity, as detected by a positive "AIDS test." (iv) AIDS follows the onset of antiviral immunity only after long and unpredictable asymptomatic intervals averaging 8 years, although HIV replicates within 1 to 2 days and induces immunity within 1 to 2 months. (v) HIV supposedly causes AIDS by killing T cells, although retroviruses can only replicate in viable cells. In fact, infected T cells grown in culture continue to divide. (vi) HIV is isogenic with all other retroviruses and does not express a late, AIDS-specific gene. (vii) If HIV were to cause AIDS, it would have a paradoxical, country-specific pathology, causing over 90 percent of Pneumocystis pneumonia and Kaposi sarcoma in the U.S. but over 90 percent slim disease, fever, and diarrhea in Africa. (viii) It is highly improbable that within the last few years two viruses (HIV-1 and HIV-2) that are only 40 percent sequence-related would have evolved that could both cause the newly defined syndrome AIDS. Also, viruses are improbable that kill their only natural host with efficiencies of 50–100 percent, as is claimed for HIVs. It is concluded that HIV is not sufficient for AIDS and that it may not even be necessary for AIDS because its activity is just as low in symptomatic carriers as in asymptomatic carriers. The correlation between antibody to HIV and AIDS does not prove causation, because otherwise indistinguishable diseases are now set apart only on the basis of this antibody. I propose that AIDS is not a contagious syndrome caused by one conventional virus or microbe. No such virus or microbe would require almost a decade to cause primary disease, nor could it cause the diverse collection of AIDS diseases. Neither would its host range be as selective as that of AIDS, nor could it survive if it were as inefficiently transmitted as AIDS. Since AIDS is defined by new combinations of conventional diseases, it may be caused by new combinations of conventional pathogens, including acute viral or microbial infections and chronic drug use and malnutrition. The long and unpredictable intervals between *infection with HIV and AIDS would then reflect the thresholds for these pathogenic factors to cause AIDS diseases, instead of an unlikely mechanism of HIV pathogenesis.*

The important thing is to not stop questioning.

ALBERT EINSTEIN

In 1981, acquired immunodeficiency was proposed to be the common denominator of a newly defined syndrome (AIDS) of diseases that were on the rise in promiscuous male homosexuals and intravenous drug users, referred to as "AIDS risk groups."[1,2] Since then, about 70,000 persons have developed AIDS in the U.S., of whom over 90 percent are still from these same risk groups.[3,4] The hallmark of AIDS is a severe depletion of T cells.[5-7] By definition, this immunodeficiency manifests itself in over 20 previously known degenerative and neoplastic diseases, including Kaposi sarcoma, Burkitt and other lymphomas, *Pneumocystis* pneumonia, diarrhea, dementia, candidiasis, tuberculosis, lymphadenopathy, slim disease, fever, herpes, and many others.[7-11] The frequent reference to AIDS as a new disease,[12-14] instead of a new syndrome composed of old diseases, has inspired a search for a single new pathogen. However, it is debatable whether a single pathogen can explain over 20 diseases, whether a clustering of old diseases in risk groups that only recently became visible signals a new pathogen, and whether an AIDS pathogen must be infectious. Indeed, compared to conventional infectious diseases, AIDS is very difficult to acquire and has a very selective host range, usually manifesting only in individuals who have taken AIDS risks for an average of 8 years (see below).

The Virus—AIDS Hypothesis

About 40 percent of the AIDS patients in the U.S.,[5] and many of those who are at risk for AIDS, have been confirmed to have neutralizing antibodies to a retrovirus that was discovered in 1983.[15] These antibodies are detected by the "AIDS test." Less than a year later, in 1984, this virus was adopted as the cause of AIDS by the U.S. Department of Health and Human Services and the AIDS test was registered as a patent, even before the first American study on the virus was published.[16] The epidemiological correlation between these antibodies and AIDS is the primary basis for the hypothesis that AIDS is caused by this virus.[3,7,12,14,17,18] AIDS is also believed to be caused by this virus because AIDS diseases appear in a small percentage (see below) of recipients of blood transfusions that have antibodies to this virus.[19-22] In view of this the virus has been named human immunodeficiency virus (HIV) by an international committee of retrovirologists and antibody to HIV became part of the definition of AIDS. If confirmed, HIV would be the first clinically relevant retrovirus since the Virus-Cancer Program called for viral carcinogens in 1971.[23,24]

The virus–AIDS hypothesis holds that the retrovirus HIV causes AIDS by killing T cells in the manner of a cytocidal virus and is transmitted by sex and parenteral exposure. Early evidence for a T-cell-specific HIV receptor lent support to this hypothesis.[25] Recently, however, the presumed T-cell specificity of HIV has lost ground, as HIV is only barely detectable in T cells and often is detectable only in monocytes[26-28] and other body cells,[29-32] displaying the same lack of virulence and broad host range toward differentiated cells as all other human and animal retroviruses. In about 50 percent of those who habitually practice risk behavior or regularly receive transfusions, AIDS is estimated to occur after an average asymptomatic period of about 8 years from the onset of antiviral immunity, and in up to 100 percent after about 15 years.[33-38] Therefore, HIV is called a "slow" virus, or lentivirus. It is on the basis of the relatively high conversion rates of these risk groups that every asymptomatic infection by HIV is now being called "HIV disease,"[39] and that some are subjected to chemotherapy.[40] Nevertheless, individual asymptomatic periods are unpredictable, ranging from <1 to >15 years. Once AIDS is diagnosed, the mean life expectancy is about 1 year.

The early adoption of the virus–AIDS hypothesis by the U.S. Department of Health and Human Services and by retrovirologists is the probable reason that the hypothesis was generally accepted without scrutiny. For instance, the virus is typically referred to as deadly by the popular press[41,42] and public enemy number 1 by the U.S. Department of Health and Human Services.[43] In view of this, it is surprising that the virus has yet to cause the first AIDS case among hundreds of unvaccinated scientists who have propagated it for the past 5 years at titers that exceed those in AIDS patients by up to 6 orders of magnitude (see below) with no more containment than is required for marginally pathogenic animal viruses.[44] It is also surprising that despite 2,000 recorded (and probably many more unrecorded) parenteral exposures to HIV-infected materials, unvaccinated health care workers have exactly the same incidence of AIDS as the rest of the U.S. labor force.[45,186] Further, it is difficult to believe that a sexually transmitted virus would not have caused more than 1,649 sex-linked AIDS cases among the 125 million American women in 8 years—and this number is not even corrected for the antibody-negative women who might have developed such diseases over an 8-year period. Morever, it is paradoxical for a supposedly new viral epidemic that the estimates of infected persons in the U.S. have remained constant at 0.5 to 1.5 million[46,47] or even declined to <1 million since the "AIDS test" became available in 1985.

About 2 years ago I proposed that HIV is not likely to be the cause of AIDS.[48–50] This proposal has since been fiercely challenged or defended at meetings and in publications.[51–65,180] Here I respond to these challenges.

HIV Does Not Meet Koch's Postulates

HIV Cannot Account for the Loss of T Cells and the Clinical Course of AIDS

The causative agent of an infectious disease is classically defined by the postulates of Robert Koch and Jacob Henle.[66,67] They were originally formulated a priori by Henle about 50 years before bacteria and viruses were discovered to be pathogens. However, their definitive text was formulated by Koch to distinguish causative from other bacteria at a time when bacteriologists applying newly developed tools in the search for pathogenic microbes found all sorts of bacteria in humans. This situation was quite similar to our current increasing proficiency in demonstrating viruses.[68] The first of these postulates states that "the parasite must be present in every single case of the disease, under conditions that can account for the pathological lesions and the clinical course of the disease." However, there is no free virus in most—and very little in some—persons with AIDS, or in asymptomatic carriers.[69,70] Virus titers range from 0 to 10 infectious units per milliliter of blood. Viral RNA is found in a very low percentage (see below) of blood cells of 50–80 percent of antibody-positive persons.[71–74] Further, no provirus is detectable in blood cells of 70–100 percent of symptomatic or asymptomatic antibody-positive persons, if tested by direct hybridization of cellular DNA with cloned proviral DNA[75,187] at the limit of detection by this method.[76] Antibody to HIV is confirmed in only about 40 percent of the U.S. cases and in only 7 percent of the AIDS cases from New York and San Francisco, which represent one-third of all U.S. cases. In some cases, even the antibody to HIV disappears, due to chronic dormancy or loss of the HIV provirus[77,78]—

analogous to the loss of antibody to other viruses long after infection. Indeed, the Centers for Disease Control publishes specific guidelines for AIDS cases in which laboratory evidence for HIV is totally negative. Thus, although viral elements can be traced in many AIDS patients, and antibody to HIV is, at least by definition, present in all of them, HIV violates Koch's first postulate in terms of a tangible presence, of being "under conditions that can account for" the loss of T cells, and of the "clinical course of the disease" that lags 8 years behind infection.

The absence of free virus in most AIDS cases and in antibody-positive asymptomatic carriers explains why HIV is not casually transmitted. For example, the probability of transmission of the virus from an antibody-positive to an antibody-negative person by heterosexual intercourse is estimated to be 1 in 500.[79,80]

Due to Extremely Low Titers, HIV Can Be Isolated Only with Great Difficulty from AIDS Patients

Koch further postulated that it must be possible to isolate and propagate the etiological agent from all cases of the disease. However, virus isolation, although possible in up to 80 percent of AIDS cases, is technically very difficult and is perhaps best described as maieutic.[81–84] It depends on reactivation of dormant proviruses from one or a few latently infected lymphocytes among millions of uninfected lymphocytes from AIDS patients. This is only possible by culturing these cells for several weeks in vitro, away from the suppressive, virus-neutralizing immune system of the host. Even then success sometimes comes only after 15 (!) trials.[85] These difficulties and the often over 20 percent failure rate in isolation of HIV from AIDS patients are consistent with the extremely low titers of HIV in such patients. Thus, HIV does not meet Koch's second postulate.

In vitro reactivation of latent HIV from antibody-positive persons is exactly analogous to the in vitro reactivation of latent Epstein–Barr virus (EBV) from healthy persons with antibody to EBV.[86] As in the case of HIV (see below), acute EBV infections occasionally cause mononucleosis.[86–88] Subsequent antiviral immunity restricts EBV to chronic latency.[87,88] Since latent EBV, again like latent HIV, is present in only 1 of 10^7 lymphocytes, millions of these cells must be cultivated in vitro to reactivate the virus.

HIV Does Not Reproduce AIDS
When Inoculated into Animals or Humans

Animal Infections

Koch's third postulate calls for inducing the disease by experimental infection of a suitable host with pure pathogen. Chimpanzees infected with pure HIV develop antibodies, indicating that they are susceptible to HIV. However, all attempts to cause AIDS in chimpanzees have been unsuccessful, even after they have been antibody-positive for 4 to 5 years. Thus, Koch's third postulate has not been fulfilled in animals.

Accidental Human Infections

Due to extremely low titers of HIV in all antibody-positive materials, very few infections have occurred. Four women who received infected donor semen in 1984 developed antibody to HIV. Yet none of them developed AIDS or transmitted the virus to their husbands, although insufficient time has elapsed for the average latent period that the virus is thought to require to cause AIDS (see below). Moreover, three of these women subsequently became pregnant and gave birth to healthy infants.[89] Further, 15 to 20 accidental infections of health care workers and scientists propagating HIV were identified during the last 4 years on the basis of antiviral antibodies, and none of these people have developed AIDS.[90]

Recently, a single conversion to AIDS of such an antibody-positive health care worker was reported anonymously without data on gender, latent period, or AIDS symptoms. This case was claimed to prove Koch's third postulate. However, 2,586 health care workers got AIDS without occupational infection. About 95 percent of these fall into the conventional risk groups and 5 percent are without verifiable AIDS risks—which are notoriously difficult to verify.[91,92] From the 135 (5 percent of 2,586) health care workers who developed AIDS without verifiable risks, the one who contracted an occupational infection was selected to prove that such infections, rather than other risks, caused AIDS. It is arbitrary to base a hypothesis on 1 case when 134 cases do not support the hypothesis. To prove the hypothesis, it is necessary to show that the percentage of health care workers with AIDS who do not belong to the known risk groups exceeds that of the rest of the population and reflects their sexual distribution. However, the incidence and even the sexual distribution of AIDS cases among health care workers are exactly the same as that of AIDS in the general population, namely 92 percent males, although 75 percent of the health care workers are female. Moreover, a subsequent study that included this case described only transient, mononucleosis-like symptoms but not one AIDS case among occupationally infected health care workers.

Blood transfusions are another source of iatrogenic infections. The best-documented cases are the 10,000 to 14,000 U.S. hemophiliacs with antibody to HIV,[93,94] of whom only 646 developed symptoms of AIDS between 1981 and August 1988. During the year that ended in August 1988, 290 developed AIDS, whereas 178 developed AIDS in the previous year. This corresponds to annual conversion rates of about 1–3 percent. Higher rates, of up to 25 percent, have been observed in certain groups of hemophiliacs. However, the view that AIDS in recipients of transfusions is due to HIV transmission is presumptive on several grounds. (i) Blood transfusion does not distinguish between HIV and other undetected viruses, microbes, and blood-borne toxins. This is particularly true since HIV-positive blood was never knowingly transfused. (ii) It is presumed that the recipients had no AIDS risks other than HIV during the average of 8 years between HIV infection and AIDS symptoms. The transfusion evidence would be more convincing if AIDS appeared in step with virus replication (see below) soon after a singular transfusion. (iii) Transfusion-related AIDS cases occur primarily in persons with other health risks, such as hemophilia, that are not representative of healthy individuals. (iv) Above all, the transfusion cases are all anecdotal.[95,96] There are no controlled studies to show that recipients of transfusions with antibody to HIV have more of the diseases now called AIDS than those without antibody to HIV.

The assertion that HIV causes AIDS is also contained in the erroneous claims that new cases of transfusion AIDS have virtually ceased appearing since the AIDS test became available in 1985, due to a factor-of-40 reduction of transfusions with antibody-positive blood. In fact, adult transfusion AIDS cases have doubled and pediatric cases have tripled in the year ending August 8, compared to the previous year. The increase in adult cases could be expected if one were to accept the assumptions that HIV requires 8 years to cause AIDS (see below) and that there was a rapid increase in unconfirmed HIV transfusions 8 years ago, which stopped 3 years ago. However, the increase in pediatric cases in the face of a 40-fold reduction of antibody-positive transfusions argues directly against HIV as the cause of AIDS, because the average latent period in children is only 2 years.

HIV Does Not Meet Established Epidemiological, Biochemical, Genetic, and Evolutionary Criteria of a Viral Pathogen

Epidemiologies of AIDS and HIV Are Not Consistent

Epidemiology has been proposed as adequate to identify causative agents, particularly in human diseases where Koch's postulates are difficult to meet, as in the case of HIV. Nevertheless, even a consistent correlation with virus—not with antibody—would fulfill only the first postulate. However, the epidemiologies of AIDS and HIV are not consistent in different risk groups and countries.

About 10 percent of the 30 million people in Zaire have been reported since 1985 to be antibody-positive.[98,184] However, only 335 AIDS cases have been reported in Zaire as of 1988.[97,99] This corresponds to an annual conversion rate of 0.004 percent. Also, since 1985, 6 percent of the 6 million Haitians have been reported to be antibody-positive,[100] but only 912 had developed AIDS by 1988. This corresponds to an annual conversion rate of 0.1 percent. Of 0.5 to 1.5 million antibody-positive Americans, about 29,000 (including 9,000 who meet only the 1987 definition for AIDS developed AIDS in the year ending August 1988, and, according to earlier definitions, 16,000 to 17,000 developed AIDS in each of the previous 2 years. This corresponds to an annual conversion rate of about 1.5 percent for the average antibody-positive American. Thus, the AIDS risk of an antibody-positive person varies with the country of residence. These calculations all assume that the pools of short- and long-term HIV carriers in each of these countries are comparable. This assumption is based on the claims that HIV was newly introduced into all countries with AIDS about 10 to 20 years ago.

Moreover, the AIDS risk of an antibody-positive American varies a great deal with his or her risk group. For example, 3–25 percent of antibody-positive Americans who habitually practice risk behavior or are hemophiliacs develop AIDS annually. Thus, the 1.5 percent annual conversion rate of antibody-positive Americans is an average of minorities with high conversion rates of 3–25 percent and a majority with a conversion rate close to 0 percent.

Since the incidence of AIDS among antibody-positive persons varies from 0 to over 10 percent depending on factors defined by lifestyle, health, and country of residence, it follows that HIV is not sufficient to cause AIDS.

AIDS Occurs Despite Minimal Viral Activity

During replication, viruses are biochemically very active in the host cell. If they replicate in more cells than the host can spare or regenerate, they typically cause a disease.

Paradoxically, HIV is very inactive even when it is said to cause fatal immunodeficiency. Viral RNA synthesis is detectable in only 1 of 10^4 to 10^6 mononuclear lymphocytes, including T cells. Frequently, virus can only be found in monocytes, and not in T cells. Virus expression recorded in monocyte-macrophages is at the same low levels as in other lymphocytes. Thus, there is as yet no experimental proof for the suggestion, based on experiments in cell culture, that monocyte-macrophages may be the reservoirs of the virus in vivo. Also, very few lung and brain cells ever express HIV.[101,102] At this level of infiltration HIV cannot account by any known mechanism for the loss of T cells that is the hallmark of AIDS, even if all actively infected T cells died. During the 2 days it takes for a retrovirus to replicate, the body regenerates about 5 percent of T cells[103] more than enough to compensate for presumptive losses due to the virus. Hence, HIV cannot be sufficient to cause AIDS.

Although there is virtually no free virus, and HIV RNA synthesis is extremely low, both in AIDS patients and in asymptomatic carriers, it has been argued that the viral core protein p24 is produced at higher levels in AIDS patients than in asymptomatic carriers.[104–108, 183] However, all studies on p24 report AIDS cases that occur without p24 antigenemia, indicating that p24 is not necessary for AIDS. They also report antigenemia without AIDS, indicating that p24 is not sufficient for AIDS. Moreover, antigenemic carriers are not viremic because they always maintain an excess of virus-neutralizing antibodies directed against the viral envelope, a positive AIDS test. In addition, the colorimetric antibody test used to measure p24 protein raises unresolved questions. Reportedly, the assay's detection limit is 50 pg/ml, and up to 100 times more p24 than that is found in some HIV carriers. Five hundred picograms of p24 is the protein equivalent of 10^6 HIV particles, given 10^{-3} pg per retrovirus, half of which is core protein.[110] Yet such high concentrations of p24 cannot be reconciled with the extremely low numbers of cells in AIDS patients that are engaged in viral RNA synthesis, nor can the failure to isolate virus from 20–50 percent of p24-antigenemic patients. Based on my 24-year experience with retroviruses, only large numbers of infected cells growing in the absence of antiviral immunity in vivo or in vitro produce such high titers of virus or viral protein. Thus, the assertions that HIV becomes activated during AIDS or that p24 antigenemia is necessary for the syndrome are without experimental support.

AIDS Occurs Despite Antiviral Immunity

Viruses typically cause disease before virus-neutralizing antibodies and cellular immunity appear. Antiviral antibodies signal a successful rejection of the virus and a lasting protection (vaccination) against diseases by the same or related viruses. Immunity is the only weapon against viral disease.

Paradoxically, HIV is said to cause AIDS, by definition, only years after inducing very active antiviral immunity. If this assertion were correct, HIV would be the first virus to cause a disease only after antiviral immunity. Yet the effectiveness of this immunity is the reason that provirus remains dormant and that free HIV cannot be found in AIDS patients. In view of this, vaccination of antibody-positive HIV was the cause of AIDS.[111–113] The claims of some scientists that antiviral antibodies fail to neutralize HIV[113–115] are incompatible with the efficient immunity in vivo and with experimental evidence for virus-neutralizing activity in vitro.[115–119]

Although most viruses are eliminated by immunity, some, such as the retroviruses and the herpesviruses, may persist—severely restricted by antiviral immunity—as latent infections. Such viruses can again become pathogenic, but only when they are reactivated. For example, upon reactivation, the herpesviruses cause fever blisters or zoster even in the presence of serum antibody.[120] Reactivation may follow a decline of cellular immunity in response to other parasitic infections, radiation, or immunosuppressive therapy. Further, it has been claimed that 8 years after primary infection and immunity, latent measles virus may cause subacute sclerosing panencephalitis[121] in about 1 case per million and that another latent paramyxovirus may cause multiple sclerosis. However, these viruses could be isolated from each system in only 2 of 8 cases after cultivating millions of patient cells in vitro. Moreover, multiple sclerosis has since been suggested to be caused by a latent retrovirus closely related to HIV[122] and subacute encephalitis by HIV. Thus, there is no proven precedent for the hypothesis that HIV causes AIDS only years after the onset of antiviral immunity and yet remains as inactive as it is in asymptomatic infections.

It has been proposed that pathogenic HIV mutants arise during the long intervals between infection and AIDS and that these mutants might escape antiviral immunity by losing specific epitopes[123,124] or even by changing their host range from T cells to macrophages. However, there is no report of a mutant HIV present at high titer in AIDS. Further, it is very unlikely that a mutant could escape an existing immunity, because it would share most variable and, of necessity, all constant determinants with the parent virus. Even though all retroviruses, including HIV,[125-128] mutate at a frequency of 1 in 10^4 nucleotides per replicative cycle, they have never been observed to escape an existing antiviral immunity. It has also been proposed that HIV escapes immunity by spreading via cell-to-cell transmission.[129] However, consistent with the syncytium-blocking function of natural antibodies there is no spread of HIV in vivo.

Intervals of 2 to 15 Years Between Infection and AIDS Are Incompatible with HIV Replication

If cytocidal viruses or retroviruses cause disease, they do so within 1 to 2 months of infection. By that time, the host's immune system either eliminates the virus or restricts it to latency, or the virus overcomes the immune system and kills the host. Indeed, clinicians have reported that, in rare cases, HIV causes a disease like mononucleosis prior to immunity, presumably due to an acute infection.[130] Since this disease correlates with viral activity and disappears within weeks as the body develops antiviral immunity, it may reflect the true pathogenic potential of HIV.

Considering that HIV replicates within 2 days in tissue culture and induces antiviral immunity within 1 to 2 months, the inevitably long and seemingly unpredictable intervals, ranging from 1 to 15 years, between the onset of antiviral immunity and AIDS are bizarre. The average latent period is reported to be 8 years in adults and 2 years in children. Indeed, at least 2 years of immunity is required before AIDS appears in adults. If one accepts that 50–100 percent of antibody-positive Americans eventually develop AIDS, the average 1.5 percent annual conversion corresponds to grotesque viral latent periods of 30 to 65 years. These intervals between HIV infection and AIDS clearly indicate all genes of HIV are expressed during the early immunogenic phase of the infection. AIDS should occur at that time, rather than years later when it is latent.

In an effort to rationalize the long intervals between infection and AIDS, HIV has been classified as a slow virus or lentivirus, a type of retrovirus that is thought to cause disease only after long incubation periods. Yet there are no "slow" viruses. Since viral nucleic acids and proteins are synthesized by the cell, viruses must replicate as fast or faster than cells (i.e., within hours or days) to survive.

Nevertheless, as pathogens, viruses may be (i) fast in acute infections that involve many actively infected cells, (ii) slow in subacute infections that involve moderate numbers of actively infected cells, or (iii) asymptomatic and latent. Retroviruses provide examples of each different pathogenic role. Acute infections with the "slow" Visna/ Maedi retrovirus of sheep, a lentivirus, rapidly cause pneumonia,[131] and those with equine anemia lentivirus cause fever and anemia within days or weeks of infection.[132] Such infections typically generate titers of 10^4 to 10^5 infectious units per milliliter or gram of tissue.[132,133] The caprine arthritis-encephalitis lentivirus is also pathogenic within 2 months of inoculation.[134] Acute infections with other retroviruses also rapidly cause debilitating diseases or cancers. This includes retrovirus infections that are now considered to be animal models of AIDS, termed simian or feline AIDS.[135] Unlike HIV in AIDS, these viruses are all very active when they cause diseases, and the respective diseases appear shortly after infection. In rare cases, when antiviral immunity fails to restrict Visna/Maedi or other retroviruses, they persist as subacute symptomatic infections. Under these conditions, Visna/Maedi virus causes a slow, progressive pulmonary disease[136] by chronically infecting a moderate number of cells that produce moderate titers of 10^2 to 10^5 virus particles per gram of tissue. However, in over 99 percent of all Visna/Maedi or caprine arthritis-encephalitis virus infections, and in most equine anemia virus infections, the retrovirus is either eliminated or restricted to latency by immunity, and hence asymptomatic, exactly like almost all other retroviruses in mice, chickens, cats, and other animals. For instance, 30–50 percent of all healthy sheep in the U.S., Holland, and Germany have asymptomatic Visna/Maedi virus infections,[137,138] and 80 percent of healthy goats in the U.S. have asymptomatic caprine arthritis-encephalitis virus infections in the presence of antiviral immunity.

Thus, the progressive diseases induced by active retroviruses depend on relative tolerance to the virus due to rare native or acquired immunodeficiency or congenital infection prior to immune competence. Since tolerance to HIV that would result in active chronic infection has never been observed and is certainly not to be expected for 50–100 percent of infections (the percentage of infections said to develop into AIDS [reference 7 and above]), the rare retrovirus infections of animals that cause slow, progressive diseases are not models for how HIV might cause AIDS. Indeed, not one acute retrovirus infection has ever been described in humans.

The Paradox of How HIV, a Noncytocidal Retrovirus, Is to Cause the Degenerative Disease AIDS

Unlike cytocidal viruses, which replicate by killing cells, retroviruses need viable cells for replication.[139] During retroviral infection, proviral DNA becomes a cellular gene as it is integrated into the DNA of the cell. Such a mechanism is superfluous for a cytocidal virus. Virus reproduction from then on is essentially gene expression in viable cells, often stimulating hyperplastic growth. Alternatively, retroviruses survive as latent proviruses, like latent cellular genes. The very distinction of not killing the host cell is the reason that scientists have for so long considered retroviruses to be the most plausible viral carcinogens.[140]

Yet HIV, a retrovirus, is said to behave like a cytocidal virus, causing AIDS by killing billions of T cells. This is said even though some infected T-cell lines remain immortal, and primary umbilical-cord blood cells may continue to divide in culture while propagating up to 10^6 infectious units per milliliter, much more than in AIDS patients. Also, there are no cytopathic changes or cell death in cultures of HIV-infected monocytes and macrophages[141-146] and B cells.[147] As is typical of retroviruses, HIV does not kill its host cells.

The cytocidal effects that are occasionally observed in HIV-infected cultures (but as yet, never in humans) soon after infection do not break this rule. These early effects result from fusions of HIV-infected and uninfected cells that depend on virus isolates and cell culture conditions, and are completely inhibited by antiviral antibody. They are not HIV-specific, because many animal and human retroviruses show conditional, but never absolute, cytocidal effects in cell culture. Thus, the fusion effect in culture might be relevant for the mononucleosis observed in some patients soon after infection, when free virus (but no fusion-inhibitory antibody) is present. However, the effect cannot be relevant to AIDS because there is plenty of fusion-inhibitory antibody and because the virus isolates from some patients fuse, and those from others don't. Thus, HIV is not sufficient to kill even the few T cells it infects in AIDS.

HIV Is a Conventional Retrovirus, Without an AIDS Gene

The virus–AIDS hypothesis proposes that HIV is an unorthodox retrovirus containing specific suppressor and activator genes that control the 2- to 15-year intervals between infection and AIDS.[188]

However, the two known HIVs (see below) are profoundly conventional retroviruses. They have the same genetic complexity of about 9,150 nucleotides, the same genetic structure, including the three major essential retrovirus genes linked in the order *gag–pol–env*, the same mechanism of replication, and the same mutation frequency[148] as all other retroviruses. Humans carry between 50 and 100 such retroviruses in their germ line, mostly as latent proviruses.[149,150] The presumably specific genes of the HIVs are alternative reading frames of essential genes shared by all retroviruses.[151] Their apparent novelty is more likely to reflect new techniques of gene analysis than to represent HIV-specific retroviral functions. Indeed, analogous genes have recently been found in other retroviruses, including one bovine and at least three other human retroviruses that do not cause AIDS.[152] Because HIV and all other retroviruses are isogenic, the newly discovered genes cannot be AIDS-specific. Moreover, it is unlikely that these genes even control virus replication. In vivo, HIV lies chronically dormant, although the presumed suppressor genes are not expressed. In vitro, HIV is propagated at titers of about 10^6 per ml in the same human cells in which it is dormant in vivo, although the presumed suppressor genes are highly expressed. Therefore, I propose that antiviral immunity rather than viral genes suppress HIV in vivo, as is the case with essentially all retroviruses in wild animals. Further, I propose that the multiplicity of AIDS diseases are caused by a multiplicity of risk factors (see below), rather than by one or a few viral activator genes, since viral gene expression in AIDS is just as low as in asymptomatic carriers. Also, the extremely low genetic complexity of HIV can hardly be sufficient to control the inevitably long times between infection and AIDS, and the great diversity of AIDS diseases. Thus, there is neither biochemical nor genetic evidence that HIV genes initiate or maintain AIDS.

The Paradoxes of an AIDS Virus with Country- and Risk-Specific Pathologies and Host Ranges

It is yet another paradox of the virus–AIDS hypothesis that HIV is said to cause very different diseases in different risk groups and countries. For example, in the U.S. over 90 percent of AIDS patients have *Pneumocystis* pneumonia or Kaposi sarcoma. However, Kaposi sarcoma is found almost exclusively in homosexuals. By contrast, in Africa over 90 percent of the AIDS cases are manifested by slim disease, fever, and diarrhea. Moreover, it is paradoxical that the prevalence of Kaposi sarcoma among U.S. AIDS cases has shifted down from 35 percent in 1983[156] to 6 percent in 1988 (see below and references 190 and 191), and *Pneumocystis* pneumonia has shifted up from 42 percent to 64 percent, while the alleged cause, HIV, has remained the same.

One explanation of these facts is that HIV is not sufficient to cause AIDS but depends critically on country- and risk-specific cofactors. However, the simplest explanation proposes that HIV is a harmless, idle retrovirus that is not the cause of AIDS.

In view of the claims that AIDS is a sexually transmitted viral syndrome, it is surprising[154,155] that, in the U.S., about 90 percent of all HIV carriers and AIDS patients are male. Even if one assumes that the virus was originally introduced into the U.S. through homosexual men, this epidemiology is hard to reconcile with the spread of a sexually transmitted virus 8 years later. In order to survive, a virus must infect new hosts, which it does most readily when it is at the highest titer.[153] In the case of HIV, this would be before antiviral immunity, or 1 to 2 months after infection. Thus, the 8 years of AIDS in the U.S. represent about 50 to 100 human passages of HIV, enough time for the virus to equilibrate between the sexes. By contrast, the uniform sexual distribution of HIV in Africa appears consistent with a sexually transmissible virus, underscoring the paradox of the U.S. epidemiology, particularly since the viruses and the epidemics of both countries are thought to be equally new.

A solution of the paradox is that HIV is not new but is endemic in Africa and, like most retroviruses, is transmitted perinatally rather than sexually. Accordingly, 10 percent of healthy Zairians are antibody-positive, and not more than 30 percent of the Kaposi sarcoma patients in Africa are infected with HIV.[157,158] Indeed, perinatal transmission between mother and child occurs with an efficiency of 30–50 percent while sexual transmission is extremely inefficient. Since the virus is not endemic in the U.S., it is transmitted more often by parenteral exposures associated with risk behavior (see below) than perinatally.

Evolutionary Arguments Against AIDS Viruses

It is now claimed that there are at least two new retroviruses capable of causing AIDS, HIV-1 and HIV-2, which differ about 60 percent in their nucleic acid sequences. Both allegedly evolved only 20 to <100 years ago. Since viruses, like cells, are the products of gradual evolution, the proposition that, within a very short evolutionary time, two different viruses capable of causing AIDS would have evolved or crossed over from another species is highly improbable.[159] It is also improbable that viruses evolved that kill their only natural host with efficiencies of 50–100 percent as is claimed for the HIVs.

Conclusions and Perspectives

It is concluded that HIV is not sufficient to cause AIDS because HIV meets neither Koch's postulates nor established epidemiological, biochemical, genetic, and evolutionary criteria of a viral pathogen. Further, it is concluded that HIV may not even be necessary for AIDS because there is neither biochemical nor genetic evidence that it initiates or maintains AIDS. HIV infiltration and activity are just as low in symptomatic carriers as in asymptomatic carriers, and HIV lacks an AIDS gene. The association between AIDS and antibody to HIV—now part of the definition of AIDS—does not prove causation because otherwise indistinguishable diseases are now set apart only on the basis of this antibody. According to this view, HIV is an ordinary harmless retrovirus that, in rare acute infections, may cause a mononucleosis-like disease before immunity.

Antibody to HIV Is a Surrogate Marker for Risk of AIDS

Although HIV does not appear to cause AIDS, it may serve in the U.S. and Europe as a surrogate marker for the risk of AIDS for the following reasons. (i) In these countries, HIV is not widespread but is one of the most specific occupational infections of persons at risk for AIDS.[160] (ii) Since HIV is extremely difficult to transmit, like all latent viruses, it would specifically identify those who habitually receive transfusions or intravenous drugs or are promiscuous. Indeed, the probability of being antibody-positive correlates directly with the frequency of drug use, transfusions,[161] and male homosexual activity. (iii) Since HIV is not cytocidal, it persists as a minimally active virus in a small number of cells, which will chronically boost antiviral immunity to produce a positive AIDS test. Latent EBV, cytomegalovirus, or other herpes-virus infections will likewise maintain a chronic immunity, although less specific for AIDS risk. By contrast, antibodies against viruses and microbes, which cannot persist at subclinical levels, tend to disappear after primary infection.

Epidemiology Is Not Sufficient to Prove Etiology

It has been argued that Koch's postulates can be abandoned as proof for etiology in favor of epidemiological correlations,[162] most recently in the case of HIV. However, adherence to this epidemiological concept as a substitute for biochemical and genetic proof of etiology has resulted in some of the most spectacular misdiagnoses in virology. (a) Based on epidemiological correlations, EBV was thought to be the cause of Burkitt lymphoma—until Burkitt lymphomas free of the virus were discovered.[163] (It is ironic that HIV is currently a proposed cause of Burkitt lymphoma.) (b) Also on the basis of seroepidemiological evidence, retroviruses were thought to cause human and bovine leukemias after bizarre latent periods of up to 40 years in humans,[164] until the discovery of these viruses in billions of normal cells of millions of asymptomatic carriers cast doubt on this hypothesis. It is scarcely surprising that the particular T cell from which a rare clonal leukemia originated was also infected. It is consistent with this view that these tumors are clonal and not contagious, like virus-negative leukemias, and that the presumably causative viruses are biochemically inactive in the human and bovine leukemias. Instead of viruses, the only specific markers of such tumors are clonal chromosomal abnormalities. (c) Likewise, slow viruses have gained acceptance as causes for such diseases as kuru, Creutzfeld–Jacob disease, and Alzheimer disease on the basis of epidemiological evidence,[165] although these viruses have never been detected.

Proof of Etiology Depends on Evidence for Activity

Regrettably, the hasty acceptance of the virus as the cause of AIDS, signaled by naming it HIV, has created an orthodoxy whose adherents prefer to discuss "how" rather than "whether" HIV causes AIDS. They argue that it is not necessary to understand HIV pathology, or how a latent virus kills, in order to claim etiology. Therefore, many different mechanisms, including ones in which HIV is said to depend on cofactors to cause AIDS, have been discussed to explain how the virus supposedly kills at least 10^4 times more T cells than it actively infects. Yet all speculations that HIV causes AIDS through cofactors cast doubt on HIV as a cause of AIDS, until such factors are proven to depend on HIV.

In contrast to what is claimed for HIV, there is unambiguous genetic evidence that biochemical activity in or on more cells than the body can spare or regenerate is absolutely necessary for viral or microbial pathogenicity. Examples are transformation-defective mutants of rous sarcoma virus[166] and replication-defective mutants of cytocidal viruses. If latent viruses or microbes were pathogenic at the level of activity of HIV, most of us would have *Pneumocystis* pneumonia (80–100 percent),[167] cytomegalovirus disease (50 percent), mononucleosis from EBV (50–100 percent) (see above; reference 88), and herpes (25–50 percent) all at once, and 5–10 percent also would have tuberculosis,[168] because the respective pathogens are latent, immunosuppressed passengers in the U.S. population at the percentages indicated. Since we can now, through molecularly cloned radioactive probes, detect latent viruses or microbes at concentrations that are far below those required for clinical detectability and relevance, it is necessary to reexamine the claims that HIV is the cause of AIDS.

In response to this, it has been argued that a biochemically inactive HIV may cause AIDS indirectly by a mechanism(s) involving new biological phenomena. This is argued even though HIV is like numerous other retroviruses studied under the Virus–Cancer Program during the last 20 years, which are only pathogenic when they are biochemically active. Nevertheless, some retroviruses[23] and DNA viruses (e.g., hepatitis virus in hepatomas[169]) are thought to cause tumors indirectly by converting, by means of site-specific integration, a specific gene of a rare infected cell to a cancer gene. Such a cell would then grow autonomously to form a monoclonal tumor, in which the virus may be inactive and often defective. However, such highly specific and hence rare virus–cell interactions cannot explain the loss of billions of cells during a degenerative disease like AIDS. It is also hard to accept that HIV could cause AIDS through a T-cell autoimmunity,[170] because it reaches far too few cells to function as a direct immunogen and because it is unlikely to function as an indirect immunogen since it is not homologous with human cells. Further, it is extremely unlikely that any virus could induce autoimmunity, which is a rare consequence of viral infection, as efficiently as HIV is thought to cause AIDS, namely in 50–100 percent of all infections.

Not All AIDS Diseases Can Be Explained by Immunodeficiency

Clearly, immunodeficiency is a plausible explanation for the microbial and viral AIDS diseases and *Pneumocystis* pneumonia. However, the effective immunity against HIV, which defines AIDS, together with those against cytomegalovirus, herpes simplex virus, hepatitis virus, and other viruses, is hard to reconcile with acquired immuno-deficiency. One would have to argue that T-cell depletion in AIDS is highly selective in order to allow *Pneumocystis* but not HIV or other viruses to become active. If HIV were able to induce T-cell immunodeficiency against itself, its titer during AIDS should be as high as it is in cultures of infected human monocytes—namely, up to 10^6 infectious units per milliliter (see above), just as high as the titers of all other retroviruses when they are pathogenic in animals.

Moreover, immunodeficiency does not explain AIDS neoplasias such as lymphomas or Kaposi sarcoma, which may be a hyperplasia.[175,178] The hypothesis that cancers reflect a defective immune system, the immune-surveillance hypothesis,[176] has been disproven through athymic (nude) mice, which develop no more cancers than other laboratory mice.[177] In fact, no immunodeficiency was observed in HIV-infected African patients who had Kaposi sarcomas.[157,158] In addition, Kaposi sarcoma tissue does not contain any HIV.[178,179] Immunodeficiency also cannot explain dementia; nor can dementia be explained by HIV infection of neurons, because retroviruses are dependent on mitosis for infection and neurons do not divide. HIV would indeed be a mysterious virus[31] to kill T cells and neurons that are not infected and, at the same time, to induce hyperplastic or neoplastic growth of other cells that are also not infected.

HIV Is Not a Rational Basis for AIDS Therapy

Since there is no proven mechanism of HIV pathogenesis, HIV is not a rational basis for the control of AIDS. Thus the treatment of symptomatic and even asymptomatic HIV carriers with azidothymidine (AZT) cannot be justified in terms of its original design, which is to inhibit HIV DNA synthesis by chain determination.[171] Even if HIV were to cause AIDS, it would hardly be a legitimate target for AZT therapy, because in 70–100 percent of antibody-positive persons proviral DNA is not detectable without amplification, and its biosyn-thesis has never been observed.

Nevertheless, AZT has been claimed to have beneficial effects for AIDS patients on the basis of a 16- to 24-week double-blind trial. However, AZT, originally developed for chemotherapy by terminat-ing cellular DNA synthesis, efficiently kills dividing blood cells and other cells,[172–174] and is thus directly immunosuppressive. Moreover, the immediate toxicity of AZT suggests that this trial could hardly have been double-blind and hence unbiased.

What Are the Causes of AIDS?

I propose that AIDS is not a contagious syndrome caused by one conventional virus or microbe, because no such virus or microbe would average 8 years to cause a primary disease, or would selectively affect only those who habitually practice risk behavior, or would be able to cause the diverse collection of over 20 degenerative and neoplastic AIDS diseases. Neither could a conventional virus or microbe survive if it were as inefficiently transmitted as AIDS, and killed its host in the process. Conventional viruses either are highly pathogenic and easy to transmit or are nonpathogenic and latent and hence very difficult to transmit. Conventional viruses or microbes also exist that cause secondary—or even primary—diseases long after infection, but only when they are activated from dormancy by rare acquired deficiencies of the immune system. Such opportunistic infections are the consequence rather than the cause of immunodeficiency.

Since AIDS is defined by new combinations of conventional diseases, it may be caused by new combinations of conventional pathogenic factors. The habitual administration of factor VIII or blood transfusions or of drugs,[190-192] chronic promiscuous male homosexual activity that is associated with drugs, numerous acute parasitic infections, and chronic malnutrition—each for an average of 8 years—are factors that appear to provide biochemically more tangible and plausible bases for AIDS than an idle retrovirus. Indeed, the correlation between AIDS and such factors is 95 percent. Among these factors, EBV, cytomegalovirus, herpes simplex virus, and administration of blood components and factor VIII have all been identified as causes of immunodeficiency not only in HIV-positive, but also in HIV-negative, hemophiliacs. In fact, the dose of factor VIII received was found to be directly proportional to subsequent immunodeficiencies. The habitual admission of narcotic toxins appears to play a major immunosuppressive role in the U.S. and Europe. About 30 percent of the American AIDS patients are confirmed users of injected drugs. Because of the difficulties in assessing drug data, it is probable that the percentage who use injected and/or noninjected drugs is even higher. For example, nine different drugs were used in combination by a cohort of antibody-positive homosexuals in San Francisco. Again there are quantitative drug-AIDS correlations. For example, the decreased use of nitrite inhalants was shown to correlate with the decreased incidence of Kaposi sarcoma in homosexuals.[190,191] Moreover, that the Kaposi sarcoma cases decreased exactly with the use of nitrites, rather than lagging behind it by 8 years as would be expected from the presumed 8-year latent period of HIV, argues directly against a role of HIV in Kaposi sarcoma. Further, it has been documented that protein malnutrition and parasitic infections are the most common causes of T-cell immunodeficiency worldwide, particularly in developing countries.[181] Unlike HIV, the specifics of these risk factors provide a plausible explanation for the risk specificity of AIDS diseases. The long and unpredictable intervals between the appearance of antibody to HIV and the onset of AIDS would then reflect the thresholds for these factors to cause AIDS diseases, rather than an unlikely mechanism of HIV pathogenesis.

In response to this view it is often pointed out that AIDS risks have existed for a long time, whereas AIDS is said to be a new syndrome. However, this argument fails to consider that the major risk groups—male homosexuals and intravenous drug users—have only become visible and acceptable in the U.S. and in Europe during the last 10 to 15 years, about the same time that AIDS became visible. Acceptability facilitated and probably enhanced risk behavior, and thus the incidence of the many diseases now called AIDS. Increased consumption of drugs was reported to have increased the number of drug-related deaths, although unconfirmed HIV infections were the preferred interpretation.[190,192] Moreover, the particular permissiveness toward these risk groups in metropolitan centers encouraged the clustering of cases that was necessary to detect AIDS. Further, it has been pointed out that slim disease, fever, and diarrhea in Africa are not a new epidemic, but old diseases under a new name, caused by previously known infectious agents and malnutrition.[182]

This analysis offers several benefits. It ends the fear of infection by HIV, and particularly of immunity to HIV, because it proves that HIV alone is not sufficient to cause AIDS. To determine whether HIV is necessary for AIDS, controlled, randomized analyses[196] either of risk takers who differ only by the presence of antibody to HIV or of antibody-positive individuals who differ only in taking AIDS risks must be carried out. Moreover, assessment of a pathogenic potential of HIV would depend on evidence that the life-span of antibody-positive risk takers is shorter than that of antibody-free controls. In addition, it should be determined whether, prior to 1981, AIDS-risk takers ever developed what are now called AIDS diseases. This analysis also suggests studies on how the nature, frequency, and duration of AIDS risks generate risk-specific diseases. Such studies should include persons treated with AZT before or after AIDS symptoms to assess the AIDS risks of AZT. To this end, diseases should be reported by their original names, rather than as AIDS because of their association with antibody to HIV. Finally, this analysis suggests that AIDS prevention efforts be concentrated on AIDS risks rather than on transmission of HIV.

This article is dedicated to the memory of Charlotte Friend. I am very grateful to Klaus Cichutek, Dawn Davidson, Thelma Dunnebacke-Dixon, David Goodrich, Steve Martin, Seth Roberts, Harry Rubin, Russell Schoch, Gunter Stent, and Ren-Ping Zhou (Berkeley); Jad Adams and Mike Verney-Elliott (London); Ruediger Hehlmann (Munich); George Miller (New Haven); Nicholas Regush (Montreal); and Harvey Bialy, Celia Farber, John Lauritsen, Nathaniel Lehrman, Katie Leishman, Anthony Liversidge, Craig Schoonmaker, and Joseph Sonnabend (New York) for encouragement, critical information, discussions, or reviews of this manuscript and, above all, for common sense. Further, the Chairman of the *Proceedings* Editorial Board is acknowledged for providing critical reviews and comments. P.H.D. is supported by Outstanding Investigator Grant 5-R35-CA39915-03 from the National Cancer Institute and Grant 1547AR1 from the Council for Tobacco Research.

NOTES

1. Gottlieb, M. S., Schroff, R., Schamber, H. M., Weisman, J. D., Fan, P. T., Wolf, R. A., & Saxon, A. (1981) *N. Engl. J. Med.* 305, 1425–1431.

2. Centers for Disease Control (1981) *Morbid. Mortal. Wkly. Rep.* 30, 305–308.

3. Institute of Medicine (1986) *Confronting AIDS* (N.A.S., Washington, D.C.).

4. Centers for Disease Control (1988) *AIDS Weekly Surveillance Report* (August 8).

5. Centers for Disease Control (1987) *J. Am. Med. Assoc.* 258, 1143–1154.

6. A. Fauci (1988) *Science* 239, 617–622.

7. Institute of Medicine (1988) *Confronting AIDS-Update 1988* (N.A.S., Washington, D.C.).

8. Selik, R., Starcher, E. T., & Curran, J. (1987) *AIDS* 1, 175–182.

9. Colebunders, R., Mann, J., Francis, H., Bila, K., Izaley, L., Kakonde, N., Kabasele, K., Ifoto, L., Nzilambi, N., Quinn, T., van der Groen, G., Curran, J., Vercauteren, B., & Piot, P. (1987) *Lancet* i, 492–494.

10. Pallangyo, K. J., Mbaga, I. M., Mugusi, F., Mbena, E., Mhalu, F. S., Bredberg, U., & Biberfeld, G. (1987) *Lancet* ii, 972.

11. Holub, W. R. (1988) *Am. Clin. Prod. Rev.* 7 (5), 28–37.

12. Gallo, R. C. & Montagnier, L. (1988) *Sci. Am.* 259 (4), 41–48.

13. Gallo, R. C. & Montagnier, L. (1987) *Nature (London)* 362, 435–436.

14. Blattner, W., Gallo, R. C., & Temin, H. (1988) *Science* 241, 514–517.

15. Barre-Sinoussi, F., Chermann, J. C., Rey, F., Nugeyre, M. T., Chamaret, S., Gruest, J., Dauguet, C., Axler-Blin, C., Vezinet-Brun, F., Rouzioux, C., Rosenbaum, W., & Montagnier, L. (1983) *Science* 220, 868–870.

16. Connor, S. (1987) *New Sci.* 113 (1547), 49–58.

17. Weiss, R., Teich, N., Varmus, H., & Coffin, J. (1985) *RNA Tumor Viruses* (Cold Spring Harbor Lab., Cold Spring Harbor, NY), 2nd Ed.

18. Coffin, J., Haase, A., Levy, J. A., Montagnier, L., Oroszlan, S., Teich, N., Temin, H., Toyoshima, K., Varmus, H., Vogt, P., & Weiss, R. (1986) *Science* 232, 697.

19. Friedland, G. H. & Klein, R. S. (1987) *N. Engl. J. Med.* 317, 1125–1135.

20. Rees, M. (1987) *Nature (London)* 326, 343–345.

21. Eyster, M. E., Gail, M. H., Ballard, J. O., Al-Mondhiry, H., & Goedert, J. J. (1987) *Ann. Int. Med.* 107, 1–6.

22. Curran, J. W., Jaffe, H. W., Hardy, A. M., Morgan, W. M., Selik, R. M., & Dondero, T. J. (1988) *Science* 239, 610–616.

23. Duesberg, P. H. (1987) *Cancer Res.* 47, 1199–1220.

24. Rettig, R. A. (1977) *Cancer Crusade: The Story of the National Cancer Act of 1971* (Princeton Univ. Press, Princeton, NJ).

25. Sattentau, Q. J. & Weiss, R. A. (1988) *Cell* 52, 631–633.

26. Gartner, S., Markovits, P., Markovitz, D., Kaplan, M., Gallo, R., & Popovic, M. (1986) *Science* 233, 215–219.

27. Popovic, M. & Gartner, S. (1987) *Lancet* ii, 916.

28. Ho, D. D., Pomerantz, R. J., & Kaplan, J. C. (1987) *N. Engl. J. Med.* 317, 278–286.

29. Khan, N. C., Chatlynne, L. G., & Hunter, E. (1988) *Am. Clin. Proc. Rev.* 7(5), 12–19.

30. Baum, R. M. (1988) *Chem. Eng. News* 66 (13), 29–33.

31. Levy, J. (1988) *Nature (London)* 333, 519–522.

32. Booth, W. (1988) *Science* 239, 1485–1488.

33. Moss, A. R., Bacchetti, P., Osmond, D., Krampf, W., Chaisson, R. E., Stites, D., Wilber, J., Allain, J.-P., & Carlson, J. (1988) *Br. Med. J.* 296, 745–750.

34. Goedert, J. J., Biggar, R. J., Weiss, S. H., Eyster, M. E., Melbye, M., Wilson, S., Ginzburg, H. M., Grossman, R. J., DiFiola, R. A., Sanchez, W. C.,

Giron, J. A., Ebbsen, P., Gallo, R. C., & Blattner, W. A. (1986) *Science* 231, 992–995.

35. Anderson, R. M. & May, R. M. (1988) *Nature (London)* 333, 514–519.

36. Medley, G. F., Anderson, R. M., Cox, D. R., & Billard, L. (1988) *Nature (London)* 333, 505.

37. Liu, K.-J., Darrow, W. W., & Rutherford, G. W. (1988) *Science* 240, 1333–1335.

38. Osmond, D. & Moss, A. (1989) in *1989 AIDS Clinical Review*, eds. Volberding, P. & Jacobson, M. (Dekker, New York), in press.

39. Patlak, M. (1988) *Discover* 9 (10), 26–27.

40. Gonda, M., Wong-Staal, F., Gallo, R., Clements, J., Narayan, O., & Gilden, R. (1986) *Science* 227, 173–177.

41. Kolata, G. (1988) *N.Y. Times* 137, June 10.

42. Hager, M. & Monmaney, T. (1988) *Newsweek* 111 (24), 66–67.

43. Centers for Disease Control (1988) *Understanding AIDS*, HHS Publ. No (CDC) HHS-88-8404 (GPO, Washington, D.C.).

44. Barnes, D. M. (1988) *Science* 239, 348–349.

45. Anonymous (1988) *Morbid. Mortal. Wkly. Rep.* 37 (15), 229–239.

46. Curran, J. W., Morgan, M. W., Hardy, A. M., Jaffe, H. W., Darrow, W. W., & Dowdle, W. R. (1985) *Science* 229, 1352–1357.

47. Booth, W. (1988) *Science* 239, 253.

48. Duesberg, P. (1987) *Bio/Technology* 5, 1244.

49. Duesberg, P. (1988) *Science* 241, 514–517.

50. Duesberg, P. (1988) *New Sci.* 118 (1610), 34–35.

51. Liversidge, A. (1988) *Spin* 3 (11), 56–57, 67, 72.

52. Farber, C. (1988) *Spin* 4 (2), 71–72.

53. Leishman, K. (1988) *Wall St. J.* 118 (39), Feb. 26.

54. AIDS Monitor (1988) *New Sci.* 118 (1603), 34.

55. Ward, R. (1988) *Nature (London)* 332, 574.

56. Lauritsen, J. (1988) *N.Y. Native* 264, 14–19.

57. Miller, J. (1988) *Discover* 9 (6), 62–68.

58. Werth, B. (1988) *N. Engl. Monthly* 5 (6), 38–47.

59. Weber, J. (1988) *New Sci.* 118 (1611), 32–33.

60. Hall, S. (1988) *Hippocrates* 2 (5), 76–82.

61. Schwartz, K. F. (1988) *Ärtztliche Praxis* 45, 1562–1563.

62. Rubin, H. (1988) *Science* 240, 1389–1390.

63. Rubin, H. (1988) *Nature (London)* 334, 201.

64. Rappoport, J. (1988) *AIDS INC.* (Human Energy Press, San Bruno, CA).

65. Matsumura, K. (1988) *Heterosexual AIDS: Myth or Fact?* (Alin Found. Press, Berkeley, CA).

66. Stewart, G. T. (1968) *Lancet* i, 1077–1081.

67. Evans, A. (1976) *Yale J. Biol. Med.* 49, 175–195.

68. Huebner, R. J. (1957) *Ann. N.Y. Acad. Sci.* 67, 430–438.

69. Albert, J., Gaines, H., Sönnerborg, A., Nyström, G., Pehrson, P. O., Chiodi, F., von Sydow, M., Moberg, L., Lidman, K., Christensson, B., Åsjö, B., & Fenyö, E. M. (1987) *J. Med. Virol.* 23, 67–73.

70. Falk, L. A., Paul, D., Landay, A., & Kessler, H. (1987) *N. Engl. J. Med.* 316, 1547–1548.

71. Harper, M. E., Marselle, L. M., Gallo, R. C., & Wong-Staal, F. (1986) *Proc. Natl. Acad. Sci. USA* 83, 772–776.

72. Ranki, A., Valle, S.-L., Krohn, M., Antonen, J., Allain, J.-P., Leuther, M., Franchini, G., & Krohn, K. (1987) *Lancet* ii, 589–593.

73. Richman, D., McCutchan, J., & Spector, S. (1987) *J. Infect. Dis.* 156, 823–827.

74. Biberfeld, P., Chayt, K. J., Marselle, L. M., Biberfeld, G., Gallo, R. C., & Harper, M. E. (1986) *Am. J. Pathol.* 123, 436–442.

75. Shaw, G. M., Hahn, B. H., Arya, S. K., Groopman, J. E., Gallo, R. C., & Wong-Staal, F. (1984) *Science* 226, 1165–1167.

76. Kahn, N. C. & Hunter, E. (1988) *Am. Clin. Prod. Rev.* 7 (5), 20–25.

77. Farzadegan, H., Polis, M. A., Wolinsky, S. M., Rinaldo, C. R., Sninsky, J. J., Kwok, S., Griffith, R. L., Kaslow, R. A., Phair, J. P., Polk, B. F., & Saah, A. J. (1988) *Ann. Int. Med.* 108, 785–790.

78. Groopman, J. E., Hartzband, P. I., Shulman, L., Salahuddin, S. Z., Sarngadharan, M. G., McLane, M. F., Essex, M., & Gallo, R. (1985) *Blood* 66, 742–744.

79. Hearst, N. & Hulley, S. (1988) *J. Am. Med. Assoc.* 259, 2428–2432.

80. Peterman, T. A., Stoneburner, R. L., Allen, J. R., Jaffe, H. W., & Curran, J. W. (1988) *J. Am. Med. Assoc.* 259, 55–58.

81. Gallo, D., Kimpton, J., & Dailey, P. (1987) *J. Clin. Microbiol.* 25, 1291–1294.

82. von Briesen, H., Becker, W. B., Henco, K., Helm, E. B., Gelderblom, H. R., Brede, H. D., & Rübsamen-Waigmann, H. (1987) *J. Med. Virol.* 23, 51–66.

83. Paul, D. A., Falk, L. A., Kessler, H. A., Chase, R. M., Blaauw, B., Chudwin, D. S., & Landay, A. L. (1987) *J. Med. Virol.* 22, 357–362.

84. Jackson, G. G., Paul, D. A., Falk, L. A., Rubenis, M., Despotes, J. C., Mack, D., Knigge, M., & Emeson, E. E. (1988) *Ann. Int. Med.* 108, 175–180.

85. Weiss, S. H., Goedert, J. J., Gartner, S., Popovic, M., Waters, D., Markham, P., di Marzo Veronese, F., Gail, M. H., Barkley, W. E., Shaw, G. M., Gallo, R. C., & Blattner, W. A. (1988) *Science* 239, 68–71.

86. Mims, C. & White, D. O. (1984) *Viral Pathogenesis and Immunology* (Blackwell, Oxford, U.K.).

87. Fenner, F., McAuslan, B. R., Mims, C. A., Sambrook, J., & White, D. O. (1974) *Animal Viruses* (Academic, New York).

88. Evans, A. S., ed. (1982) *Viral Infection of Humans: Epidemiology and Control* (Plenum, New York/London).

89. Stewart, G. J., Tyler, J. P. P., Cunningham, A. L., Barr, J. A., Driscoll, G. L., Gold, J., & Lamont, B. J. (1985) *Lancet* ii, 581–584.

90. Baum, R. M. (1987) *Chem. Eng. News* 65 (47), 14–26.

91. Abramson, P. R. & Rothschild, B. (1988) *J. Sex Res.* 25 (1), 106–122.

92. Abramson, P. R. (1988) *J. Sex Res.* 25 (3), 323–346.

93. Barnes, D. (1987) *Science* 236, 1423–1425.

94. Sullivan, J. L., Brewster, F. E., Brettler, D. B., Forsberg, A. D., Cheeseman, S. H., Byron, K. S., Baker, S. M., Willitts, D. L., Lew, R. A., & Levine, P. H. (1986) *J. Pediatr.* 108, 504–510.

95. Ward, J. W., Holmberg, S. D., Allen, J. R., Cohn, D. L., Critchley, S. E., Kleinman, S. H., Lenes, B. A., Ravenholt, O., Davis, J. R., Quinn, M. G., & Jaffe, H. W. (1988) *N. Engl. J. Med.* 318, 473–478.

96. Jaffe, H. W., Sarngadharan, M. G., DeVico, A. L., Bruch, L., Getchell, J. P., Kalyanaraman, V. S., Haverkos, H. W., Stoneburner, R. L., Gallo, R. C., & Curran, J. W. (1985) *J. Am. Med. Assoc.* 254, 770–773.

97. Tinker, J. (1988) *Issues Sci. Technol.* IV (1), 43–48.

98. Editorial (1987) *Lancet* ii, 192–194.

99. Fleming, A. F. (1988) *AIDS-Forschung* 3, 116–138.

100. Koenig, R. E., Pittaluga, J., Bogart, M., Castro. M., Nunez, F., Vilorio, I., Devillar, L., Calzada, M., & Levy, J. A. (1987) *J. Am. Med. Assoc.* 257, 631–634.

101. Chayt, K. J., Harper, M. E., Marselle, L. M., Lewin, E. B., Rose, R. M., Oleske, J. M., Epstein, L. G., Wong-Staal, F., & Gallo, R. C. (1986) *J. Am. Med. Assoc.* 256, 2356–2371.

102. Stoler, M. H., Eskin, T. A., Been, S., Angerer, R. C., & Angerer, L. M. (1986) *J. Am. Med. Assoc.* 256, 2360–2364.

103. Sprent, J. (1977) in *B and T Cells in Immune Recognition*, eds. Loor, F., & Roelants, G. E. (Wiley, New York), pp. 59–82.

104. Goudsmit, J., Lange, J. M. A., Paul, D. A., & Dawson, G. A. (1987) *J. Infect. Dis.* 155, 558–560.

105. Forster, S. M., Osborne, L. M., Cheingsong-Popov, R., Kenny, C., Burnell, R., Jeffries, D. J., Pinching, A. J., Harris, J. R. W., & Weber, J. N. (1987) *AIDS* 1, 235–240.

106. Pederson, C., Nielsen, C. M., Vestergaard, B. F., Gerstoft, J., Krogsgaard, K., & Nielsen, J. O. (1987) *Br. Med. J.* 295, 567–569.

107. Wittek, A. E., Phelan, M. A., Well, M. A., Vujcic, L. K., Epstein, J. S., Lane, H. C., & Quinnan, G. V. (1987) *Ann. Int. Med.* 107, 286–292.

108. de Wolf, F., Goudsmit, J., Paul, D., Lange, J. M. A., Hooijkaas, C., Schellekens, P., Coutinho, R. A., & van der Noordaa, J. (1987) *Br. Med. J.* 295, 569–572.

109. Bialy, H. (1988) *Bio/Technology* 6, 121.

110. Vogt, P. K. (1965) *Adv. Virus Res.* 11, 293–385.

111. Baum, R. M. (1987) *Chem. Eng. News* 65 (47), 27–34.

112. Barnes, D. M. (1988) *Science* 240, 719–721.

113. Seligmann, M., Pinching, A. J., Rosen, F. S., Fahey, J. L., Khaitov, R. M., Klatzmann, D., Koenig, S., Luo, N., Ngu, J., Reithmüller, G., & Spira, T. (1987) *Ann. Int. Med.* 107, 234–242.

114. Weiss, R. A., Clapham, P. R., Cheingsong-Popov, R., Dalgleish, A. G., Carne, C. A., Weller, I. V. D., & Tedder, R. S. (1985) *Nature (London)* 316, 69–72.

115. Robinson, E., Montefiori, D. C., & Mitchell, W. M. (1988) *Lancet* i, 790–794.

116. Weiss, R. A., Clapham, P. R., Weber, J. N., Dalgleish, A. G., Lasky, L. A., & Berman, P. W. (1986) *Nature (London)* 324, 572–575.

117. Ho, D. D., Sarngadharan, M. G., Hirsch, M. S., Schooley, R. T., Rota, T. R., Kennedy, R. C., Chanh, T. C., & Sato, V. L. (1987) *J. Virol.* 61, 2024–2028.

118. Robey, G., Arthur, L. O., Matthews, T. J., Langlois, A., Copeland, T. D., Lerche, N. W., Oroszlan, S., Bolognesi, D. P., Gilden, R. V., & Fischinger, P. J. (1986) *Proc. Natl. Acad. Sci. USA* 83, 7023–7027.

119. Rusche, J. R., Lynn, D. L., Robert-Guroff, M., Langlois, A. J., Lyerly, H. K., Carson, H., Krohn, K., Ranki, A., Gallo, R. C., Bolognesi, D. P., Putney, S. D., & Matthews, T. J. (1987) *Proc. Natl. Acad. Sci. USA* 84, 6924–6928.

120. Douglas, R. G., Jr., & Couch, R. B. (1970) *J. Immunol.* 104, 289–295.

121. Koprowski, H. (1977) in *Slow Virus Infections of the Central Nervous System*, eds. ter Meulen, V. & Katz, M. (Springer, New York), pp. 152–158.

122. Koprowski, H., DeFreitas, E. C., Harper, M. E., Sandberg-Wollheim, M., Sheremata, W. A., Robert-Guroff, M., Saxinger, C. W., Feinberg, M. B., Wong-Staal, F., & Gallo, R. C. (1985) *Nature (London)* 318, 154–160.

123. Hahn, B. H., Shaw, G. M., Taylor, M. D., Redfield, R. R., Markham, P. D., Salahuddin, S. Z., Wong-Staal, F., Gallo, R. C., Parks, E. S., & Parks, W. P. (1986) *Science* 232, 1548–1553.

124. Cheng-Mayer, C., Seto, D., Tateno, M., & Levy, J. A. (1988) *Science* 240, 80–82.

125. Preston, B. D., Poiesz, B. J., & Loeb, L. A. (1988) *Science* 242, 1168–1171.

126. Takeuchi, Y., Nagumo, T., & Hoshino, H. (1988) *J. Virol.* 62, 3900–3902.

127. Coffin, J. M., Tsichlis, P. N., Barker, C. S., Voynow, S., & Robinson, H. L. (1980) *Ann. N. Y. Acad. Sci.* 54, 410–425.

128. Temin, H. M. (1988) *Cancer Res.* 48, 1697–1701.

129. Haase, A. T. (1986) *Nature (London)* 322, 130–136.

130. Kessler, H. A., Blaauw, B., Spear, J., Paul, D. A., Falk, L. A., & Landay, A. (1987) *J. Am. Med. Assoc.* 258, 1196–1199.

131. Lairmore, M. D., Rosadio, R. H., & DeMartini, J. C. (1986) *Am. J. Pathol.* 125, 173–181.

132. Perryman, L. E., O'Rourke, K. J., & McGuire, T. E. (1988) *J. Virol.* 62, 3073–3076.

133. Narayan, O. & Cork, L. C. (1985) *Rev. Infect. Dis.* 7, 89–98.

134. Crawford, T. B. & Adams, D. S. (1981) *J. Am. Vet. Med.* 178, 713–719.

135. Lackner, A. A., Rodriguez, M. H., Bush, C. E., Munn, R. J., Kwang, H.-S., Moore, P. F., Osborn, K. G., Marx, P. A., Gardner, M. B., & Lowenstine, L. J. (1988) *J. Virol.* 62, 2134–2142.

136. DeBoer, G. F. & Houwers, J. (1979) in *Aspects of Slow and Persistent Virus Infections*, ed. Tyrrell, D. A. J. (ECSC, Brussels-Luxembourg), pp. 198–220.

137. DeBoer, G. F., Terpstra, C., & Houwers, D. J. (1978) *Bull. Off. Int. Epizoot.* 89, 487–506.

138. Cutlip, R., Lehmkuhl, H. D., Brodgen, K. A., & Sacks, J. M. (1986) *Vet. Microbiol.* 12, 283–288.

139. Rubin, H. & Temin, H. (1958) *Virology* 7, 75–91.

140. Tooze, J., ed. (1973) *The Molecular Biology of Tumor Viruses* (Cold Spring Harbor Lab., Cold Spring Harbor, NY).

141. Ho, D. D., Rota, T. R., & Hirsch, M. S. (1986) *J. Clin. Invest.* 77, 1712–1715.

142. Nicholson, J. K. A., Gross, G. D., Callaway, C. S., & McDougal, J. S. (1986) *J. Immunol.* 137, 323–329.

143. Salahuddin, S. Z., Rose, R. M., Groopman, J. E., Markham, P. D., & Gallo, R. C. (1986) *Blood* 68, 281–284.

144. Hoxie, J. A., Haggarty, B. S., Rachowski, J. L., Pilsbury, N., & Levy, J. A. (1985) *Science* 229, 1400–1402.

145. Walker, C. M., Moody, D. J., Stites, D. P., & Levy, J. A. (1986) *Science* 234, 1563–1566.

146. Anand, R., Siegal, F., Reed, C., Cheung, T., Forlenza, S., & Moore, J. (1987) *Lancet* ii, 234–238.

147. Dahl, K., Martin, K., & Miller, G. (1987) *J. Virol.* 61, 1602–1608.

148. Clavel, F. (1987) *AIDS* 1, 135–140.

149. Duesberg, P. H., Vogt, K., Beemon, K., & Lai, M. (1974) *Cold Spring Harbor Symp. Quant. Biol.* 39, 847–857.

150. Wang, L.-H., Galehouse, D., Mellon, P., Duesberg, P., Mason, W. S., & Vogt, P. K. (1976) *Proc. Natl. Acad. Sci. USA* 73, 3952–3956.

151. Martin, M. A., Bryan, T., Rasheed, S., & Khan, A. S. (1981) *Proc. Natl. Acad. Sci. USA* 78, 4892–4896.

152. Weiss, R. A. (1988) *Nature (London)* 333, 497–498.

153. Andrewes, C. H. (1965) *J. Gen. Microbiol.* 49, 140–156.

154. Gould, R. E. (1988) *Cosmopolitan* 204 (1), 146–147, 204.

155. Brecher, E. M. (1988) *Columbia Journalism Rev.* 26 (6), 46–50.

156. Centers for Disease Control (1985) *Morbid. Mortal. Wkly, Rep.* 34, 245–248.

157. Craighead, J., Moore, A., Grossman, H., Ershler, W., Frattini, U., Saxinger, C., Hess, U., & Ngowi, F. (1988) *Arch. Pathol. Lab. Med.* 112, 259–265.

158. Kestens, L., Melbye, M., Biggar, R. J., Stevens, W. J., Piot, P., DeMuynck, A., Taelman, H., DeFeyter, M., Paluku, L., & Gigase, P. L. (1985) *Int. J. Cancer* 36, 49–54.

159. Sonnabend, J. (1989) in *The Acquired Immune Deficiency Syndrome and Infections of Homosexual Men*, eds. Ma, P. & Armstrong, D. (Butterworth, Stonehan, MA), 2nd Ed., in press.

160. Darrow, W. W., Echenberg, D. F., Jaffe, H. W., O'Malley, P. M., Byers, R. H., Getchell, J. P., & Curran, J. W. (1987) *Am. J. Publ. Health* 77, 479–483.

161. Ludlam, C. A., Tucker, J., Steel, C. M., Tedder, R. S., Cheingsong-Popov, R., Weiss, R., McClelland, D. B. L., Philip, I., & Prescott, R. J. (1985) *Lancet* ii, 233–236.

162. Evans, A. (1978) *Am. J. Epidemiol.* 108, 249–258.

163. Pagano, J. S., Huang, C. H., & Levine, P. (1973) *N. Engl. J. Med.* 289, 1395–1399.

164. Gallo, R. C. (1986) *Sci. Am.* 255 (6), 88–98.

165. Gajdusek, D. C. (1977) *Science* 197, 943–960.

166. Martin, G. S. & Duesberg, P. H. (1972) *Virology* 47, 494–497.

167. Pifer, L. L. (1984) *Eur. J. Clin. Microbiol.* 3, 169–173.

168. Evans, A. S. & Feldman, H. A., eds. (1982) *Bacterial Infections of Humans: Epidemiology and Control* (Plenum, New York/London).

169. Watson, J. D., Hopkins, N. H., Roberts, J. W., Steitz, J. A., & Weiner, A. M. (1987) *Molecular Biology of the Gene* (Benjamin/Cummings, Menlo Park, CA), 4th Ed.

170. Stricker, R. B., McHugh, T. M., Moody, D. J., Morrow, W. J. W., Stites, D. P., Schuman, M. A., & Levy, J. A. (1987) *Nature (London)* 327, 710–713.

171. Yarchoan, R., Weinhold, K. J., Lyerly, H. K., Gelmann, E., Blum, R. M., Shearer, G. M., Mitsuya, H., Collins, J. M., Mayers, C. E., Klecker, R. W., Markham, P. D., Durack, D. T., Lehman, S. N., Barry, D. W., Fischl, M. A., Gallo, R. C., Bolognesi, D. P., & Broder, S. (1986) *Lancet* i, 575–580.

172. Dagani, R. (1987) *Chem. Eng. News* 65 (47), 35–40.

173. Richman, D. D., Fischl, M. A., Grieco, M. H., Gottlieb, M. S., Volberding, P. A., Laskin, O. L., Leedom, J. M., Groopman, J. E., Mildvan, D., Hirsch, M. S., Jackson, G. G., Durack, D. T., Nusinoff-Lehrman, S., & the AZT Collaborative Working Group (1987) *N. Engl. J. Med.* 317, 192–197.

174. Gingell, B. D. (1988) *Issues Sci. Technol.* IV (2), 17–18.

175. Brown, R. K. (1987) *Am. Clin. Pro. Rev.* 6 (11), 44–47.

176. Pitot, H. (1979) *Fundamentals of Oncology* (Dekker, New York).

177. Duesberg, P. H. (1987) *Proc. Natl. Acad. Sci. USA* 84, 2117–2124.

178. Bovi, P. D., Donti, E., Knowles, D. M., II, Freidman-Kien, A., Luciw, P. A., Dina, D., Dalla-Favera, R., & Basilico, C. (1986) *Cancer Res.* 46, 6333–6338.

179. Salahuddin, S. K., Nakamura, S., Biberfeld, P., Kaplan, M. H., Markham, P. D., Larsson, L., & Gallo, R. C. (1988) *Science* 242, 430–433.

180. Duesberg, P. H. (1988) *Science* 242, 997–998.

181. Seligmann, M., Chess, L., Fahey, J. L., Fauci, A. S., Lachmann, P. J., L'Age-Stehr, J., Ngu, J., Pinching, A. J., Rosen, F. S., Spira, T. J., & Wybran, J. (1984) *N. Engl. J. Med.* 311, 1286–1292.

182. Konotey-Ahulu, F. I. D. (1987) *Lancet* ii, 206–208.

183. Andrieu, J. E., Eme, D., Venet, A., Audroin, C., Tourani, J. M., Stern, M., Israel-Biet, D., Beldjord, K., Driss, F., & Even, P. (1988) *Clin. Exp. Immunol.* 73, 1–5.

184. N'Galy, B., Ryder, R., Bila, K., Mwandagalirwa, K., Colebunders, R. L., Francis, H., Mann, J., & Quinn, T. (1988) *N. Engl. J. Med.* 319, 1123–1127.

185. Raymond, C. A. (1988) *J. Am. Med. Assoc.* 259, 329, 332.

186. Marcus, R. & CDC Needlestick Surveillance Group (1988) *N. Engl. J. Med.* 319, 118–123.

187. Shaw, G. M., Harper, M. E., Hahn, B. H., Epstein, L. G., Gajdusek, D. C., Price, R. W., Navia, B. A., Petito, C. K., O'Hara, C. J., Cho, E.-S., Oleske, J. M., Wong-Staal, F., & Gallo, R. C. (1985) *Science* 227, 177–182.

188. Haseltine, W. A. & Wong-Staal, F. (1988) *Sci. Am.* 259 (4), 52–62.

189. Kolata, G. (1987) *Science* 235, 1462–1463.

190. Haverkos, H. W. (1988) in Health Hazards of Nitrate Inhalants, eds. Haverkos, H. W. & Dougherty, J. A., National Institute on Drug Abuse Monograph 83, pp. 96–105.

191. Lange, W. R., Haertzen, C. A., Hickey, J. E., Snyder, F. R., Dax, E. M., & Jaffe, J. H. (1988) *Am. J. Drug Alcohol Abuse* 14 (1), 29–40.

192. Stoneburner, R. L., Des Jarlais, D. C., Benezra, D., Gorelkin, L., Sotheran, J. L., Friedman, S. R., Schultz, S., Marmor, M., Mildvan, D., & Maslansky, R. (1988) *Science* 242, 916–919.

193. Sonnabend, J. (1989) *AIDS Forum*, ed. Callen, M. 1, 9–15.

194. Fischl, M. A. & the AZT Collaborative Working Group (1987) *N. Engl. J. Med.* 317, 185–191.

195. Dournon, E. & the Claude Bernard Hospital AZT Study Group (1988) *Lancet* ii, 1297–1302.

196. Feinstein, A. R. (1988) *Science* 242, 1257–1263.

HIV Infection
and Its Epidemiology

HIV: The Etiologic Agent of AIDS

Early in the epidemic, epidemiological analysis of the pattern of the spread of AIDS showed it to be reminiscent of that for hepatitis B virus, an observation that pointed scientists in the right direction in their search for an etiologic agent. In 1983 and 1984 several researchers identified a retrovirus that is now understood to be HIV as the cause of AIDS. *The committee believes that the evidence that HIV causes AIDS is scientifically conclusive.*

That a particular organism causes a disease is demonstrated by a confluence of evidence linking the two: HIV and AIDS have been so linked in time, place, and population group. For example, in San Francisco, the examination of frozen blood from a cohort of homosexual men showed the appearance of antibodies to HIV as early as 1978. At that time, the prevalence of HIV infection was probably less than 5 percent in the population of male homosexuals in San Francisco. The first cases of AIDS in homosexual men in San Francisco were detected in 1981 (CDC, 1981). This association between the cumulative incidence of HIV infection and of AIDS cases is the epidemiological pattern that must exist if HIV and AIDS are causally associated: the virus must be newly introduced into the

National Academy of Sciences, "HIV Infection and Its Epidemiology," Chapter 2 of *Confronting AIDS: Update 1988* (National Academy of Sciences Press, 1988), pp. 33–55. Reprinted by Permission of the National Academy of Sciences, Washington, D. C.

population, it must become widely prevalent, and its dissemination must precede the incidence of AIDS (Winkelstein, 1988).

The conjunction heralded by the joint appearance of HIV and AIDS has been confirmed by their continued association. HIV seropositivity rates in defined subpopulations of homosexual men in San Francisco and New York City and in IV drug abusers in New York City are associated with later cases of AIDS in the same groups (Curran et al., 1988). In San Francisco, these subpopulations can be further broken down by neighborhood of residence, in which the association between HIV seropositivity and AIDS is also high (Winkelstein et al., 1987b). Conversely, AIDS is unknown in populations that are free of HIV antibodies.

The virus has been isolated from persons with AIDS; as assay techniques have improved, close to 100 percent of affected individuals can be found to harbor the virus (Booth, 1988). The virus is not found in persons who are not at risk for infection. These points are supported by epidemiological data from the ongoing San Francisco Men's Health Study, which began in 1984. Among 374 homosexual men who remained uninfected with HIV during the first 30 months of follow-up, no cases of AIDS occurred. Among 36 homosexual men who became infected with HIV during this period, 3 cases of AIDS (8 percent) occurred. Among 399 study subjects who were infected with HIV when they entered the study, 52 (13 percent) developed AIDS. None of the heterosexual men in the study acquired HIV infection, and none developed AIDS. The probability that this distribution might have occurred by chance is less than one in a million (Winkelstein, 1988).

Perhaps the clearest evidence linking HIV to AIDS is to be found in the tragic results of blood transfusions in the United States and around the world. The transmission of HIV in contaminated blood and blood products has been clearly linked to AIDS (Curran et al., 1984); in the United States, over 1,500 reported cases of AIDS are associated with blood transfusions. Since routine screening of the blood supply for antibodies to HIV began in 1985, HIV transmission by this route has practically disappeared. Nevertheless, 13 recipients from 7 donors who initially tested negative for HIV antibodies are known to have acquired HIV infection between March 1985 and October 1987 (Ward et al., 1988). The 7 donors, who were tested at the time of donation, probably had negative test results because testing occurred soon after infection and before the development of detectable antibodies. On later retesting, however, all 7 donors were found to have detectable HIV antibodies in their blood. Of the 13 recipients, 1 developed AIDS, and 3 developed HIV-related illnesses.

Of the 3 developing illness, 1 was an infant twin who received transfusions shortly after birth; her fraternal twin, who received no transfusions, remained healthy. Thus, 13 people with no other risk factors became infected, and 4 of them developed the illness after receiving transfusions from donors who were initially thought to be free of infection. After careful investigation, the donors were found, in fact, to have HIV infection.

The causal role of HIV in AIDS is also supported by the high risk (30 to 50 percent) of perinatal HIV transmission from an infected mother to her infant (CDC, 1987b) and the subsequent diagnosis of AIDS in the infected infants.

The pathogenesis of HIV infection—how the organism causes disease—is still incompletely understood. Several mechanisms have been proposed for the profound immunodeficiency that results from HIV infection, including the aggregation of uninfected and infected T lymphocytes into multinucleated syncytia that subsequently die, the infection of stem cells, and the inhibition of lymphocyte functions by viral products. A complete understanding of a disease's pathogenesis, however, is not a prerequisite to knowing its etiology.

Proportion of Infected Individuals Who Will Develop AIDS

As epidemiological cohorts of HIV-infected individuals are observed over time, a larger and larger proportion of seropositive persons has been seen to develop AIDS. The available data suggest that the great majority of HIV-infected persons will eventually progress to AIDS in the absence of effective therapy to slow or halt the infection's progression.

The cohort of individuals that has been studied longest in relation to AIDS is a group of gay men in San Francisco who were enrolled in a study of hepatitis B virus vaccine in the late 1970s. As part of the study, blood samples were collected, from which serum was saved and frozen. Because this group of men was later found to be at high risk for AIDS, samples of the frozen serum were analyzed for HIV infection, and infected individuals have been followed for clinical and laboratory evidence of AIDS. Almost no cases of AIDS occurred during the first 2 years after infection was discovered. After 8½ years, more than 40 percent of the infected cohort has developed AIDS; a similar proportion has developed symptoms of HIV infection and is expected to progress to AIDS. Statistical modeling of the incidence of AIDS in this cohort predicts the possibility that 100 percent will develop AIDS within 13 years after initial infection (G. W. Rutherford, San Francisco Department of Public Health, personal communication, 1988).

The analysis of another cohort of 288 seropositive homosexual men in San Francisco who were seropositive when the study began shows that 22 percent have developed AIDS after 3 years of observation. Another 19 percent have clinical symptoms of infection, and an additional 24 percent demonstrate laboratory evidence of immunologic compromise. Projections for this cohort are that 50 percent of the men will develop AIDS within 6 years of observation (or probably 9 years of infection) and that many more will develop the disease in subsequent years (Moss et al., 1988).

Data from individuals infected with HIV through blood transfusions and data from persons with hemophilia suggest that the rate of progression from HIV infection to AIDS increases with age. The exception to this pattern is newborns, who have the highest progression rate of all age groups (Eyster et al., 1987; Medley et al., 1987). The progression rate in adults with hemophilia appears to be similar to that in male homosexuals (Goedert and Blattner, in press).

The Spectrum of HIV Infection

In grappling with a new disease, especially one that quickly assumes epidemic proportions, terminology and definitions become vital for clinical management of patients, data gathering and research, and decisions about coverage and reimbursement. In 1982 CDC developed a definition of AIDS for surveillance purposes that relied on the presence of opportunistic infections and malignancies; in August 1987 the definition was revised to incorporate two other syndromes indicative of AIDS: dementia and wasting syndrome. Yet fairly early in the epidemic, it became apparent that many infected individuals who suffered from clinical symptoms and laboratory abnormalities signaling the presence of HIV infection did not meet the CDC criteria for the disease. For example, persistent generalized lymphadenopathy (PGL) was thought to be associated with an increased risk of developing AIDS, especially when combined with oral candidiasis and certain laboratory abnormalities. Another group of patients displayed other chronic symptoms of AIDS—fever, weight loss, night sweats, chronic diarrhea, and fatigue—and a high proportion of this group also exhibited laboratory abnormalities. Even so, these patients did not fit what had become the standard definition of the disease, although some of them seemed to develop AIDS at a rapid pace. They were described as having AIDS-related complex (ARC), and the ARC clinical syndrome was eventually incorporated in a CDC definition (although it was never used as a basis for case reporting). Clinicians noted, however, that even this definition failed to include some patients who appeared to be at high risk for progressing to AIDS. A third, more broadly defined syndrome was termed the AIDS-related condition.

Today, with a better understanding of the natural history of HIV infection and with more precise laboratory assessments of disease progression, *the committee believes that the term ARC is no longer useful, either from a clinical or a public health perspective, and that HIV infection itself should be considered a disease.* It is more accurate to describe HIV infection as a continuum of conditions, ranging from the acute, transient, mononucleosis-like syndrome associated with seroconversion, to asymptomatic HIV infection, to symptomatic HIV infection, and, finally, to AIDS, a spectrum that encompasses a great variety of clinical symptomatology. The terms ARC and PGL do not have the precise prognostic implications they were once thought to have. For instance, it is now known that the presence of persistent, generalized lymphadenopathy in and of itself does not imply a worse prognosis than HIV seropositivity. For clinical (treatment or research) purposes, a patient can be more accurately described by a combination of a description of symptoms and laboratory evidence of immune dysfunction rather than by terms such as ARC or PGL.

Experience with cohorts of infected individuals indicates that a majority of HIV-infected individuals shows some evidence of progressive immunodeficiency and is likely to develop AIDS in the absence of effective therapy. AIDS, a dramatic and devastating syndrome, caught the attention of physicians and public health officials earlier than the milder manifestations of HIV infection, but it is now clear that AIDS is end-stage HIV infection. Like many other progressive disease processes, both infectious and noninfectious, HIV has an asymptomatic period that varies in length.

Viewing HIV infection as a disease is important because it may eventually be amenable to treatment. The drug zidovudine (i.e., AZT) has been shown to prolong the life of AIDS patients; it and other drugs are currently being tested to determine whether they also halt or slow disease progression in infected asymptomatic individuals. If an effective therapy is found, HIV infection will need to be treated early, just as diseases such as gonorrhea are often diagnosed and treated in asymptomatic infected patients. Even though no treatment is available, diagnosing HIV infection is still important now so that opportunistic infections and malignancies can be recognized as early as possible. Many treatments for these complications are more effective and less toxic when initiated early.

Considering HIV infection a disease is important to other aspects of the AIDS crisis. From a public health perspective, the population of most interest is the group infected with the virus, because these persons are capable of infecting others. In addition, medical care coverage should be based on symptoms associated with HIV infection rather than on arbitrary definitions of when "disease" begins. A terminology that reflects the progression of the disease from the initial, acute stage of infection to asymptomatic HIV infection and finally to symptomatic HIV infection and AIDS would be useful for clinical treatment and for society's management of the disease. CDC has developed a classification system that might form the basis for such a terminology.

Modes and Efficiencies of HIV Transmission

Epidemiological data continue to support the observation that HIV transmission is limited to sexual contact, the sharing of contaminated needles and syringes, exposure to infected blood or blood products, transplantation of infected organs or tissue, and transmission from mother to child either across the placenta or during delivery. A recent follow-up investigation of more than 1,100 AIDS cases that were initially reported to CDC as having no identified risk factors has shown that transmission in these individuals was also limited to the recognized routes (Castro et al., 1988). Finally, additional data from studies of health care workers (CDC, 1988d), nonsexual household contacts (Friedland and Klein, 1987), and insect bites (CDC, 1986) all support the conclusion that HIV is not transmitted by casual contact or insect bites. A change in HIV transmission modes would be biologically unprecedented in a virus. There is no evidence that HIV is capable of such a change.

Heterosexual Transmission

It has been clearly documented that HIV infection can be transmitted from men to women and from women to men through vaginal and anal intercourse (Fischl et al., 1987; Goedert et al., 1987; Padian et al., 1987a; Peterman et al., 1988). So far, however, the heterosexual spread of the virus in the United States has been confined mainly to persons whose sexual partners acquired HIV by other means—for example, by sharing contaminated needles and syringes or from blood transfusions.

Evidence to date shows that the spread of infection among heterosexuals has been rather slow in instances in which neither partner can be classified in a known risk category (CDC, 1988b). In nine seroprevalence surveys of heterosexual men and women attending sexually transmitted disease (STD) clinics in six cities, the prevalence of HIV infection ranged from 0 to 2.6 percent (CDC, 1987b). STD clinics treat individuals in the community who, because of their sexual behavior, are most likely to be infected with HIV. In studies conducted in clinics in which data were collected during personal interviews and not through self-administered questionnaires, and in which seropositive individuals were reinterviewed to obtain better information about their risk status, the prevalence of HIV infection ranged from 0 to 1.2 percent among persons with no known risk factors. The results obtained from large-scale studies of over 36 million blood donations and 1.5 million military personnel (in which there are indications of the self-exclusion of persons at high risk) show that the overall prevalence of HIV has been less than 1 percent in these populations for the period 1985 to 1987. This low prevalence among heterosexuals (compared to the 20 to 50 percent prevalence among male homosexuals) appears to indicate that the virus is not spreading rapidly in populations that are considered to be primarily low-risk groups.

To become complacent in the face of this apparent trend would be a mistake, however. Heterosexual transmission of the virus is an established fact; although the numbers are small, cases acquired through heterosexual transmission are the fastest-growing group of AIDS cases in the United States. Indeed, in parts of Africa, heterosexual transmission of HIV is great enough to sustain AIDS in an epidemic status. It is useful to review the African experience with AIDS and attempt to pinpoint conditions that may augur changes in the patterns of disease spread in the United States.

It is believed that, in Africa, HIV infection appeared in great numbers first in the heterosexual community and that prostitution has played a major role in its spread. Prostitution is not uncommon in some urban areas in central and east Africa, and the prevalence of HIV infection is quite high (25 to 88 percent) among the prostitutes tested in some of those areas (Kreiss et al., 1986; Piot et al., 1988). Case-control studies have also shown that sexual activity with female prostitutes is more common among men with AIDS than among controls; African patients with AIDS also report contact with more heterosexual partners than do controls (Quinn et al., 1986). On the other hand, homosexuality and IV drug abuse do not play a major role in HIV transmission in Africa (Piot et al., 1988). In addition, STDs, in particular genital ulcers, are fairly prevalent in some sexually active populations in Africa and are associated with an increased risk of infection, perhaps by providing a more direct portal of entry into the bloodstream. The contamination of the African blood supply and frequent exposure to unsterilized needles and syringes in both medical settings and ritual practices may also be important factors in the spread of AIDS among the African heterosexual population. Furthermore, African heterosexual adults show chronically activated immune systems more frequently than American heterosexual men, which may be a factor that increases their susceptibility to HIV infection (Quinn et al., 1987).

The pattern of disease spread in the United States has been much different. Here, the epidemic began in a few cities and within a closed community—male homosexuals—in which high-risk behaviors were practiced (multiple partners and receptive anal intercourse). These behaviors enhanced the rapid spread of HIV infection within that community, which also had high STD rates, another factor that may have increased the risk for HIV infection. The observation that the spread of HIV infection into the heterosexual community appears to be much slower suggests that one or more of the following may be true: (1) there has been relatively little sexual contact between this pool of infected men and heterosexuals; (2) heterosexuals probably change partners less frequently than homosexual men; and (3) vaginal intercourse may not spread the virus as easily as anal intercourse. Consequently, HIV infection in the heterosexual population in the United States has been somewhat contained.

Similarly to the appearance of disease among homosexual men, HIV infection also became pronounced in communities of IV drug abusers who practiced high-risk behaviors—in this instance, frequent drug injections and the sharing of contaminated drug injection equipment. These behaviors are the functional equivalent of frequent receptive anal intercourse and multiple sexual partners among homosexual men. Here also, the spread of infection was rapid but contained (Robertson et al., 1986; Des Jarlais et al., 1988). The potential for the spread of infection beyond the IV drug-abusing population is discussed below.

Will HIV infection reach epidemic proportions in the "general" heterosexual population in the United States, and are the conditions necessary for such an epidemic already in place? Sustaining the spread of the disease requires a "chain of transmission" from individuals practicing high-risk behaviors to their partners and from them to individuals with no known risks. This chain of transmission would have to include sufficient numbers of infected women interacting with men who would not otherwise be at high risk. Such a reservoir of infected women might be created in several ways: one mechanism is bisexuality; another probably more significant avenue is IV drug abuse (Guinan and Hardy, 1987; Moss et al., 1987). Of all IV drug abusers, 90 percent are heterosexuals, and 30 percent are women. Moreover, between 30 and 50 percent of female IV drug abusers have engaged in prostitution. Thus, there exists the possibility that a pool of infected prostitutes might be created (whose source of infection is the sharing of contaminated needles and syringes). HIV infection could then enter the heterosexual community from male customers of female prostitutes.

To date, most of the cases of AIDS among heterosexuals have resulted from IV drug abuse, and the number of infected addicts is growing. Moreover, seroprevalence among heterosexuals with no known risk factors is higher in areas of the country in which seroprevalence among IV drug abusers is high. This correspondence means that IV drug abusers play a pivotal role in the spread of HIV to adults through heterosexual transmission (and to infants through perinatal transmission).

For 1987, a 30 percent increase in syphilis was reported in the United States (CDC, 1988c), primarily among heterosexuals. Higher rates were reported for blacks and Hispanics than for whites. In addition, the areas reporting the largest absolute increases in syphilis cases (i.e., Florida, New York City, and California) were also areas that have high rates of HIV infection. The increases in syphilis cases suggest that behavior that increases the probability of HIV infection among heterosexuals is not being effectively curtailed.

In sum, the evidence to date is that heterosexual HIV transmission occurs from men to women and from women to men through vaginal and anal intercourse. The virus is capable of spreading among heterosexuals, but so far the prevalence of infection in the heterosexual population with no known risks for infection is low. Yet the extent of future heterosexual spread is uncertain. A "window of opportunity" apparently exists for preventing the further spread of infection to the heterosexual population.

Efficiencies of Transmission

The modes of HIV transmission are well documented. What is not as clear is how easily or how "efficiently" HIV is transmitted by a particular route if an individual is exposed. Specially designed epidemiological studies provide information that helps to estimate the probability of HIV transmission by the various known routes.

Blood Transfusions

The efficiency of this transmission route can be estimated using studies of the recipients of blood from donors who were subsequently found to have AIDS or HIV antibodies. Between 66 and 100 percent of blood transfusion recipients became infected if donors either tested positive for antibodies to HIV or later became antibody positive or developed AIDS (Ward et al., 1987). Furthermore, recipients were more likely to become infected if the transfusion occurred close to the time the donor developed symptoms. All recipients of blood transfusions became infected if the donors developed AIDS within 23 months of the donation (Ward et al., 1987). Thus, the large dose of the virus a transfusion represents, coupled with this particular route, appears to be quite efficient as a transmission path.

Perinatal Transmission

Risk of transmission can also be estimated from studies that evaluate the risk that an HIV-infected pregnant woman will deliver an infected infant. The results from such studies suggest that the probability of HIV transmission from mother to infant ranges from 30 to 50 percent (CDC, 1987b). Some studies suggest that the risk of transmission is higher for infants born to mothers who have symptoms of HIV infection during pregnancy or who show evidence of immunosuppression (Mok et al., 1987; Nzilambi et al., 1987; Piot et al., 1988).

IV Drug Abuse

Information on HIV transmission through the sharing of contaminated needles and syringes is hard to gather because of the illicit nature of IV drug abuse. However, several studies have shown that once HIV is introduced into a community, its spread is rapid among IV drug abusers and a majority of them soon becomes infected (Novick et al., 1986; Robertson et al., 1986; Des Jarlais et al., 1988). In New York City, where there are large numbers of infected IV drug abusers, the patterns of needle-sharing behavior include the practice of renting used needles and other drug paraphernalia in "shooting galleries" in which IV drug abusers gather (Friedland and Klein, 1987). Studies of IV drug abusers have shown an association between HIV seropositivity and both the frequency of drug injections and the sharing of drug injection equipment (Chaisson et al., 1987b; Marmor et al., 1987).

Homosexual Transmission

The risk of HIV transmission from receptive anal intercourse between homosexual men has been estimated, although partner tracing among homosexuals can be difficult in situations in which there have been multiple sexual partners (Grant et al., 1987). Cohort and case-control studies of homosexual men (Darrow et al., 1987; Kingsley et al., 1987; Moss et al., 1987; Winkelstein et al., 1987) show that the risk of HIV infection is greatest for persons who engage in receptive anal intercourse. The risk of infection is less for partners who engage in insertive anal intercourse, and the risk appears even lower for oral receptive intercourse.

Heterosexual Transmission

Estimates of the risk of heterosexual transmission have been derived from studies of the sex partners of infected persons. In this study design, an index case (the infected person) is identified, and the antibody status of his or her sexual partner is determined at entry and observed over time. In several studies of female partners of IV drug abusers, the risk of infection was reported to be about 50 percent (Curran et al., 1988). Studies of the male sex partners of female IV drug abusers found similarly large risks of infection, although the numbers of male partners tested were small. In these studies, HIV transmission by the sharing of contaminated needles and syringes cannot be ruled out.

The risk of transmission is lower for female partners of hemophiliacs and bisexual men and for partners of transfusion-infected persons than it is for male or female partners of IV drug abusers (Padian, 1987; Padian et al., 1987a; Curran et al., 1988; De Gruttola and Mayer, 1988; Johnson, 1988). In studies of the wives or female partners of hemophiliacs, the risk of infection was about 10 percent. Studies of female partners of bisexual men reported a risk of transmission of around 25 percent. Risks of similar magnitude have been found in studies of the spouses of transfusion-infected persons. In a recent study, of the 55 wives who had sexual contact with their infected partners, 10 (18 percent) became seropositive (Peterman et al., 1988). In this study, the risk of infection was not related to the number of sexual contacts a woman had with her infected spouse; in fact, seropositive wives reported fewer sexual contacts and were somewhat older than seronegative wives. This result suggests that, in addition to behavioral factors, biological factors probably play a role in determining how easily HIV is transmitted. There may be differences in transmissibility as a result of changes in the infectiousness of the infected individual over time. Thus, heterosexual contact during periods of high infectiousness may be more likely to transmit the virus than contact during periods of low infectiousness. A similar finding has been reported from a cohort study of partners of infected hemophiliacs. In this study, the best predictor of HIV transmission was the absolute number of T-helper lymphocytes in the hemophiliacs, suggesting that, as their immune systems became more suppressed, they were more likely to infect their sex partners, regardless of the frequency of sexual contact or the duration of their infection (Goedert et al., 1987).

Another finding from the investigation of spouses of transfusion-infected persons was a higher rate of transmission from men to women than from women to men. Whereas 10 of 55 wives (18 percent) became seropositive through sexual contact with their infected husbands, only 2 of 25 husbands (8 percent) became seropositive through sexual contact with their infected wives. Although this difference was not statistically significant, the finding that HIV transmission may be more efficient from men to women than from women to men has been reported in other studies (Padian, 1987; De Gruttola and Mayer, 1988).

Needle-Stick Transmission

Studies among health care workers of accidental needle-stick injuries or cuts with sharp objects provide information on the risk of HIV infection by this route. As of December 31, 1987, a collaborative surveillance study conducted by CDC had followed 489 health care workers who sustained needle-stick exposures to infected blood and for whom both acute- and convalescent-phase serum samples were obtained. Three of the 489 health care workers (0.6 percent) had seroconverted within 6 months of exposure. Two other prospective studies of health care workers in the United States are also assessing the risk of HIV transmission from accidental needle-stick exposure. As of April 15, 1988, a similarly designed study at the University of California at San Francisco had reported that 1 of 180 health care workers (0.5 percent) seroconverted after at least 6 months of follow-up (J. L. Gerberding and H. F. Chambers, personal communication [updating Gerberding et al., 1987], 1988). As of April 30, 1988, the National Institutes of Health had obtained both acute and convalescent serum samples at least 6 months after exposure for 108 health-care workers with needle-stick injuries; none had seroconverted (D. K. Henderson, personal communication [updating Henderson et al., 1986], 1988). The results from these studies, as well as from studies conducted in England and Canada, suggest that the risk of transmission from needle-stick exposure is less than 1 percent and probably closer to 0.5 percent. In most instances, these risks are associated with *one episode* of exposure, in contrast to the studies of sexual partners, which involve multiple exposures over time.

Relative Efficiencies of HIV Transmission

Several investigators have estimated the probability of HIV transmission for different modes of transmission (e.g., per episode of heterosexual intercourse or per screened blood transfusion), but these estimates are uncertain because the calculations are based on very limited information (Grant et al., 1987; Padian et al., 1987b; Hearst and Hulley, 1988; Ward et al., 1988). Neither is it possible to rank routes of transmission from the greatest to the least efficient with complete certainty. Factors other than the route appear to determine whether transmission of the virus occurs; these factors include the dose (inoculum size) of virus transferred, the frequency of exposure, differences in host susceptibility, variation in infectiousness of an infected person over time, possible differences in virulence among HIV isolates, and the presence of other sexually transmitted diseases or other cofactors. In addition, study designs differ, which makes it difficult to compare results.

However, some preliminary conclusions can be drawn. The recipients of infected blood transfusions are at very high risk of infection, as are children born to infected mothers. Studies of infected IV drug abusers also report high rates of infection for this group, suggesting that the sharing of contaminated needles and syringes combined with frequent injections carries a high risk of infection. The sexual partners of IV drug abusers have a greater risk of becoming infected than the sexual partners of individuals who were infected by other routes, suggesting that the mode of transmission may be either heterosexual transmission or the unacknowledged sharing of contaminated needles and syringes. Studies of the sex partners of individuals who were infected by routes other than IV drug abuse show much lower risks of infection, as do studies of the risk of infection from accidental needle-stick exposure. It is important to note that, although the risk of infection from one episode of heterosexual sex and one needle-stick injury may be roughly equivalent, studies of sexual transmission involve repeated exposures over the course of years, whereas needle-stick injury studies usually involve one or a few episodes. Although it seems intuitively correct that risk increases with increased exposure, other factors (for instance, the apparent inability of a particular infected person to transmit the virus) may intervene.

In sexual transmission, the risk of infection is greater for the receptive partner in anal intercourse than for the insertive partner. Vaginal intercourse is probably less efficient than receptive anal intercourse as a transmission route; preliminary evidence also suggests that, in vaginal intercourse, infectivity from men to women is somewhat greater than from women to men.

Prevalence and Incidence of HIV Infection in the United States

The importance of accurate descriptions of the prevalence and incidence of HIV infection, both at present and for the future, cannot be overstated. Defined cases of AIDS are only the clinical end stage of the devastating effects produced by HIV infection. The description of HIV infection by demographic characteristics and other distinguishing features helps determine which groups to target for intervention strategies to prevent the further spread of infection.

HIV Prevalence in Groups at Recognized Risk

In November 1987, CDC summarized current knowledge of the prevalence and incidence of HIV infection for various segments of the United States population according to age, sex, race or ethnic group, and geographic area (CDC, 1987b). The report reviewed data obtained from several sources (including federal agencies, health departments, and medical centers) on the prevalence of HIV infection as measured by the presence of HIV antibodies in the blood (i.e., seroprevalence).

The observed prevalence of HIV infection is highest in those risk groups that account for the majority of AIDS cases reported to CDC. Still, caution is needed in interpreting prevalence data. For example, the prevalence of HIV infection may be seen to vary in STD clinics in different geographic areas because the background prevalence in any two communities may be different. Other problems in comparing data arise from differences in questionnaire design, the inclusion or exclusion of symptomatic individuals in reports of seroprevalence, and differences in the demographic characteristics of the individuals being tested. Further, reported prevalence may be higher or lower than the true prevalence for a given group depending on who "walked in the door" (i.e., most of these surveys are based on self-selected samples).

Estimates of the prevalence of HIV infection in homosexual and bisexual men based on data from 23 cities range from 10 to 70 percent, with most estimates falling between 20 and 50 percent (CDC, 1987b). Prevalence is highest in cohorts of homosexual men in San Francisco. Yet the data probably overestimate the true prevalence of HIV infection in this group because most of the respondents to these surveys were persons who were either seeking medical attention for STDs or who were concerned that their past or present sexual behavior had placed them at risk (Curran et al., 1988).

The populations of IV drug abusers appear to be less mobile than the population of homosexual men, as larger differences in HIV prevalence are reported by geographic area. Surveys consistently show very high prevalence (50 to 60 percent) in major East Coast cities with geographic or close cultural connections to New York City and northern New Jersey; prevalence is much lower (less than 5 percent) in other areas of the country (CDC, 1987b). Most of the surveys measuring prevalence in IV drug abusers are conducted at facilities for chronic heroin abuse treatment. It is thought that only 10 to 20 percent of the estimated 1.2 million drug abusers in the United States are currently in treatment and that those not in treatment may be habitual users whose risk for HIV infection is even greater (CDC, 1987b).

The prevalence of HIV infection for persons with hemophilia ranges from 15 percent to more than 90 percent, depending on the type and severity of hemophilia and, in turn, the amount of clotting factor received (CDC, 1987b). Persons with severe hemophilia A have the highest prevalence (approximately 70 percent), whereas persons with hemophilia B or mild hemophilia A have a somewhat lower prevalence (approximately 35 percent). Within these clinical categories, however, prevalence is uniform throughout the country, reflecting the distribution of clotting factor concentrate received before 1985. Only hemophiliacs who seek treatment are tested; consequently, the prevalence reported here may be an overestimate of the true prevalence for hemophiliacs as a group (CDC, 1987b).

The prevalence of HIV in female prostitutes in the United States varies from 0 percent to more than 50 percent. Seropositivity is higher in black and Hispanic prostitutes than in white prostitutes. The differences in prevalence appear to be related to the extent of IV drug abuse in the groups tested and the background HIV prevalence in IV drug abusers in the area (CDC, 1987b).

In studies of seroprevalence conducted among persons who are heterosexual sex partners of HIV-infected persons but who have no other identifiable risk factors for HIV infection, prevalence ranged from less than 10 percent to 60 percent (CDC, 1987b). As noted earlier in this chapter, surveys in STD clinics of heterosexual men and women who do not belong to any risk group and who do not have partners in any risk group report prevalences ranging from 0 percent to 2.6 percent, depending on the population studied and the method of data collection. Seroprevalence is higher among heterosexuals in areas in which seroprevalence in IV drug abusers is high. However, such studies may overrepresent the true prevalence of HIV among heterosexuals because people surveyed in STD clinics may be more sexually active than the "general" heterosexual population.

HIV Prevalence Among Selected Segments of the General Population

The prevalence of HIV infection in the population at large has been estimated primarily from studies of various special populations: blood donors, civilian applicants to the military, Job Corps entrants, sentinel hospital patients, and newborn infants (whose antibody status at birth reflects the presence or absence of antibodies in their mothers) (CDC, 1987b). More than 36 million blood or plasma donations in the United States have been tested for HIV antibodies since 1985. HIV prevalence among first-time donors for the period 1985 to 1987 was 0.04 percent. Prevalence was much higher for men than for women and higher for blacks and Hispanics than for whites. Since October 1985, blood samples from over 1.5 million applicants for military service have also been tested for HIV antibodies. The prevalence of HIV infection increases with age for applicants between the late teens and late twenties. Prevalence by birth year cohorts also increased from the first screening period (1985–1986) to the second (1986–1987). As with blood donors, seropositivity was higher for men than for women and higher for blacks and Hispanics than for whites. The overall prevalence (for October 1985 to September 1987), adjusted for the age, sex, and racial and ethnic composition of the U.S. adult population aged 17 to 59 years, was 0.14 percent. Since March 1987, HIV antibody screening has been conducted for new members of the Job Corps who participate in residential training programs. This program recruits rural and inner-city disadvantaged youths aged 16 to 21. Provisional data from the first 25,000 entrants showed a seroprevalence of 0.33 percent. The prevalence of infection in the nation as a whole is probably higher than what has been observed in blood donors, applicants to the military, and Job Corps entrants, as persons at highest risk for infection are probably underrepresented.

To avoid the self-selection bias associated with volunteer programs, anonymous HIV antibody testing has also recently begun on selected hospital patients (excluding AIDS cases and other conditions related to HIV infection) at sentinel hospitals. Based on the first 8,668 test results, the age- and sex-adjusted prevalence of infection was 0.32 percent. This sample represents hospitalized patients who are at low risk for infection. In addition, the hospitals selected to participate in the program may service specialized segments of the community; therefore, the data collected are not representative of all hospitalized patients.

Several states have begun programs to assess the prevalence of HIV infection in women of childbearing age by testing for HIV antibodies in their newborns. Maternal antibodies against HIV cross the placenta and are therefore present in the baby's blood. A baby with antibodies to HIV may or may not itself be infected; however, the presence of antibodies in the baby's blood always indicates that the mother is infected. Neonatal blood specimens are routinely collected in hospitals to test for metabolic disorders; the test for HIV antibodies has been added to this program. A recent study has reported that 1 of every 476 women (0.2 percent) giving birth in Massachusetts was antibody positive during the period December 1986 to June 1987. The prevalence of HIV infection differed according to the type and location of the maternity hospitals. Prevalence was highest in inner-city hospitals (0.8 percent), lower in mixed urban and suburban hospitals (0.25 percent), and lowest in suburban and rural hospitals (0.09 percent) (Hoff et al., 1988). In New York, the prevalence of HIV infection among women delivering babies in hospitals in the five New York City boroughs between November 1987 and February 1988 was 1.45 percent; the prevalence of HIV infection among women delivering babies in hospitals outside the metropolitan area was 0.18 percent (Novick et al., 1988).

Incidence of New Infections

Data on the incidence (the number of new infections over time) of HIV infection are more difficult to obtain than prevalence data, but they are crucial for longer term projections of the course of the epidemic. Evidence from eight cohort studies of gay men suggest a lower HIV incidence rate in that population for 1985–1987 than in the earlier part of the decade (CDC, 1987b). This observed decline in the incidence of infection may be attributed to several factors, but it is consistent with reports of a decline in other sexually transmitted diseases in this group (CDC, 1988c) as well as changes in sexual behavior (Winkelstein et al., 1987a). Serologic screening of blood and plasma donors and heat treatment of factor concentrate, as well as efforts to exclude donors at high risk, have also reduced the rate of new infection among transfusion recipients and hemophiliacs since 1985. In contrast, HIV incidence appears to be increasing in IV drug abusers in New York City and San Francisco (Chaisson et al., 1987a; Des Jarlais et al., 1987; Schoenbaum et al., 1987). These data suggest that the epidemic of HIV infection in the United States may be viewed as a series of overlapping smaller epidemics, each with its own dynamics and time course (Curran et al., 1988).

National Estimates of HIV Infection

In 1986, CDC estimated the size of various segments of the population that were known to be infected (i.e., male homosexuals, IV drug abusers, hemophiliacs, heterosexuals with no known risks), as well as the prevalence of HIV infection for each of these groups. It then calculated from these estimates that 1 to 1.5 million people in the United States were currently infected with HIV. In November 1987, CDC reviewed these estimates and modified them slightly based on new information about the size of the various populations and new seroprevalence data for these groups. In retrospect, the 1986 estimates made by CDC appear to have been too high. CDC now estimates that between 945,000 and 1.4 million Americans currently are infected with HIV. The major limitation of both the original and the revised estimates is the unknown size of the homosexual population that engages in at-risk behaviors (CDC, 1987b). CDC will continue to update national estimates of the prevalence of HIV infection as more information is gathered. Other groups and investigators have also estimated the prevalence of HIV infection in the United States; these estimates have been both higher and lower than those made by CDC, ranging from 400,000 to 2.2 million for the end of 1987 (De Gruttola and Lagakos, 1987; Harris, 1987). Such estimates provide an overall picture of the magnitude of the epidemic; however, seroprevalence and incidence data on specific groups at risk are more important because they offer the necessary information to target prevention strategies and evaluate their effectiveness in curbing the epidemic.

The Program of HIV Surveys and Studies

CDC has responded to the urgent need to monitor the spread of HIV infection by instituting a series of seroprevalence studies and surveillance systems (Dondero et al., 1988). In approximately 30 metropolitan areas in the United States, blood samples will be routinely collected from persons treated at STD clinics, drug abuse treatment centers, family planning and women's health clinics, and tuberculosis clinics, as well as from selected hospital admissions and newborns. These studies will provide local officials with information on HIV prevalence so that interventions can be designed to control HIV infection in specific settings. The surveys of newborns will provide some of the most valuable information because sample selection is unbiased; the entire population of childbearing mothers is included. As noted earlier, testing for HIV antibodies, which will occur in approximately 30 states, will be added to already existing programs that routinely test newborns for metabolic disorders. These surveys will, therefore, be population based and, by providing information on the antibody status of newborns, will reflect the prevalence of infection in mothers delivering in these hospitals.

In addition to these activities, studies of HIV infection will continue in civilian applicants to the military services, active duty military personnel, blood donors, and Job Corps entrants. Surveys of HIV prevalence will also be conducted in other populations of special interest such as patients from emergency rooms, patients using other hospital services, students on college campuses, and prisoners. The National Center for Health Statistics (NCHS) will also conduct a study to determine the feasibility of a nationwide household seroprevalence survey. In addition, NCHS also plans to include anonymous HIV antibody testing of an estimated 17,000 blood specimens collected from adults over a 6-year period as part of the National Health and Nutrition Examination Survey.

It is important to note that some of these surveys will be "blinded" (i.e., HIV antibody testing will be done on blood specimens collected for other purposes with personal information on the individual permanently removed) to avoid the uninterpretable impact of self-selection bias. Other surveys, however, will be nonblinded. In these settings, volunteer participants will be interviewed to evaluate risk factors for HIV transmission.

AIDS Cases in the United States

In October 1986, when *Confronting AIDS* was published, approximately 24,500 cases of AIDS had been reported to CDC. As of May 1988, 62,200 cases of AIDS had been reported since June 1981, and 35,051 of these had ended in death (CDC, 1988a). An additional 10 to 20 percent of cases are believed to have been missed by the surveillance system. The number of cases reported each year continues to increase, although the rate of increase is less steep than it was earlier in the decade. Cases have been reported from all 50 states and the District of Columbia.

Since the publication of *Confronting AIDS*, the distribution of cases by risk group as well as by sex, race, age, and geographic area has not changed substantially: 63 percent of cases are homosexual or bisexual men not known to have abused IV drugs, 19 percent are heterosexual IV drug abusers, 7 percent are both male homosexuals and IV drug abusers, 1 percent are patients with hemophilia and related disorders, 4 percent are persons who acquired the disease through heterosexual contact, 3 percent are recipients of blood transfusions, and 3 percent are cases in which risk information is undetermined because it is incomplete (patients have died, refused to be interviewed, or have been lost to follow-up) or the patients are still under investigation. This 3 percent also includes men reporting contact with a prostitute and patients with no identifiable risk factor. Of the 981 cases of AIDS among children that had been reported to CDC by May 1988, 77 percent are offspring of a parent with AIDS or at high risk for AIDs. Of the remaining pediatric cases, 6 percent are children with hemophilia, 14 percent are transfusion recipients, and 4 percent are children for whom risk information cannot be determined.

Over the past 2 years, the largest increases in new cases have been observed in two groups: heterosexual partners of HIV-infected individuals and children whose mothers abuse IV drugs or are sexual partners of men at high risk. There is an overrepresentation of blacks and Hispanics in both of these groups. The only group showing a steady decline in AIDS incidence over the past 2 years has been children with transfusion-associated AIDS. This decline is attributed to the screening of blood and blood products that began in early 1985 and to the rather short incubation period of 12 months or less observed for children with transfusion-associated AIDS. It is now thought that more than 80 percent of HIV infection in children can be directly linked to IV drug abuse in the mother or father.

The Demographic Impact of AIDS

AIDS has already begun to alter the demographic characteristics of New York City and San Francisco. A disease that was virtually unknown to Americans 8 years ago, AIDS is now the leading cause of death in New York City among men aged 25 to 44 and women aged 25 to 34. In 1986, mortality from AIDS was the eighth leading cause of years of potential life lost before the age of 65 in the United States (CDC, 1988b). Recent data from New York City indicate that 1 of every 66 infants born between November 1987 and February 1988 tested positive for HIV antibodies, reflecting the prevalence of HIV infection in women of childbearing age in that city (Novick et al., 1988). In San Francisco, approximately 50 percent of the male homosexual population is infected with the virus, suggesting the possible future devastation of a large component of the city's population. In 1986, New York City and San Francisco accounted for approximately 40 percent of all AIDS cases; by 1991 these two cities will account for less than 20 percent of cases nationwide (Morgan and Curran, 1986), suggesting that other metropolitan areas will soon face major economic and demographic losses.

AIDS cases occur in higher proportions in black and Hispanic populations than in white populations (on the West Coast, the proportion is 3 times higher in black and Hispanic than in white populations and 12 times higher on the East Coast), mainly as a result of higher HIV prevalence in black and Hispanic IV drug abusers and their sex partners and offspring. Recent data also suggest that the virus is spreading more rapidly among blacks and Hispanics at risk than among other population groups, especially in northeastern cities, suggesting that the future composition of AIDS cases will consist primarily of poor, urban minorities.

Future Research Needs

Epidemiological studies are the main source of information on the prevalence and incidence of HIV infection and AIDS, the modes and efficiencies of HIV transmission, the proportion of infected individuals who progress to AIDS, serologic markers of disease progression, and the distribution of behaviors associated with increased exposure to HIV. Epidemiological studies have also provided some of the strongest evidence for the association between HIV infection and AIDS. Whether or not these studies are prevalence or incidence surveys, cohort or case-control in design, they provide essential data to understand and control the epidemic.

Although much has been learned about the epidemiology of HIV infection, more research is needed to address its many unanswered questions. *The committee therefore strongly urges continued epidemiological research in support of appropriate prevention and control measures.* CDC must be provided with the necessary funding to ensure that personnel, space, and technical resources are adequate to the task of continuing epidemiological research.

REFERENCES

Booth, W. 1988. A rebel without a cause of AIDS. Science 239:1485–1488.

Castro, K. G., A. R. Lifson, C. R. White, T. J. Bush, M. E. Chamberland, A. M. Lekatsas, and H. W. Jaffe. 1988. Investigations of AIDS patients with no previously identified risk factors. J. Am. Med. Assoc. 259:1338–1342.

CDC (Centers for Disease Control). 1981. Kaposi's sarcoma and *Pneumocystis* pneumonia among homosexual men—New York City and California. Morbid. Mortal. Wkly. Rep. 30:305–308.

CDC. 1986. Acquired immunodeficiency syndrome (AIDS) in western Palm Beach County, Florida. Morbid. Mortal. Wkly. Rep. 35:609–612.

CDC. 1987a. Antibody to human immunodeficiency virus in female prostitutes. Morbid. Mortal. Wkly. Rep. 36:157–161.

CDC. 1987b. Human immunodeficiency virus infection in the United States: A review of current knowledge. Morbid. Mortal. Wkly. Rep. 36(suppl. 6):1–48.

CDC. 1987c. Revision of the CDC surveillance case definition for acquired immunodeficiency syndrome. Morbid. Mortal. Wkly. Rep. 36(suppl. 1):3S–15S.

CDC. 1988a. AIDS weekly surveillance report—United States, May 16. Atlanta, Ga.: CDC.

CDC. 1988b. Changes in premature mortality—United States, 1979–1986. Morbid. Mortal. Wkly. Rep. 37:47–48.

CDC. 1988c. Continuing increase in infectious syphilis—United States. Morbid. Mortal. Wkly. Rep. 37:35–38.

CDC. 1988d. Update: Acquired immunodeficiency syndrome and human immunodeficiency virus infection among health-care workers. Morbid. Mortal. Wkly. Rep. 37:229–239.

Chaisson, R. E., D. Osmond, A. R. Moss, H. W. Feldman, and P. Bernacki. 1987a. HIV, bleach, and needle sharing. Lancet 1:1430.

Chaisson, R. E., A. R. Moss, R. Onishi, D. Osmond, and J. R. Carlson. 1987b. Human immunodeficiency virus infection in heterosexual intravenous drug users in San Francisco. Am. J. Public Health 77:169–172.

Curran, J. W., D. N. Lawrence, H. Jaffe, J. E. Kaplan, L. D. Zyla, M. Chamberland, R. Weinstein, K.-J. Lui, L. B. Schonberger, T. J. Spira, W. J. Alexander, G. Swinger, A. Ammann, S. Solomon, D. Auerbach, D. Mildvan, R. Stoneburner, J. M. Jason, H. W. Haverkos, and B. L. Evatt. 1984. Acquired immunodeficiency syndrome (AIDS) associated with transfusions. N. Engl. J. Med. 310:69–75.

Curran, J. W., H. W. Jaffe, A. M. Hardy, W. M. Morgan, R. M. Selik, and T. J. Dondero. 1988. Epidemiology of HIV infection and AIDS in the United States. Science 239:610–616.

Darrow, W. W., D. F. Echenberg, H. W. Jaffe, P. M. O'Malley, R. H. Byers, J. P. Getchell, and J. W. Curran. 1987. Risk factors for human immunodeficiency virus (HIV) infections in homosexual men. Am. J. Public Health 77:479–483.

De Gruttola, V., and S. W. Lagakos. 1987. The value of doubling time in assessing the course of the AIDS epidemic. Paper prepared for the Institute of Medicine Workshop on Modeling the Spread of Infection with Human Immunodeficiency Virus and the Demographic Impact of Acquired Immune Deficiency Syndrome, Washington, D.C., October 15–17.

De Gruttola, V., and K. H. Mayer. 1988. Assessing and modeling heterosexual spread of the human immunodeficiency virus in the United States. Rev. Infect. Dis. 10:138–150.

Des Jarlais, D. C., S. R. Friedman, M. Marmor, H. Cohen, D. Mildvan, S. Yancovitz, U. Mathur, W. El-Sadr, T. J. Spira, J. Garber, S. T. Beatrice, A. S. Abdul-Quader, and J. L. Sotheran. 1987. Development of AIDS, HIV seroconversion, and potential cofactors for T4 cell loss in a cohort of intravenous drug users. AIDS 1:105–111.

Des Jarlais, D. C., S. R. Friedman, and R. L. Stoneburner. 1988. HIV infection and intravenous drug use: Critical issues in transmission dynamics, infection outcomes, and prevention. Rev. Infect. Dis. 10:151–158.

Dondero, T. J., M. Pappaioanou, and J. W. Curran. 1988. Monitoring the levels and trends of HIV infection: The Public Health Service's HIV Surveillance Program. Public Health Rep. 103:213–220.

Eyster, M. E., M. H. Gail, J. O. Ballard, H. Al-Mondhiry, and J. J. Goedert. 1987. Natural history of human immunodeficiency virus infections in hemophiliacs: Effects of T-cell subsets, platelet counts, and age. Ann. Intern. Med. 107:1–6.

Fischl, M. A., G. M. Dickinson, G. B. Scott, N. Klimas, M. A. Fletcher, and W. Parks. 1987. Evaluation of heterosexual partners, children, and household contacts of adults with AIDS. J. Am. Med. Assoc. 257:640–644.

Friedland, G. H., and R. S. Klein. 1987. Transmission of the human immunodeficiency virus. N. Engl. J. Med. 317:1125–1135.

Gerberding, J. L., C. E. Bryant-LeBlanc, K. Nelson, A. R. Moss, D. Osmond, H. F. Chambers, J. R. Carlson, W. L. Drew, J. A. Levy, and M. A. Sande.

1987. Risk of transmitting the human immunodeficiency virus, cytomegalovirus, and hepatitis B virus to health care workers exposed to patients with AIDS and AIDS-related conditions. J. Infect. Dis. 156:1–8.

Goedert, J. J., and W. A. Blattner. In press. The epidemiology and natural history of human immunodeficiency virus. In AIDS: Etiology, Diagnosis, Treatment and Prevention, 2nd ed., V. T. DeVita, S. Hellman, and S. A. Rosenberg, eds. Philadelphia: Lippincott.

Goedert, J. J., M. E. Eyster, R. J. Biggar, and W. A. Blattner. 1987. Heterosexual transmission of human immunodeficiency virus: Association with severe depletion of T-helper lymphocytes in men with hemophilia. AIDS Res. Hum. Retrovir. 3:355–361.

Grant, R. M., J. A. Wiley, and W. Winkelstein. 1987. Infectivity of the human immunodeficiency virus: Estimates from a prospective study of homosexual men. J. Infect. Dis. 156:189–193.

Guinan, M. E., and A. Hardy. 1987. Epidemiology of AIDS in women in the United States: 1981 through 1986. J. Am. Med. Assoc. 257:2039–2042.

Harris, J. E. 1987. The AIDS epidemic: Looking into the 1990s. Technol. Rev. 90:59–64.

Hearst, N., and S. B. Hulley. 1988. Preventing the heterosexual spread of AIDS. Are we giving our patients the best advice? J. Am. Med. Assoc. 259:2428–2432.

Henderson, D. K., A. J. Saah, B. J. Zak, R. A. Kaslow, H. C. Lane, T. Folks, W. C. Blackwelder, J. Schmitt, D. J. LaCamera, H. Masur, and A. S. Fauci. 1986. Risk of nosocomial infection with human T-cell lymphotropic virus type III/lymphadenopathy-associated virus in a large cohort of intensively exposed health care workers. Ann. Intern. Med. 104:644–647.

Hoff, R., V. P. Berardi, B. J. Weiblen, L. Mahoney-Trout, M. L. Mitchell, and G. F. Grady. 1988. Seroprevalence of human immunodeficiency virus among childbearing women. Estimation by testing samples of blood from newborns. N. Engl. J. Med. 318:525–530.

Johnson, A. M. 1988. Heterosexual transmission of human immunodeficiency virus. Br. Med. J. 296:1017–1020.

Kingsley, L. A., R. Kaslow, C. R. Rinaldo, Jr., K. Detre, N. Odaka, M. VanRaden, R. Detels, B. F. Polk, J. Chmiel, S. F. Kelsey, D. Ostrow, and B. Visscher. 1987. Risk factors for seroconversion to human immunodeficiency virus among male homosexuals. Lancet 1:345–349.

Kreiss, J. K., D. Koech, F. A. Plummer, K. K. Homles, M. Lightfoote, P. Piot, A. R. Ronald, J. O. Ndinya-Achola, L. J. D'Costa, P. Roberts, E. N. Ngugi, and T. C. Quinn. 1986. AIDS virus infection in Nairobi prostitutes. Spread of the epidemic to east Africa. N. Engl. J. Med. 314:414–418.

Marmor, M., D. C. Des Jarlais, H. Cohen, S. R. Friedman, S. T. Beatrice, N. Dubin, W. El-Sadr, D. Mildvan, S. Yancovitz, U. Mathur, and R. Holzman. 1987. Risk factors for infection with human immunodeficiency virus among intravenous drug abusers in New York City. AIDS 1:39–44.

Medley, G. F., R. M. Anderson, D. R. Cox, and L. Billard. 1987. Incubation period of AIDS in patients infected via blood transfusion. Nature 328:719–721.

Mok, J. Q., C. Giaquinto, A. De Rossi, I. Grosch-Worner, A. E. Ades, and C. S. Peckham. 1987. Infants born to mothers seropositive for human immuno-deficiency virus. Preliminary findings from a multicentre European study. Lancet 1:1164–1168.

Morgan, W. M., and J. W. Curran. 1986. Acquired immunodeficiency syndrome: Current and future trends. Public Health Rep. 101:459–465.

Moss, A. R. 1987. AIDS and intravenous drug use: The real heterosexual epidemic. Br. Med. J. 294:389–390.

Moss, A. R., D. Osmond, P. Bacchetti, J.-C Chermann, F. Barre-Sinoussi, and J. Carlson. 1987. Risk factors for AIDS and HIV seropositivity in homo-sexual men. Am. J. Epidemiol. 125:1035–1047.

Moss, A. R., P. Bacchetti, D. Osmond, W. Krampf, R. E. Chaisson, D. Stites, J. Wilber, J.-P. Allain, and J. Carlson. 1988. Seropositivity for HIV and the development of AIDS or AIDS related condition: Three-year follow-up of the San Francisco General Hospital cohort. Br. Med. J. 296:745–750.

Novick, D. M., M. J. Kreek, D. C. Des Jarlais, T. J. Spira, E. T. Khuri, J. Ragunath, V. S. Kalyanaraman, A. M. Gelb, and A. Miescher. 1986. Abstract of clinical research findings: Therapeutic and historical aspects. Pp. 318–320 in Proceedings of the 47th Annual Scientific Meeting, Committee on Problems of Drug Dependence (1985), L. Harris, ed. Rockville, Md.: National Institute on Drug Abuse.

Novick, L. F., D. Berns, R. Stricof, and R. Stevens. 1988. New York State Department of Health newborn seroprevalence study. Interim report draft. Albany. March 15.

Nzilambi, N., R. W. Ryder, F. Behets, H. Francis, E. Bayende, A. Nelson, J. M. Mann, et al. 1987. Perinatal HIV transmission in two African hospitals. P. 158 in Abstracts of the Third International Conference on AIDS, Washington, D.C., June 1–5.

Padian, N. S. 1987. Heterosexual transmission of acquired immunodeficiency syndrome: International perspectives and national projections. Rev. Infect. Dis. 9:947–960.

Padian, N., L. Marquis, D. P. Francis, R. E. Anderson, G. W. Rutherford, P. M. O'Malley, and W. Winkelstein, Jr. 1987a. Male-to-female transmission of human immunodeficiency virus. J. Am. Med. Assoc. 258:788–790.

Padian, N., J. Wiley, and W. Winkelstein. 1987b. Male-to-female transmission of human immunodeficiency virus (HIV): Current results, infectivity rates, and San Francisco population seroprevalence estimates. P. 171 in Abstracts of the Third International Conference on AIDS, Washington, D.C., June 1–5.

Peterman, T. A., R. L. Stoneburner, J. R. Allen, H. W. Jaffe, and J. W. Curran. 1988. Risk of human immunodeficiency virus transmission from hetero-sexual adults with transfusion-associated infections. J. Am. Med. Assoc. 259:55–58.

Piot, P., F. A. Plummer, F. S. Mhalu, J.-L. Lamboray, J. Chin, and J. M. Mann. 1988. AIDS: An international perspective. Science 239:573–579.

Quinn, T. C., J. M. Mann, J. W. Curran, and P. Piot. 1986. AIDS in Africa: An epidemiologic paradigm. Science 234:955–963.

Quinn, T. C., P. Piot, J. B. McCormick, F. M. Feinsod, H. Taelman, B. Kapita, W. Stevens, and A. S. Fauci. 1987. Serologic and immunologic studies in patients with AIDS in North America and Africa. The potential role of infectious agents as cofactors in human immunodeficiency virus infection. J. Am. Med. Assoc. 257:2617–2621.

Robertson, J. R., A. B. V. Bucknall, P. D. Welsby, J. J. K. Roberts, J. M. Inglis, J. F. Peutherer, and R. P. Brettle. 1986. Epidemic of AIDS related virus (HTLV-III/LAV) infection among intravenous drug abusers. Br. Med. J. 292:527–529.

Schoenbaum, E. E., P. A. Selwyn, D. Hartel, R. S. Klein, K. Davenny, and G. H. Friedland. 1987. HIV seroconversion in intravenous drug abusers: Rate and risk factors. P. 117 in Abstracts of the Third International Conference on AIDS, Washington, D.C., June 1–5.

Ward, J. W., D. A. Deppe, S. Samson, H. Perkins, P. Holland, L. Fernando, P. M. Feorino, P. Thompson, S. Kleinman, and J. R. Allen. 1987. Risk of human immunodeficiency virus infection from blood donors who later developed the acquired immunodeficiency syndrome. Ann. Intern. Med. 106:61–62.

Ward, J. W., S. D. Holmberg, J. R. Allen, D. L. Cohn, S. E. Critchley, S. H. Kleinman, B. A. Lenes, O. Ravenholt, J. R. Davis, M. G. Quinn, and H. W. Jaffe. 1988. Transmission of human immunodeficiency virus (HIV) by blood transfusions screened as negative for HIV antibody. N. Engl. J. Med. 318:473–478.

Winkelstein, W., Jr. 1988. Epidemiological observations on the causal nature of the association between infection by the human immunodeficiency virus and the acquired immunodeficiency syndrome. Paper presented at the Scientific Forum on the Etiology of AIDS, American Foundation for AIDS Research, Washington, D.C., April 9.

Winkelstein, W., Jr., M. Samuel, N. S. Padian, J. A. Wiley, W. Lang, R. E. Anderson, and J. A. Levy. 1987a. The San Francisco Men's Health Study. III. Reduction in human immunodeficiency virus transmission among homosexual/bisexual men, 1982–86. Am. J. Public Health 76:685–689.

Winkelstein, W., Jr., D. M. Lyman, N. Padian, R. Grant, M. Samuel, J. A. Wiley, R. E. Anderson, W. Lang, J. Riggs, and J. A. Levy. 1987b. Sexual practices and risk of infection by the human immunodeficiency virus. The San Francisco Men's Health Study. J. Am. Med. Assoc. 257:321–325.

The Terrifying Normalcy of AIDS

Stephen Jay Gould

DISNEY'S EPCOT CENTER IN Orlando, Florida is a technological tour de force and a conceptual desert. In this permanent World's Fair, American industrial giants have built their versions of an unblemished future. These masterful entertainments convey but one message, brilliantly packaged and relentlessly expressed: Progress through technology is the solution to all human problems. G.E. proclaims from Horizons: "If we can dream it, we can do it." A.T.&T. speaks from on high within its giant golf ball: We are now "unbounded by space and time." United Technologies bubbles from the depths of Living Seas: "With the help of modern technology, we feel there's really no limit to what can be accomplished."

Yet several of these exhibits at the Experimental Prototype Community of Tomorrow, all predating space disaster, belie their stated message from within by using the launch of the shuttle as a visual metaphor for technological triumph. The *Challenger* disaster may represent a general malaise, but it remains an incident. The AIDS pandemic, an issue that may rank with nuclear weaponry as the greatest danger of our era, provides a more striking proof that mind and technology are not omnipotent and that we have not canceled our bond to nature.

In 1984, John Platt, a biophysicist who taught at the University of Chicago for many years, wrote a short paper for private circulation.

Stephen Jay Gould, "The Terrifying Normalcy of AIDS," *New York Times Magazine*, April 19, 1987. Reprinted by Permission of the Author.

At a time when most of us were either ignoring AIDS, or viewing it as a contained and peculiar affliction of homosexual men, Platt recognized that the limited data on the origin of AIDS and its spread in America suggested a more frightening prospect: we are all susceptible to AIDS, and the disease has been spreading in a simple exponential manner.

Exponential growth is a geometric increase. Remember the old kiddy problem: If you place a penny on square one of a checkerboard and double the number of coins on each subsequent square—2, 4, 8, 16, 32 . . .—how big is the stack by the 64th square? The answer: about as high as the universe is wide. Nothing in the external environment inhibits this increase, thus giving to exponential processes their relentless character. In the real, noninfinite world, of course, some limit will eventually arise, and the process slows down, reaches a steady state, or destroys the entire system: the stack of pennies falls over, the bacterial cells exhaust their supply of nutrients.

Platt noticed that data for the initial spread of AIDS fell right on an exponential curve. He then followed the simplest possible procedure of extrapolating the curve unabated into the 1990's. Most of us were incredulous, accusing Platt of the mathematical gamesmanship that scientists call "curve fitting." After all, aren't exponential models unrealistic? Surely we are not all susceptible to AIDS. Is it not spread only by odd practices to odd people? Will it not, therefore, quickly run its short course within a confined group?

Well, hello 1987—worldwide data still match Platt's extrapolated curve. This will not, of course, go on forever. AIDS has probably already saturated the African areas where it probably originated, and where the sex ratio of afflicted people is 1-to-1, male-female. But AIDS still has far to spread, and may be moving exponentially, through the rest of the world. We have learned enough about the cause of AIDS to slow its spread, if we can make rapid and fundamental changes in our handling of that most powerful part of human biology—our own sexuality. But medicine, as yet, has nothing to offer as a cure and precious little even for palliation.

This exponential spread of AIDS not only illuminates its, and our, biology, but also underscores the tragedy of our moralistic misperception. Exponential processes have a definite time and place of origin, an initial point of "inoculation"—in this case, Africa. We didn't notice the spread at first. In a population of billions, we pay little attention when 1 increases to 2, or 8 to 16, but when 1 million becomes 2 million, we panic, even though the *rate* of doubling has not increased.

The infection has to start somewhere, and its initial locus may be little more than an accident of circumstance. For a while, it remains confined to those in close contact with the primary source, but only by accident of proximity, not by intrinsic susceptibility. Eventually, given the power and lability of human sexuality, it spreads outside the initial group and into the general population. And now AIDS has begun its march through our own heterosexual community.

What a tragedy that our moral stupidity caused us to lose precious time, the greatest enemy in fighting an exponential spread, by downplaying the danger because we thought that AIDS was a disease of three irregular groups: minorities of lifestyle (needle users), of sexual preference (homosexuals), and of color (Haitians). If AIDS had first been imported from Africa into a Park Avenue apartment, we would not have dithered as the exponential march began.

The message of Orlando—the inevitability of technological solutions—is wrong, and we need to understand why.

Our species has not won its independence from nature, and we cannot do all that we can dream. Or at least we cannot do it at the rate required to avoid tragedy, for we are not unbounded from time. Viral diseases are preventable in principle, and I suspect that an AIDS vaccine will one day be produced. But how will this discovery avail us if it takes until the millennium, and by then AIDS has fully run its exponential course and saturated our population, killing a substantial percentage of the human race? A fight against an exponential enemy is primarily a race against time.

We must also grasp the perspective of ecology and evolutionary biology and recognize, once we reinsert ourselves properly into nature, that AIDS represents the ordinary workings of biology, not an irrational or diabolical plague with a moral meaning. Disease, including epidemic spread, is a natural phenomenon, part of human history from the beginning. An entire subdiscipline of my profession, paleopathology, studies the evidence of ancient diseases preserved in the fossil remains of organisms. Human history has been marked by episodic plagues. More native peoples died of imported disease than ever fell before the gun during the era of colonial expansion. Our memories are short, and we have had a respite, really, only since the influenza pandemic at the end of World War I, but AIDS must be viewed as a virulent expression of an ordinary natural phenomenon.

I do not say this to foster either comfort or complacency. The evolutionary perspective is correct, but utterly inappropriate for our human scale. Yes, AIDS is a natural phenomenon, one of a recurring class of pandemic diseases. Yes, AIDS may run through the entire population, and may carry off a quarter or more of us. Yes, it may make no *biological* difference to *Homo sapiens* in the long run: there will still be plenty of us left and we can start again. Evolution cares as little for its agents—organisms struggling for reproductive success—as physics cares for individual atoms of hydrogen in the sun. But *we* care. These atoms are our neighbors, our lovers, our children and ourselves. AIDS is both a natural phenomenon and, potentially, the greatest natural tragedy in human history.

The cardboard message of Epcot fosters the wrong attitudes; we must both reinsert ourselves into nature and view AIDS as a natural phenomenon in order to fight properly. If we stand above nature and if technology is all powerful, then AIDS is a horrifying anomaly that must be trying to tell us something. If so, we can adopt one of two attitudes, each potentially fatal. We can either become complacent, because we believe the message of Epcot and assume that medicine will soon generate a cure, or we can panic in confusion and seek a scapegoat for something so irregular that it must have been visited upon us to teach a moral lesson.

But AIDS is not irregular. It is part of nature. So are we. This should galvanize us and give us hope, not prompt the worst of all responses: a kind of "new-age" negativism that equates natural with what we must accept and cannot, or even should not, change. When we view AIDS as natural, and when we recognize both the exponential property of its spread and the accidental character of its point of entry into America, we can break through our destructive tendencies to blame others and to free ourselves of concern.

If AIDS is natural, then there is no *message* in its spread. But by all that science has learned and all that rationality proclaims, AIDS works by a *mechanism*—and we can discover it. Victory is not ordained by any principle of progress, or any slogan of technology, so we shall have to fight like hell, and be watchful. There is no message, but there is a mechanism.

THE SOCIAL CONTEXT OF HIV INFECTION

Introduction

IN WHATEVER WAY WE as a culture finally come to terms with the HIV epidemic, AIDS will nonetheless always be associated with what it has disclosed about America in the latter part of the twentieth century: that its racism was pervasive; that its homophobia was cruel and self-righteous, and that its health care system was practically incapable of accommodating its chronically ill, much less those made ill by an epidemic. Only the twin reactions of homophobia and racism can sufficiently explain the national neglect at the heart of the official response to the epidemic. Larry Kramer, playwright and founder of ACT/UP, is a chronicler of the epidemic and has consistently expressed the horror that the HIV-affected felt as they grew sicker and were shunned and abandoned in the first years of the crisis. In the first eight years of the epidemic, the majority of those who died were gay men. It is important to understand that the struggle over AIDS was and is not only a demand for money, for services, for access to health care and influence over research agendas. It was and still is a fight over who shall define what the epidemic is. Because of America's reaction to homosexuality, AIDS was associated with irresponsibility and with abnormality. It was only when the gay community itself fought back and required a medical definition for the HIV-affected that the AIDS epidemic became a medical phenomenon. The struggle is not over yet.

As "HIV Infection and Its Epidemiology" in the preceding section indicates, the populations at increasing risk of HIV infection are those who share needles in intravenous drug use or are sexual partners of intravenous drug users who share needles. With the intravenous drug user, the social characteristics of medical needs and medical resources change from those needs and resources as they were met initially by the gay population. The actual material situation of the person with AIDS (PWA) who is a gay male and the intravenous drug user may not be that different. Fifty percent of PWAs in New York City have no home to go to upon release from the hospital. It is, however, unclear whether this kind of economic destitution accompanies the PWA through the course of many episodes of acute illness that marks the profile of AIDS, whether it preceded the disease, or whether it is the *coup de grâce* of a health care system unable to respond to the housing needs of those severely incapacitated. Nonetheless, at least initially, the needs of those who are ill and also drug-addicted look quite different from those who are ill and stigmatized for their sexual preference.

This section deals in the most detail with the different ways in which HIV has affected Americans who are poor. Drug use, particularly intravenous drug use, unlike male-to-male sex, is usually accompanied by economic need, either as a cause of addiction or as a result. Hence, case studies of the newly affected bring into relief a group of people with different needs and resources than those represented by earlier patterns of transmission. The distinctions are somewhat academic, however. When we are describing intravenous drug use this does not rule out any particular kind of sexual activity and when we concentrate on homosexual transmission we are not ruling out economically deprived men. But as a general sociological rule of the epidemic—that we concentrate on *where* infection emerges and look at the medical and social resources of those people— those who do intravenous drugs and share needles, as well as their sexual partners, have a different economic context than the bulk of those whose *only* social categorization is that they engage in male-to-male sexual intimacy.

What we see in the material in this section is the degree to which people already vulnerable economically are doubly jeopardized by the virus. Increasingly the people most affected are black and Hispanic. "AIDS in Blackface" by Harlon Dalton, professor of law at Yale University and member of the President's Commission on AIDS, directly addresses this difficult issue. Dalton outlines the ways in which the epidemic, which has fostered the development of a large network of "AIDS advocates," has been resisted by the black community and gives an argument for why this is so. He tries to explain not only the hesitancy of the black community to take on the epidemic as an explicit political issue, but how and in what ways intervention by white public health officials strikes a dissonant chord in a population so long neglected by the system of health care in America. Dalton asks the reader to concentrate upon some features of African-American life that make the black community hesitant to get involved in a public health campaign orchestrated by mainstream health officials and one where the African-American bears the brunt of drug addiction and the early designation as a "vector" of the HIV virus—a hesitancy that is as tragic as it is understandable.

More than any other section, "The Social Context of HIV Infection" tries to give the true contours of the epidemic. As Dalton points out, the issue of HIV is entangled with the issue of drug addiction in the black and Hispanic communities. Rarely, however, do investigators document the extent to which the intravenous-drug-use community is affected by the epidemic. Dr. Ernest Drucker, director of the Division of Community Health in the Department of Social Medicine at Montefiore Hospital ("Drug Users with AIDS in the City of New York: A Study of Dependent Children, Housing, and Drug Addiction Treatment"), documents the types and extent of need among the more than 100,000 intravenous drug users currently thought to be HIV-antibody-positive in New York City. Dr. Drucker includes in his report the minimal extent to which the current health care system can respond to the needs of those who are sick. He also makes it quite clear that without drug rehabilitation programs, what resources there are are practically useless. One fascinating part of Dr. Drucker's survey is a kind of frontline report from those people who advocate for AIDS patients in the health care imbroglio of New York City—the social workers who themselves work within structures that are essentially worn out.

One of the consequences of HIV coupled with intravenous drug use for the majority of those affected is relative or absolute homelessness. For those who are treated without proper social service resources, released without drug treatment, and stigmatized by drug use *and* AIDS, an intact life is difficult to maintain. In "Housing, Homelessness, and the Impact of HIV Disease," the Citizens Commission on AIDS addresses this truly monstrous aspect of the epidemic, and it does so by disclosing the downside of a crumbling urban health care system. AIDS, if one is affected and yet is able to retain one's job, one's private insurance, and one's home, is devastating. AIDS to the person not perched securely above the risks of unemployment and medical indigence is a slippery slope. There is a very quick descent from a marginal and stressful existence as, perhaps, an underpaid and uneducated worker, or an unemployed intravenous drug user, or single mother on public assistance, to homelessness and destitution.[1] We have no places in hospitals or residential facilities for the destitute sick. More often than not, they walk the streets or reside precariously (the technical term for them) in unsanitary city shelters. In a city where the poor are the most at jeopardy for HIV infection and where on average they pay 78 percent of their earnings for housing, it is clear what happens when they get sick. In its report the Commission cites various studies of the number of homeless PWAs, citing figures that include those with marginal AIDS diagnosis [5,000] and those that include the HIV affected altogether [10,000].[2] Focusing from the institutional direction, these figures outline a health catastrophe of mammoth proportions. The following figures are taken from New York State's Division of Adult Service's study of patients with HIV-related illness or AIDS in 20 New York City hospitals: "Just over 50 percent of these patients had *no* home to which they could return. Of that 50 percent, 36 percent had been undomiciled prior to admission; 48 percent had houses or apartments but couldn't return for reasons such as eviction, failure to pay rent, increased clinical needs, or the exhaustion or rejection of essential support persons."

The Citizens Commission on AIDS report ends, importantly, with a list of specific needs that must be addressed by all urban cities immediately. The specter of 10,000–20,000 homeless PWAs in New York City or double and triple that by 1991 is a specter of a country bereft of civic virtue.

Special focus on the impact of HIV infection upon women and children is necessitated not only by their relative invisibility in the "numbers" describing the HIV-affected but by the urgency due to two factors only recently emphasized: Women and children are the fastest-growing groups of new cases; the impact on women and children is, perhaps, greater than upon men (if one can state degrees of tragic suffering) given the number of physical, mental, familial, and social factors that form the context of women's lives.

Although the first U.S. case of AIDS in a woman was reported in 1981, the epidemic's history has fostered a false perception of AIDS as a disease of men. In "Women—The Missing Persons in the AIDS Epidemic," physicians Kathryn Anatos and Carola Marte describe how HIV-related infections often manifest themselves differently in women than in men, and as a result, the women with these infections are not considered to have AIDS. Because symptoms in both men and women are interpreted, investigated, and treated differently, underdiagnosis becomes a significant bias in epidemiological data on women with AIDS and these "missing women" often do not get the treatment they need. But they are disregarded from another perspective. The fact that women have children provides a complication that, as Anastos and Marte point out, often predominates in the medical profession's response to their HIV infection. It also complicates the legal rights they have since the prospect of HIV infection in a fetus brings up reproductive decision issues. (Some treatment of these issues is offered in the Introduction to Section Five.)

The Citizens Commission report, "The Special Needs of Women, Children, and Adolescents," highlights the complicated social issues surrounding women with AIDS. Most women affected by the HIV virus are mothers. Most women are at an economic and social disadvantage in comparison to men, and most women have responsibility not only for their own health but that of their families, often including an HIV-affected male partner and equally as often between 1 and 3 children, 1 or more of whom may be HIV-antibody-positive. Because women with HIV-related illnesses are most often *already* caretakers of others with HIV-related illnesses, their partners and their children make it almost impossible for them to focus upon their own health. The prospect of their children ending in foster care accompanies their illness. According to the National Women's Health Network quoted in the study, there are between 32,000 and 45,000 infected women in New York City. If 80 percent of them develop an HIV-related illness, 26,000 to 36,000 will die. If each of these women on average have at least two children, 52,000 to 72,000 children will be orphaned, since in many or most cases the father has died, is absent, or is unable to take the children. This description does not include the numbers of HIV-antibody-positive infants born to mothers who are HIV-antibody-positive or sick with an HIV-related illness. The issue of "boarder babies" is wrenching, and the Commission has many recommendations to deal with the growing numbers of these children, as well as the over 10 percent of adolescents now thought to be HIV-antibody positive in New York City.

NOTES

1. As indicated earlier, one does not have to begin one's HIV illness with economic marginality. But one most probably ends there. The Gay Men's Health Crisis, serving over 3,000 clients each year, reports that 90 percent of their clients use their financial advocacy division, which helps with private and public entitlement procurement.

2. According to a recent report from the Coalition for the Homeless in New York City, there are currently 10,000 AIDS-diagnosed homeless individuals, with 15–20,000 HIV-infected altogether. (Virginia Schubert, Coalition for the Homeless, "AIDS and Homelessness," [Paper presented at the VI International AIDS Conference, San Francisco, June 1990].)

The Plague Years

Larry Kramer

TONIGHT, THE PRESIDENT OF all the American people is finally going to make his first real AIDS speech.

He will address a fund-raising dinner of the American Foundation for AIDS Research. He will speak on the eve of the Third International Conference on AIDS, which is expected to draw 6,000 attendees to Washington, twice last year's attendance in Paris.

He will tell us that AIDS is awful and that it's his administration's number one health priority, hollow assertions that have been voiced by somebody or other in his administration since 1983. He may talk about his new advisory commission on AIDS, about "education" and about testing.

But what will really count is how long and how seriously Ronald Reagan addresses the issues of research and treatment—the launching of an all-out federal war to find a cure for this plague. Even if he mentions these subjects, it is perfectly clear to me that no matter what Reagan says tonight, it's not going to alter the sorry journal of these plague years.

As a Reagan AIDS bureaucrat told me recently: "God help us with the AIDS epidemic, because the U.S. government won't. Washington, D.C., is not interested in AIDS." The aide spoke in a very low voice—obviously ill at ease. "Why are you so nervous talking about AIDS?" I asked him.

Larry Kramer, "The Plague Years," *Newsday*, May 31, 1987. Reprinted by Permission of St. Martin's Press.

"Are you kidding?" he replied. "If you don't say what they want you to say, you get reassigned to the Indian reservations."

Choose your favorite horror movie:

The World Health Organization estimates a total of 100 million will test positive for Human Immunodeficiency Virus (the presumed cause of AIDS) in five to 10 years. Estimates vary on how many of the infected will succumb to AIDS, but there's increasing evidence that almost all infected people will fall ill, and the great majority will die.

The federal Department of Health and Human Services says that in three years our annual health care bill for AIDS alone will be $16 billion. In a one-year span, full-blown AIDS cases attributed to heterosexuals who aren't intravenous drug users rose from 1 percent of all AIDS cases to 4 percent.

The numbers of AIDS patients hospitalized increased from 10,000 in 1984 to 23,000 in 1985. Fifty percent of all acute-care hospital beds could be AIDS-occupied in 4 years, according to Rodger McFarlane, the head of Professional AIDS Education at the Memorial Sloan-Kettering Cancer Center in Manhattan

Says Dr. Mathilde Krim, co-chair of the American Foundation for AIDS Research: "Everything about this epidemic has been utterly predictable, utterly, utterly and completely predictable, from the very beginning, from the very first day. But no one would listen. There are many people who knew exactly what was happening, what would happen and has happened, but no one of importance would listen. They still won't listen. This is an epidemic that could have been contained. We definitely could have contained it."

But now the AIDS epidemic is 7 years old, has killed 20,798 in the United States alone, is spreading uncontrollably throughout the population—heterosexual as well as homosexual—and will soon bankrupt the American health care system.

And now Ronald Reagan is finally making a speech about AIDS.

Will he finally explode the myth that most Americans need not fear AIDS?

"A virus does not discriminate. A virus does not know the difference between black and white or straight and gay or male and female," McFarlane tells each and every class. "Why doesn't anyone believe that," even now?

One answer is offered by a congressional aide who deals with health issues: "Never has such a bunch of second-rate people been put in charge of such a first-rate problem."

One of those in charge is Gary Bauer, 41, a former undersecretary of education, who is now assistant to the President for domestic policy and head of the Office of Policy Development. He has been in his White House office a scant few months and is credited with helping Reagan put on the new makeup that's going to be worn tonight.

Recently, I asked Bauer if there had been a conscious decision to ignore AIDS. "I've never heard anyone," he answered, "or even seen anybody wink, or even with body language, suggest that—look, if a lot of people die, hey, you know.... Now maybe when I'm not around, they let their true emotions hang out ..."

I begged Bauer to ask Reagan to consider his place in history, to institute some noble action before it was too late. Bauer's answer was: "I have not seen enough evidence that this is the Black Plague ... I think only time will tell ..."

Why isn't there a forceful, clear-headed administrator in charge of combatting AIDS—of coordinating research into its causes and developing a vaccination against it, and a cure for it, and of educating the public?

"Our belief is that the President is that already, the AIDS-czar," is Bauer's answer.

The boss of the several contending government agencies that deal with AIDS is Dr. Otis R. Bowen, the Health and Human Services secretary. His flock includes HHS, the Food and Drug Administration, the National Institutes of Health, and the Centers for Disease Control.

It's the CDC that charts the numbers. The CDC's leaps to conclusions about who is vulnerable to AIDS delayed an attack on AIDS for years. Since the syndrome (it was not yet named AIDS) was first seen in 1980 and first described in the CDC's Morbidity and Mortality Weekly Report on June 5, 1981, the CDC has been the source of continually changing dicta about who is at risk. (First, it was gays and Haitians. Now, it's everybody.)

I asked Bauer why Reagan hadn't met with Surgeon General C. Everett Koop, the administration figure who is most outspoken about AIDS.

Bauer replied: "I saw a story where Koop was quoted as saying he had not been able to meet with the President. Let me tell you this: Dr. Koop would not normally meet with the President ... The fact that Dr. Koop has not met with the President is really not significant, although it's become some sort of symbol of something, I'm not sure what." Koop is a born-again Christian. His insistence that AIDS be dealt with as a medical, not a moral, problem, has made him a pariah not only at the White House, but also to his former brethren in Christ who now boycott dinners in his honor.

Reagan has admitted that he hasn't read the forceful AIDS report that he asked Koop to prepare for him and that was published last October, just ahead of the equally discouraging report of the National Academy of Sciences.

It is Bowen who talks to the President about the state of the nation's health. Bowen declined to be interviewed for this essay.

Jim Gottlieb, staff director to Rep. Ted Weiss (D-N.Y.), said of Bowen: "I can't recall anything substantial he has said on AIDS."

The congressional aide I spoke with said Bowen's pet interest is catastrophic health insurance, which would be available only to those over 65 or those disabled for more than two years—qualifications AIDS patients don't live long enough to meet. "A messenger can go to the (presidential) well only so often," the aide said. "Bowen has chosen not to carry AIDS."

The next highest-ranking federal health official is Dr. Robert Windom, the assistant secretary of health. Windom, in office less than a year, had never before worked in Washington, or in government, or directed a large bureaucracy. A successful Sarasota, Florida, internist in private practice, Windom was chairman of the Reagan-Bush 1984 reelection committee in Florida, Georgia, and Alabama. Federal records show that Windom gave about $55,000 to Republican candidates between 1979 and 1984.

Bowen has handed Windom the AIDS crisis. Earlier this month, I asked Windom why more drugs weren't being tested. "We have a task force for that." was his answer. I asked why appropriated AIDS treatment money wasn't being spent. He answered, "We have a committee for that." I asked him about the most talked-about AIDS treatment, AL 712. "I'm not familiar with the details on that," he replied.

Such responses may be why a leading AIDS lobbyist called Windom "just plain dumb." A congressional aide says, "If his IQ were any lower, you'd have to water him." One of his coworkers did describe him as a "warm, affable, back-slapping fellow." Then his colleague sighed, "But he's out of his league."

Next "in command" of AIDS is Dr. Lowell Harmison, who is Windom's deputy assistant secretary for health and who also declined to be interviewed. One of Harmison's own colleagues explained Harmison's inaction on AIDS thusly: "Lowell's philosophical framework is more 'how do we keep the bastards from getting us' instead of 'how can we maximize our influence.' "

It took the CDC six years to admit that it was dealing with an equal-opportunity virus. It has taken the FDA the same amount of time to accomplish something positive.

AIDS drugs are to be given "fast-track" attention when it comes to authorizing their use, FDA chief Frank Young announced this month. (It usually takes six to nine years for a drug to be approved.)

Criticizing the FDA speedup, Dr. Jerome Groopman of Boston's New England Deaconess Hospital said, "They'll destroy the entire clinical investigatory process."

S. Jay Plager, counselor to the undersecretary of Health and Human Services, explained a new FDA rule that he said would allow "desperately ill patients" the chance to decide by themselves "whether they would take an experimental drug or die of the disease untreated."

Huge drug companies such as Burroughs Wellcome (the owners of the antiviral drug AZT) seem to have an advantage at the FDA. Small, undercapitalized, or inexperienced companies that might be in the possession of potentially first-rate treatments may not get first-rate treatment from the FDA.

An example is Praxis Pharmaceuticals of Los Angeles. Praxis has the world license to produce AL 721, which was developed by the prestigious Weizmann Institute in Israel. It has taken two years for the FDA to take notice of AL 721, which is derived from egg yolks and could just as easily be distributed without FDA approval as a health food.

There's obviously more potential profit for Praxis in waiting to please the FDA; the price of AZT has gone from $8,000 to $14,000 per patient per year in less than four months since FDA approval. Before approval, Burroughs Wellcome had to give the stuff away.

Patients are now so tired of waiting for AL 721 (it's been two years since a favorable mention in the *New England Journal of Medicine*—and supplies in Israel have been mysteriously cut off) that they've had it analyzed, have passed around the recipe from coast to coast, and now whip it up in their own kitchens. A New York group has ordered $200,000 worth of a Japanese knockoff (one kilo, good for about a month, cost $200), and it's now being consumed. Dr. Craig Metroka of St. Luke's-Roosevelt Hospital Center has advised some of his patients to get it wherever they can: NIH trials of AL 721 are at least six months away.

Patients are also learning to duplicate or obtain other drugs that haven't received FDA approval. They include DTC, a French drug, Foscarnet from Sweden and ribavirin, on sale legally in over 20 countries, including Mexico.

There are plenty of other reasons for patients to go drug-shopping: The few drugs that the NIH and FDA have elected to test have either been busts, like Surinam, or, like AZT, have toxic side effects for many.

(Bauer, by the way, didn't seem well-acquainted with AZT—which he mistakenly calls "ACT," although it has received more media attention than all the other drugs combined.)

It's no wonder that patients have more faith in their own underground information network than in any establishment sources. There is still no official central computerized registry of AIDS information. A doctor in Santa Barbara, California, recently lost a patient to cytomegalovirus, one of the many opportunistic infections that afflict AIDS sufferers, according to Dr. Nathanial Pier, an AIDS specialist. The California doctor could have learned to treat CMV by calling a doctor in New York.

The NIH is currently everybody's least favorite place. *Newsday, The New York Times,* and *The Wall Street Journal* have questioned why some $47 million appropriated a year ago for the testing of AIDS drugs has actually remained unspent, and why 19 AIDS Treatment Evaluation Units, established with great hoopla almost two years ago, are either not functioning or are greatly underutilized.

For example, most of the 150 beds at the Institute for Immunological Disorders in Houston, this country's first hospital devoted solely to AIDS, are empty because none of the $47 million has trickled down to Texas. (Additionally, Texas is the only state in the Union that does not reimburse hospitals for taking care of indigent patients. Administrators of the profit-making Houston institute say it's too costly to hospitalize uninsured AIDS patients.)

"The honeymoon with the NIH is over," is how Representative Weiss put it, as his office prepares to instigate congressional oversight hearings on NIH-delays.

The NIH may be in charge of medical research in this country but it was none too eager to embrace AIDS. One of the first evidences of the deadly syndrome were unusual cancers in otherwise healthy young men. For this reason, the AIDS question was first tossed to Dr. Vincent T. Devita, director of the National Cancer Institute at NIH. (Neither Devita nor his boss, Dr. James Wyngaarden, who is lord of the 12 institutes of the NIH, had time to speak to me.)

In 1981, Devita was in the possession of almost a billion dollars of research money; nevertheless, he decided that the as-yet unnamed AIDS, which includes such cancers as Kaposi's sarcoma and various lymphomas, really belonged to the National Institute of Allergy and Infectious Diseases (NIAID), which had one-quarter the budget of the cancer institute. NIAID's director then, Richard Krause, didn't want AIDS either, but Allergies didn't have as much power as Cancer.

Today, major and painful rivalries between the cancer institute and NIAID and inside both institutes are hampering the AIDS fight. Two figures at the cancer institute, Dr. Robert Gallo and Dr. Samuel Broder, have certainly found new meanings in competitiveness. According to one pharmacologist involved, Broder attempted to disparage Gallo's championing of AL 721 (in that *New England Journal* report) mainly because Broder, who's in charge of developing new treatments, hadn't noticed it first. This gave rise to the NIH being condemned by the pharmaceutical community for rarely championing anything "Not Invented Here."

It's also said that Broder and Dr. Anthony Fauci aren't on such hot terms either. Fauci is director of NIAID and chief administrator of the 19 AIDS Treatment Evaluation Units and of AIDS research and testing for the entire country, and no major decision can be made without him. He is being asked to do more than any human is capable of doing, with predictably human results.

He works 18-hour days; he must summon committees, preside over meetings, supervise the selection of drugs to test, monitor their results, deal with pharmaceutical companies, keep up on all the latest information (a new drug application can run to 100,000 pages of evidence), attend conferences all over the world, and put up with complaints from absolutely everyone.

Instead of screaming and yelling for help as loud as he can, he tries to make do, to negotiate quietly.

Only after intense questioning does Fauci quietly admit that he desperately needs "somebody to cut through all the government red tape." But he doesn't want a larger research staff.

"I've got no place to put them," he explained.

It is apparently *verboten* for a new lab to be built on the supremely manicured campus of NIH.

It should also be noted that the beds in Fauci's AIDS ward are, save two, empty. A whole floor in America's state-of-the-art hospital, $47 million given him to fund the testing of new treatments, and his beds are empty. Critics charge that Fauci is so in love with AZT, which he administers on an outpatient basis, that he is not interested in testing other drugs.

The battling over who's going to get the credit in the AIDS fight extends to the international arena. French scientists at the Pasteur Institute announced that they had isolated the AIDS virus and developed a test to detect it during 1983. A year later, NCI's Gallo claimed the same discovery as his own.

A recent British television documentary questioned the honesty of Gallo's assertions and research. The Granada TV documentary also said: "The effects of the row are far-reaching. Senior scientists are refusing to talk to one another. Laboratories fear to exchange samples without watertight legal guarantees. The search for a cure has inevitably been set back."

The bitter U.S.-French dispute over the AIDS virus discovery was resolved in March with an agreement to share the patients for the AIDS blood test. But the aftertaste lingers on the international scene, and few European scientists will attend this week's NIH-sponsored meetings.

Dr. Don Francis, a CDC scientist who was reassigned from the CDC headquarters in Atlanta after criticizing Gallo, told Granada TV that the fight "has truly inhibited the progress necessary to combat this really, really dangerous virus that's now all over the world. Now there are two camps that are divided and therefore make the field a relatively unpleasant one to get into—and that keeps some of the best scientists out."

"You have smart men out there," said Krim, of the American Foundation for AIDS Research, "who know certain things are not working at the NIH; but it's difficult to expect an investigator to bite the hand that feeds him—the NIH."

Outspoken AIDS doctors have a difficult time at institutions beyond NIH, too. Take the case of Dr. Michael Gottlieb, cochair of the American Foundation. Gottlieb, who has been working with AIDS since 1980, recently quit a full-time post at UCLA because, he said, he couldn't obtain tenure. The university claims he resigned before a tenure decision was reached.

The quality of NIH research and American research overall can be judged by the recognition that most AIDS breakthroughs have come from abroad: the discovery of the virus at the Pasteur Institute in Paris; the discovery of a second (West African) AIDS virus at the Pasteur Institute; the vaccine studies and experiments under way by Dr. Daniel Zagury at the University of Paris; the possible genetic predisposition toward AIDS susceptibility announced in London by Dr. Anthony Pinching; AL 721 from Israel; CSF, a new immune-stimulating drug, controlled by Sandoz, a Swiss company; and, indeed, AZT itself. Although American-discovered, it is now owned by Burroughs Wellcome, a British bunch.

Who is fighting all this American inertia?

Only two elected officials in Washington sounded the alarm early and have been courageous enough not to run away: Reps. Henry Waxman (D-Calif.) and Ted Weiss. They've been joined by Sen. Lowell Weicker (R-Conn.).

Sens. Daniel Patrick Moynihan and Alfonse M. D'Amato as elected representatives of the state most under siege by AIDS, New York, have betrayed their constituents by the banality of their response. Nor has the occupant of Gracie Mansion been a Profile in Courage. "It is disgraceful that the mayor of New York does not provide sufficient leadership on this issue," says Nathan Kolodner, president of Gay Men's Health Crisis.

Edward I. Koch was so roundly booed at the recent GMHC Walkathon (which raised $1.6 million to help defray costs of services the city should be providing, but isn't) that he ripped up his speech and sat glaring out at the audience, facing signs that proclaimed him "the Worst." "Would you trust this man?" one of the signs asked, under his picture.

The city recently announced that it has drafted, but not implemented, a 5-year plan to deal with AIDS by expanded care for those already afflicted, promotion of research and expansion of education programs and voluntary testing.

This sounds like the plan Koch announced 3 years ago that never happened.

Reagan will talk tonight about mandatory testing and "education," and there will be much yelling and screaming from opponents and supporters of both.

It is imperative that the American people realize that while all the heat and fury from the religious right and its equally vocal supporters on the political right continue about the naughtiness of condoms and sex education and homosexuality and intravenous drug use, the virus continues to spread and kill.

Every stalling tactic costs lives.

They know this. Anyone who watched the numbers of dead grow and grow knows this.

The record convinces me that no matter what Reagan says tonight, no substantial battle for a cure will be mounted while he is in office. There's only one word to describe his monumental disdain for the dead and dying: genocide.

AIDS in Blackface

Harlon L. Dalton

MY AMBITION IN THE pages that follow is to account for why we African-Americans have been reluctant to "own" the AIDS epidemic, to acknowledge the devastating toll it is taking on our communities,[1] and to take responsibility for altering its course. By the end, I hope to convince you that what may appear to the uninitiated to be a crazy, self-defeating refusal to stand up and be counted is in fact sane, sensible, and determinedly self-protective. The black community's impulse to distance itself from the epidemic is less a response to AIDS, the medical phenomenon, than a reaction to the myriad social issues that surround the disease and give it its meaning. More fundamentally, it is the predictable outgrowth of the problematic relationship between the black community and the larger society, a relationship characterized by domination and subordination, mutual fear and mutual disrespect, a sense of otherness, and a pervasive neglect that rarely feels benign.

If I am right, then there is a profound need to reorient the public health enterprise so that it can succeed in a multicultural society. Public health officials cannot simply wander uptown (or wherever the local black ghetto is situated), their expertise in one hand, their goodwill in the other, and expect to slay the disease dragon. They must first discern just who this particular public is and how it sees itself in relation to them. How does the black community see its

Harlon L. Dalton, "AIDS in Blackface," *Living with AIDS*, Part 2, *Daedalus*, Journal of the American Academy of Arts and Sciences, Summer 1989. Reprinted by Permission of *Daedalus*.

own health needs, and how do they stack up against its other concerns? And, not least, just what has been the black community's prior experience in dealing with government do-gooders?

Answering these questions is not an impossible task, even in the midst of an epidemic. Consider, for example, the extent to which the relationship between the white gay community[2] and the public health establishment changed in the mid-1980s. Much has been written about the latter's failure to intervene in a timely and sensitive way early on, when the AIDS epidemic might have been successfully contained.[3] I do not quarrel with the explanations usually proffered for this failure—the health establishment's inability to identify with or care about the gay men who were viewed as the disease's principal targets, bureaucratic ineptitude and infighting, and an administration in Washington mindlessly committed to reducing social spending no matter what. I do, however, want to highlight an additional factor, the fact that initially most public health officials approached AIDS as solely a biomedical phenomenon and exhibited little comprehension of the many ways in which culture, politics, and disease intersect. Thus they failed to realize how much freight would attach to their well-intentioned attempts to safeguard the public's health and did not anticipate that both the gay community and the larger society would react in ways reflective of the social distance between the two.

The moment of truth arrived shortly after the Food and Drug Administration approved the first HIV antibody test for the screening of the nation's blood supply. Many health officials advocated that the test be used diagnostically as well, to determine whether persons in so-called high-risk groups had been exposed to the virus. The officials were surprised to discover that most gay organizations and AIDS support organizations took the opposite view and strongly recommended that gay men, including those who had engaged in high-risk activity, *not* take the test.[4]

At first, the public health establishment saw this resistance as misguided, irresponsible, and self-destructive. In fairly short order, however (thanks largely to the efforts of "bridge" people who served, in effect, as bicultural interpreters), key officials began to see past the bare fact that their recommendations were being opposed, to the concerns underlying the gay community's opposition: that the test was not sufficiently accurate to be used for diagnostic purposes; that testing would produce needless mental anguish for many; that persons seeking the test might thereby open themselves to criminal liability by admitting to having engaged in sodomy or the use of illicit drugs; that testing would facilitate the quarantining of persons who tested positive; that absent strict confidentiality, testing would lead (at least for seropositives) to the loss of insurance, employment, and housing, and to social isolation and vilification as well. These concerns, the officials realized, were as much the lived reality of AIDS as helper-T cells and transmission routes.

It became apparent that to reach the gay community, public health officials had to learn to view the epidemic from the perspective of the gay community. Consequently, today even the most control-minded health officials take care to involve the gay community in decision-making and emphasize the need for a high degree of test accuracy, for strict confidentiality, and for enhanced laws against discrimination.[5] The moral of this story is plain. The public health establishment *can* take account of community differences if it has to. It *can* take account of the sociopolitical contexts in which it operates. It *can*, if pressed, recognize that its targets are, in an important sense, its teachers. My hope is that the failure of New York's needle-exchange program, together with other failures to reach the black community, will, like the white gay opposition to testing in the mid-1980s, provoke thoughtful reconsideration of how the public health enterprise should operate in a society deeply divided along racial lines.

I have arrived at the conclusions in this essay in much the same way a reporter, or perhaps a biographer, would. Rather than engage in rigorous empirical research, I have relied on my store of impressions formed over several years of communicating about AIDS with the black community and, more important, listening to concerns voiced outside that community. The comparison to reporting and biography is less than perfect inasmuch as I do not claim to be neutral. I do not pretend to be solely a channel for the experiences and expressions of others. On the contrary, as a member of the black community I have personally experienced most of the sentiments and dynamics about which I report, and like human beings in general, tend to view others' experience through the prism of my own. My hope is that the texture and depth of the result will more than offset any distortions.

My approach rests on two assumptions—that an African-American subculture exists (marked by shared sentiments, sensibilities, experiences, and history) and that I am sufficiently linked to it (by virtue of upbringing, kinship ties, and spirit) to be qualified to interpret it.

The first proposition is, I should think, relatively unproblematic so long as we remain near the subculture's core and resist the temptation to specify its precise contours. As for the second proposition, you are, I am afraid, going to have to trust me, at least provisionally. The true test of my entitlement to speak about (not for) the black community will be whether my words resonate for the majority of its members (and for the small set of others who know it well).

On occasion I will take the liberty of treating you, dear reader, as a stand-in for white America. That is to say, I will speak directly to *it* through *you*. My goal in so doing is not to artificially divide (though that is certainly a risk I take), but rather to speak in a way that captures the timbre as well as the pitch of the community sentiments I seek to convey.

The Impact of AIDS

Unquestionably, AIDS has hit the black community hard. We are losing our sons and daughters at an alarming rate. Twenty-five percent of all persons with AIDS in the United States are African-American.[6] Among the newly diagnosed, the figure exceeds 36 percent.[7] In many eastern cities, blacks and Latinos constitute a majority of the AIDS cases.[8] In New York City, where AIDS is the number-one killer of women between the ages of twenty-five and thirty-four,[9] black women, with their Latina sisters, account for 84 percent of the adult female AIDS cases.[10] Nine out of ten children with AIDS in New York City are black or Latino.[11] In the Bronx one baby in forty-three is born infected.[12] Across the board, black people are disproportionately represented. Thus, even among gay and bisexual men and intravenous drug users, blacks are more likely to be infected than are their white counterparts.[13] On average, black persons with AIDS (PWAs) are sicker at time of diagnosis than white PWAs and die nearly five times as rapidly.[14]

Notwithstanding this bleak picture, public health officials and AIDS organizations around the country have been frustrated in their efforts to organize the black community to deal with AIDS.[15] While the vast majority of such people and organizations are predominantly white, even black and Latino officials and activists have run into more than their fair share of walls.[16] Resistance within the community ranges from the simple refusal to acknowledge that AIDS is a problem for black people (an increasingly difficult position to maintain in the face of the overwhelming numbers) to the rejection of programs designed to stem the transmission of HIV. In between these extremes, our leaders, however defined, seem to run away from the issue of AIDS. They talk about it as little as possible and even more rarely involve themselves in efforts to develop constructive solutions.[17]

Perhaps the most dramatic example of the black community's resistance to AIDS intervention involves New York City's pilot needle-exchange program. The goal of the program is to test whether addicts will, if given a chance, exchange used needles for clean ones, and if so, whether that step will appreciably lower the incidence of HIV infection in the addict population. Originally designed to operate in neighborhoods where drug abuse is prevalent, the program was located instead, thanks to pressure from black and Latino community leaders, in a downtown government office building, far away (geographically and otherwise) from its target population. This concession of city officials (a move that, in the view of most observers, severely compromised the program's prospects for success) did not, however, dampen community opposition. On the contrary, word of the program's grand opening "ignited," in the words of one reporter.[18]

Typical of the reaction was Harlem city council member Hilton B. Clark, who characterized the program as a "genocidal campaign."[19] A key opponent was New York's police commissioner, Benjamin Ward, who explained that as a black person, he had "a particular sensitivity to doctors conducting experiments, and they too frequently seem to be conducted against blacks." One month after needle exchange began, the New York City Council, led by its black and Hispanic caucus, urged the health commissioner to cancel the program. In commenting on the nonbinding resolution, which passed on a vote of 31–0, caucus chair Enoch Williams explained that "the city is sending the wrong message when it distributes free needles to drug addicts while we are trying to convince our children to say no to drugs."[20]

City officials were not the only ones to join the chorus. For example, the Reverend Reginald Williams of the Addicts Rehabilitation Center in East Harlem promised that "there will never be a needle-exchange program here. I think the communities and neighborhoods would rise up in opposition. They tell me this is what we must try. . . . Why must we again be the guinea pigs in this genocidal mentality?"[21] To the surprise of many, the needle-exchange program was even opposed by the likes of Dr. Beny J. Primm, a highly respected leader in the field of substance abuse and a belated addition to former President Reagan's AIDS Commission. Primm took issue with the claim that needle exchange would lower the incidence of HIV transmission and, as an alternative, pushed for a more rational system of assigning addicts to available treatment program openings.[22] There were, of course, some blacks and Latinos who lined up in favor of the program, most notably the Brooklyn-based Association for Drug Abuse Prevention and Treatment (ADAPT), led by Yolanda Serrano.[23] For the most part, however, the community response was exceedingly negative.

The Reluctance to "Own" AIDS

Already, a set of stock explanations for this reluctance has emerged. We are told that for too long the media have inaccurately portrayed AIDS as a disease that almost exclusively afflicts white gay men,[24] that for too long public health officials have failed to use media appropriate to the black community,[25] and that the black church has stood in the way of effective AIDS education because of its opposition on moral grounds to homosexuality and drug use.[26] While valid to a point, these explanations have, in my opinion, been very much overblown. First, the mass media are scarcely the only avenues of communication in the black community (a point made by some of the same people who seek to pin the misrepresentation tail on the media).[27] Moreover, we have long since learned to view the media with suspicion and to discount their distortions when our own experiences contradict them. Second, even though the public health establishment has relied on media not well suited to reaching the black population (too many pamphlets and not enough radio spots, for example), by and large health officials have used the same media that arguably have succeeded at presenting a distorted picture of who has AIDS.

As for the third stock explanation, it does a disservice, in my view, to the black church. It is, of course, true that much of the church is doctrinally fundamentalist and socially conservative. These characteristics, however, are constraints not so much on what can be done in the realm of social action as on how to do it. In practice, the church has proved adaptable, pragmatic, and even crafty when need be. To paraphrase former President Nixon, if you want to understand the black church, watch what it does, not what it says. Time and again, the church has demonstrated its awareness of the variability of human existence and the fragility of the soul under siege. Time and again, the church has been responsive to the needs, spiritual and nonspiritual, of the community. The civil rights movement of the 1950s and 1960s is simply the most dramatic example in recent memory.

What else, then, accounts for the black community's reluctance to grapple with AIDS? I have isolated five overlapping factors that I think explain a great deal. The first is that many African-Americans are reluctant to acknowledge our association with AIDS so long as the larger society seems bent on blaming us as a race for its origin and initial spread. Second, the deep-seated suspicion and mistrust many of us feel whenever whites express a sudden interest in our well-being hampers our progress in dealing with AIDS. Third, the pathology of our own homophobia hobbles us. Fourth, the uniquely problematic relationship we as a community have to the phenomenon of drug abuse complicates our dealings with AIDS. And fifth, many in the black community have difficulty transcending the deep resentment we feel at being dictated to once again.

Blame

Early on in the AIDS epidemic, and continuing for some time, scientists, the press, and the public seemed curiously fixated on the origins of the virus associated with AIDS. From the perspective of the black community, interest in HIV's possible African roots seemed insatiable. Article after article appeared, recirculating identical hypotheses. The discovery of a similar virus in the African green monkey stirred the pot and prompted endless speculation about how it might have traveled from an "animal reservoir" into the human species. When pressed to explain why so much time and energy were being devoted to so marginal a concern, white people usually responded that determining where the virus originated might lead to the discovery of ways to slow it down or eliminate it altogether. Perhaps. Black folks, however, offer a different explanation. We understood in our bones that with origin comes blame. The singling out of Haitians as a so-called risk group simply confirmed our worst fears.

Although the society's fixation with the origin of AIDS has faded and Haitians are no longer officially viewed as synonymous with AIDS, for us the memory dies hard. Our exasperation and sometimes rage lingers just below the surface. Were I to go out tomorrow and speak about AIDS to a black audience anywhere in this country, I guarantee you that once the discussion gets going, someone would ask about the disease's origins. The question "Is it true that it started in Africa?" would quickly become "Why do they keep trying to pin it on Africa?" "Why do they keep trying to pin it on us?" and eventually I would be asked the clincher: "What are they trying to say we *did* with that monkey?"

More than insult and affront are at issue here. So long as we African-Americans continue to worry that any hint of connection with AIDS will be turned against us, we will remain leery of accepting responsibility for its impact on our community.

Suspicion and Mistrust

It is difficult to overemphasize the extent to which the black community, qua community, reflexively responds with suspicion and mistrust to what are perceived as "white" initiatives. Just as Jews admonish each other to "never forget," we do not wish to forget the bitter lessons we have been taught since being brought to these shores. Slavery, a subject one does not bring up in polite company, exists within our extended memory; my father used to sit around the dinner table with his grandmother, a former slave. Segregation was upon us only yesterday. Today we must deal with Ed Koch, David Duke, and political campaigns that showcase people like Willie Horton. Push just a little bit and you will tap into wellsprings of mistrust even in those of us who live much of our lives within the ambit of the larger society and negotiate it with apparent ease (though not without cost).

Frequently, our acute mistrust manifests itself as resistance, as sparring, as buying time until we are sure we are safe. The early "negotiations" with the black community regarding AIDS seem largely to have followed this pattern. Given enough time, we can together work our way out of the pattern by building up trust, but time is at a premium where AIDS is concerned. A second way out is for black people to reconceptualize AIDS as not something white America is insisting we deal with but rather as a set of issues we ourselves want to take on. In other words, in order to "own" AIDS even in part, we may need to own it outright.

Homophobia

A third reason the black community has been slow in responding to AIDS is that many of us do not want to be associated with what is widely perceived as a gay disease. More than once I have heard of black parents readily volunteering, so as to forestall even more embarrassing speculation, that their HIV-infected children are addicts. Homophobia is not, of course, unique to the black community, but it takes on a particular character within the context of African-American history and culture. Precious little has been written on the subject. Straight black authors tend to ignore the subject altogether. A notable exception is Bell Hooks, who deftly captures the complexity of black attitudes toward homosexuality and the imperfect connection between those attitudes and actual behavior.[28] Gay black writers seem to find it easier to train their fire on racism within the white gay community than on homophobia within the straight black community.[29] Recently a small but hardy band of academics has begun extensive research on the life experiences of black gay men and lesbians.[30] In time, this work will provide a rich base from which a fuller picture of the character and consequences of black homophobia can be drawn.

If we in the black community are to make progress coping with AIDS, we must deal simultaneously with our homophobia. As a first step, we must name the problem, map its contours, and develop an understanding of how it is detrimental to us as a community. I will not attempt to advance this enterprise very far here, in part because I am not sure that this essay is the best vehicle for doing so. I feel obliged, however, having flagged the issue, to at least say a bit more.

First, let me distinguish between homophobia that is directed at whites and homophobia that is internal to the black community. As we seek to understand the former, it will be difficult, I suspect, to disentangle it from an animus based on race. That is to say, gay whites who encounter hostility from blacks may be the target of antigay sentiment, antiwhite sentiment, or both. Even the originators of the hostility may not know where one motivation ends and the other begins. Moreover, racial prejudice and homophobia may well activate or reinforce each other. It stands to reason that someone who is viewed as an "other" along one dimension will more easily be viewed as an "other" along a second and third. Internal homophobia does not suffer this complication, but it scarcely lacks complexity. Like most aspects of the African-American subculture, its roots are dual. The black community has doubtless been influenced by the larger society's attitudes toward sexual minorities even as its historical experience has produced a distinctive set of attitudes and practices. I would like to focus briefly on the latter.

In the manner in which homosexuality is spoken about, the black community differs markedly from the larger society. In our denunciation of homosexuality and of persons thought to be gay, blacks (including closeted gays) tend to be much more open and pointed than whites.[31] Our verbal attacks seem tinged with cruelty and are usually delivered with an offhandedness that many white observers find unnerving. At the same time, there is, within the black community, an enormous gulf between talk and action, or for that matter, between talk and belief.[32] What we say and what we think, or do, need not be congruent. In fact, a cruel tongue is often used to hide a tender heart. Bell Hooks tells of a "straight black male in a California community who acknowledged that though he often made jokes poking fun at gays or expressing contempt as a means of bonding in group settings, in his private life he was a central support person for a gay sister." "Such contradictory behavior," she adds, "seems pervasive in black communities."[33]

On reflection, none of this is surprising. We, as a people, are given to verbal excesses, to hyperbole, to putdowns meant for sport rather than wounding. People of my generation and older grew up "playing the dozens," verbal horseplay that involved the most scandalous imaginable accusations about the families and acquaintances of the other participants. So long as you stayed within certain well-understood (albeit unwritten and unspoken) bounds of propriety, you could say vicious things without anybody thinking you really meant it. A similar dynamic attends verbal gay bashing. There is a common understanding of which nasty things are acceptable to say, and as long as one stays within the canon, one can claim an absence of malice.[34]

There is, however, a key difference. In the dozens, the participants stand on equal footing; typically they alternate between the role of the slanderer and the role of the slanderized. In addition, there is no necessary relationship between the calumnies heaped on an individual and those heaped on her or his real-life position. In fact, one of the unwritten rules is that you tread lightly around areas of true vulnerability.

In practice, black communities across the country have knowingly and sometimes fully embraced their gay members. But the price has been high. In exchange for inclusion, gay men and lesbians have agreed to remain under wraps, to downplay, if not hide, their sexual orientation, to provide their families and friends with "deniability." So long as they do not put the community to the test, they are welcome. It is all right if everybody knows as long as nobody tells.[35] That is more easily accomplished than you might imagine. For the most part, even the pillars of the black community are content to let its gay members be, and to live alongside them in mutual complicity. This is true even within the church. Indeed, it is a well-kept secret, or more precisely, it is well-denied knowledge, that gays are disproportionately represented within the ministry, including (and perhaps especially) the ministry of many of the more fundamental denominations.[36]

This complex relationship works most successfully when gay men and lesbians are willing to carry on appearances, to live, in effect, straight lives. Many gay black men seek the ultimate cover and become ostentatiously involved with women. One noteworthy consequence of this phenomenon is that their female sexual partners may unknowingly be exposed to an increased risk of HIV infection.[37]

What accounts for the way in which the black community has approached homosexuality—boisterous homophobic talk, tacit acceptance in practice, and a broad-based conspiracy of silence? I have a theory (and it is no more than that) that within the black community, internal homophobia has less to do with regulating sexual desire and affectional ties than with policing relations between the sexes. In this view, gay black men and lesbians are made to suffer because they are out of sync with a powerful cultural impulse to weaken black women and strengthen black men. They are, in a sense, caught in a sociocultural cross fire over which they have little control.

Among the many horrors of slavery is the havoc it wreaked on relations between black men and women. Slave couples were not allowed to form stable bonds, and those relationships that did develop were burdened in ways painful to recount. Men were torn away from their families, women were subjected to the slavemasters' bidding, and both were, on occasion, bred like animals. As a result, men were unable to provide for, much less protect, "their" women and women were unable to rely on their men. This emasculation of black men (when measured against traditional gender role expectations and concepts of male prerogative) boded ill for male-female relations in the postslavery era in the absence of a fundamental redefinition of gender. The near century of Jim Crow that followed—legalized discrimination backed up and surrounded by powerfully disintegrative social forces—simply added to the strain. Black people in general, and black men in particular, were "kept in their place," routinely excluded from places that would bring them honor and respect or that would allow them to serve as family providers. While women could usually find employment as domestics, black men frequently drifted and did not, could not, come close to pulling their own weight.

For me, this reality is best captured by something that happened on the old Art Linkletter show during the 1950s, I believe. The show included a segment entitled "Kids Say the Darnedest Things," in which Linkletter interviewed children about whatever was on their minds. Somehow the word spread that on this particular day Linkletter would have a black kid on the show, a rare occurrence. Like hundreds of thousands of other black folk, I eagerly tuned in and watched with fascination and horror as this little kid, who looked a lot like me, answered the question "What do you want to be when you grow up?" "I want to be a white man," he answered quickly and confidently. Linkletter gulped, paused, and then plunged ahead. "Why?" he asked. "Because," answered the kid, "my momma says that black men aren't worth shit!"

The network instantly broke for a commercial, and when the show returned, the little black kid had been whisked off the set, but no commercial break could stanch the psychic wound opened up in an entire community in that moment of childlike innocence. Black people talked about that show for months, amidst much handwringing and headshaking. Yet, despite the countless retellings and postmortems, the message implicit in the little boy's answer—that relations between black men and women had reached a parlous state—was never disputed.

What does this have to do with homophobia? My suspicion is that openly gay men and lesbians evoke hostility in part because they have come to symbolize the strong female and the weak male that slavery and Jim Crow produced. More than even the mother quoted on the Linkletter show, lesbians are seen as standing for the proposition that "black men aren't worth shit." More than even the "no account" men who figure prominently in the repertoire of female blues singers, gay men symbolize the abandonment of black women. Thus, in the black community homosexuality carries more baggage than in the larger society. To address it successfully, we may have to take on such larger issues as the social construction of gender and the nature of male-female relations.

Drug Abuse

A fourth impediment to our efforts to grapple with AIDS is the association of the disease with drug abuse. We as a community have a complex relationship with illicit drugs, a relationship that often paralyzes us. On the one hand, blacks are scared to even admit the dimensions of the problem for fear that we will all be treated as junkies and our culture viewed as pathological. On the other, we desperately want to find solutions. For us, drug abuse is a curse far worse than you can imagine. Addicts prey on our neighborhoods, sell drugs to our children, steal our possessions, and rob us of hope. We despise them. We despise them because they hurt us and because they *are* us. They are a constant reminder of how close we all are to the edge. And "they" are "us" literally as well as figuratively; they are our sons and daughters, our sisters and brothers. Can we possibly cast out the demons without casting out our own kin?

We know that white America cannot comprehend our dilemma. We know that you do not truly share our concerns. Your interest in drug abuse has always been episodic and shallow. During the 1960s, you focused briefly on the problem when you became convinced that most street crime and petty theft are drug related. Although some of you saw this opening as an opportunity to broaden the nation's commitment to drug prevention and treatment, most energy went into keeping white people from being victimized. Meanwhile, the plight of black victims "uptown" didn't even merit lip service. During the 1970s, drug abuse once again briefly took center stage as suburban high school students began to experiment and addicted GIs returned home from Viet Nam. Left in the shadows as usual was the civilian drug problem in our nation's inner cities.

Now, as the 1980s draw to a close, a combination of factors, including the rise of the social right, the highly visible fall of dozens of professional athletes, the intertwining of drug trafficking and foreign policy, the emergence of crack as the drug of choice among many communities, and, not least AIDS, has made drug abuse a hotter social issue than at any time in recent history. Yet for all the *Sturm und Drang*, the white community has shown little concern that day by day, drugs are eating away at the heart and soul of the black community. When school children were gunned down by a maniac in Stockton, California, you furiously debated the wisdom of allowing private citizens to purchase semiautomatic weapons; at the same time, you appeared oblivious to the fact that every day in the inner city *our* children are being gunned down by such armaments in the never-ending struggle over drug turf and profits.

And so we find ourselves paralyzed, caught up in our own conflicting emotions—guilt, anger, shame, horror, fear, sympathy, aversion, affinity—and your uncertain commitment. We know that to deal with AIDS we must deal with drugs. If only we knew how.

Neocolonialism

Although most of my 1960s rhetoric is safely stored away in my mental attic, I was forced to resurrect this trusty old friend, for try as I might, I couldn't come up with a post-postmodern phrase that captures the one-sided relationship now existing between the black community and the larger society, a relationship built on power and control. When we want help, white America is nowhere to be found. When, however, *you* decide that we need help, you are there in a flash, solution in hand. You then seek to impose that solution on us, without seeking our views, hearing our experiences, or taking account of our needs and desires. We tell you that we fear genocide, and you quarrel with our use of the term. Then you try to turn our concerns back on us. "Don't you know," you ask us in an arch tone of voice, "that while you are standing on ceremony, thousands of the very people you say you care about are dying from AIDS?" Struggling to ignore the insulting implication that we are either profoundly retarded or monumentally callous, we respond, "Don't *you* know that they are already dying from drug overdoses, Uzis and Ak-47s, joblessness, despair and societal indifference?" And, white America, you sigh and say, "What's one thing got to do with the other?" Then we sigh and wonder if you truly do not understand.

In the silence that follows, none of our real concerns gets voiced. Why can't *we* choose which of the many problems facing us to tackle first? Suppose we think that crack is more of a menace than AIDS? Are you willing to help us take on that one? Why do you want *us* to take all the risks? You say that making drug use safer (by giving away bleach or distributing clean needles) won't make it more attractive to our children or our neighbors' children? But what if you are wrong? What if as a result we have even more addicts to contend with? Will you be around to help us then, especially if the link between addiction and AIDS has been severed? Why do you offer addicts free needles but not free health care? Why do you show them how to clean their works but not how to clean up their lives? Why not provide immediate treatment for every addict who wants it? Why not provide us with job training so that our youth will have realistic alternatives to the street? Instead of asking us to accept on faith that we won't be abandoned and possibly worse off once you move on to a new issue, why not demonstrate your commitment by empowering us to carry on the struggle whether you are there or not?

Where To From Here?

Quite simply, we have to learn how to stop talking past each other. We have to figure out a way to communicate across the racial chasm. Our language is the same, but our frames of reference are so different. Admittedly, part of the blame for recent failures to connect rests with the black community. We have been so intent on trying to get your attention that we have occasionally forgotten why. We have been so busy expressing our fears that we have failed to express our hopes. We have been so focused on past fiascos that we have been unwilling to test whether this time we can work together. We have been afraid to say straight out what is on our minds. And too often when we speak, we do so cryptically, metaphorically, or in a code undecipherable by outsiders.

This concern brings me to the term *genocide*. Although I understand its appeal, I regret the use of the term in conversations about AIDS. My regret stems from the fact that *genocide* tends to be a conversation stopper, and I am desperately anxious for genuine conversation to begin. It is so hard to get past the term itself to the sentiments and experiences that animate its use. Yet those sentiments and experiences reveal a good deal about why efforts to organize the black community around AIDS have been disappointing, so let me take a run at it.

What do community leaders (and followers) mean when they accuse seemingly well-intentioned public health officials of engaging in genocide? Admittedly, the term is a useful club, the kind one uses to get a mule's attention. But that is not its sole function. After all, black folks use it meaningfully even when talking among ourselves. It speaks to us. It resonates. It is shorthand for a wide range of fears and expectations, all of which are backed up by shared experience.

In its strong form, the term *genocide* reflects the genuine suspicion of many that the AIDS virus was developed in a government laboratory for the express purpose of killing off the unwanted. This belief is helped along by HIV's curious affinity for those whom the larger society disdains. Lest you judge this a fringe concern, I must tell you that whenever I speak about AIDS to a grass-roots audience in a black neighborhood, at some point during the question-and-answer session someone invariably asks me whether I think AIDS was purposefully developed as a means of wiping out black people or, alternatively, whether black people are being used as guinea pigs to test this new form of biological warfare. Others in the room usually murmur their agreement with the statement within the question or wait expectantly for my answer.

Although I answer no, I understand full well where the question comes from and recognize that it must be heard against the backdrop of the larger society's historic disregard for the sanctity of black people's lives. We need not go back to slavery. There are examples aplenty within my lifetime, or that of my parents, of black people's lives being treated casually or worse. Take, for example, the infamous experiment at Tuskegee Institute in which the government purposefully exposed black men to syphilis so as to study the natural course of the disease. Although an effective treatment was developed mid-experiment, the men were never told about it and were never treated, lest the research be compromised.[38] Another well-documented example is the forced sterilization of women on welfare, many of whom were black or brown. In some states, the practice continued unabated into the 1970s.[39] The recent election of former Klansman David Duke to the Louisiana legislature suggests that this unlovely practice, a key element of his platform, has not altogether lost its appeal.[40] A third example, relatively recently come to light, is the FBI's attempt to pressure Dr. Martin Luther King, Jr., into committing suicide.[41] To these highly visible stories someone in every black audience can add dozens more, stories of people who found themselves the unwitting object of experimentation or the target of government persecution.

Two assumptions underlie the strong claim of genocide. The first is that the hostility of white America toward black America is so powerful, or the disregard so profound, that no depredation is unthinkable. This view is rooted in racial strife and feeds on the storehouse of sins visited upon blacks by whites. The second assumption is that under the right circumstances, the government is not above compromising the lives of innocent citizens. The grist for such a view is considerable. Time and again the government has demonstrated a willingness to jeopardize the lives of even its most favored in order to expand its knowledge or advance its policies. The purposeful exposure of American soldiers to radiation in the Nevada desert comes readily to mind.[42] For black people, the realization that even white skin does not protect one from being expendable is chilling indeed.

Less strongly, the term *genocide* reflects a widespread belief that the federal government willingly let AIDS spread as long as it was confined to populations that straight white America would rather do without. The grist for this view is provided by the government's own spokespersons, among others. At a press conference following her keynote address at the International Conference on AIDS held in Atlanta in 1985, then Health and Human Services secretary Margaret Heckler caused considerable consternation among people at society's margins when she implored: "We must conquer [AIDS] ... before it affects the heterosexual population and threatens the health of our general population."[43] Her parallel statement, that we must also conquer AIDS for the sake of "individuals in every country who fall within the risk categories"[44] was perceived as, at best, a sop. In similar fashion, when called on to explain on a nationally telecast interview show why President Reagan did not speak publicly about AIDS until late 1985, White House chief domestic policy adviser Gary Bauer responded that until then AIDS had not been a problem worth commenting on because "it hadn't spread into the general population yet."[45]

In its weakest form, *genocide* signifies a reckless indifference to, or deliberate disregard of, the black community's vital interests, or at a minimum the subordination of those interests to the distinct concerns of the larger society. Let me illustrate by once again turning to New York City's needle-exchange program. No one, I take it, would quarrel with the proposition that the black community has a legitimate interest in discouraging its young people from using illicit drugs. Yet that very same interest is directly threatened if the fears expressed by the program's many black critics are warranted, that is to say if providing clean needles to addicts creates a substantial risk that the number of young people willing to experiment with intravenous drugs will rise significantly. The fact that the city pressed forward with the program in the face of such concerns contributed to the charge of genocide.

In fairness, it cannot be said that New York City's health commissioner simply disregarded the issue of whether free needles would encourage addiction. Rather, after thoughtfully considering the issue, he concluded that the risk was minimal.[46] The rub is that most black critics of needle exchange rejected that conclusion.[47] Given this disagreement over a matter of fundamental importance to the black community, to proceed anyway looks a lot like indifference or disrespect.

My overriding goal in writing this essay has been to spur conversation about how a country as racially polarized as ours can hope to deal with a virulent disease that, as fate would have it, manifests itself differentially. It is in the pursuit of that goal that I have struggled to give content to a charge that usually produces more heat than light. I have no particular investment in the term *genocide*; I simply want to jumpstart the conversation that usually dies out whenever the word is deployed.

My vision is of a conversation that takes place both on the streets and in the academy, by design and by chance. My hope is for conversation characterized by mutual risk taking and mutual candor. In the spirit of candor, I must warn you that not all will be pleasant. For most Americans of African descent, our history, especially our trials and tribulations—slavery, discrimination, malign neglect—is a lived thing, something we experience and feel even when we do not know its particulars. We wear Jim Crow like our skin, with precious little choice in the matter. Because our history is ever with us, we can never consider the slate wiped clean. It is, for example, difficult for us to divorce our dealings with white persons as individuals from our dealings with whites who preceded them.

When you extend a hand in friendship, we can't help wondering whether you carry trouble in the other one. When you invite us to dinner, we can't help wondering why. If your manner of speech reflects considerable training and education, we wonder whether you are putting us down. If, instead, you speak in the vernacular, we wonder if you are being condescending. No matter how pure your motives, we will question why you are in our midst. No matter how deep your commitment, we will wonder what you are getting out of it.

My point, then, is that even as I invite you to bridge the chasm, I know it won't be easy. While we insist that you respectfully come calling, we aren't quite ready to put out the welcome mat. When you predictably bridle at our lack of hospitality, we will peer into your soul to determine whether you are simply one more white person who can't stand to see black folks asserting themselves. But even if we decide that your pique is justified (in the sense that you truly have embraced our concerns and are anxious to work with us), we will expect you to be sympathetic to our predicament while we argue that you cannot expect us to be sympathetic to yours.

Perhaps that is a lot to ask. But we as a nation must play the hand that slavery has dealt us. We cannot undo history, except through long, hard struggle. Meanwhile, we must learn to live with AIDS here and now, in the present that we find so bewildering.

In so doing, we must recognize that the face of AIDS is rapidly changing, from mostly white to predominantly black and brown. The implications of this shift for public health policy and practice are profound; we have just begun to explore them. But this much is clear already. As the drama unfolds, we cannot simply ask white actors to put on blackface and favor us with their best rendition of "life in de ghetto." We must increasingly turn to black actors, and to black directors and producers as well, if we are to really capture the social meaning of the darkening epidemic. Nor can we treat as bothersome background noise black America's complex attitudes toward white America, and vice versa. Only by acknowledging such disconcerting realities do we have a prayer of a chance of escaping their constraining force.

NOTES

1. Throughout, I use the term *black community* to refer both to geographic areas in which African-Americans are concentrated and to a subculture with which African-Americans may be originally linked no matter where they reside. I trust that it will be evident from the context which of the two meanings (if not both) I intend.

2. Unless the context suggests otherwise, I use the terms *gay community* and *white gay community* interchangeably to refer to the community of interests and support formed by gay men and lesbians who identify as such. I characterize the gay community as white because of its historical unwillingness to embrace fully its sisters and brothers of color. See, for example, Thom Beame, "Racism from a Black Perspective," in Michael J. Smith, ed., *Black Men/White Men: A Gay Anthology* (San Francisco: Gay Sunshine Press, 1983).

3. Perhaps the best known and most comprehensive account of this early history is in Randy Shilts's *And the Band Played On* (New York: St. Martin's Press, 1987).

4. Ibid., 540–43.

5. See, for example, Franklyn N. Judson and Thomas M. Vernon, Jr., "The Impact of AIDS on State and Local Health Departments: Issues and a Few Answers," *American Journal of Public Health* 78 (4) (1988):387–93.

6. Centers for Disease Control, *HIV/AIDS Surveillance Report* (Atlanta: Centers for Disease Control, March 1989).

7. Ibid.

8. See, for example, AIDS Surveillance Unit, *AIDS Surveillance Update* (New York: New York City Department of Health, 29 March 1989); AIDS Section, *Surveillance Report: AIDS in Connecticut* (Hartford, Conn.: State of Connecticut Department of Health Services, 31 December 1988).

9. René Sabatier, *Blaming Others: Prejudice, Race and Worldwide AIDS* (Washington, London, Paris: The Panos Institute, 1988), 8.

10. AIDS Surveillance Unit.

11. Ibid.

12. B. Lambert, "Study Finds Antibodies for AIDS in 1 in 61 Babies in New York City," *New York Times*, 13 January 1988.

13. S. R. Friedman et al., "The AIDS Epidemic among Blacks and Hispanics," *Milbank Quarterly* 65 (suppl. 2) (1987): 477–80.

14. Sabatier, 19; V. M. Mays and S. D. Cochran, "Acquired Immunodeficiency Syndrome and Black Americans: Special Psychosocial Issues," *Public Health Reports* 102 (2) (1987):228; and Friedman et al., 476.

15. See generally Veneita Porter, "Minorities and HIV Infection," *New England Journal of Public Policy* 4 (1) (1988): 371. For an account of public health officials' efforts to overcome racial barriers in educating Detroit's black community about AIDS, see generally L. S. Williams, "AIDS Risk Reduction: A Community Health Education Intervention for Minority High Risk Group Members," *Health Education Quarterly* 13 (4) (1986): 407–21; see also J. Kosterlitz, "'Us,' 'Them' and AIDS," *National Journal* 20 (27) (1988):1742; and J. L. Peterson and G. Marin, "Issues in the Prevention of AIDS among Black and Hispanic Men," *American Psychologist* 43 (11) (1988):872–73.

16. Sabatier, 134–37; E. Hammonds, "Race, Sex, AIDS: The Construction of 'Other,'" *Radical America* 20 (6) (1987):35–36.

17. Friedman et al., 490–93; and Hammonds, 31–34.

18. Michel Marriott, "Needle Exchange Angers Many Minorities," *New York Times*, 7 November 1988.

19. Ibid.

20. "Council Calls for End to Free-Needles Plan," *New York Times*, 7 December 1988.

21. Marriott.

22. Ibid.

23. Ibid.

24. Sabatier, 134–35; Friedman et al., 491. Note that this argument assumes either that black gay men do not exist or that they do not have sex with white gay men. For a multidimensional refutation of both assumptions, see Michael J. Smith. For an analysis of the silence of the white (and black) media on the racial dimension of AIDS, see Hammonds.

25. Peterson and Marin, 872–73; Williams, 413; and Hammonds, 34–35.

26. Kosterlitz, 1742; Mays, 227; Hammonds, 35–36; and Friedman et al., 491.

27. See, for example, Friedman et al., 487; see also Peterson and Marin, 872–73.

28. Bell Hooks, "Homophobia in Black Communities," *Zeta* 1 (3) (March 1988):35–38.

29. Notable exceptions include Leonard Patterson, "At Ebenezer Baptist Church," and James S. Tinney, "Struggles of a Black Pentecostal," both in Michael J. Smith.

30. These include psychologists Susan D. Cochran of California State University-Northridge, Vickie M. Mays, and Letitia Anne Peplau of UCLA, and Julius M. Johnson. See C. Craig and G. Harris, "Black Lesbians and Gays: Empirically Speaking," *Black/Out: The Magazine of the National Coalition for Black Lesbians and Gays* 2 (1) 1988:9.

31. My experiences in this regard parallel those described by Bell Hooks (see note 28).

32. Ibid.

33. Ibid.

34. To be sure, the words may still wound, particularly if one's "acceptance" of the terms of cruel discourse is coerced by circumstance, in particular by the felt need to remain closeted. For an interesting refutation of the old adage that "sticks and stones may break my bones, but names can never hurt me," see Richard Delgado, "Words that Wound: A Tort Action for Racial Insults, Epithets, and Name Calling," *Harv. C.R.-C.L.L. Rev.* 17 (1982): 133.

35. For moving accounts of this phenomenon, see Patterson, and Tinney (in note 29).

36. Ibid.

37. The risk that a black woman will be infected by a bisexual man is 4.6 times as great as for a white woman. Richard M. Selik, Kenneth G. Castro, and Marguerite Pappaioanou, "Racial/Ethnic Differences in the Risk of AIDS in the United States," *American Journal of Public Health* 78 (12) (1988):1540. To be sure, the principal means by which women in this country contract HIV is through sharing intravenous needles and "works." A distant second transmission route is sexual contact with straight male sex partners who themselves become infected via needles. Far back in third place is sexual contact with non-drug-using bisexual males. Institute of Medicine, *Confronting AIDS: Update 1988* (Washington, D.C.: National Academy Press, 1988); and William L. Heyward and James W. Curran, "The Epidemic of AIDS in the U.S.," *Scientific American* 259 (4) (1988):79.

38. J. Jones, *Bad Blood: The Tuskegee Syphilis Experiment* (New York: Free Press, 1981); A. M. Brandt, "Racism and Research: The Case of the Tuskegee Syphilis Study," *Hastings Center Report* 8 (21) (December 1978).

39. See general Note, "Coerced Sterilization Under Federally Funded Family Planning Programs," *New England Law Review* 11 (1976):589–614.

40. P. Reynolds, "Ex-Klan Leader Riding White Fear Toward Louisiana Legislature," *Boston Globe*, 5 February 1989.

41. David J. Garrow, *The FBI and Martin Luther King, Jr.: From "Solo" to Memphis* (New York: W. W. Norton, 1981).

42. Howard L. Rosenberg, *Atomic Soldiers: American Victims of Nuclear Experiments* (Boston: Beacon Press, 1980).

43. Quoted in Sandra Panem, *The AIDS Bureaucracy* (Cambridge: Harvard University Press, 1988).

44. Ibid.

45. Grover, "AIDS Keywords," *October* 43 (1987):17.

46. Bruce Lambert, "Study Supports New York's Needle Plan," *New York Times*, 6 June 1988. See also Bruce Lambert, "Ethics and Needles," *New York Times*, 13 August 1988.

47. A notable exception is Dr. Beny Primm, who sidesteps the issue by focusing on a different question: whether the data from other countries reliably establish that the provision of clean needles reduces the incidence of HIV infection. See M. Marriott, "Needle Exchange Angers Many Minorities," *New York Times*, 7 November 1988.

Drug Users with AIDS in the City of New York: A Study of Dependent Children, Housing, and Drug Addiction Treatment

Ernest Drucker, Ph.D.

Project Overview

The initial experience of New York-area hospitals treating AIDS patients with histories of intravenous drug use makes it apparent that this group has substantial needs that extend far beyond the provision of acute medical care for AIDS itself. The presence of dependent children, the poor quality (or absence) of housing, and the character of untreated addiction all generate needs that are not easily met through hospital-based care programs. As New York's hospitals try to prepare to meet the needs of large numbers of these patients, they face an unusual challenge. The case-management model for AIDS, devised in San Francisco for the care of a different population, is mandated in the New York State AIDS Center guidelines and forms the framework for service provision in all designated AIDS programs. But for those areas with a high proportion of IV-drug-using AIDS patients, this model must address needs which differ dramatically from those of the San Francisco patient population. Consequently a revision of the model may be in order. This project attempts to specify and evaluate the baseline level of needs

Ernest Drucker, Ph.D., Principal Investigator, Montefiore Medical Center, "Drug Users with AIDS in the City of New York: A Study of Dependent Children, Housing, and Drug Addiction Treatment" ("Overview," "Principal Findings" and "Interviews"), July 1988, pp. 2–4, 11–26, 40–56. Reprinted by Permission of the Author.

of 174 IV-drug-using AIDS patients during the initial phase of operation of designated AIDS Centers in 5 New York City hospitals. By specifying these areas in some detail it is hoped that this study will set a process in motion for responding more quickly to these needs by the development and evaluation of new program initiatives and capabilities.

Areas Investigated

We studied needs related to three factors: dependent children, housing, and drug addiction treatment. In every instance our intent was to establish the patient's status with respect to each factor just prior to the onset of AIDS.

Dependent Children

Over 50 percent of IV drug users are involved in some kind of steady relationship,[1, 2] and the majority have children.[2] In this regard, the family constellations and parental responsibilities of the IV-drug-using AIDS patients are distinctly different from those of the male homosexual population for which the current case-management model was designed. We evaluated several variables pertinent to the maintenance of parental households and the provision for the care of dependent children, including the presence of partners, age of children, and current custody arrangements for their children.

Housing

The high prevalence of homelessness, shelter residency, and precarious housing arrangements among New York City residents requires little additional documentation, yet drug users often have even more unstable housing situations with frequent turnover, doubling up, and recurrent episodes of homelessness and shelter use.[3] Even those with more stable lives may tip over into homelessness after an episode of severe illness. Further, stigmatizing conditions such as AIDS can make it virtually impossible to find replacement housing near the network of friends and family who might provide the social support necessary between periods of hospitalization. These factors place great pressure on hospitals by delaying discharge when it would otherwise be appropriate. This element of the study tried to determine housing status and characteristics prior to the first hospitalization leading to the diagnosis of AIDS and evaluated the suitability of the housing arrangement for discharge of the patient following acute episodes.

Addiction Treatment

Finally, there is the usually long-standing problem of the patient's addictive disorder itself, and its related social, psychological and physical features. In this group, diagnosis with AIDS is superimposed on an already existing and major secondary diagnosis, i.e., addiction or chronic drug use. In New York City there are inadequate and incomplete services currently available for addiction treatment—even without the added problems imposed by the diagnosis of AIDS. While it is estimated that there are over 200,000 addicted individuals in New York City,[4] only 35,000 are currently enrolled in drug treatment programs.[5] There is a severe shortage of drug detoxification beds and few outpatient detoxification services available.[6] Thus, a drug-using AIDS patient entering the hospital for the first time with an opportunistic infection may be discharged after a few weeks with that infection under control but may still be actively shooting drugs or practicing unprotected sexual intercourse, thereby exposing others. Yet he or she will not be enrolled in any ongoing drug treatment program. In the case of those using IV heroin, with or without other drugs, methadone treatment may be suitable, but such programs are currently operating beyond their capacity and cannot assure ready access for new patients. For that large group of younger users of drugs who are not principally intravenous heroin users (e.g., cocaine users), methadone treatment has little relevance to their care. Far more ambitious treatment services are required, e.g., day programs, residential care, intensive group therapy, and peer support, but these are not readily available for the drug user with or without AIDS. In this study we sought evidence of current enrollment in drug treatment programs and specification of the type of treatment.

Principal Findings

Dependent Children

Over half of the patients had children under 18 years of age: 67 percent of the women (32/48) and 46 percent of the men (58/126). The number of children, younger than 18, born to these patients averaged 2 per patient with children (184/90) or 1.1 if calculated for all patients. The patient-fathers, 59 percent of whom were *older* than 34, had dependent children with a median age of 11, the patient-mothers, 59 percent *younger* than 34, had younger children, median age 8. The dependence of the children's age upon the sex of the patient is clear (Table 2). Two-thirds of the children of patient-mothers were under 10, while the pattern is reversed among children of patient-fathers—56 percent over 10 years old.

Table 1:
Patients with Children Younger than 18

Sex of patient	Patients with children under 18	All patients
Female	32 (67%)	48 (100%)
Male	58 (46%)	126 (100%)
Total	90 (52%)	174 (100%)

Table 2:
Number of Children by Age

Sex of patient	Child's age in years				All ages
	0–5	6–10	11–15	16–17	
Female	17 (27%)	25 (40%)	11 (18%)	9 (15%)	62 (100%)
Male	21 (17%)	32 (26%)	44 (36%)	25 (20%)	122 (100%)
Total	38 (21%)	57 (31%)	55 (30%)	34 (18%)	184 (100%)

One in six of all of the patients in this study, and a third of those who are patients (28/90), had custody* of at least one child under 18 at the time of their admission for AIDS (Table 3). This reflects the child care arrangements prior to hospitalization. The picture, however, varies dramatically by the sex of the patient. Patient-mothers were more likely to have custody of their children: 56 percent (18/32) were caring for at least one child. By contrast, only 17 percent (10/58) of the fathers had one or more of their children living with them when hospitalized.

*The term *custody* is used here to indicate with whom dependent children were living. Children were listed as in the custody of the patient if living in the same household, even if in the apartment of someone else, the patient's mother for example.

Table 3:
Patient-Parents with Custody of Dependent Children

Sex of Patient	Patients with Children under 18	Patients with Custody
Female	32 (100%)	18 (56%)
Male	58 (100%)	10 (17%)
Total	90 (100%)	28 (32%)

Children of these patients were largely in the care of family members, 92 percent living with the patient or a relative, when the patient was first hospitalized. Relatively few (2 percent) were in foster care, and these only where the mother was the patient (Table 4).

Table 4:
Number of Children in Family's Care

| Sex of patient | Number of children living with | | | Custody known | All children |
	Family[1]	Nonrelative[2]	Foster care		
Mother	51 (86%)	4 (7%)	4 (7%)	59 (100%)	62
Father	103 (93%)	8 (7%)	0	111 (100%)	122
Total	154 (91%)	12 (7%)	4 (2%)	170 (100%)	184

NOTES: 1. Family includes patient and/or partner living in the same household, other parent in separate household, mother of patient (not living in the same household with patient) or other relative.
2. Does not include foster care, tabulated separately, regardless of family relationship.

The corresponding disposition of the children shows that a third of all children with known living arrangements (52/170) were in the custody of the patient and/or their current partner at the time of hospitalization, i.e., they were living in the same household as the patient (Table 5).

Table 5:
Children in the Care of Family Members

| Sex of patient | Number of children living with | | | | Children with known custody |
	Patient or partner[1]	Other parent[2]	Mother of patient[2]	Other relative[2]	
Female	30 (51%)	1 (2%)	9 (15%)	11 (19%)	59 (100%)
Male	22 (30%)	68 (61%)	8 (7%)	5 (5%)	111 (100%)
Total	52 (31%)	69 (41%)	17 (10%)	16 (9%)	170 (100%)

NOTES: 1. Patient and/or partner living in the same household.
2. Not living with patient in the same household.

Table 6 shows the range of household and family members caring for the patient's children prior to the disruptive impact of AIDS. Again women were most frequently caring for their children within their own households (60 percent); in the case of male patients, their children's mother was most often the caretaker (65 percent).

Table 6:
Households Caring for Patient's Children

| Sex of patient | Family members with at least one child | | | | Families with known custody |
	Patient or partner[1]	Other parent[2]	Mother of patient[2]	Other relative[2]	
Female	18 (60%)	1 (3%)	6 (20%)	5 (17%)	30 (100%)
Male	10 (18%)	37 (65%)	6 (11%)	4 (7%)	57 (100%)
Total	28 (32%)	38 (44%)	12 (14%)	9 (10%)	87 (100%)

NOTES: 1. Patients and/or partner living in the same household.
2. Not living with patient in the same household.

In the case of patient-mothers who did not have custody, the alternate custody arrangement of their children were evenly divided three ways: foster or institutional care (28 percent), the patient's own mother (31 percent), and other relatives (38 percent) (Table 7). Children of male patients were generally in the custody of their mother, who was living separately from the patient (either divorced or separated). These children living with a separated mother accounted for 76 percent of those not living with their patient-father, or 65 percent of all dependent children of male patients whose custody is known.

Table 7:
Care of Children Not in Custody of Patient

| Sex of patient | Number of children living with | | | | Children not living with patient |
	Other parent[1]	Mother of patient[1]	Other relative[1]	Non-relative[2]	
Female	1 (3%)	9 (31%)	11 (38%)	8 (28%)	29 (100%)
Male	68 (76%)	8 (9%)	5 (6%)	8 (9%)	89 (100%)
Total	69 (58%)	17 (14%)	16 (14%)	16 (14%)	118 (100%)

NOTES: 1. Not living with patient in the same household.
    2. Including foster care.

Younger children are more likely to be in the custody of their patient-parents: 37 percent (35/95) of those younger than 11, but only 19 percent (17/89) of those older than 10. A similar pattern exists where the grandmother (patient's mother) has custody: 13 percent (12/95) versus 6 percent (5/89). Overall, mothers with AIDS are three times as likely as fathers to have custody of their children (18/32 versus 10/58, Table 3).

Table 8:
Number of Children in Patient's Custody

| Sex of patient | Child's age in years | | | | All ages |
	0–5	6–10	11–15	16–17	
Female	9 (53%)	12 (48%)	7 (64%)	2 (22%)	30 (48%)
Male	9 (43%)	5 (16%)	6 (14%)	2 (8%)	22 (18%)
Total	18 (47%)	17 (30%)	13 (24%)	4 (12%)	52 (26%)

NOTE: Relative distribution is expressed as percent of all children in that age and parent sex group, see Table 6.

Housing

The extent of homelessness or precarious housing among this group prior to hospitalization is striking: 44 percent of men and 28 percent of women were inadequately housed (Table 9). The trend is most pronounced among men, of whom 20 percent were either in shelters or homeless. Only 60 percent of the study population were "securely housed" in their own apartment or private home (72 percent of the women, 56 percent of the men). Precarious housing is defined as those living in rooming houses, single room occupancy hotels (SRO), temporarily housed in welfare hotels, or doubling up with relatives. These are all circumstances which impede discharge.

Table 9:
Housing of Patients before Hospitalization

Housing status of patient	Number of patients		
	Females	Males	Both sexes
Homeless or insecure	13 (28%)	52 (44%)	65 (40%)
Homeless	4 (9%)	23 (20%)	27 (17%)
(In shelters)[1]	2 (4%)	4 (3%)	6 (4%)
(No shelter)[2]	2 (4%)	19 (16%)	21 (13%)
Insecure	9 (20%)	29 (25%)	38 (23%)
(Jail)	2 (4%)	11 (9%)	13 (8%)
(Institutions)[3]	2 (4%)	7 (6%)	9 (6%)
(SRO)[4]	5 (11%)	11 (9%)	16 (10%)
Secure housing	33 (72%)	65 (56%)	98 (60%)
(House)	3 (7%)	4 (3%)	7 (4%)
(Apartment)	30 (65%)	61 (52%)	91 (56%)
Housing Status known	46 (100%)	117 (100%)	163 (100%)
All PWAs	48	126	174

NOTES: 1. Municipal shelters.
2. Living in the street or other public space.
3. Drug treatment or other residences, and hospitals.
4. Single room occupancy hotels, boarding houses, emergency family housing.

This study also included a prison unit (at St. Clare's), as well as discharged prisoners at other institutions. A substantial number of these (11) are included and many of these are scheduled for early release due to their illness. These will, in turn, represent a serious disposition problem for the hospitals, as they often do not have a home to which they may return.

Drug Addiction Treatment

Only 29 percent of patients (51/174) were identified as being in a drug addiction treatment program at the time of admission (Tables 10 and 11). Women in our population were twice as likely to be enrolled in treatment as men (44 percent versus 24 percent). It seems likely that most of those whose drug addiction treatment status was unknown were in fact not in treatment since those in treatment could be expected to seek some sort of assistance, e.g., methadone.

Table 10:

Patients in Drug Addiction Treatment when Admitted

Sex of patient	In treatment	Not in treatment	Status known	All patients
Females	21	18	39	48
Males	30	62	92	126
Total	51	80	131	174

Table 11:

Percentage of Patients in Drug Addiction Treatment

Sex of patient	Patients in drug treatment		Patients with known status as percentage of all patients of same sex
	As percentage of patients with known drug status	As percentage of all patients	
Females	54%	44%	81%
Males	33%	24%	73%
Total	39%	29%	75%

Conclusions

This study was conducted to help service providers better appreciate the scope and characteristics of problems associated with the AIDS epidemic among drug users in New York City. These problems are by now all too familiar to those involved in the care of such patients. They include inadequate housing and virtually nonexistent residential care; insufficient and underskilled child support services; and a severe shortage of space in even the minimally effective addiction treatment programs currently available. By augmenting the wide awareness of these problems with concrete data which documents their full extent and details their nature, we hoped to accomplish several objectives:

- To arm advocates for the development and improvement of these services
- To assist social and health planners in specifying the types and quantity of services needed over the next few years
- To educate the public at large about important aspects of the AIDS epidemic that often remain invisible

The 174 patients in the 5 hospitals included in this study represent only about 1 percent of the AIDS cases seen in New York City so far. By its nature, this type of study is blind to the most important human experience of the epidemic—the pain and loss of the patients and their families and the dedication and immense labor of the caregivers. But it does provide data that can help both patients and caregivers construct a more humane and comprehensive response to a terrible epidemic.

Children

These findings reinforce previous observations and research findings indicating the extent of family and social disruption in those inner city communities with high rates of drug addiction—the same communities now being struck by the AIDS epidemic. This is most dramatically evident in the impact of AIDS on families with dependent children. On the average, each IV drug user with AIDS has 1 child under the age of 18. For women (the fastest growing group of AIDS patients in NYC) 2 or more children under 18 years of age are the norm and more than half of these are in the female patient's custody at the time she is diagnosed with AIDS. Hence, the impact of the illness and likely death of the patient before these children

grow up predetermines a substantial additional impact of the illness. This must be taken into account in our approach to AIDS in
NYC.

For people with AIDS who are also parents there is the additional
responsibility of making provision for the custody of their child
either for a time when they are no longer capable of providing that
care themselves or for after their death. Although in many cases
IV-drug-using AIDS patients have little if any family support for
themselves, relatives will often come forward and commit themselves to the care of the patient's dependent children. This situation
is not unusual, and finding a family member to take custody is seen
as a priority by AIDS patients and their families. In the case of these
families, alternate arrangements for child care must be made early
in order to assure coverage during the multiple periods of hospitalization and increasing disability when the patient is at home between hospitalizations.

Family members assuming custody receive little or no financial
or emotional support. If the appointed guardian is on public assistance, Aid to Families with Dependent Children (AFDC) funds can
be obtained and the child put on the budget, but only after providing extensive documentation concerning the dependent and their
relationship to the child. Foster care funds are usually not available
for guardians who are employed, and any request for assistance
initiates an intrusion into the life of the family by a system that is
often viewed as unfeeling, abrupt and untrustworthy. In these instances the children of AIDS patients are simply absorbed into their
new families without access to counselling regarding the illness or
death of their parent, or the changes it brings in their young lives.

The young age of these children (most below 10 years) suggests
that almost a decade of responsibility will have to be assumed for
each such child. The mothers of IV-drug-using women appear to be
the most likely candidates for assuming this role, and already do so
in 75 percent of the cases of patient-mothers. Means must be
developed to better support these caretakers in meeting this responsibility and new mechanisms developed for helping to finance
and otherwise assist such arrangements, since they provide an
invaluable dimension of family continuity and commitment—the
best assurance of decent care.

Finally, the child of an IV-drug-using AIDS patient must deal with
the double stigma of having a parent who is both a drug user and
has AIDS. As the parent becomes debilitated, the child confronts
uncertainty about the outcome of the parent's illness and where and
with whom he or she will live. Some of these children must also

cope with their parent's inability to communicate honestly about his or her circumstances thus increasing the degree of uncertainty experienced. In the aftermath of a parent's death, these children will often find themselves caught in custody battles, shunted from one family member to another while trying to come to terms with the loss of a parent and the image of the disease of which the parent died. They must also deal with their own fears of contracting the disease. For the child who is too young to fully comprehend the parent's illness and death, many of these issues will be postponed until the child is older, at which time they will surely surface as a locus of shame, guilt and confusion if not properly dealt with.

Even for male parents who are less likely to have custody of their offspring (a phenomenon that goes beyond drug addiction or AIDS), the impact of the illness and loss should not be minimized. First, since there are so many more male IV drug users (about 4:1 male to female) the lower likelihood of child custody for the male and his current partner (about 18 percent) still translates into a large number of children in their parent's custody who will be displaced or orphaned by the epidemic's impact. It is estimated that there are 200,000 IV drug users in NYC, half of whom are infected. It is likely, therefore, that over 100,000 children will lose at least one parent— and, in the case of 35,000 children, the parent with whom that child lives. Probably over 10,000 children in NYC will lose both parents to AIDS.

Housing

The extent of the housing problem for the poor of NYC, a group that contains most IV drug users, is evident. However, the conjunction of this pattern with drug addiction and AIDS creates a new and most devastating expression of its severity. Many AIDS patients are already homeless, living in shelters, or precariously housed at the onset of their illness—our study indicates 40 percent in this condition. The inevitable progression of HIV disease further degrades the housing status of those afflicted and thus large numbers of patients are difficult to discharge from the hospital at the end of their need for acute care. Even among those securely housed, discharge is often delayed due to inadequacies in home care. Regardless of their initial status, the AIDS patient finds him- or herself with sharply reduced housing options and a system totally unprepared to deal with the need for an appropriate place to live while sick with AIDS. Fully 25 percent of the IV-drug-using patients identified in this study cannot return or will not return to the housing from which they were admitted. Seventeen percent are completely undomiciled, i.e., homeless in the street or living in shelters or residences that expressly bar people diagnosed with AIDS or ARC. These constitute the "boarder adults" who occupy between 10 and 20 percent of acute-care hospital beds devoted to AIDS in New York City—often for long periods beyond their need for the level of care provided by the hospital. Frequently these patients remain there until they become sick once again and die. Eighteen percent of all AIDS hospitalizations in NYC end in death and, of these, approximately half were in the hospital only because they had no home to which to be discharged.

Male drug-using AIDS patients are most likely to be inadequately housed—fully 20 percent being homeless or in shelters at admission. We know that the disincentives to revealing one's AIDS diagnosis in the shelter system (or on the streets) leads to late admission and late diagnosis so this figure may not represent the condition of all male IV drug users without AIDS. However, the high rate of shelter residency (4 percent for both sexes), institutional residency (4 percent and 6 percent for females and males respectively), and single-room occupancy hotel (SRO) residency (11 percent for women, 9 percent for men) bespeak a large population on the edge of homelessness well before the ravages of AIDS have ever begun.

In the case of those with precarious arrangements at the time of admission, e.g., doubling up with a friend or relative, or living in isolated unsupportive conditions (SRO or hotel), the likelihood of being able to return after the first bout of PCP, toxoplasmosis, or CMV is slight. The weakened condition and consequent symptoms (e.g., weight loss, diarrhea) make it difficult to conceal one's status in what are often cruel and predatory environments. Even in a situation where friends and neighbors would be willing to help, the means to do so may extend beyond their capabilities. In the case of those with friends or relations willing to help out, the new dependency that AIDS signals will further compromise their capacity to sustain the supportive relationship.

Drug Addiction Treatment

At any given time fewer than 20 percent of the city's 200,000 IV drug users are in addiction treatment programs. While many transit through treatment programs (about 90,000 in methadone since 1969), only about 50 percent of those currently enrolled in treatment (fewer than 10 percent of the city's addicts) can be said to be stably engaged; that is, the dropout rate in methadone treatment is at least

20 percent in the first year and is believed to be higher in drug free therapeutic communities.

The finding of this study is that a somewhat higher proportion than average of IV-drug-using AIDS patients report enrollment in drug treatment at the time of admission—54 percent of the women and 33 percent of those men whose status was known to the social worker or recorded in the hospital record. If, however, we take all cases (including the 25 percent whose drug addiction treatment status was unknown) and factor these in, we get a lower figure: 44 percent of females and 24 percent of males. In New York City, women are more likely than men to be enrolled in drug treatment relative to their proportion in the total IV drug using population. While only 20 percent of IV drug users are women (and 20 percent of IV-drug-use-related AIDS cases are among women), these are overrepresented in methadone treatment, that is, in New York City about 30 percent of all methadone patients are women. Thus our finding of drug treatment enrollment is roughly consistent with drug treatment enrollment patterns citywide.

Most significantly, however, the vast majority (80 percent) of the AIDS patients surveyed in this study are not known to be enrolled in any drug treatment at the time of initial diagnosis with AIDS and their first hospital admission. This means that, in addition to the complexities of AIDS patient care, most of these patients must be found a drug treatment "slot" in order to make an effective discharge plan possible. In New York City, the drug treatment system is currently operating at 110 percent of capacity and no new methadone program has been opened in over a decade. Expansion of treatment slots by 3,000–4,000 is planned but can only take place by jamming more patients into already overcrowded facilities. Most recently even this planned expansion is jeopardized by state budget shortages.

Recommendations

Children

It appears that the AIDS epidemic in New York City may lead to the death of over 100,000 parents and orphan over 35,000 dependent children. Greatly expanded and skilled child care services will be needed during the course of the parent's illness and more permanent arrangements needed after the parent's death. In addition, children of these AIDS patients will require special consideration due to the multiple stigmas of a parent who has an addiction and who is sick or has died of AIDS. For these, the consequences of the parent's illness do not conclude with the parent's death. Counselling services appropriate to the ages of the children must be provided during the parent's illness and after the parent has died.

Housing

Over 40 percent of the drug-using AIDS patients are either homeless or precariously housed at the time of diagnosis and hospitalization. This will translate over the next five years into the need for housing thousands of such individuals for periods ranging from six months to several years. New York City currently has housing programs for fewer than 100 people with AIDS, and these must serve the gay population as well as IV drug users—the total need will probably exceed 30,000 in the next 5 years. For IV drug users a network of residential, intermediate care, and scattered-site housing must be made available and the design of these facilities and their programs must take cognizance of these patients' addictions and include drug treatment personnel in their staffing.

Drug Addiction Treatment

Addiction treatment upon demand has been identified as a broad need for slowing the spread of the epidemic among those IV drug users not yet sick with AIDS. At the very least, however, addiction treatment services must be made available to those already stricken. The appearance of an untreated drug user in an AIDS unit should assure referral and follow-up care through a local drug program. Every AIDS treatment center should have a network of associations for placement of such patients. Each AIDS unit in a hospital requires addiction specialists for counselling and referral, and medical care personnel must extend themselves to drug treatment programs to help cover the medical care needs of their patients. Finally, hospitals must devote more beds to detoxification—especially for cocaine users who represent the highest risk group for HIV infection among IV drug users.

Family Supports

The emergence of family support networks suggests an important avenue of intervention, namely the provision of support (financial and otherwise) to the patient's family members to enable them to help care for these AIDS patients and their children. This may take place in the household of the patient (if this exists) or in the household of the relative—most likely (in our study) to be the patients' mother. Models of adult foster care and paid family home care may be supplemented by other provisions of paid personnel (e.g., home care attendants) to relieve the family member periodically and by adult and child day care programs to also provide relief.

The family member, so engaged, should not have to fight welfare and Medicaid bureaucracies to help the sick family member. Rather, special assistance ought to be available in the form of additional liaison personnel in HRA and in training and peer support groups through the clinical AIDS care centers. Similar models have been employed for family members in cancer care and Alzheimer's disease.

Community-Based Care

The problems outlined in this report suggest that there must be serious consideration given to extending the locus of AIDS case management beyond the hospital. Community-based AIDS care models must be developed both to provide services and to create a framework for the recruitment, training, and employment of additional health care providers and assistants drawn from the very communities most heavily affected by the AIDS epidemic. Even if adequate funds were made available, it is grossly unrealistic to expect large infusions of human resources from outside these communities. Each area so stricken will have to find the people to help from within. The role of government and the health professions must be to facilitate and support this natural process.

Need for Further Study

This study merely scratches the surface of a set of issues and problems that are becoming increasingly apparent as the AIDS epidemic deepens and builds in intensity. Further study should therefore be focused on the most pressing and practical matters related to coping with AIDS in our local communities. These issues would include:

- Mechanisms that encourage and support the emergence of family and neighborhood support networks for the care of the sick
- Programs that enhance family and community resources for child care and counselling
- Decentralized housing and residential care programs staffed appropriately for IV drug users with AIDS

- Programs that recruit, educate and employ local people in AIDS care

Learning how to cope with the AIDS epidemic in New York City will be a painful and difficult task. It may, however, teach us much about ourselves and the communities in which we live— knowledge we will surely need even after AIDS has passed.

Appendix: Social Worker Interviews

These interviews were conducted during the course of the study in order to provide a fuller and more open-ended opportunity for the AIDS unit social workers to address the same set of issues covered in the survey questionnaire. Their observations closely parallel the principal findings and conclusions of the study itself and add an important dimension of personal experience and individual insight to the data presented in the body of this report.

Monnie Callan, C.S.W.
Department of Social Services
AIDS Treatment Unit
Montefiore Medical Center

Housing

"There was the burning of the Bronx in the seventies. This led to homelessness. The drug epidemic was already there, it started in the 1940s. Racism is also a factor. All these factors are the underlying building blocks of AIDS epidemics.

"All along, buildings in the city were milked. No building repairs were made. No plumbing repairs were made. Faucets were left to drip. There were no allocations for housing or repairs. 'People' became 'the homeless.' Our present circumstances are the product of 20 years of neglect.

"The people we see are predominantly black and Hispanic people whose extended families include members in Puerto Rico as well as New York.... All of them need support.... All of them are going through a crisis.... Whom do they tell?

"AIDS patients go in and out of the hospital very rapidly and therefore don't require the average social work, that is, the discharge of one patient and the picking up of the next.... These patients need help at home.... They're still sick when they leave the hospital and then they come back.... They need continuity of care. The social worker remains with the patient and the patient's family for the patient's life and beyond—with the family after the patient dies ...

"There are the homeless—no nursing home will take demented persons or PWAs. Generally, there is limited chronic care. There are long waiting lists ...

"HPD city-owned housing is particularly bad. No codes are followed. Things like heat and hot water are neglected or nonexistent.... And many patients are living in multiple-floor walkups. In these cases, the patient can't go out even with the help of an aide or a family member. Many patients wait in the hospital for lack of suitable home care ...

"And homes are terrible in general. Some patients' homes are comfortable but likely to be crowded. The patient or the patient's mother may sleep on the sofa and the children may sleep on the floor.... Even when they're sick!... And then there are problem behaviors such as the patient vomiting, things like that.... Things that are difficult for the grandmother to deal with. And difficult for the children to deal with. Clothes become drenched with sweat and that means increased laundry costs and more time spent by the grandmother doing the wash.... The patient is often sick at night which means the cost of utilities is increased....

"The patient loses weight and therefore clothing no longer fits. AZT produces gains! Frequent clothing changes are necessary because of vomiting. Many people need more clothing.

"There are other problems of cost. If the patient is in the hospital, SSI is reduced and Medicaid may even be cut off. This reopens family problems because the rent must still be paid. Welfare provides less than cost. If there is an AIDS diagnosis, there is a supplement but if the patient dies, the funding to the family is cut off ...

"Most help available to these people comes from volunteers. Aides cannot be sent to the home of a patient without family members present to supervise medication and work.... What do you do for a patient living in a fifth-floor walkup? What do you do if a patient is sick and at home and his wife works?

"The MAP office is supposed to coordinate things.... They're trying to be humane but the PWA must be clearly diagnosed and must require Medicaid to get help. The diagnosis is often shaky.... The doctor is often uncertain and the patient picks up on that.... Why don't we just grade HIV infection? Diagnosis is a serious barrier to help!

"And when the patient dies, the costs of burial are extreme. Public Assistance and SSI are available if the funeral costs less than $1,200. Most families want a better funeral than that but they get no financial aid. Families often make hasty decisions and end up in a mess.

"At the root of all this is the fabric of poverty and a lack of housing. These people are generally poor people. They are the result of the country's attitude toward the poor. IV drug users are the result of this attitude. We need to pay attention to the social causes of drug addiction.

Children

"Children are another problem. Who will care for them during their parent's illness and after? Their feelings and emotions are at risk. How can you conceal things from them? Playmates may find out about their parent's illness. Then they may exclude them.... Neighbors may do the same.

"There should be homemakers for children. Grandparents carry the load, particularly with the bereaved children. Usually there is an extended family but teenagers are often not assimilated.... Many are out there by themselves. For example, a grandmother came here from Puerto Rico to care for her child, who was a PWA. The child died, leaving teenage daughters. The grandmother couldn't get along with the teenage girls so she took the patient's body back to Puerto Rico for burial and left the girls here by themselves.... One got pregnant ... I lost contact with them ...

"Often family members become critical because the teenagers don't act as they should. After a parent dies, they still want to hang out ... see their friends.... They don't sit down all day with a sad expression. They're too full of life.

Staff

"The staff goes crazy with all this. They do what they can. A period of multiple deaths may lead to feelings of depression. Just trying to keep up with what needs to be done is impossible. The staff has an investment in these families. There aren't enough supports. We need HIV+ groups, family support groups, bereavement groups.... There is a need to cope with death and dying issues ... Child care.... We have to work with the family as a whole ... and then the amount of paperwork increases.... There is a pressure to get patients out of the hospital, but often there's inadequate support in the community."

Diane Pincus Strom, C.S.W.
Social Work Supervisor
Bronx Lebanon Hospital

Housing

"Housing is way up on the list of important issues. Because IV drug users have a paucity of social supports, they often don't have stable housing.... They're often living in abandoned buildings, shelters, a friend's room here, some space there ... some live with their mothers ... some of these people aren't completely without shelter but their housing is certainly precarious.

"The problem we have with housing is that there's no place to send people. Many hotels are inadequate places. And in many of these hotels, patients end up sharing bathrooms. Infections are present in the environment, jeopardizing others, too.

"According to city policy, a person with an AIDS diagnosis can't be returned to a shelter. A person with an ARC diagnosis can, a person who is HIV positive can, too. The only thing the policy of not sending people with AIDS to shelters does is prevent some very sick people from being in shelters. In some sense, we play with the AIDS diagnosis.... We know if we can document the diagnosis is AIDS, we'll succeed in keeping that person out of the shelters.... And that's often a good thing to do.

"If a patient has an AIDS diagnosis, MAP will provide housing but the person can spend months waiting. Poor housing in general contributes to these people's problems.

"Children are not being raised in places which indicate they are respected—places that are clean and healthy. These children are living in places where there are rats and roaches, and a lack of heat and hot water. These are things which affect children in very profound ways.

"Many of the men we see with AIDS grew up in that kind of environment. Consequently, we have patients upstairs here in the hospital who tell us this is the most wonderful place they've ever been. It's heartbreaking!

"I'd like to add, too, that something goes on in this treatment situation. A kind of behavior is modeled where the patients are made to feel that they have something important to say. Patients have the need to grieve when someone dies here. They see staff grieve, too. They then identify with that. In the hospital, people—drug-using people who come from backgrounds which lack respect, are learning to care for each other. A patient who hears someone call out for help goes to see what he can do.

"We've been finding out that even when patients have been isolated from their families for long periods of time, we have reconciled them with their mothers and fathers.... Many people go to their mothers, sometimes siblings take them in. Many of these family members find they have a feeling of competence, a feeling of being able to manage something well when they take care of their sick relatives.

"It seems to me that we are going to have to build institutions, chronic hospitals for the treatment of really sick people. It's true that the AIDS epidemic has produced an "us and them" mentality—a mindset which promotes taking a group "them" and putting them away. I'm hopeful that quarantine or encampment never becomes a reality in this country like it was during the Second World War for Japanese citizens. There are too many organizations like the Civil Liberties Union that are vigilant about people's civil liberties, and I think we can count on them for protection against that possibility.

"The 'us and them' attitude that we see in the population means that we don't want to integrate AIDS patients into society. But we need housing in Harlem. We need it here in the Bronx. The middle class needs housing, too. It's a big problem!

"So we're confronted with a situation in which just finding a place for well enough people is hard. We have to keep prevention in mind, and housing is a piece of that issue. There has to be a place for sick people and a place for well people with AIDS.

Children

"From what I can glean, a lot of the impact of the disease depends on whether the parent is male or female. If a person is a male IV drug user, he may not have been in a stable relationship with his wife and children for many years. In that case, the ramifications may not be as disastrous for the children. On the other hand, if the HIV-infected person is a woman, the consequences may well be a disaster for the children. If the AIDS person is male and hasn't been around, the situation is tragic. But if the person is a woman with children ... It's tragic and then some ...

"One mother who has AIDS was thrown out of her home, and dragged a 3-year-old around the streets with her. She's been in the hospital for 3 months now. The child is living with the patient's mother. The child's grandmother doesn't bring the child in to see her mother. It was certainly a terrible thing for that child to be living in the streets with her mother, but at least she knew her mother loved her and wanted her with her. Now, she doesn't see her mother. What will happen to that child?

"These women love their kids. It's not that they don't give a damn. That woman who dragged her kid around in the streets loved that kid! It may not be the kind of love we like to think we feel. It may be a bit narcissistic. But it's love nonetheless. It would be a mistake not to understand that.

"One of the roles of the social worker is to find a place for the children. But if you remember, if a grandmother has the children of an AIDS patient, and it was she, the grandmother, who was the very person responsible for the AIDS patient's personality in the first place—you know some people think drug use proceeds from a lack of something emotional—well, in that case, the same person who raised the drug-using person is raising those children.... These children, the children of IV-drug-using AIDS patients, aren't in vastly different circumstances from other children in the ghetto.

"And then we deal with the decision whether or not to test the children of AIDS patients. It's not always so simple. For example, we've been following one woman who is an IV-drug-using AIDS patient. Her husband died 3 weeks ago of AIDS.... He weighed 70 pounds.... She has an 8-year-old daughter living in Puerto Rico with her maternal grandmother and she has another child, a baby less than two years old. The baby looks ill; he has colds all the time, he's pale. She brought him in and he tested negative. But what does that tell us? He could convert.

"The dilemma is: Do we keep bringing him in and testing him? Or do we leave him and not test him? What we do here is monitor him until his medical situation is clear. The stigma is considerable. We don't want to burden these children more than they are already burdened.

"The whole issue of mandatory testing brings with it a very significant question: What are we going to do with the results? Why test if there is nothing we can do once we know what the HIV status of the child is?

"There are other issues, too. For example, a child's mother dies. But from what? Do we tell the child the truth? Do we lie? We try to bring the child in to see the mother so the woman can say good-bye, I love you, or whatever to her child. The social worker needs to help people to say I love you. Sometimes staff and the patient's family are against the child coming but we feel it's important. And I can tell you, this is the most painful thing I can think of.... To bring a child to say good-bye to a dying mother. I don't believe ever in telling a child a lie but you have to think about all of these things.

We need to stay in touch with the caretakers of these kids ... and we need to tell the children what's appropriate for them to know at the time . . . and stay in touch so that when they need more information we can give it to them.

Drug Treatment

"Well, first of all, there are such long waiting lists for programs. There's no place to send these people. I would, if it were up to me, create every conceivable kind of treatment: methadone, drug-free, whatever. In theory, distributing clean needles is a good idea but in the midst of getting high people don't always remember to get clean needles.... And then there are other aspects, too. One woman noticed that when she nodded out, her husband's other girlfriend used her needles. So I'm feeling kind of pessimistic about the needle campaign ...

"And there's another reality. How do you tell someone who's dealing with a second bout of PCP, who's depressed and feeling hopeless, don't go out and use drugs? There's the problem of what he's going to do when he's out there. Some people take care ... some die the way they've lived.

"If you make a commitment to help people who are involved in drugs, you have to recognize that these people are frequently borderline personalities, narcissistic personalities, very self-involved.... Why should AIDS change that? How could it? You have to deal with all that if you're going to work with these people.... Some people try to reclaim their lives ... others can't.

"It's important to recognize that the reason AIDS patients are not being taken in by their families frequently has to do with the patient's drug-related behavior prior to the diagnosis, not necessarily the fact they have AIDS. Often mothers are afraid the patient will be the target of retribution for past behavior if he or she comes home. Drug-related behavior is often the basic problem for the family, not AIDS.

Staff

"My staff is burning out. Not because patients are dying but because the state comes in and goes over and over and over our work. If one of my social workers is running a group and 15 people come, how can she go into 15 charts and document in depth the group process in addition to the rest of her work?

"Yes, the state request is legitimate. I understand there needs to be some kind of control if the state is providing funding and managing quality, but if the worker is covering 20 in-house patients, plus 30 outpatients, plus counselling families, and doing all the paperwork involved in all that work, how can we expect her to write 15 additional notes each time she runs a group? One of my workers recently said it very well: 'Maybe we should stop seeing patients and just make notes!'

"Dying of AIDS is different from dying of other diseases because there's a stigma and an exposure—your life is out there for everyone to see—that's not associated with other diseases like cancer or heart disease. If you die of cancer, people say poor thing.... If you die of AIDS, people say you got what you deserved. The sympathy level is different. There is no contagion issue attached to those diseases, transmission isn't a problem. But you've got to say that people who struggle with these things are at least working it through.

"Part of the case manager's job, the social worker's job is to help the person with AIDS do a life review ... to look at what can be fixed before it's too late.... It's hard for many people to do this, and it's hard for staff helping them, too.

"The kinds of things we do are very specific, too. For example, a man with AIDS who, faced with dying wants to have a child before he dies.... He wants to leave something behind, something that he made. That's a powerful feeling and it's also clearly a situation we have to deal with and counsel.

"When people ask me what I do for a living lately I say I'm a social worker in a hospital. Social workers who work with AIDS patients are stigmatized within the professional community, too. One social worker, not in our unit, said to me, 'I don't know how you do your job ... a job where you accomplish nothing.'

"In this job, you have to deal directly with people's angers. There's a lot of irritability in an AIDS staff. Obviously, the patients are angry ... and lately there's evidence that there are subtle neurological disturbances about which we weren't aware before. Everyone is in the same quandary in this unit. That mother who was dragging her 3-year-old around had a 1-year-old who died of AIDS a month or so ago.... My worker holds that woman when she sobs.... She sits on her bed and holds her."

George La Fountain, M.S.W.
Supervisor of Clinical Services/Social Work
St. Clare's Hospital

Housing

"One of the biggest problems is getting people out of the hospital. We brag about our psychosocial work, our phone counselling, our HIV testing clinic and the counselling we do in it, and our groups and all that, but when it comes right down to it, referral is the real job. We have to figure out where to send people, how to help them find a place to live when they leave the hospital.

"Often patients we have are homeless, they have no medical insurance, no financial resources. They may have had Medicaid back in New Jersey, or in Pennsylvania, but not here in New York where we're treating them ...

"I saw a guy today, he's got ARC, and he comes from New Jersey.... His wife died of AIDS.... He has no Medicaid.... Where do you start? What do we do first to help the guy?... We talked about Medicaid application ... he was put off by the lines and the waiting.... We talked about shelters ... he didn't want to go to a shelter.... We got in touch with the Neighborhood Coalition for the Homeless ... I don't know yet what we'll be able to do ... we'll see what happens ...

"Theoretically, we begin discharge planning as soon as we meet the patient and that's somewhere between 24 and 48 hours after admission. What happens, of course, is that, in spite of our efforts, we can't identify housing for AIDS patients and they stay a lot longer than they need to. Although we can't prove it, some of the infections they come down with are hospital contracted, infections they've picked up during their stay with us.... Once sick again, their stay is extended."

"The thing to remember about discharge is that the critical question is how ambulatory is the patient?... There are a lot of indigent people without benefits of any kind. Often we don't even ask if there are benefits, but we're lucky here at St. Clare's. The hospital doesn't require us to turn those people away. The answer to indigent people who come to us for care and have no benefits or resources doesn't have to be no, we won't take you ...

"So, we take them and then we scramble to find help for them. We, that is the social workers, do the initial work up and then we refer them to our resource coordinators. The resource coordinators get people Medicaid, SSI, try to get them into an AZT program ...

or other drug treatment. Of course, prisoners are a special case.... The application process has to start while the person is in prison ...

"Getting people out of the hospital when they're medically stable. That's the real problem. Getting them out and into some place that's comfortable, safe, and reasonably free from infection!

"We can't discharge AIDS patients to shelters. We don't discharge high-level ARC patients to shelters either.... The reason for that is as much for the person as for the others in the shelter ... the high level ARC patient is very susceptible to infection.... Frankly, the irony is that there're more options for AIDS patients than there are for someone who has ARC.

"Another chronic problem is taking care of the neurologically impaired patient, usually coupled with psychomotor problems. There's Coler Hospital ... and the waiting list. We used to get people into Coler, but not recently ...

"Then there's Bailey House.... But we haven't gotten anyone into Bailey House for six months ...

"And the Gift of Love. The Sisters are the Missionaries of Charity, based in Calcutta. They're the order that's willing to take care of AIDS patients. They work with the lepers abroad. They're not scared ... they have been wonderful. We do the intake for Gift of Love as well as sending patients there. The Sisters aren't selective, if someone's homeless and they have a place for him, they take him.

"We can't solve all the problems ... and the home needs are the most critical. There aren't any ad hoc agencies willing to get out there and do something. In the private sector, especially relative to residence, there aren't many efforts like the Gay Men's Health Crisis, vested in services, willing to get out there and do the work. Most of the groups are dealing with this epidemic and the housing problems as though it was business as usual. And the point is, it's not.... It might not be a bad idea if the city were to make available to willing groups facilities which could be renovated or fixed up for AIDS patients.

Drug Treatment

"As far as drug treatment is concerned, we need more detox beds. People are requesting detox more and more.... More beds would be a big help!

"It's rare that we get a patient into a drug treatment facility.... We try to work with receptive programs ... we try to work with people who are HIV-positive ... we sometimes turn to the therapeutic communities but there aren't very many we can rely on. Project

Return takes people readily without too much focus on HIV status. Others aren't as cooperative. They don't want to deal with HIV-positive people.

Prisoners

"St. Clare's was the first designated AIDS unit in the state. In 1985, there were 13 or 14 patients. At the present time, there are more than 60 patients and plans to increase the number of beds for AIDS patients but we're a little different from other AIDS units because we have a prison unit. It started as an 8 bed unit, went to 15 beds and will be 27 or so in the near future. Otherwise, when we have too many patients, we juggle people in the hospital.

"Awhile ago, Mother Teresa came and saw how we were treating these dying men and convinced the state that dying patients should be medically furloughed. After she pleaded their cases, some were medically furloughed to an open unit. Then they were kept here in a locked facility in this hospital.

"The prison authorities are cooperative when it comes to diagnosis and treatment when one of the AIDS inmates is in acute distress. Inmates are sent to infirmaries or private hospitals nearby. However, when the inmates need a high level of infectious disease treatment, then they're sent here to us.

"There are problems we deal with that are specific to the prison population. For example, a prisoner who's an AIDS patient here in St. Clare's might be discharged from jail while he's in the hospital. He might not have housing, and he might not have other entitlements. He has to have those things applied for before we discharge him. If he were being discharged directly from jail the parole people would do this work for him. But if he's discharged from jail while he's here, we have to do the work and that's a problem because all his important papers are up there in the jail. Of course, it would be easier for the parole officer to do that work. Sometimes it's hard to coordinate these efforts.

Staff

"The job was overwhelming when I first got here, I hired someone, as soon as that person came, we needed another ...

"And things have continued to escalate. We're bombarded daily with the needs of the community. We have a hotline at St. Clare's. We get calls, men, middle-income people who're afraid of AIDS infection. We do a lot of telephone counselling. We staff outpatient clinics, full HIV testing clinic (which includes counselling), and then we're running around the hospital all the time from one inpatient to another. We also run therapy groups for various categories of needy persons suffering in some way from the HIV infection plague. Each social worker has at least one group. One of our workers has a woman's group. The problem is that we are short-staffed. Right now we have 3½ social workers. We haven't been able to replace the ½ staff we're missing and I have ended up with a caseload of my own.... We're out straight all the time, trying to meet the needs.

"In an overall sense, there's an absence of social support and resources. You don't have a lot of people to do the work for you. People who are willing to do the legwork. And the burden falls on the social worker. Everyone else washes his or her hands of the problems. The social worker is often both responsible and ineffectual in bringing about quality discharge planning.

"The most important matter, however, is that this whole process, caring for people, and housing them, and providing services for them ... this whole process that we social workers and health care workers are involved in, in a sense insulates the larger community from the problem. They simply aren't involved. As it is now, AIDS isn't the caring community's responsibility, it's the responsibility of the hospital authorities.... Changing that would help a lot."

Veronica Toomer, C.S.W.
Social Work Supervisor
AIDS Center Program
St. Luke's Hospital
St. Luke's/Roosevelt Hospital Center

Housing

"For most patients, housing is a major problem. What we have to continuously keep in mind is that the issue for the patients is taking care of themselves. Their energy levels vary and this fact, coupled with limited resources, impacts on how creative social workers have to be to supply resources that don't exist!...

"I had a patient who was homeless. That patient spent 8 months in the hospital waiting for housing. That's how long it took the city to find housing for this patient ... they tried.... But it was 8 months.

"Once in a while, if the family and the patient are estranged, we can reunite them, but even if they're reconciled, it doesn't mean the family will take the patient into their home."

"Secondly entitlements need to be delivered in a timely way. In terms of housing, for example, we make applications for people for

Bailey House, to the YMCA, to SROs, to hotels.... But it's up to the city. We can only make the applications ...

"There are external lacks such as housing and entitlements and then there are internal tensions. The symptoms of stress on workers are often subtle. One becomes robotlike, angry. You have to listen for it. You have to build new ways into the system for the social workers to do the work. The social workers, confronted with so much need and so little external support, need to be reminded that if they structure the crisis, it will diminish. It can be dealt with. You've got to assess people's time and realize that their long-term clinical work is more rewarding than one-shot therapy sessions ... both for the worker and the patient.

Drug Treatment

"It's easy to get burned out dealing with IV-drug-using AIDS patients. These are people who have very limited social support. And because of that, the hospital staff becomes the extended support system. When we discharge a patient, we never fully say good-bye to them. Sure, they come back for medical appointments, but they also come back for friendship, for nurturing.

"And then there is the problem of staff perceptions of IV drug users within the hospital, on the part of social work and medical staff. You know, it's the same old stuff. They think we baby the drug-abusing population.... They insist the disease is the fault of the people who have it.... They resent the fact that there's a program.... They think the patients have brought the disease upon themselves. That means we have to do a lot of in-hospital advocacy on behalf of our patients.

Staff

"During 1985 I started seeing an increase in AIDS patients. There would be 2 or 3 on any given floor. Most of the social workers in the hospital didn't want to work with AIDS patients. A 'them and not me' attitude. I believe what was being expressed really was fear. They were scared, but that's not what was being stated. During that time, there were 2 other social workers who occasionally worked with AIDS patients. One left and the other only took care of those who were on her floor.

"Now we have two full-time social workers and one intern in social work from Hunter College. We have trouble finding people from within the social work department of the hospital. We put ads in the paper, we conducted workshops. We had a job fair. We got 22 responses. Thirteen or 14 of those responses requested the AIDS program but only 6 followed up on when contacted.

"Right now we're understaffed. Just this week we saw 8 new patients ... not readmissions, new patients.... We can't keep up with them. My staff carries a caseload of 20 to 25 patients. And we need more staff. Our unit is therapy focused. We see inpatients and outpatients. We provide ongoing support groups and family groups and we provide individual therapy if it's needed. I'm looking forward to funding from the state for another social worker. We've requested the funding. We really need someone.

"For example, there's the case of a female IV-drug-using patient who comes back to the ER all the time in the midst of one crisis or another. She gets to the ER, the doctors examine her and don't find a medical problem, and then the woman refuses to leave. The social worker is called and she rushes down to the woman only to find that the crisis isn't really medical. There's nothing to be done medically at the moment. The woman is in need of emotional care ... and after this has happened enough times, the worker, overworked and worried about the patient, becomes furious ... frustrated ... and angry ...

"My thought is this: We have to look carefully at how the woman's needs are being inappropriately met both by the ER and the social worker who drops what she's doing and runs down every time the patient comes in with a crisis. Wouldn't it be better to get the woman into a weekly therapy group where she'd have the benefit of the social worker's help plus the additional support from the group? The social workers need to be directed toward these solutions because the job has many problems built into it and it gets very overwhelming. And we need to fund more jobs so that the workers have time to run these groups and provide this kind of care."

Suzanne Hill, M.S.W.
Bernstein Pavillion
Beth Israel Medical Center

Housing

"Finding housing in New York is hard to begin with, but if you're a PWA, it's much harder. We keep patients in the hospital for so long because there aren't enough resources. People become infected with hospital-acquired infections after they've been stable and afebrile. People who are stable and afebrile need normal family situations and recreation. Things which don't exist in the hospital. And so, because there is a lack of resources, they end up staying in the hospital. . . . And they end up dying in the hospital.

"Coler Hospital had two openings recently. We had two patients, both of whom had been waiting for several months. One of them died the day before the space opened up after waiting for such a long time. If you have a compromised immune system and you're post-infection, that is, you're out of an acute situation . . . when you have a little more mobility you want to resume your old habits . . . Do the things that you're accustomed to doing. You want to eat a hot dog! That's what keeps people going.

"Basically, there are four places we can try to help people find housing in. There's Bailey House. There's scattered housing administrated by the AIDS Resource Center in Chelsea. They're not supposed to discriminate between risk groups. But no matter what your risk group is or how competent you are, you've got to have a strong social worker behind you, to guide you and advocate for you, to make you aware of the options and alternatives, limited as they are. And then there's MAP, run by the HRA. MAP contracts with hotels in various parts of the city. Basically it's the SROs. If a person is homeless they can be referred to MAP. They can be referred if they have ARC as well, especially if they need home care. . . . And the fourth place is Coler/Goldwater, part of the city hospital system . . .

"There is a need for transitional housing for both drug users and non-drug users who are PWAs. . . . When resources are less limited than they are right now, we can find housing for drug users . . . but when resources are scarce, drug users who are PWAs are more difficult to find housing for. . . . There just aren't adequate resources.

Children

"We see grandparents and relatives fighting over the children of AIDS patients. For example, a dying mother wants her sister to have her children . . . or maybe her next door neighbor who has been taking care of them for years and knows them well, and loves them. But the children's father, serving a sentence on Riker's Island, doesn't want them to go either to her sister or to the neighbor. He wants the children, he'll be getting out soon, he says. But he might not have seen these children for years! So the courts are involved and the children suffer . . . and often the person who is least equipped to take care of the children gets them.

Drug Treatment

"In 1971, I went to the Bernstein Institute. At that time Bernstein was a very interesting place to be. New things were happening in drug treatment ... people were working in dance, music, theater, plays, children's plays.... There was a mixed staff, there were nurses with a holistic bent. We were primarily a detox facility. Our patients went through detox and were referred to methadone maintenance. TCs like Phoenix House and Day Top Village, and drug-free daytime programs like Greenwich House. The primary methodologies were encounter and confrontation.

"There's a difference between that time and this. Today drug-using people have fewer family resources, fewer cultural resources, neighborhood resources, community resources. They are more alone today than they were, less connected. And then there is more poly-drug abuse and that complicates the situation.

"Then, along with the closing down of day centers and other forms of community drug treatment, reimbursement to detox shrunk and the hospitals started to abbreviate detox. We used to keep people from 21 to 26 days. After 5 to 7 days, when their heads were clearer, their families were involved, too. And we gave them counselling, and they went to group. Now, with the shrinking of government funding, we keep people 14 days and we have very strict guidelines re: Medicaid reimbursement. We're short-staffed, we need more social workers. We don't have any recreation workers ...

"Along with these government cut backs in detox, there were cut backs in the funding for smaller agencies, day programs, and residential treatment programs that were not so well situated, those in poorer neighborhoods. They started losing their funding and then there were fewer and fewer of them operating.

"Now, drug users see methadone as pretty much the only drug treatment. But drug users frequently have other illnesses, problems with child abuse, nutrition problems, job problems. The staff needs to see the person, and his or her family. There needs to be follow-up. Has the intervention worked? How are things going? There needs to be follow-up on housing, education, children's welfare, finances ...

"The central issue is that community drug treatment funding has dried up for teens and people in their early twenties. The street is their community now."

NOTES

1. J. Gross, "The Devastation of AIDS," *New York Times*, March 16, 1987.

2. S. Deren, "Parents in Methadone Treatment and Their Children," New York State Division of Substance Abuse Services, Bureau of Research and Evaluation, February 1986.

3. H. Joseph, "AIDS and Homelessness in New York City," Narcotic and Drug Research Institute, New York State Division of Substance Abuse Services, May 1988.

4. E. Drucker and S. Vermund, "A Model of Estimating the Number of IV Drug Users in Urban Areas," *American Journal of Epidemiology*, July 1989.

5. New York State Division of Substance Abuse Services, "Report of Treatment Services," 1987.

6. New York City Health Systems Agency, "Addiction Services Treatment Plan, 1986."

Housing, Homelessness, and the Impact of HIV Disease

Peter Arno, Ph.D.

> Homelessness is a great tragedy. AIDS is another. No words are sufficient to describe the plight of those facing both afflictions, strewn amidst the gleaming towers of our greatest of cities in this land of plenty.

JUSTICE EDWARD H. LEHNER, in his New York State Supreme Court preliminary injunction of January 11, 1989, urged New York City and State into action with these words. Unless local and state governments, as well as the private sector, step in to alleviate the tragedy of those with HIV-related illness who have no homes, we may soon witness an unravelling of the social fabric in our city. A plan of action for dealing with AIDS and homelessness is clearly vital.

The numbers of men, women, adolescents and children suffering from AIDS and other HIV-related illnesses who lack adequate housing are growing, while the importance of permanent supportive homes for them and their families is becoming ever more clear. As the epidemic shifts increasingly toward intravenous drug users, their sexual partners and children, many of the assumptions regarding patterns of care developed for gay men may be inappropriate

Peter Arno, Ph.D., "Housing, Homelessness and the Impact of HIV Disease," *The Crisis in AIDS Care: A Call to Action*, Working Group of the Citizens Commission on AIDS, March 1989, pp. 49–60. Reprinted by Permission of the Citizens Commission on AIDS for New York City and Northern New Jersey.

for a patient population who a) have different HIV-related clinical syndromes; b) are 30-40% female; c) are primarily low income blacks or Hispanics; and d) often lack insurance, and material resources, including access to stable housing.[1,2,3,4]

The crisis in housing for HIV-infected persons is part of the nationwide homeless tragedy. Much of the blame rests directly on the policies of the Reagan Administration, which slashed annual Federal housing subsidies from $30 billion to $8 billion over the past decade. The typical poor family is now forced to spend an unheard-of 78 percent of its income on housing.

The city and state's reliance on the outdated AIDS surveillance definition used by the Centers for Disease Control (CDC) also contributes to the tragedy of homelessness. It has been official government policy to house or provide rental subsidies only to those persons with a CDC-defined AIDS diagnosis. Those with HIV-related illnesses, which can be as debilitating as AIDS itself, have not been eligible for any special housing benefits. The New York City Department of Health is reconsidering this policy; both the city and state should act quickly to bring housing eligibility criteria in line with medical knowledge about the spectrum of HIV illness.

The number of homeless people with HIV disease cannot easily be determined. Estimation problems include uncertainty over both the total numbers of homeless and the number of people infected with HIV, as well as confusion over the arbitrary distinctions along the clinical spectrum of illness. The Partnership for the Homeless estimates that there are 5,000 homeless with AIDS or ARC now in the city and that the number will rise to 30,000 over the next 3 to 4 years. Andrew Stein, president of the City Council, adopted that estimate as the subtitle for his hearings of December 1988, "Sick and No Place to Go: 5,000 Homeless People with AIDS and AIDS-related Illness." The AIDS Resource Center puts the number slightly lower—citing a rough estimate of 2,000–5,000 with projections for a large increase by 1991.[5] The Coalition for the Homeless, which has filed a class action suit to force New York City and State to house HIV-infected persons who do not meet the criteria for CDC-defined AIDS, estimates that population group at 10,000.[6]

In New Jersey, the state health department has been collecting data from its AIDS Health Services Program, which provides case management services to persons with HIV disease in hospitals in Newark and Jersey City. Of the program's 1,903 clients, 197 are in need of "housing assistance" (approximately 10 percent). These clients include those with "CDC-defined" AIDS, ARC, and mildly symptomatic HIV infection. Applying that same 10 percent figure to the 2,300 people living with AIDS in New Jersey, one can estimate there are about 230 homeless PWAs in the state.[7]

In New Jersey, the majority of AIDS cases are related to intravenous drug use. Those affected are generally residents of poor, minority communities. Most of the drug abusers had housing problems even before the AIDS crisis. Although the major urban areas of Newark, Jersey City, and Paterson are especially affected, recent trends show growing problems in coastal areas including Asbury Park and Atlantic City.

The increasing number of homeless PWAs in New Jersey is the result of several factors: (1) an increase in the number of AIDS-related evictions; (2) eviction by family members who are either unwilling or unable to provide care for the individual; (3) loss of employment and income; and (4) the impoverishment that many PWAs were already struggling with prior to their illness; and (5) loss of eligibility for Aid to Families with Dependent Children (AFDC) when a mother with AIDS loses custody of her children because they have been placed in foster care.

In addition, the rate of HIV infection among homeless adolescents is high and rising according to a New York State Department of Health study of youths tested at Covenant House between October 1987 and October 1988. That study concluded that 10 percent of adolescents then resident at Covenant House and almost 7 percent of all homeless adolescents in the street survey were HIV-seropositive—a statistic that must challenge any optimistic predictions for a drop in the rate of HIV infection in the future.[8]

Although all New Yorkers recognize the existence of homelessness on our streets, the problem is not limited to the most visible homeless, those on the streets, on subways, and in bus stations. For HIV-infected IV drug users, precarious housing has become almost the norm.[9] The city agencies also place men and women in single room occupancies (SROs) unsuitable for those who are HIV-infected and, despite official denials, hundreds (and perhaps thousands) are also "housed" in city-owned or operated shelters. Here again, the distinction among HIV-related illnesses is used to excuse inappropriate housing. Many persons, particularly those in the shelters, have not received a "full-blown" diagnosis of AIDS or are afraid to pursue medical attention for fear of social or economic repercussions, according to Dr. Stephen C. Joseph, New York City Commissioner of Health.[10]

A report prepared by the New York State Division of Substance Abuse Services (the DSAS Report) states clearly that it is impossible to determine the number of homeless AIDS or ARC patients in the shelters because they fear intimidation and violence and are afraid to come forward.[11]

Appearing before the Assembly Committee on Health, New York State Department of Social Services Division of Adult Services Deputy Commissioner Judith Berek described a joint city/state study of the post-discharge needs of 269 clinically stable patients with HIV-related illness or AIDS in 20 New York City hospitals. She testified: "Just over 50 percent of these patients had *no* home to which they could return. Of that 50 percent, 36 percent had been undomiciled prior to admission; 48 percent had had houses or apartments but couldn't return for reasons such as eviction, failure to pay the rent, increased clinical needs, or the exhaustion or rejection of essential support persons."[12]

Jo Ivey Boufford, president of New York City's Health and Hospital Corporation, has a lower estimate. She reports that 15 percent of patients in public hospitals are homeless.[13] Many of those homeless patients are otherwise self-directing and functionally independent and could be helped by rent subsidies and visiting home care in scattered-site apartments—if more such housing were available.

The lack of appropriate, affordable housing—a tragedy in any circumstance—multiplies astronomically as HIV disease progresses. All treatments, whether medicinal, nutritional, or holistic, assume the availability of basic necessities, including access to a clean kitchen, bathroom, bed, and heat. Most obvious, but worth emphasizing: a patient cannot receive home health care without a home. Visiting nurse services and home-care practitioners cannot provide medical care without, at a minimum, hot running water and sanitary facilities. The control over one's life that is vital for wellness becomes virtually impossible without stable housing.[14]

Ginny Shubert of the Coalition for the Homeless has stated: "Infection with HIV is becoming a primary cause of homelessness in New York City. Persistent and recurring illness and episodic hospitalizations result in the loss of jobs and housing and leave HIV-infected persons without the resources to fight their way back into the housing market. For those HIV-infected persons already homeless, progression to serious illness and death will likely be hastened by life on the streets or in City barrack shelters, where infectious disease is rampant and violence toward HIV-infected persons is common."[15]

The DSAS Report identifies not only medical but managerial problems of homeless AIDS patients: They are unable to complete diagnostic tests, they lose prescriptions, and they break outpatient appointments. Many of these problems are clearly due to living conditions in shelters, SROs, or on the streets.[16]

At the Assembly Health Committee hearing, Manhattan Borough President David Dinkins provided a consensus report detailing the criteria for supported housing for HIV-infected persons that specified a minimum of 120 square feet per person, single rooms with private bathrooms, cots for health aides and care providers, staff and support services, and adaptive physical access (see Appendix A).[17] Advocacy groups serving the homeless and the AIDS community have demanded housing that is not only sanitary and physically adequate but also "supportive." Douglas Dornan, executive director of the AIDS Resource Center, defined supported housing as subsidized housing and support services (such as case management, mental health and substance abuse counseling, home health care services, recreational therapy, transportation, etc.) provided on-site or through agreement and affiliation with other community agencies.[18]

The lack of adequate housing with these or lesser standards is also affecting the hospitalization patterns of AIDS patients, adding to the length of their stay in acute care beds and, therefore, increasing the cost of providing care. Based on a survey of 174 hospitalized IV drug users with HIV disease, Ernest Drucker and his colleagues report that an estimated 40 percent of patients are homeless (living on the streets or in shelters) or are precariously housed (i.e., living doubled-up or at some place where they are unlikely to return following a hospital stay) at the onset of their illness.[19] Borrowing a term previously reserved for infants with no place to go, Drucker described 10–20 percent of the hospitalized IV drug-using AIDS patients as "boarder adults." In August, 1988, Emmaus House, a community organization based in Harlem, which has provided a range of services to the homeless for more than 20 years, cited even more alarming statistics for Harlem Hospital. Emmaus House reported that "50 percent to 60 percent of that daily flow of [AIDS and ARC] patients have no home or have very tenuous living situations."[20]

Government Response: New York City

A summary of AIDS services available in New York City published in *The New York Times* on January 3, 1989, cited a 1985 memorandum by then-Mayoral Assistant Victor Botnick recommending that the city "work to develop viable housing options" and "offer community and voluntary groups assistance in locating and finding congregate facilities and rehabilitating in-rem housing" (tax delinquent housing taken over by the City). In the last four years, the City cannot reasonably claim to have fulfilled either of these goals.

At legislative hearings held by City Council President Andrew Stein and State Assemblyman Richard Gottfried, representatives of government, AIDS advocacy groups, the medical community, and the homeless have all decried the lack of speed in the city's response. New York's two leading advocacy groups for the homeless—the Coalition for the Homeless and the Partnership for the Homeless—have reported on housing problems for the HIV-infected population in the context of a citywide shortage of affordable housing. All sides emphasize that the city's response has been inadequate, that funds have been improperly targeted and in short supply, and that the reliance on the CDC definition of AIDS for determining housing assistance eligibility criteria has misdirected efforts to solve the dual tragedies of AIDS and homelessness. The city has recently begun to work with some community and voluntary groups, but its progress has been limited by two major factors: First, these small community-based groups are ill-equipped to deal with governmental bureaucracies; and second, these groups have been denied funds if they overstep the arbitrary boundary between HIV illness and CDC-defined AIDS.

In a class action suit brought against the city and state by the Coalition for the Homeless, Dr. Stanley R. Yancovitz, director of clinical AIDS activities for Beth Israel Medical Center in Manhattan, testified that:

> The known prevalence of infectious disease in the municipal shelters poses a substantial health risk to ... anyone infected with HIV. Persons who are HIV infected are highly susceptible to the types of infectious disease rampant in shelters, and the crowded conditions and shared use of sanitary facilities further increase the risk of infection. Once an infectious disease is contracted, one who is HIV-infected is more likely to become seriously ill than a non-infected person. Moreover, a weakened immune system, coupled with the stress of living in an environment such as that found on the streets or in the municipal shelters makes recovery from infection difficult or impossible.[21]

Government Response: New York State

New York State's response to AIDS and homelessness has focused on the creation of a two-pronged plan for the future—the building or rehabilitation of facilities to provide supportive care and the use of federal funds to establish and finance them. Judith Berek outlined the state's plan at the Gottfried Hearings, where she stated that AIDS not only "compounds" the problems of homelessness, but prevents progress in "developing housing models that will improve, or at least maintain, the quality of life of a person or family with HIV infection."[22] The state's initial effort has been to maintain self-directed people with AIDS and ARC and their families in their own homes by providing home relief, social security disability insurance, Aid to Families with Dependent Children, food stamps, homemaker services and housekeeper/chore services, personal care services, and home health care services. Emergency shelter allowances of up to $480 per month for a single adult and up to $333 for each additional person living in the house or apartment can serve as a supplement to rent. This money can be used for scattered-site housing as available. Berek testified that, as of July 1988, "1,080 clients in New York City were receiving that assistance and that, according to the City's Human Resources Agency, about 52 percent of the cases served by their management unit were getting the rental supplement."[23] She added that Tier II family shelter programs, developed for the general population and funded by various government programs, may eventually be made available to HIV-affected families.

The population of single adults with AIDS and HIV-related diseases form the core of the housing problem in New York State as it does in New York City. The state, however, has focused its attention on AIDS-specific health-related facilities. The state appears to endorse residential health care for the future, based on two factors: First, its demographic analysis of AIDS patients who are most often fairly young (average age 35), with a history of drug use, without a suitable home support system or home, and second, its perception of the progress of medical care, specifically "chemotherapeutic advances for HIV infection."[24] Berek praised this approach for its efficient physical plant and for its funding capabilities. Medicaid will reimburse the state for each patient's care under existing legislation.

Berek specified four models of adult care that the State considered both appropriate and economically feasible under current SSI (Supplemental Security Income) levels: (1) family-type homes for 1 to 4 residents; (2) enriched housing programs operated by not-for-profit corporations or public agencies for five or more residents; (3) adult homes for 5 to 200 residents; and (4) multilicensed facilities.[25] The latter, called the most preferable congregate care option, presents a way to provide the different levels of care required by the episodic nature of the disease and at the same time bring in Medicaid dollars. Given the extent of the problem, all of these models may be adopted by the state, but it is highly unlikely that any of them will be operational until the end of 1991. (For more on the state's plan to build residential care beds, see Section 3, "Long-term Care: A Long-term Commitment.")

Although New York State has based its housing plan on the availability of federal Medicaid funds, state planners may have overlooked another grant source. Catholic Charities in San Francisco recently received a $2 million federal grant under the Stewart B. McKinney Homeless Assistance Act of 1987 (PL10-77) to provide Section 8 rent subsidy vouchers for up to 35 HIV-infected residents in a supported housing program over a 10-year period. The funds are funneled through the Departments of Public Health of the City and County of San Francisco.[26] We know of no attempt on the State or City level to utilize federal funds in a similar manner.

Government Response: New Jersey

Although the New Jersey Department of Health has made some efforts to create some medically related housing for PWAs, there are no programs that provide supported housing.

At present, a PWA can apply to the county or municipal welfare office for emergency assistance and shelter; this is normally provided in congregate shelters, which are a less expensive option but are often inappropriate for PWAs. Such settings are closed during the day, and PWAs need a place to stay round the clock. Proper diet, rest, and administration of medication are practically impossible in such settings. Overcrowding also places individuals at serious risk of infections such as tuberculosis.

Advocates are often needed to insure that the welfare office provides a separate room in a sanitary facility for the individual. Furthermore, municipal shelter has been available for a 5-month period only. However, a recent appellate court decision found that this time limit violated state law because homeless individuals, some of whom are PWAs, were being evicted at 5 months without being provided with any alternatives.[27]

The Response of Community-based Organizations

AIDS advocacy groups in New York have developed financial, legal, pastoral, and medical support networks since the onset of the epidemic. They have been joined by religious and community-based organizations, and by advocates for the homeless in the fight to provide housing for all. A number of housing programs have been established, and while limited in scope, they show that solutions are possible. On December 27, 1988, the City's Human Resources Administration solicited proposals from qualified community-based organizations to manage supportive, scattered-site housing for homeless persons with AIDS. The Request for Proposals required each agency to secure, furnish, operate, and maintain a total of at least 100 scattered-site apartments with counseling, referral services, and advocacy specified as contracted services.

Community-based, religious, and advocacy organizations have developed or proposed a number of other projects. Emmaus House now includes men, women and infants with AIDS within its continuing programs. Currently, 55 homeless men and women live at Emmaus House on a long-term basis and 16 additional men can be housed in an emergency shelter. Emmaus House has applied to the city for title to 20 city-owned apartments in clustered sites, preferably in East Harlem, in order to expand its programs. Its AIDS housing proposal includes orientation, counseling, advocacy for those dealing with entitlement applications, and participation in community meals programs.

The AIDS Resource Center maintains both the only supported residence for AIDS patients, Bailey House, a 44-bed residential facility, and a group of 20 scattered-site apartments that have served more than 100 persons through the end of 1988. Bailey House will be enlarged to a capacity of 52 beds and will be made wheelchair-accessible through a $600,000 grant from the United States Public Health Service and a $1 million award from the State's Homeless Housing Assistance Program. The Task Force on Homeless PWAs has endorsed the scattered-site model and is proposing to establish small group homes for no more than 10 people, each with an entitlements advocacy program, visiting nurses, and city-funded home health aides. The Task Force's proposal emphasizes that with the scattered-site program no community would be asked to carry a disproportionate burden of housing homeless PWAs/ARC. By renovating available housing stock, such a project could expand with a relatively small infusion of capital funds and could be completed far more quickly than the time required to construct new facilities.

New Jersey, unlike New York City, does not have community-based organizations focused on housing comparable to the AIDS Resource Center in New York City. Since hospital social workers are often unwilling to discharge homeless patients, and since the cost of a hospital bed can reach up to $700 per day, the failure to develop housing for PWAs continues to be a financially devastating problem. Moreover, although New Jersey does have a Medicaid community-care waiver program in place, the lack of housing at the time of discharge results in ineligibility for community-based services.

Conclusions

Any solution to the overlapping problems of homelessness and AIDS will require commitments from the city, state, and federal governments that recognize the continuum of HIV disease. Unless HIV disease is redefined in light of medical realities, immunocompromised people are destined for death in shelters or on the streets. Advocacy, whether from AIDS activist groups, religious institutions, or community-based institutions, is vital to guiding the HIV-infected through the maze of bureaucratic entitlement programs. Appropriate treatment and concomitant social services must be provided to patients struggling with the burdens of illness, many of whom are substance abusers.

Scattered-site supported housing, which generally does not alarm the residential communities in which it is placed or ghettoize the HIV-infected, is one cost-efficient and humane way to provide care. The Partnership for the Homeless has recommended a "1 percent" program in which 1 percent of the currently habitable 225,000 apartments owned, subsidized or controlled by New York City would be set aside to provide supported housing for homeless and near-homeless people with HIV illness. These apartments would be passed into scattered-site programs operated by nonprofit sponsors over three years at the rate of about 750 units per year from the normal annual vacancies of over 10,000 apartments.[28] The AIDS Resource Center has created an important model for supported housing that provides a full range of counseling, food, medical care, and other services. Adequate public funding will enable other nonprofit sponsors to duplicate that model and ensure that genuinely supported housing—not barracks—are actually constructed. Health-related facilities (HRF) clearly have some drawbacks, notably the fact that they create an institutional, rather than a homelike environment, and traditionally require residents to be discharged when their health status changes. Further, the state will not be able to complete construction on them for several years. However, an HRF solution has the advantage of not requiring a change in existing regulations and allowing the state to access federal funds through the Medicaid program.

In order to meet the needs of homeless HIV-infected individuals or PWAs in New Jersey, leadership is essential. Local resistance to the siting of residential facilities and the lack of technical assistance available to nonprofit organizations attempting to develop housing alternatives are also serious problems.

Rather than attempting to squeeze solutions into existing funding streams, however, we should be looking closely at what the actual problems are and what it will take to solve them. As a nation, we have been painstakingly slow to develop appropriate responses to the triple tragedies of AIDS, homelessness, and drug abuse. Increasingly, these issues are intertwined. We cannot afford to allow fear, indifference, or even budget deficits to shape our response to an epidemic that poses a real danger to the social fabric of our communities.

Appendix A
Criteria for Supported Housing
for People with AIDS
Prepared by Manhattan
Borough President's Office

Size and Configuration
- Facilities should house no more than 50 people
- Minimum of 120 square feet per person in sleeping area
- No more than 1 person per room
- Private bathroom for each person
- Physical access issues unique to this population must be adequately addressed
- Common lounge space
- Common kitchenette on every floor
- Refrigerator in each room
- Three meals a day as individually necessary
- Capacity to open a cot for an additional person, to accommodate a health aide or other care provider

Support Services
- Bilingual staff capacity in the delivery of services
- Case manager/client ratio of 1:15 maximum should be maintained
- Mental health/counseling staff should include: psychiatrist, social worker, substance abuse counselor, case manager
- Recreational therapist
- Home health care services (aides) attached to facility or personal care assistants (2 per shift)
- 24-hour nursing
- 24-hour security
- 24-hour transportation available according to need
- Elevator service in building at all times

NOTES

1. A. R. Moss, "AIDS and Intravenous Drug Use: The Real Heterosexual Epidemic," *British Medical Journal* 294 (1987): 389–90.

2. D. C. Des Jarlais and S. R. Friedman, "HIV Infection Among Intravenous Drug Users: Epidemiology and Risk Reduction," *AIDS* 1 (1987): 67–76.

3. P. S. Arno, "The Future of Voluntarism and the AIDS Epidemic," in D. E. Rogers and E. Ginzberg, eds., *The AIDS Patient: An Action Agenda* (Boulder and London: Westview Press, 1988), 65–70.

4. P. S. Arno and R. G. Hughes, "Local Policy Responses to the AIDS Epidemic: New York and San Francisco," *New York State Journal of Medicine* 87 (1987): 264–272.

5. D. Dornan, "Supportive Housing for Homeless People with AIDS and AIDS-Related Illnesses," Testimony before the New York State Assembly Committee on Health, 5 December 1988.

6. *Mixon v. Grinker*, Index No. 14932/88 (Sup Ct NY Cty) (Opinion granting preliminary injunction Lehner, J.) (1989).

7. Personal communication with Stephen Young of the New Jersey Department of Health, 26 January 1989.

8. Covenant House. A blind seroprevalence study done at Covenant House in conjunction with New York City and New York State Departments of Health. Presented at the Annual Meeting of the American Public Health Association, Boston, 14–16 November 1988.

9. E. Drucker et al., *IV Drug Users with AIDS in the City of New York: A Study of Dependent Children, Housing and Drug Addiction Treatment* (The AIDS Service Delivery Consortium/NYC: July 1988), 15.

10. G. Kolata, "Many with AIDS Said to Live in Shelters in New York City," *New York Times*, 4 April 1988: B1.

11. New York State Division of Substance Abuse Services, *The Homeless Intravenous Substance Abuser and the AIDS Epidemic* (May 1988): 11.

12. J. Berek, "Residential Care and Housing Services for Persons with AIDS," Testimony before the New York State Assembly Committee on Health, 5 December 1988.

13. Jo Ivey Boufford, "What Needs to Be Done on the Hospital Front," in D. E. Rogers and E. Ginzberg, eds., *The AIDS Patient: An Action Agenda* (Boulder and London: Westview Press, 1988), 20.

14. AIDS Resource Center. "More than Just a Place to Live," *News from the AIDS Resource Center* (November/December 1988): 1.

15. G. Shubert, Coalition for the Homeless, Press release, 12 January 1989.

16. DSAS Report, op cit., 13.

17. D. Dinkins, Testimony before the New York State Assembly Committee on Health, 5 December 1988.

18. D. Dornan, "Supportive Housing for Homeless People with AIDS and AIDS-related Illnesses," *AIDS Resource Center*, 29 September 1988: 1.

19. Drucker et al., op cit.

20. Emmaus House, "A Proposal for Housing Homeless Persons with AIDS," August 1988.

21. S. R. Yancovitz, Medical Affidavit in *Mixon v. Grinker* (September 1988).

22. Berek, op cit.

23. Ibid, 6–7.

24. New York State, *AIDS, New York's Response: A 5-Year Interagency Plan* (January 1989): 71–77.

25. Berek, op cit., 12–13.

26. D. Werdegar et al., *AIDS in San Francisco: Status Report for Fiscal Year 1987–1988 and Projections of Service Needs and Costs for 1988–93*. (San Francisco: San Francisco Department of Public Health, 15 March 1988), 5.117.

27. *Williams vs. New Jersey Department of Human Services*, ——— N.J. Super. ———, (App. Div. 15 November 1988) dkt. A-4317-87T1F. Companion case was *Jimperson vs. New Jersey Department of Human Services*.

28. The Partnership for the Homeless, *AIDS—The Cutting Edge of Homelessness in New York City* (January 1989), 23–26.

Women—The Missing Persons in the AIDS Epidemic

Kathryn Anastos and Carola Marte

OUR CURRENT UNDERSTANDING OF the public health problem posed by the acquired immunodeficiency syndrome (AIDS) in women is seriously distorted by the underrepresentation of women in official data and the misrepresentation of their disease. Through November 1989, 10,369 women in the United States were reported to have the acquired immunodeficiency syndrome—9 percent of the total number of AIDS cases.[1] In urban areas on the East and West coasts, the numbers are higher; for example, 13 percent of all people who have been diagnosed with AIDS in New York City are women. The percentage is higher still in the most recently diagnosed cases—18 percent of New York City cases since January 1988 are in women.[2]

It is unlikely, however, that these numbers accurately reflect the number of women who in fact have serious manifestations of HIV (human immunodeficiency virus) infection, for several reasons. The diagnosis of AIDS depends not only upon demonstrated infection with HIV, but also upon the clinical manifestations of the disease—that is, the ways in which those infected become sick. Because those affected first were almost exclusively men, the case definition of AIDS is centered in how the disease has manifested in men, and gynecologic conditions are not included as manifestations of HIV infection. If women's disease manifests with the same infec-

Kathryn Anastos and Carola Marte, "Women—The Missing Persons in the AIDS Epidemic," *Health/Pac Bulletin*, Winter 1989. Reprinted by Permission of *Health/Pac Bulletin*.

tions as it does in men, it may be recognized and reported as AIDS; if the infections, still HIV related, are different, the women are not considered to have AIDS.

For example, HIV-infected women with severe infections of their fallopian tubes (pelvic inflammatory disease or PID) are not categorized as having AIDS. This is in spite of the fact that many doctors have found that these infections are worse in HIV-infected women: treatment is more difficult and less likely to be successful.[3] This resistance to cure by ordinary therapy is the sign of a failing immune system.

Similarly, vaginal yeast infections in HIV-infected women are more severe and less likely to be cured by ordinary therapy.[4] A woman may suffer from vaginal yeast infections even before she has thrush, a yeast infection of the mouth that affects both women and men and that is officially used as one of the criteria for a pre-AIDS condition (AIDS-related complex or ARC). Does it make sense that the same infection in another orifice—an orifice not present in men—is not categorized as an AIDS-related condition?

Moreover, and most seriously, a number of published reports indicate dramatically higher rates of abnormal Pap smears and cervical cancer in HIV-infected women compared to uninfected women.[5] Cervical cancer in immune-suppressed women is known to be more severe and life-threatening than in women with healthy immune systems. It may advance with dangerous rapidity and often requires special treatment.[6] Given the many years between the time a person becomes infected with HIV and the time he or she becomes ill with full-blown AIDS—now thought to average nine years— many HIV-infected women may die from cervical cancer, a potentially treatable disease, before they die from AIDS as officially defined. Clearly, the case definitions of AIDS and ARC should be revised to include those women whose severe infections and malignancies are obvious manifestations of immune system failure induced by HIV infection.

Another major problem is that similar symptoms in both women and men are interpreted, investigated, and treated differently, because women are not expected to have AIDS. Underdiagnosis is thus a significant bias in epidemiologic data on women with AIDS. For example, one study showed that women with pneumocystis carinii pneumonia (PCP), the most common opportunistic infection in AIDS patients and a major cause of AIDS deaths, were more likely to be treated for minor respiratory ailments and not for PCP.[7] The result was life-threatening respiratory failure and a higher death rate than in men who had the same symptoms and whose PCP was recognized and treated. The potential magnitude of this problem may be seen in recent statistics showing unexplained and dramatic increases in deaths of women from a variety of respiratory and infectious diseases. For example, in New York City and Washington, D.C., there were, respectively, a 154 percent and a 225 percent increase in deaths in young women (aged 15 to 45 years) from 1981 to 1986. Idaho, in contrast, has experienced no such increase in mortality rates in women.[8] Chris Norwood of the National Women's Health Network, who compiled these statistics, has suggested that because these increased numbers of deaths in women are found in geographic areas with heavy concentrations of AIDS cases, they may in fact be uncounted HIV-related deaths.

A better understanding of the true scope of the AIDS epidemic in women requires us to reconsider all these factors. The case definition of AIDS must be changed to include gynecologic conditions. Some estimate must be made of the proportion of the observed increase in respiratory and infection-related deaths that is caused by HIV-induced immunosuppression. In addition, health care providers need to develop an increased clinical awareness of AIDS in women in order to achieve more accurate diagnoses of full-blown AIDS, even by the current case definition.

The problem of the "missing women" in the AIDS epidemic goes well beyond the epidemiology. Women have been forgotten in every aspect of AIDS medicine. Fundamental questions about the progression of this disease in women have not been asked or answered. Is cervical cancer more common in HIV-infected women? How does HIV infection affect pregnancy and childbirth? Do the different hormones in women and men affect the course of HIV infection? Do women fall prey to different opportunistic infections than men do? Do women respond differently to treatment regimens established for male patients? Do women suffer different side effects and toxicities from AIDS medications? Do women survive a shorter time after the diagnosis of AIDS has been made? Are the causes of death in women different than in men? In particular, gynecologic disease has until recently been entirely ignored in discussions of HIV-related conditions, and current guidelines for medical management do not include recommendations for gynecologic care.[9] We have little information to indicate how often Pap smears should be done, and common symptomatic conditions such as vaginal yeast infections are not routinely discussed with patients or treated prophylactically, as are comparable oral or anal conditions.

The neglect of women with HIV disease extends to other important areas. Very few women have been included in drug trials. The original studies of AZT in 282 patients included only 13 women,[10] and many drug trials have specifically excluded women. The potential importance of gender differences in response to HIV infection is rarely addressed in current medical publications, and this lack allows only the most rudimentary understanding of AIDS in women. Physicians find little information available to help them understand HIV-related gynecologic conditions in women.

Women at Risk

In the United States, AIDS declared itself first in gay men and subsequently among intravenous drug users, who are predominantly men. This history has led to our false perception of AIDS as a disease of men. This fallacy is quickly dispelled by the observation that in large areas of the world, for example, African and Caribbean nations where the dominant mode of transmission is heterosexual contact, women and men are infected with equal frequency.[11] In addition, the increasing importance of heterosexual transmission in the United States has already produced a faster rate of increase in the numbers of women who have become sick through heterosexual transmission compared to any other group.[12] For gay men in particular, massive educational efforts have been effective in decreasing the rate of new infections.

One factor in this epidemiologic shift is the crack epidemic and its associated hypersexuality and exchange of sex for drugs. Young women and adolescent girls have multiple sexual partners in a day in exchange for a dollar or a hit, and their "clients" are frequently older men with a history of intravenous drug use. As Willard Cates of the Centers for Disease Control observed, the crack houses are for heterosexual transmission to women what the bath houses were for transmission among gay men.[13]

Of the 3,668 cases of AIDS reported in American women in the single year ending November 30, 1989, 51 percent are attributed to transmission by intravenous drug use; 32 percent are attributed to heterosexual transmission; 9 percent to transfusion; and 9 percent to "undetermined means of acquiring infection" (compared to 2 percent in this category for men).[14] The higher rate of "undetermined" risk in women is assumed to reflect heterosexual transmission in which the woman is not aware of her partner's risk-taking behaviors. The category of women at double risk—those who are both intravenous drug users and partners of infected men or men at risk—is not calculated separately for women as it routinely is for men, even though these women are at substantially increased risk for infection. This matters because it subjects them to the victim-blaming attitude held by many: their source of infection is seen to justify their second-class treatment and care.

It is not clear how many of the estimated 1,000,000 HIV-infected individuals in the United States are women. Among women who are HIV-infected, many are unaware that they are at risk. In a CDC study of HIV-infected blood donors, 44 percent of 34 infected women studied could not identify a risk factor associated with their source of infection, and an equal number were known to have become infected through heterosexual contact.[15] Other studies also indicate an increasing number of infected women who do not know how they acquired the infection. For example, 15 of 26 HIV-positive mothers in a South Bronx hospital and 5 of 12 mothers in a Brooklyn hospital had no history of intravenous drug use or other identifiable risk behavior.[16]

In fact, for many women, their address alone places them at risk. Although area of residence is not officially viewed as a risk factor, data on seroprevalence make clear that, in fact, it constitutes a risk because it is so strongly associated with acknowledged risk factors. Epidemiologic data collected by the Centers for Disease Control (CDC) documents that seroprevalence rates in inner-city hospitals are high even when people with known risks are not counted. Recent CDC data show that as many as 8 percent of women and 18 percent of men visiting emergency rooms in some inner-city hospitals are HIV-infected.[17] Similarly, available information about women giving birth suggests that in some inner-city areas as many as 4 to 9 percent of deliveries are to women who are HIV-infected.[18] Breakdown of New York City data by zip code area also reveals that the most socially and economically devastated inner-city areas are those with the most HIV disease, whereas contiguous affluent areas may have much less HIV disease. For example, in 1988 the Upper East Side of Manhattan below 96th Street reported an AIDS case mortality rate of 27 per 100,000 people, compared to 48 per 100,000 for East Harlem on the east side of Manhattan above 96th Street.[19]

A woman who lives in an inner-city area and follows a conventional lifestyle of marriage and raising a family, who does not use drugs and is monogamous, nonetheless runs a high risk of becoming infected because her partner has a high probability of being infected, usually because of drug use. In many cases, these women are not aware that their partner is at risk. This means again that poor black and Latina women are at unduly high risk for infection, whatever their life-style, because poverty and lack of resources and opportunity keep them in areas of high HIV seroprevalence.

Women as "Vectors"

Deeply ingrained societal sexism as well as racism and classism have skewed the public perception of AIDS and HIV infection in women in the United States. Since the first case of a woman with AIDS was reported in the United States in 1981 in the Bronx, women have remained a forgotten group in the AIDS epidemic. They are regarded by the public and studied by the medical profession as vectors of transmission to their children and male sexual partners rather than as people with AIDS who are themselves frequently victims of transmission from the men in their lives. Until recently, one could gain epidemiologic information concerning women and AIDS mainly from perinatal studies and, to a lesser extent, from studies of prostitutes. Women have been defined primarily in terms of childbearing activities, despite the facts that pregnancy lasts a relatively short period of time and most of the serious AIDS-related illnesses in women occur outside of pregnancy.

Both in clinical practice and public discussion, pregnant women with HIV infection are perceived as incubators of sick babies who are destined to become a burden to society, not as individuals with a life-threatening illness, nor as mothers in struggle and in pain. Mothering, which for most women is an intense and perhaps the strongest emotional bond of their lives, is seen as an irresponsible and selfish act if the woman is HIV-infected and especially if she is also poor and of color. Many doctors and other health care providers feel that it is not only their right but their responsibility to counsel and persuade an HIV-infected woman to abort her pregnancy, even in the face of clear statements by the woman that she does not want to choose an abortion.

Such providers are poorly educated about, or choose to ignore, the reasons that their HIV-infected patients may wish to carry a pregnancy to term. A woman's choice is made in the context of cultural attitudes in which bearing children may be seen as the most valuable contribution a woman can make to her family and community. Families often exert pressure to plan pregnancies or to continue pregnancies already conceived. For many women, children may be the only means of attaining a sense of identity and status. In addition, poor women may perceive as favorable the risk described to them of transmitting HIV infection to their offspring. A 20 to 40 percent chance of bearing an infected child is a 60 to 80 percent chance of bearing a healthy child. This is a risk they may be willing to take; these odds seem better than those they routinely face in other aspects of their lives.

Several studies have suggested that HIV-infected women make decisions about pregnancy for the same reasons that uninfected women do. For instance, a study of decisions about pregnancy and abortion made by women on methadone maintenance found that a woman's HIV status was not the best predictor of her decision to terminate a pregnancy.[20] These choices were more readily predicted by factors directly related to the pregnancy, such as the woman's feelings about it and whether it was planned. HIV-infected women in this study who chose to continue their pregnancies cited family pressure, religious beliefs, and the desire to have a child as important factors in making their decision—in other words, the same factors considered by women who are not infected.

Male Prerogative, Female Risk

Discussions of heterosexual HIV transmission in the United States are also frequently permeated with sexist assumptions. For example, there are a number of studies on HIV infection in prostitutes,[21] presumably because this affects heterosexual transmission to men. In contrast, there has been no discussion in the professional literature of how women's lack of empowerment affects heterosexual transmission to women. Prostitutes are frequently seen as the guilty parties in the infection of women whose husbands or steady partners are the clients and the major support of the sex industry. This shifts the responsibility away from the man who engages in risk-taking sexual encounters. How many men inform their steady partners that they are exposing them to the risk of HIV transmission? The underlying inequity between women and men, at the level of individual relationships as well as in the culture at large, contributes to much of the transmission of HIV infection, particularly to women who do not perceive that they are at risk. The prevailing ethic that it is a man's prerogative to have multiple sexual encounters without condemnation has been uncritically integrated into official attitudes and research.

Sexist and classist attitudes allow the sweeping condemnation of prostitutes as transmitters of HIV infection. Studies have clarified that intravenous drug use by prostitutes, and not the prostitution itself, places women at high risk of HIV infection.[22] The prevalence of HIV infection is low in prostitutes who don't use intravenous drugs. For example, the CDC compiled statistics from several previous studies demonstrating a seroprevalence of 3.5 to 45.3 percent in drug-using street prostitutes, whereas none of the call girls who did not use drugs were HIV-infected.[23]

Lack of empowerment is a problem for all women, and especially poorer women, in protecting themselves against HIV infection. Education is only the first step in successful prevention, and even when a woman does recognize the risk of contracting HIV infection from her sexual partner, she may not be able to protect herself adequately. A heterosexual woman is usually not an equal partner in the bedroom, and her requests that her partner use a condom may be met with refusal or even physical abuse. Many providers involved in counseling women about safe sex have had experience with patients who have been beaten because they asserted the need to use condoms. Both the woman and her health care provider must weigh the immediate risk of battering against the long-term risk of HIV infection and AIDS. Similarly, women in the sex industry often omit the use of condoms because of clients' threats or offers of higher payment to do so. It is reportedly a widespread practice among prostitutes to be more careful about condom use with their clients than with their steady partners, although the steady partners are often intravenous drug users and may represent a far greater risk to the prostitute than her clients.[24]

Sexism and the lack of empowerment it causes are having a serious impact on the AIDS epidemic. Women are unable to protect themselves adequately from infection because they are frequently unaware that they are at risk; and even when they are aware, they are unable to assert their need for protection. When women are infected with HIV, they frequently do not receive appropriate medical care because of underdiagnosis, a flawed case definition, and insufficient information about manifestations of HIV disease in women. Sexism feeds on itself with the false perception of women as vectors rather than victims of HIV transmission. When classism and racism join with sexism, as they do for inner-city women, the impact of AIDS is devastating.

NOTES

1. Centers for Disease Control, Division of HIV/AIDS, Atlanta, Georgia, personal communication, January 2, 1990.

2. New York City Department of Health, "AIDS Surveillance Update," November 10, 1989.

3. Hoegsberg, B., et al., "Human Immunodeficiency Virus in Women with Pelvic Inflammatory Disease," Fourth International Conference on AIDS, Stockholm, Sweden, 1988, abstract, p. 333; and personal communication.

4. Rhoads, J. L., et al., "Chronic Vaginal Candidiasis in Women with Human Immunodeficiency Virus Infection," *Journal of the American Medical Association*, 1987:257, pp. 3105–3107.

5. Provenchar, D., et al., "HIV Status and Positive Papanicolaou Screening: Identification of a High-Risk Population," *Gynecologic Oncology*, 1988:31, pp. 184–190; and Schrager, L. K., et al., "Cervical and Vaginal Squamous Cell Abnormalities in Women Infected with Human Immunodeficiency Virus," *Journal of Acquired Immunodeficiency Syndrome*, 1989:2, pp. 570–575.

6. Sillman, F. H., and A. Sedlis, "Anogenital Papillomavirus Infection and Neoplasia in Immunodeficent Women," *Obstetrics and Gynecology Clinics of North America*, 1987:14, pp. 537–558.

7. Verdegem, T. D., et al., "Increased Fatality from Pneumocystis Carinii Pneumonia in Women with AIDS," Fourth International Conference on AIDS, Stockholm, Sweden, 1988, abstract, p. 445.

8. Norwood, Chris, "Women and the 'Hidden' AIDS Epidemic," *Network News*, Newsletter of the National Women's Health Network, November-December 1988, pp. 1, 6.

9. See, for example, New York Statewide Professional Standards Review Council, "Criteria Manual for the Treatment of AIDS," Albany, NY: AIDS Intervention Management System, 1988.

10. Fischl, M. A., et al., "The Efficacy of Azidothymidine (AZT) in the Treatment of Patients with AIDS and AIDS-Related Complex: A Double-Blind Placebo-Controlled Trial," *New England Journal of Medicine*, 1987:317, pp. 185–191.

11. Haverkos, H. W., and R. Edelman, "The Epidemiology of Acquired Immunodeficiency Syndrome Among Heterosexuals," *Journal of the American Medical Association*, 1988:260, pp. 1922–1929; and Quinn, T. C., et al., "AIDS in Africa: An Epidemiologic Paradigm," *Science*, 1986:234, pp. 955–963.

12. Guinan, M. E., and A. Hardy, "Epidemiology of AIDS in Women in the United States: 1981–1986," *Journal of the American Medical Association*, 1987:257, pp. 2039–2042; and Centers for Disease Control, "Update:

Heterosexual Transmission of Acquired Immunodeficiency Syndrome and Human Immunodeficiency Virus Infection—United States," *Morbidity and Mortality Weekly Report*, 1989:38, pp. 423–424.

13. Cates, W., quoted in M. F. Goldsmith, "Sex Tied to Drugs = STD Spread," *Journal of the American Medical Association*, 1988:260, p. 2009.

14. Centers for Disease Control, personal communication, January 2, 1990.

15. Ward, J. W., et. al., "Epidemiologic Characteristics of Blood Donors with Antibody to Human Immunodeficiency Virus," *Transfusion*, 1988:28, pp. 298–301.

16. Checola, R. T., et al., "Maternal Drug Abuse and HIV Seropositivity," Fifth International Conference on AIDS, Montreal, Quebec, Canada, 1989, abstract, p. 313; and Landesman, S., et al., "Serosurvey of Human Immunodeficiency Virus Infection in Parturients," *Journal of the American Medical Association*, 1987:258, pp. 2701–2703.

17. Ernst, J. A., et al., "HIV Sero-Prevalence at the Bronx-Lebanon Hospital Center—A CDC Sentinel Hospital," Fifth International Conference on AIDS, Montreal, Quebec, Canada, 1989, abstract, p. 79.

18. Hand, I. L., et al., "Newborn Screening for HIV Seropositivity in the South Bronx," Fifth International Conference on AIDS, Montreal, Quebec, Canada, 1989, abstract, p. 120; and Novick, L. F., et al., "HIV Seroprevalence in Newborns in New York State," *Journal of the American Medical Association*, 1989:261, pp. 1745–1750.

19. *New York City Community Health Atlas* (New York: United Hospital Fund, 1988).

20. Selwyn, P. A., et al., "Prospective Study of Human Immunodeficiency Virus Infection and Pregnancy Outcomes in Intravenous Drug Users," *Journal of the American Medical Association*, 1989:261, pp. 1289–1294.

21. Cohen, J., et al., "Prostitutes and AIDS: Public Policy Issues," *AIDS and Public Policy Journal*, 1988:3, pp. 16–22; Centers for Disease Control, Survey Summaries, "Distribution of AIDS Cases by Racial/Ethnic Group and Exposure Category, June 1, 1981–July 4, 1988," *Morbidity and Mortality Weekly Report*, 1988:37 (no. SS-3), pp. 1–3; Centers for Disease Control, "Update: Heterosexual Transmission of AIDS and HIV Infection"; and Landesman, op. cit.

22. Centers for Disease Control, "Update: Heterosexual Transmission of Acquired Immunodeficiency Syndrome and Human Immunodeficiency Virus Infection."

23. Centers for Disease Control, Survey Summaries, "Distribution of AIDS Cases by Racial/Ethnic Group and Exposure Category."

24. Centers for Disease Control, "Antibody to Human Immunodeficiency Virus in Female Prostitutes," *Morbidity and Mortality Weekly Report*, 1987:36, pp. 157–161.

The Special Needs of Women, Children, and Adolescents

Carol Levine

ALTHOUGH MEDIA ATTENTION AND celebrity visits have drawn the public eye to the plight of hospitalized "AIDS babies," the concrete services that children and their families need are still inadequate in New York City and Northern New Jersey. Other sections of this report have outlined shortcomings in the health care and social service systems that affect all persons with HIV disease. This section will focus on the increasingly urgent needs of the young, which include access to primary medical care, housing, a wide range of social services, foster care, day care, and support services for natural and foster families.

The special needs of women are often neglected in systems designed for a disease that began largely in the male population. While increasing attention is being focused on women as potential vectors of HIV infection to their fetuses, women's needs should not be seen solely in that context. Women who have AIDS or HIV illness need care that is attentive to their individual situations, whether or not they have children or husbands.

Still, most women who need services do have children and face enormous obstacles in providing appropriate care for them. Services for children are in that sense services for their mothers and other family members as well.

Carol Levine, "The Special Needs of Women, Children, and Adolescents," *The Crisis in AIDS Care: A Call to Action,* Working Group of the Citizens Commission on AIDS, March 1989, pp. 63–74. Reprinted by Permission of the Citizens Commission on AIDS for New York City and Northern New Jersey.

How Many Children and Youth Are Affected?

Three main categories of children and youth are affected by HIV/AIDS: (1) those who are HIV-infected or already have AIDS; (2) infants whose HIV status is indeterminate because they are born with their mother's antibodies but may not be truly infected; and (3) those who are not infected but who are deprived of emotional and financial support because a parent or other family member has HIV-related illness or has died of AIDS.

Pediatric Cases

With 1,432 pediatric cases of AIDS, defined as children under 13 years of age, reported to the Centers for Disease Control as of February 20, 1989, New York City leads the nation with 432, or about a third of the cases. New Jersey is second with 187. Florida and California are the only other states reporting significant numbers of children with AIDS. Half of the reported cases have died.[1] The surveillance statistics probably underestimate the number of cases of full-blown AIDS and do not count children with other HIV-related diseases. A recent study of New York City hospitals identified 828 children with CDC-defined AIDS or clinically apparent HIV infection who had received care in 1988; by contrast, the New York City Department of Health Surveillance report of November 1988 listed 134 CDC-defined pediatric AIDS cases in the city.[2]

AIDS now ranks as the ninth leading cause of death nationwide among children aged 1 to 4 years, and the seventh among young people aged 15 to 24, according to Dr. Antonia Novello, deputy director of the National Institute of Child Health and Human Development. She predicts that if present trends continue, in the next 3 or 4 years AIDS will move to fifth place as a killer of Americans from birth to their twenty-fourth birthday.[3] The U.S. Public Health Service estimates that by 1991 there will be a cumulative total of between 10,000 and 20,000 children infected with HIV. Based on the current percentage distribution, this means that between 4,500 and 9,000 of these children will be in New York and New Jersey.[4]

The New York State Department of Health predicts that 700 HIV-infected infants will be born in 1988. Most of these births will occur in New York City, one-third in the Bronx, and the vast majority will be black or Hispanic. The New York Department of Health now estimates that from 1,600 to 4,400 children are HIV-infected. Many of these children will go on to develop AIDS.[5]

Some evidence about transmission comes from a New York State Department of Health HIV seroprevalence study of newborn infants. As of June 30, 1988, more than 158,000 newborn infants in the state had been tested for HIV antibodies. The confirmed presence of antibodies in the infant is a reliable predictor of infection in the mother; an estimated 25 to 40 percent of these infants will themselves be infected. The rest will lose their maternal antibodies, usually within the first year of life. This serosurvey found that one in every 150 women who gave birth in New York State during the previous six months was infected; 87 percent of them were from New York City. The ZIP code breakdown of HIV-positive births in New York City correlates with areas known to have a high prevalence of IV drug use.[6] Selected studies in some hospitals in Brooklyn, Manhattan, and the Bronx indicate rates of infection among pregnant women of ranging from 1 in 50 to 1 in 20.

A similar statewide seroprevalence study conducted over a three-month period by the Department of Health in New Jersey found that of 30,000 newborns tested, 1 in 200 was seropositive (indicating true infection in their mothers). The highest rates were found in Essex and Hudson counties, but only 6 of New Jersey's 21 counties had no antibody-positive infants at all. On the basis of this survey, Commissioner Molly Joel Coye estimates that 200 to 300 babies born each year will be truly HIV-infected.[7] Newark is particularly hard hit: A sample test conducted in University Hospital in Newark in the fall of 1988 showed an extremely high rate of infection—1 in 20 births, or 10 times higher than the state as a whole.[8]

In addition to the infants who are found to be antibody positive at birth, increasing numbers of HIV infection are diagnosed only when the child becomes symptomatic. A recent study of newborns in New York City concluded that the incubation periods between HIV infection and AIDS is longer than previously reported.[9] Therefore, children may not show signs of HIV infection until they reach the age of four or five.

Adolescents

Although the numbers of cases are still low, indications are that AIDS and HIV infection are growing among adolescents in the region. The spread of HIV is linked to drug use and sexual behavior, and young women are affected in almost the same numbers as young men.

If data about newborns and young children are sparse, information about adolescents is almost nonexistent. The CDC has only recently begun to count AIDS among adolescents as a separate category. Relatively few cases (350 through February 1989) have been reported among young people aged 13 to 19. However, it is misleading to look only at AIDS cases. Because of the long latency period between HIV infection and the onset of symptoms, many of the cases of AIDS now being seen in people in their 20s undoubtedly reflect infection in their adolescent years.

Although nationwide the ratio of male to female adolescents with AIDS is 7 to 1, in New York City it is 3 to 1. That ratio approaches the statistics in Africa, where AIDS is predominantly a disease of heterosexual men and women and equal numbers of men and women are infected.

Nationwide, 22 percent of adolescent cases are linked to hemophilia or transfusions with contaminated blood, whereas in New York City these risk factors account for just 11 percent. Twenty-three percent of the adolescents with AIDS in New York City are more likely to report drug use as a risk factor, a much higher figure than elsewhere in the country. Among young women, heterosexual transmission (usually as a result of sex with a drug-using partner) accounts for 52 percent of the adolescent AIDS cases.[10]

IV infection rates among New York City military recruits are higher than the national average. A study of HIV seroprevalence rates among military applicants in four New York counties (New York, Kings, Queens, and the Bronx) showed that "rates for any specified age group were four to ten times greater in these counties than in the rest of the United States." Furthermore, HIV seroprevalence rates among men and women in these four counties were "surprisingly similar, suggesting that infection is occurring in the male and female populations at comparable rates."[11]

Although proportionately fewer adolescents have acquired AIDS through homosexual behaviors, young gay men are clearly at special risk. Homeless youth, many of whom turn to homosexual or heterosexual prostitution and drug use, are another category of adolescents at high risk. (See Section Two, "Housing, Homelessness, and the Impact of HIV Disease.")

HIV is already spreading among adolescents; it will be facilitated by high rates of other sexually transmitted diseases in this population, and by a reluctance to change risky behavior. In the light of these facts, the inadequacy of AIDS education and services especially designed for adolescents is particularly alarming.

Healthy Children in HIV-infected Families

An estimated 10,000 children in New York City will lose both parents to AIDS within the next few years. Another 60,000 to 70,000 will lose one parent.[12] In addition to the growing numbers of children and adolescents who are HIV-infected or who have AIDS there are healthy children who have special needs because their family structure has been disrupted by HIV-related disease. Such children include the healthy siblings of HIV-infected babies. Their mothers, themselves infected and likely to become ill, are often unable to provide appropriate care for either sick or healthy children. Without supervision, nurturing, and emotional support, these healthy children may turn to risky sexual and drug-using behavior. At the very least, they are vulnerable to problems at school and must deal with the stigma associated with AIDS and drug use in their families.

The New York City AIDS Task Force has concluded that "over the next few years a minimum of 60,000 to 70,000 children in New York City will lose at least one parent to AIDS. Of these, maybe 10,000 will lose both parents to the disease."[13] Ernest Drucker and his colleagues at Montefiore Medical Center agree that 10,000 children will be orphaned; they place the number of children who will lose at least one parent at over 100,000, "and in the case of 35,000 children, it will be the parent with whom that child lives."[14]

Another study conducted by the National Women's Health Network estimates that there are between 32,000 and 45,000 infected mothers in New York City (a much higher figure than official New York City Department of Health estimates). If 80 percent of these women develop AIDS or a lethal HIV-related illness, between 26,000 and 36,000 will die. If on the average these women have two uninfected children, a total of 52,272 and 72,000 children will be motherless. Since in many cases the child's father has either died of AIDS, is not present, or is unable to take over the care, the child will be in effect orphaned. Although these figures are based on many still-unproven assumptions, they suggest at the very least a serious problem that has not been addressed at all.[15]

The Economic Impact

Current estimates of the costs of care for HIV-related disease and AIDS vary considerably, depending on the population served, the region of the country, and the services provided. But these estimates generally share one feature: They are based on the care of adults, not children.

A recent study conducted at Harlem Hospital Center suggests that hospital costs for children are different in some respects and probably higher.[16] James D. Hegarty and his colleagues note that the incubation period for pediatric HIV disease is shorter and the cumulative mortality rate higher. Infected children are particularly vulnerable to recurrent episodes of bacteremia, meningitis, and other bacterial infections, as well as to many of the same opportunistic infections that strike adults. Most of these children also experience developmental and growth delays and the social and medical problems associated with poverty and drug use in their families.

The Harlem Hospital study found that the total cost of caring for 37 HIV-infected children from 1981 to 1986 was $3,362,597, or an average lifetime cost of $90,347 per child. One-third of the total inpatient days and more than 20 percent of the cost resulted from social factors. "Boarder babies" had a mean length of stay nearly 4 times longer than those with homes (339 days versus 89 days), although their daily costs were lower ($466) than for babies with opportunistic infections ($705 per day) who required intensive medical interventions. By comparison, the average daily costs at St. Clare's Home for Children, a transitional residence in Elizabeth, New Jersey, for children with AIDS or HIV infection, are $260.[17] The key factors predicting length of stay were not medical but social: maternal intravenous drug use and the lack of a suitable home.

In reviewing 1986 data, the New York State Department of Health found that more than one-third of the pediatric AIDS cases had an average length of stay per hospitalization of more than 50 days; the longest length of stay was 129.5 days. In 1987, nearly one-third of the hospital stays was 40 or more days. Because large numbers of children have not historically needed home care or long-term care, virtually no such services exist.[18]

A study conducted at Yale–New Haven Hospital found that 54 percent of the days spent in the hospital by 34 HIV-infected children were "medically unnecessary."[19] Nearly all of the unnecessary stays over 3 weeks resulted from difficulties in placing the child after discharge. The proportion of medically unnecessary days was actually lower than those reported in 1983 and 1984, due to improved outpatient services offered by the hospital.

These studies conclude that improved outpatient medical and social services could substantially reduce the costs of care. However, they do not consider the indirect costs to society that will result from premature mortality and morbidity, or the social and human costs of inappropriate hospitalization of children.

Any assessment of indirect costs should also account for the long-term impact on the economy of the future loss of productivity among HIV-infected young people. In her report to Dr. Bowen, Dr. Novello pointed out that the current population of young people aged 11 to 24 is unusually small to begin with. "If AIDS were to make serious inroads in this group, the long-term consequences could be disastrous for the nation's economy."[20] Since adolescents in the New York City-Northern New Jersey region are most at risk, this region's economy may be the hardest hit in the nation.

The Major Needs

Several groups have already issued reports on the major needs of children and adolescents affected by HIV/AIDS, and have proposed remedies. Although some encouraging individual projects are underway or planned, none of these reports has resulted in dramatically increased services.

In April 1987 the Citizens Committee for Children of New York issued a report entitled "The Invisible Emergency: Children and AIDS in New York." The Citizens Committee found that "[HIV-infected] children and their families have intense medical and social support needs that are not being adequately met by the network of services available in New York City."[21] Services most difficult to obtain, the report concluded, are safe and decent housing, foster home placement, adequate stimulation and recreational services for the children, and counseling services for their parents.

New York City's Strategic Plan for AIDS, issued in May 1988, which covers only city agencies, included a section on pediatric AIDS prepared by the Health and Hospitals Corporation. The plan contains some specific goals and timetables but so far no reports have been issued to document progress or lack of it in meeting these goals.[22]

The New York City AIDS Task Force, a public-private collaboration organized by the New York City Department of Health, has addressed the problems of providing care for adolescents and children. Its report, entitled "Models of Care," outlines several constraints in providing care for adolescents. Specifically, the report notes that health care facilities are usually organized to provide care for adults or young children, and that the few existing adolescent health services do not have staff to accommodate new HIV-related services. Adolescents living on their own do not have access to public or private health insurance. Even when they are able to obtain medical care, they often cannot afford drugs and other medical supplies. Existing drug treatment facilities usually exclude minors, and housing for homeless youth and HIV-positive adolescents is difficult to obtain.[23]

The Task Force recommended that New York State and New York City "establish special funding for purposes of providing medical care and psychosocial support services to HIV-positive youth." It also recommended, among other things, the development of group homes for homeless youth under 18 years of age with multiple problems, and residences and shelters for homeless youth 18 to 21 years of age.

The Task Force noted that long-term care and respite services for children are severely limited, that there are tremendous difficulties in recruiting foster parents for HIV-infected children, and that there is community resistance to group homes for HIV-infected children. Among its recommendations were the provision of mental health services for children to lessen the psychological impact of AIDS, and the continuation of financial incentives to attract more foster care parents. "The aim," the Task Force said, "should be to place every abandoned or orphaned HIV-infected child who cannot be placed with relatives in a foster home." However, it stressed that natural families should be given assistance in cash and services to maintain their children at home if at all possible.[24]

The New York State 5-Year Interagency Plan calls for a broad array of services for women, children, and families, and reports that "a major Department of Health initiative is underway to augment services within the AIDS center system for children, adolescents, pregnant women and their families."[25] These initiatives, if implemented, would make an enormous difference. However, since the five-year plan does not contain any funding sources, the program goals may never be reached.

The New York City AIDS Fund issued its "Needs Assessment" in October 1988. The Fund is a private sector collaboration of the National Community AIDS Partnership, a project of the Ford Foundation, and grantmaking organizations in New York City. It found that the outstanding needs for adolescents and preadolescents are: primary prevention/education programs for those youngsters not yet sexually active and/or abusing drugs; and behavior change strategies tailored to adolescent subpopulations at especially high risk. For infants and children the priority needs are: expanded and improved family supports and foster care resources, services for uninfected children of parents and/or siblings with HIV infection or AIDS, and family-oriented prevention and care services.[26]

In a comparable effort in New Jersey, the New Jersey AIDS Fund recently completed its needs assessment. It found that private funds are particularly needed to support the recruitment of foster parents for children with AIDS and to underwrite a new transitional residence in Monmouth County and at least 2 more additional homes in southern and northern New Jersey. The Fund also identified day care for adults and children as pressing needs.

Existing Models of Care

While existing facilities and services are inadequate to meet future needs, they do provide some replicable models if the necessary funding and support were provided:

Acute Care Units

Children with AIDS and some with HIV infection need the specialized care that is available on an inpatient basis. Some hospitals have established special units offering comprehensive medical care and access to experimental drugs for pediatric patients. Such units have been established at Harlem Hospital, Albert Einstein College of Medicine, and the Newark Children's Hospital.

Transitional Pediatric Residences

St. Clare's Home in Elizabeth, New Jersey, serves as a transitional facility for children with AIDS who do not need to be hospitalized and are awaiting placement with a foster family or return to their natural family.[27] The home, located near the grounds of St. Elizabeth's Hospital, was opened with the support of the community, including volunteer labor for remodeling. St. Clare's can accommodate 5 babies at a time and provides a comprehensive set of services. Operated by a nonprofit organization called AIDS Resource Foundation for Children (ARFC), St. Clare's is funded by a grant from the New Jersey Department of Health, the State's Division of Youth and Family Services, Medicaid payments, and private contributions. ARFC has opened a second home in Jersey City and is planning a third in Monmouth County. It also operates Haller House in Newark, which provides housing as well as a variety of services for children with AIDS.

In New York City, the Association to Benefit Children is planning to open a Child Center in Yorkville. It will be the primary home for six abandoned, homeless infants diagnosed with AIDS or non-HIV-related handicapping conditions, until they can be placed in families. There are also plans to provide on-site day care for 10 other babies with similar problems. An extensive volunteer program is planned to supplement the staff efforts. Funding will come from Medicaid and the New York City Human Resources Administration.

The Children's Center, a pediatric residence, has opened in Brooklyn (after considerable community protest), and the Archdiocese of New York is also planning to open a residential facility for children.

Day Care Facilities

Many children with AIDS and HIV infection are able to attend regular day care and educational programs. However, some are too ill or too developmentally delayed to participate in these mainstream programs and need special services. The Bronx Municipal Hospital and the Albert Einstein College of Medicine operate a day care program for children with AIDS and ARC that can accommodate 25 children per day, ranging in age from infancy to age 7. Medical support is provided by a nurse on site and by the Bronx Municipal Hospital Center pediatric staff.

The Parent/Child Extension Center, a day care center that incorporates a Head Start program, broke ground in October in Newark, and is expected to begin operations shortly. Operated by the Babyland Nursery of the New Community Corporation, it will eventually care for 30 children and will receive state and federal support to provide day care, preschool programs, and medical care in a previously vacant building.[28]

Adolescent Services

Special health care services for adolescents are provided at Montefiore Medical Center in the Bronx and at The Door, an adolescent health program in Manhattan. The Hetrick-Martin Institute provides services to gay and lesbian youth. Covenant House provides temporary housing for homeless youth and has just opened a special section of their Manhattan facility for adolescents with HIV infection or AIDS.

Foster Care

Financial incentives—a monthly rate of $1,177 a month, which is at least double the standard rate—are provided in New York City to foster care families who take children with AIDS, and the problem of "boarder babies" has been somewhat ameliorated. The Leake and Watts Home in Yonkers has been a leader in providing foster care for New York City children. In New Jersey, the Children's Hospital AIDS Program of Newark has been providing comprehensive services to children and their families; by the end of 1987, 55 percent of the children receiving care at Children's Hospital were in some type of foster care setting (an increase of 20 percent over the previous year).[29] However, foster care systems have many problems of their own, and placing a child in foster care does not end the need for special services. Many of the developmental problems associated with HIV infection are discovered only when the child has been placed in a family setting.[30]

What Must Be Done

The studies and surveys so far have reached many of the same conclusions: AIDS and HIV infection present special problems among newborns, children, and adolescents. The major needs are:

1. Access to primary medical care, with an emphasis on early diagnosis and intervention and continuity of comprehensive care.
2. Housing appropriate for the child's age, family status, and health. Especially urgent is the need for transitional residences for HIV-infected children who do not need to be hospitalized but who do not have biological or foster families able to care for them. Another urgent need is for housing for homeless HIV-infected adolescents.
3. Social services that include case management, mental health services, recreational opportunities, legal advocacy, and special educational services for developmental problems.
4. Day care for children who are too ill to be able to attend regular day care facilities.
5. Family supports (whether for natural or foster families) that enable children to be raised in a nurturing environment.
6. Special services for uninfected children whose parents or siblings are ill with AIDS or HIV infection.

While the costs of providing the services and programs that meet these needs will be significant, the costs of not doing so will be even greater. A society that claims to support "family values" cannot ignore the most needy of its children.

NOTES

1. Centers for Disease Control, *AIDS Weekly Surveillance Report* (5 December 1988).

2. Citizens Committee for Children, United Hospital Fund, and Gay Men's Health Crisis, *The Invisible Emergency Continues: The Problem of Unreported Cases of HIV-Infected Children in New York City* (24 February 1989), 3.

3. Antonia Novello, report to Dr. Otis R. Bowen, Secretary of Health and Human Services, reported in *The New York Times*, 20 December 1988.

4. U.S. Public Health Service, "Report of the Second Public Health Service AIDS Prevention and Control Conference," *Public Health Reports* 103, supplement no. 1 (1988), 94.

5. New York City Department of Health, *Report of the Expert Panel on HIV Seroprevalence Estimates and AIDS Case Projection Methodologies* (New York: February 1989), 5.

6. State of New York, *AIDS: New York's Response: A 5-Year Intragency Plan* (Albany, NY: February 1989), 18.

7. Robert Schwaneberg, "One in 200 Jersey Newborns Tests Positive for AIDS Virus," *The (Newark) Star-Ledger*, 10 February 1989, 1, 38.

8. P. L. Wyckoff, "Babies Born in Newark Will Be Tested Anonymously for AIDS Antibodies," *The (Newark) Star-Ledger*, 15 March 1988, 26.

9. I. Auger et al., "Incubation Periods for Paediatric AIDS Patients," *Nature* 336, no. 8 (December 1988): 575–577.

10. Sten H. Vermund, Karen Hein, Helene D. Gayle, et al., "Acquired Immunodeficiency Syndrome among Adolescents in New York," *Journal of Diseases in Children*, 1989.

11. Donald S. Burke et al., "Demography of HIV Infections among Civilian Applicants for Military Service in Four Counties in New York City," *New York State Journal of Medicine* (May 1987): 262–264.

12. New York City AIDS Task Force, *Models of Care Report* (December 1988), 42.

13. New York City Aids Task Force, *Service Model for Persons Infected with the Human Immunodeficiency Virus* (December 1988), 42.

14. Ernest Drucker et al., "IV Drug Users with AIDS in New York City: A Study of Dependent Children, Housing and Drug Addiction Treatment," Montefiore Medical Center, Albert Einstein College of Medicine, Department of Epidemiology and Social Medicine, 20 July, 1988, 19.

15. Chris Norwood, "AIDS Orphans in New York City: Projected Numbers and Policy Demands," National Women's Health Network (September 1988).

16. James D. Hegarty et al., "The Medical Care Costs of Human Immunode-ficiency Virus—Infected Children in Harlem," *Journal of the American Medical Association* 260, no. 13 (8 October, 1988): 1901–1905.

17. Terrence P. Zealand, "St. Clare's Home for Children: A Transitional Residence for Children with AIDS," *QRB* (January 1989): 18.

18. New York State, *AIDS: New York's Response*, 88.

19. Kathi Kemper and Brian Forsyth, "Medically Unnecessary Hospital Use in Children Seropositive for Human Immunodeficiency Virus," *Journal of the American Medical Association* 260, no. 13 (8 October, 1988): 1906–1909.

20. Novello, 84–85.

21. Citizens Committee for Children of New York, Inc., *The Invisible Emergency: Children and AIDS in New York* (New York: April 1987), 50.

22. Interagency Task Force on AIDS, *New York City Strategic Plan for AIDS*, section E.2 (May 1988), 16–18.

23. New York City AIDS Task Force, *Service Model for Persons Infected with the Human Immunodeficiency Virus* (December 1988), 29–31.

24. Ibid., 42–44.

25. *AIDS: New York's Response*, 86–89.

26. New York City AIDS Fund, *AIDS, Community Needs and Private Funding: A Needs Assessment for New York City* (October 1988), 30.

27. Zealand, "St. Clare's Home for Children," 17–20.

28. Joan Whitlow, "A Caring Place," *The (Newark) Star-Ledger*, 5 October 1988, 1, 53.

29. Mary G. Boland, Patricia Evans, Edward M. O'Connor, and James M. Oleske, "Foster Care Needs of Children with HIV Infection," *AIDS & Public Policy Journal* 3, no. 1 (Winter 1988): 8–9.

30. Suzanne Daley, "Study of Foster Infants Finds New York City Failed Them," *The New York Times*, 1 February. 1989, A1, B5.

HIV AND THE RIGHT TO HEALTH CARE

Introduction

America is facing a health care crisis of mammoth proportions. This crisis has been building for at least twenty years due to three essential factors: (1) the centralization of health care in university hospitals where exotic research is funded at the expense of primary care; (2) the lopsided demographics of health care providers where those areas in most need have the fewest practitioners and those in least need have an overabundance; (3) an across-the-board decrease in both federally funded insurance under Aid to Families and Dependent Children (AFDC), Medicaid, and disability insurance in the Reagan years and an equally broad-based decrease in private insurance coverage due to both employee benefits cutbacks and a significant increase in relative unemployment (30 percent of Americans are temporary employees. As temporary employees they are not eligible for employer-paid health insurance, life insurance, or retirement benefits). Currently, America has a real unemployment rate as severe as any since the Depression of the 1930s.

Thirty-seven million Americans are without health care coverage of any kind: commercial, federal, or state. The media representation of the health care needy shows urban public hospitals with emergency room overflows so great that a 2–3 day wait for a bed is not unusual. It represents a system where there are incredible shortages of doctors for basic medicine. The kind of medicine that prevents asthma from being a life-threatening illness. Public and private hospitals are operating in such debt that no one foresees relief for the next 10 years. This debt, in fact, is seen to be one that will become critical in a few years.

The crisis is not one only of financial factors. We are faced with a crisis in "care" that involves not only the issues of deficits for hospitals, a dearth of hospital beds, a shortage of health care personnel, but the equally important obstacles to health caused by a lack of preventive, continuous, and rehabilitative care. This lack of *caretaking* has long been a fact of life for the poor and now is increasingly experienced by middle-class Americans. The crisis in care is a crisis in conception of health care. A crisis that requires us to rework our health care system to provide local and community-based care, clinic care, home care, and management of chronic disease. The crisis in health care is a crisis, more than anything else, in primary care medicine—medicine that is the entree to comprehensive basic care and that administers to long-term and debilitating disease. Nowhere are the inadequacies in the health care system more apparent than in the AIDS health care crisis.

The readings in this section attempt to accomplish two things. They are designed to acquaint the reader with the current status of health care access (benefits) for Americans by concentrating on the numbers of Americans who are uninsured and, as a result, underserved by our health care system. The second aim of the chapter is to spell out how the financial crisis affects the utilization of health care services and, as in the HIV crisis, has led to the lack of comprehensive and wide-ranging health services absolutely essential to the viability of people who are chronically ill.

The first article details the extent to which Americans are without health care due to the lack of either private or public insurance. "Uninsured and Underserved: Inequities in Health Care in the United States," completed in 1981 without cognizance of the HIV epidemic, documents the disturbing fact that 37 million Americans[1] go without health care because they cannot pay for it. Some of the study's conclusions are daunting: The uninsured population, whether covered for all or part of the year, is almost entirely under age 65. The highest rate of uninsured is in the age range of 19–24. The next highest rate is among the 25–54 year olds.[2] Rural areas of America are worse off than urban areas in terms of insurance coverage, but urban areas have appreciably higher numbers of people with health needs. Those having the greatest need of health care, blacks and Hispanics, have substantially less insurance coverage for physician visits than do whites and have the least utilization of such visits. Insured minorities, on the other hand, receive 80 to 90 percent more ambulatory care than uninsured minorities. The insured receive 90 percent more inpatient hospital care than the uninsured. In urban settings, the uninsured primarily rely on the emergency rooms of public hospitals for their entry into the health care system. Only about 50 percent of uninsured blacks and Hispanics have a physician office as their source of health care. Seventy-one percent of the insured in both metropolitan and nonmetropolitan areas have a physician's care. As the Davis and Rowland article indicates, our health care system is stratified by class. Current indicators are that fewer than 25 percent of New York City's minority community have a physician's office as their source of health care.[3]

The authors of this study indicate that the lack of insurance is the major barrier to health care. This barrier has three major consequences: unnecessary pain and suffering, disability, and death; increased financial burdens on the uninsured who struggle to budget into their household finances health care costs; increased financial strains upon hospitals, physicians, and other health care providers. Added to this lack of health care and its financial costs has been a 25 percent[4] cut in health care financing to municipalities at the federal level, replaced piecemeal by separate funding to crisis points through "targeted approaches" to overwhelmed institutions.

Davis and Rowland display the landscape of the American health care system prior to any systemic crisis like the HIV epidemic. Essentially, what they document is a two-tiered system of health care where those who need health care most are increasingly unlikely to receive it and where the public hospital system serves needs both inappropriate to it and needs overwhelming to its own ratios of beds and caretakers.

What the Davis and Rowland article does not document is the financing mechanisms available to Americans at the private and public insurance levels. America is the only developed country besides South Africa that does not have a national health system. Almost completely privately owned and operated, the American health care system is funded by a combination of public and private insurance. The major funders are private insurance companies, health maintenance organizations, and the federal and state governments. "Health Benefits: How the System Is Responding to AIDS" gives a detailed account of what programs are available to those who find themselves with a chronic disease like those exemplified by HIV affection. The work, a project of the National Health Law Program, gives a microscopic view of the relative jeopardy any person with a debilitating illness is placed in by the American health care system. It also serves as a handbook for those trying to negotiate such a system. Finally, what the article discloses is how "flexible" the levels of the system are as the federal and state governments and almost all private carriers try to cut back on funding for HIV-related illnesses while the need to increase them grows exponentially; and those in need are represented by suits brought by such networks as the National Health Law Program. One of the most frightening aspects of "Health Benefits: How the System Is Responding to AIDS" is the almost wholesale blocking of the HIV-affected from purchasing or remaining on private insurance coverage. As with the poor, a lack of insurance is not the only problem. A recent study also showed that two-thirds of new physicians in a study of 1,000 residents in the United States preferred not to treat individuals with HIV infection. One quarter expressly went into medical specialties that would allow them to avoid the HIV-affected. As one researcher revealed: "The problem that HIV patients face may well be compounded in the future by a lack of physicians willing to treat them."[5]

A look at how a crumbling health care system of New York City *begins*[6] to deal with the HIV epidemic is provided in two articles from the Citizens Commission on AIDS. "AIDS and the Future of Hospital Care" offers a detailed analysis of the hospital care system itself and the paradoxical demands that AIDS cases place on a system reliant upon hospital care as the locus of caretaking. Care for the HIV-affected individual is care that should be local and long-term. These are requirements that the health care system in New York City is not designed to meet and yet must. The urgency of this health-care imperative is discussed in "Long-term Care: A Long-term Commitment."

The final article in this section is the personal testimony of a staff attorney at a gay rights legal advocacy agency in New York City who is also a person with AIDS. What David Barr highlights is the absolutely crucial role that his physician plays in his treatment and the quality of his life with the HIV virus. Mr. Barr contrasts his own care with that of a young Hispanic woman in the Bronx, New York, who is seropositive and whose only access to medical care is through the hospital system. Barr's testimony demonstrates quite vividly the two-class system of health care that has developed in America which allows a white male to have "state of the art" health care from his private physician while a poor woman of color can only rely upon the overcrowded and overutilized resources of the public hospital system.

NOTES

1. The authors' statistic for 1981 is 24 million. The current rate is 37 million.

2. AIDS is the leading killer of people in urban environments between the ages of 25 and 40 years of age.

3. A recent study by the Community Service Society, "Building Primary Care in New York City's Low-Income Communities," 1990, shows that these utilization patterns are not only due to a lack of insurance benefits but are also due to a dearth of primary-care physicians in low-income areas. CSS found 27 physicians in private practice providing basic care to 1.7 million residents of New York City's 9 lowest-income neighborhoods.

4. Figures for the loss of general federal revenue to metropolitan areas from 1981 until the present vary greatly. The consensus is that the loss amounts to at least 50 percent. When Ronald Reagan took office, federal dollars provided 20 percent of the New York City budget. It provided only 10 percent in 1989.

5. Molly Cooke, M.D., "Which Physicians Will Provide Care?" (Paper presented at the VI International AIDS Conference, San Francisco, California, June 1990).

6. Ninety percent of the full-blown AIDS cases are yet to occur.

Uninsured and Underserved: Inequities in Health Care in the United States

Karen Davis and Diane Rowland

THE UNITED STATES HAS one of the highest-quality and most sophisticated systems of medical care in the world. Most Americans take for granted their access to this system of care. In times of emergency or illness, they can call upon a vast array of health resources—from a family physician to a complex teaching hospital—assured that they will receive needed care and that their health insurance coverage will pick up the tab for the majority of bills incurred.

For a surprisingly large segment of the United States population, however, this ease of access to care does not exist. At any point in time, over 25 million Americans have no health insurance coverage from private health insurance plans or public programs (Kasper et al., 1978). Without health insurance coverage or ready cash, such individuals can be and are turned away from hospitals even in emergency situations (U.S. Congress. House. Committee on Energy and Commerce, 1981). Some neglect obtaining preventive or early care, often postponing care until conditions have become life-threatening. Others struggle with burdensome medical bills. Many come to rely upon crowded, understaffed public hospitals as the only source of reliable, available care.

The absence of universal health insurance coverage creates seri-

Karen Davis, Ph.D., and Diane Rowland, Ph.D., "Uninsured and Underserved: Inequities in Health Care in the United States," *Milbank Quarterly:* Health and Society 61, no. 2 (1983). Reprinted by Permission of the *Milbank Quarterly*, Milbank Memorial Fund.

ous strains in our society. These strains are felt most acutely by the uninsured poor, who must worry about family members—a sick child, an adult afflicted with a deteriorating chronic health condition, a pregnant mother—going without needed medical assistance. It strains our image as a just and humane society when significant portions of the population endure avoidable pain, suffering, and even death because of an inability to pay for health care. Those physicians, other health professionals, and institutions that try to assist this uninsured group also incur serious strain. Demands typically far outstrip available time and resources. Strain is also felt by local governments whose communities include many uninsured persons, because locally funded public hospitals and health centers inevitably incur major financial deficits. In recent years, many of the public facilities that have traditionally been the source of last-resort care have closed, thereby intensifying the stresses on other providers and the uninsured poor.

As serious as these strains have been in the last five years, the years ahead promise to strain the fabric of our social life even more seriously. Unemployment levels today are the highest since the Great Depression. With unemployment, the American worker loses not only a job but also health insurance protection. As unemployment rises and the numbers of the uninsured grow, fewer and fewer resources are available to fill the gaps in health care coverage. Major reductions in funding for health services for the poor and uninsured have been made in the last year; further reductions are likely. Deepening economic recession, high unemployment, and declining sales revenues are strapping the fiscal resources of state and local governments. Their ability to offset federal cutbacks seems limited. Nor can the private sector be expected to bridge this gap. The health industry is increasingly becoming an entrepreneurial business endeavor—with little room for charitable actions.

It is especially timely, therefore, to review what we know about the consequences of inadequate health insurance coverage for certain segments of our population. The first section of this paper presents information on the number and characteristics of the uninsured, while the second section describes patterns of health care utilization by the uninsured. The third section assesses the policy implications of these facts and offers recommendations for future public policy to ensure access to health care for all.

Who Are the Uninsured?

The 1977 National Medical Care Expenditure Survey (NMCES) provides extensive information on the health insurance coverage of the U.S. population. Six household interviews of a nationwide sample of over 40,000 individuals were conducted over an 18-month period during 1977 and 1978. By following the interviewed population for an entire year, NMCES provided a comprehensive portrait of health insurance coverage, including changes in health insurance status during the course of that year.

Although the scope of the NMCES survey provides extensive information on the characteristics and utilization patterns of the uninsured, it should be noted that the profile of the uninsured presented here describes the portion of the population without insurance in 1977. Recent changes in health insurance coverage due to unemployment and cutbacks in eligibility for Medicaid have increased the size of the nation's uninsured population, but are not reflected in the statistics in this paper.

In the NMCES results, individuals classified as insured are those who were covered throughout the year by Medicaid, Medicare, the Civilian Health and Medical Program of the Uniformed Services (Champus), Blue Cross/Blue Shield or commercial health insurance, or who were enrolled in a health maintenance organization. Differences in scope of coverage among the insured were not available, although further analysis of the NMCES data will address this issue. Therefore, many individuals in the insured category may have actually had very limited health insurance coverage, leaving them basically uninsured for most services. For example, many individuals classified as insured have coverage for inpatient hospital care, but are not covered and are, therefore, essentially uninsured for primary care in a physician's office. In contrast, insured individuals also include those enrolled in a health maintenance organization offering comprehensive coverage for both inpatient and ambulatory care.

The uninsured fall into two groups: the always uninsured and the sometimes uninsured. The always uninsured are individuals without Medicare, Medicaid, or private insurance coverage for the entire year. Individuals using Veterans Administration hospitals and clinics or community health centers are classified as uninsured unless they have third-party coverage. The sometimes uninsured are those who were covered by public or private insurance part of the year but were uninsured the remainder of the year. The sometimes uninsured include the medically needy individuals who qualify for Medicaid coverage during periods of large medical expenses, but are otherwise uninsured. Changes in insurance status during the year are generally the result of loss of employment, change in employment, change in income or family situation that alters eligibility for Medicaid, or loss of private insurance when an older spouse retires and becomes eligible for Medicare.

A snapshot view of the uninsured at a given point in time understates the number of people who spend some portion of the year uninsured. At any one time, there are over 25 million uninsured Americans, but as many as 34 million may be uninsured for some period of time during the year. Approximately 18 million are without insurance for the entire year, and 16 million are uninsured for some portion of the year (Wilensky and Walden, 1981; Wilensky and Berk, 1982).

The 34 million uninsured are persons of all incomes, racial and ethnic backgrounds, occupations, and geographic locations. In some cases whole families are uninsured, while in others coverage is mixed depending on employment status and eligibility for public programs (Kasper et al., 1978). However, the poor, minorities, young adults, and rural residents are more likely than others to be uninsured. As noted in Table 1, over one-quarter of all blacks and minorities are uninsured during the year—a rate of 1½ times that of whites. This disparity holds across the demographic and social characteristics of the uninsured (Wilensky and Walden, 1981; Institute of Medicine, 1981).

Age

The uninsured population, whether covered for all or part of a year, is almost entirely under age 65. Nearly one-fifth of the non-aged population is uninsured for some or all of the year. Less than 1 percent of the aged, barely 200,000 persons, are uninsured during the year (Table 1). This is attributable primarily to Medicare, which provides basic coverage for hospital and physician services to most older Americans. The success of Medicare in providing financial access to health care for the elderly is demonstrated by the extensive coverage of the elderly today in contrast to the dramatic lack of insurance prior to implementation of Medicare in 1966 (Davis, 1982). Medicaid and private insurance help to fill the gap for those elderly persons ineligible for Medicare because they lack sufficient Social Security earnings contributions. The uninsured elderly are primarily individuals with incomes above the eligibility levels for welfare assistance and Medicaid.

Table 1

Insurance Status during Year by Age and Race, 1977

Age and Race	Total	Always uninsured	Uninsured part of year	Always insured
	Number in millions			
Total, all persons	212.1	18.1	15.9	178.1
Persons under age 65	189.8	18.0	15.8	156.0
White	163.7	14.5	12.5	136.7
Black and other	26.1	3.5	3.3	19.3
Persons age 65 and over	22.3	0.1	0.1	22.1
White	20.2	0.07	0.09	20.0
Black and other	2.1	0.03	0.01	2.1
	Percentage			
All persons	100%	8.6%	7.5%	83.9%
Persons under age 65	100	9.5	8.3	82.2
White	100	8.9	7.6	83.5
Black and other	100	13.3	12.7	74.0
Persons age 65 and over	100	0.4	0.5	99.1
White	100	0.3	0.5	99.2
Black and other	100	1.0	0.8	98.2

Source: Data from the U.S. Department of Health and Human Services, National Center for Health Services Research, National Medical Care Expenditure Survey.

Examination of the uninsured by age group reveals that young adults are the group most likely to be uninsured. As highlighted in Table 2, almost one-third of all persons aged 19 to 24 are uninsured during the course of a year. Roughly 16 percent of this age group are without coverage all year, and an additional 14 percent lack coverage at least part of the year. This rate is nearly double that of other age groups. A variety of factors undoubtedly contribute to this situation. Young adults frequently lose coverage under their parents' policies at age 18. Many young adults may elect to forego coverage when it is available, since coverage is costly and they assume themselves to be relatively healthy. High youth unemployment, as well as employment in marginal jobs without health benefits, make insurance difficult to obtain or afford for this group.

Table 2
Percent Uninsured during Year
by Selected Population Characteristics, 1977

Population characteristic	Percentage uninsured during year	Percentage always uninsured	Percentage uninsured part of year
All persons	16.1%	8.6%	7.5%
Age			
Under age 65	17.8	9.5	8.3
less than 6 years	19.6	8.3	11.3
6 to 18 years	16.1	8.6	7.5
19 to 24 years	30.3	16.0	14.3
25 to 54 years	16.1	8.7	7.4
55 to 64 years	12.6	8.2	4.4
Age 65 and over	0.9	0.4	0.5
Occupation			
Farm	22.3	15.9	6.4
Blue collar	19.8	11.3	8.5
Services	20.8	11.9	8.9
White collar	12.6	5.6	7.0
Region			
Northeast	10.7	5.4	5.3
North Central	12.5	5.7	6.8
South	20.5	11.6	8.9
West	20.8	11.7	9.1

Source: Wilensky and Walden (1981), and data from the U.S. Department of Health and Human Services, National Center for Health Services Research, National Medical Care Expenditure Survey.

Employment

Employment status and occupation are important factors in assessing the likelihood of being uninsured for all or part of a year. Most American workers receive their health care coverage through the workplace, but insurance coverage varies widely depending on the type of employer (Taylor and Lawson, 1981). Employees of small firms are less likely to be insured than employees of large firms. For example, 45 percent of employees in firms of 25 or fewer employees do not have employer-provided health insurance compared with only 1 percent of firms with more than 1,000 employees. Yet, small firms employ over 20 percent of all workers. Unionized firms are 6 times more likely to have employee health insurance than are nonunionized firms.

Insurance status varies by type of employment (Table 2). Nearly one-quarter of all agriculture workers are uninsured during the year, with 16 percent uninsured for the entire year. As expected, white-collar workers are the most likely to be insured, while blue-collar and service workers fare only somewhat better than agricultural workers (Wilensky and Walden, 1981). Among blue-collar and service workers, insurance coverage is low in the construction industry, wholesale and retail trades, and service industries, and high in manufacturing. Of manufacturing employees, 96 percent have health insurance through their place of employment (Davis, 1975).

Residence

These trends in coverage by employment are reflected in the regional picture of insurance status. In the heavily industrial and unionized Northeast and North Central regions of the country, the percentage of uninsured during the year is half that of the South and the West. In these areas where agricultural interests are strong and unionization less extensive, over 20 percent of the population is uninsured during the course of a year. Of those living in the South and West, 11 percent are uninsured throughout the year compared with 5 percent in the Northeast and North Central regions. Similarly, people in metropolitan areas are more likely to be insured than people living outside metropolitan areas (Wilensky and Walden, 1981).

Income and Race

However, while nature of employment and unionization may explain some of the regional variations, a critical underlying factor in the analysis is the distribution in the population of poverty and minorities. Residents of the South comprise 32 percent of the total population under age 65. Yet 48 percent of the nation's minorities live in the South (Department of Health and Human Services, 1982a). The higher concentration of poor and minority persons in the South in comparison with other parts of the country helps explain the high level of uninsured individuals.

Poverty and lack of insurance are strongly correlated. Of poor families with incomes below 125 percent of the poverty line, 27 percent are uninsured. The near-poor, with incomes between 125 and 200 percent of poverty, fare only slightly better, with 21 percent uninsured during the year. The poor are always more likely to be uninsured than the middle and upper income groups (Table 3) (Wilensky and Walden, 1981).

The limited health insurance coverage for the poor and near-poor demonstrates the limits of coverage of the poor under Medicaid (Wilensky and Berk, 1982). Many assume that Medicaid finances health care services for all of the poor. However, many poor persons are ineligible for Medicaid due to categorical requirements for program eligibility and variations in state eligibility policies. Two-parent families are generally ineligible for Medicaid and single adults are covered only if they are aged or disabled (Davis and Schoen, 1978). Moreover, many states have established income eligibility cutoffs well below the poverty level. Many states have not adjusted income levels to account for inflation, resulting in a reduction in the number of individuals covered over the last few years (Rowland and Gaus, 1983). As a result of the restrictions on Medicaid cover-

Table 3
Percent Uninsured during Year
by Ethnic/Racial Background and Income, 1977*

Ethnic/Racial Background	Percentage uninsured during year	Percentage always uninsured	Percentage uninsured part of year
White, all incomes	14.0	7.0	7.0
Poor	27.1	13.5	13.6
Other low income	21.0	10.9	10.1
Middle income	12.6	6.3	6.3
High income	8.8	4.2	4.6
Black, all incomes	23.2	9.7	13.5
Poor	32.2	10.6	21.6
Other low income	26.6	11.9	14.7
Middle income	17.4	8.6	8.8
High income	12.4	7.1	5.3
Hispanic, all incomes	24.3	12.8	11.5
Poor	29.6	9.5	20.1
Other low income	32.0	18.2	13.8
Middle income	17.7	12.4	5.3
High income	20.0	12.3	8.0

Source: Wilensky and Walden (1981).
* In 1977, the poverty level for a family of 4 was $8,000. Poor are defined as those whose family income was less than or equal to 125 percent of the 1977 poverty level. Other low income includes those whose income is 1.26 to 2 times the poverty level; middle income is 2.01 to 4 times the poverty level; and high income is 4.01 times the poverty level or more.

age, about 60 percent of the poor are not covered by Medicaid. Of the 35 million poor and near-poor in 1977, almost 5 million or about 15 percent had no insurance throughout 1977. Approximately 35 percent were on Medicaid for at least part of the year (Wilensky and Berk, 1982). This situation can only be expected to worsen as the recession swells the numbers of poor and near-poor while cutbacks in social programs and Medicaid further erode the health coverage available to some of the poor.

Thus, while the poor are obviously the least able to pay for care directly, they are the most likely to be without either Medicaid or private insurance. The poor are twice as likely to be uninsured as the middle class and three times as likely as those in upper income groups. Lack of insurance is inversely related to ability to bear the economic consequences of ill health.

Blacks, Hispanics, and other minorities are also more likely to be uninsured than whites regardless of their income; poor blacks are the most likely to be uninsured. As noted in Table 3, nearly one-third of poor blacks are uninsured during a year. If you are poor and a member of a minority group, your chances of being uninsured are four times as great as for a high income white.

Yet this relationship between race and income (Table 3) actually understates the situation because the aged are included in the population analyzed. The aged are overrepresented in the lower income groups, but, as noted in Table 1, almost all of the aged are insured. Thus, inclusion of the aged in Table 3 tends to overstate the insured status of the nonelderly poor.

Regional and racial differences in insurance coverage for the population under age 65 are enumerated in Table 4. When the aged are excluded from the analysis, the differentials become even more striking. Southerners are nearly 1½ times as likely to be uninsured as those from other parts of the country. But blacks in the South are 1½ times more likely to be uninsured as are whites from the South or nonsouthern blacks. Southern blacks are twice as likely to be uninsured as nonsouthern whites.

Similarly, when differences in insurance status are assessed from the perspective of metropolitan versus nonmetropolitan areas, blacks fare much worse than whites. Over 16 percent of nonelderly residents of Standard Metropolitan Statistical Areas (SMSAs) are uninsured compared with over 21 percent of those residing in non-SMSA areas. But, for minorities living outside SMSAs, almost 40 percent are uninsured—a rate twice that of whites residing in non-SMSA areas and 2½ times that of whites in SMSAs.

Thus, health insurance coverage in the U.S. is to some extent a

Table 4
Percent of Persons under Age 65 Uninsured
during Year by Race and Residence, 1977

Race and residence	Population (in millions)	Percentage uninsured during year	Percentage always uninsured	Percentage uninsured part of year
Total, all persons under 65	189.8	17.8%	9.5%	8.3%
South	60.5	22.4	12.7	9.7
White	47.9	20.4	11.8	8.6
Black and other	12.6	30.0	16.2	13.8
Non-South	129.3	15.7	8.0	7.7
White	115.8	14.9	7.7	7.2
Black and other	13.5	22.2	10.7	11.5
SMSA	132.6	16.3	8.2	8.1
White	111.3	14.9	7.6	7.3
Black and other	21.3	23.2	11.1	12.1
Non-SMSA	57.2	21.4	12.5	8.9
White	52.5	19.9	11.6	8.3
Black and other	4.7	38.2	23.3	14.9

Source: Data from the U.S. Department of Health and Human Services, National Center for Health Services Research, National Medical Care Expenditure Survey.

matter of luck. Those fortunate enough to be employed by large, unionized, manufacturing firms are also likely to be fortunate enough to have good health insurance coverage. Those who are poor, those who live in the South or in rural areas, and those who are black or minority group members are more likely to bear the personal and economic effects of lack of insurance and the consequent financial barriers to health care.

Utilization of Health Services by the Uninsured

With the investment in primary care made by federal programs in the late 1960s and 1970s, significant progress in improving access to primary care for the poor and other disadvantaged groups was achieved. Virtually all of the numerous studies examining trends in access to health care conclude that differentials in utilization of physician services and preventive service by income have narrowed (Davis et al., 1981).

In the early 1960s the nonpoor visited physicians 23 percent more frequently than the poor even though the poor, then as now, were considerably sicker than the nonpoor. By the 1970s the poor visited physicians more frequently than the nonpoor, and more in accordance with their greater need for health care services. Blacks and other minorities also made substantial gains over this period. Utilization of services by rural residents also increased relative to urban residents (Davis and Schoen, 1978).

However, use of preventive services by the poor, minorities, and rural residents continues to lag well behind use by those not facing similar barriers to health care. Some studies have also found that these differentials continue to exist for all disadvantaged groups even when adjusted for the greater health needs of the disadvantaged (Davis et al., 1981).

The major difficulty with past studies, however, is that they have not examined insurance coverage of subgroups of the poor to detect the cumulative impact of lack of financial and physical access to care. How do uninsured blacks in rural areas fare in obtaining ambulatory care services? Can nearly all disadvantaged persons get care from public hospitals or clinics, or do those facing multiple barriers to care simply do without?

Data and Methodology

New data from the 1977 National Medical Care Expenditure Survey (NMCES) shed some light on the cumulative effect of multiple barriers to care. Insured persons are those covered during the entire year; the uninsured are those uninsured for the entire year. Those insured for part of the year are excluded; presumably their utilization resembles that of the insured for the portion of the year in which they are insured and that of the uninsured for the portion of the year in which they are uninsured.

The NMCES sample was designed to produce statistically unbiased national estimates that are representative of the civilian noninstitutionalized population of the United States. Since the statistics presented here are based on a sample, they may differ somewhat from the figures that would have been obtained if a complete census had been taken. Tests of statistical significance are indicated in the tables included below (see Department of Health and Human Services, 1982d, Technical Notes, for further detail on methodology). Particular caution should be taken in interpreting those data items for which the noted relative standard error is equal to or greater than 30 percent.

The statistics presented here show utilization differentials between insured and uninsured individuals under age 65. Analysis of age-specific differentials between the insured and uninsured showed patterns similar to the general pattern of the nonelderly population. The elderly were excluded from the analysis since the majority of the elderly population is insured.

Ambulatory Care

Most striking is the extent to which insurance coverage affects use of ambulatory care. Table 5 presents data on use of physicians' services from NMCES for the population under age 65; the insured average 3.7 visits to physicians during the year compared with 2.4 visits for the uninsured. That is, the insured receive 54 percent more ambulatory care from physicians than do the uninsured. However, the differential between the insured and uninsured for physician

Table 5
Physician Visits per Person under Age 65 per Year,
by Insurance Status, Residence, and Race, 1977

Insurance status, residence, and race	Uninsured	Insured	Ratio
Total	2.4	3.7	1.54*
South	2.1	3.5	1.67*
White	2.3	3.7	1.61*
Black and other	1.5	2.8	1.87*
Non-South	2.6	3.8	1.46*
White	2.7	3.8	1.41*
Black and other	1.9	3.5	1.84*
SMSA	2.4	3.8	1.58*
White	2.6	3.9	1.50*
Black and other	1.7	3.2	1.88*
Non-SMSA	2.3	3.3	1.43*
White	2.4	3.4	1.42*
Black and other	1.6	2.9	1.81

Source: Data from the U.S. Department of Health and Human Services, National Center for Health Services Research, National Medical Care Expenditure Survey.
* Indicates values for insured and uninsured are significantly different at the .05 level.

visits may understate the actual differential because variations in scope of coverage among the insured population are not accounted for. Some of the insured may only have insurance coverage for inpatient hospital care, not ambulatory care. Thus, although their utilization pattern is considered in the insured category, such individuals are actually uninsured for physician visits. Better data on ambulatory-care insurance coverage of the insured population therefore might indicate even greater differentials in use of ambulatory care.

Residence and race also affect utilization of ambulatory services. The lowest utilization of ambulatory care occurs for uninsured blacks and other minorities, including Hispanics. These persons use far less than more advantaged groups. For example, uninsured blacks and other minorities in the South make 1.5 physician visits per person annually, compared with 3.7 physician visits for insured whites in the South. That is, to be advantaged multiply leads to a utilization rate almost 2.5 times that of individuals who are disadvantaged multiply.

These data point to the importance of financial and physical barriers to access. It is not the case that the uninsured manage to obtain ambulatory care comparable in amount to that obtained by the insured by relying on public clinics, teaching hospital outpatient clinics, nonprofit health centers, or the charity of private physicians. Without insurance, many simply do without care.

The patterns of utilization for different groups provide some insight into the relative importance of financial, physical, and racial barriers to care. Financial access to care is clearly the most important factor affecting use. Insurance coverage reduces much but not all of the differential in use of ambulatory services. Insured blacks in the South, for example, average 2.8 physician visits annually, compared with 3.7 for insured whites in the South. That is, whites average about 30 percent more ambulatory care than blacks and other minorities even if both are insured. But this differential is substantially smaller than the 2½ times greater use of physicians between insured southern whites and uninsured southern blacks.

Location remains an important determinant of use of physician services. Lack of insurance coverage is more predominant in rural areas; however, even among the insured, urban residents are more likely to receive ambulatory care than are rural residents, whether white or black (see Table 5). Among insured groups, rural whites receive 3.4 physician visits annually compared with 3.9 visits for urban whites. Rural blacks and other minorities with insurance make 2.9 physician visits compared with 3.2 visits for their insured counterparts in urban areas. That is, a 10 to 15 percent differential in use between urban and rural areas occurs even when financial access to care is not a problem. It should be noted, however, that the quality of insurance for ambulatory care may not be as good in rural areas as in urban areas.

Racial differentials in utilization of ambulatory care are also ameliorated with insurance coverage. Insurance is particularly helpful in improving access to care for minorities. Insured minorities receive 80 to 90 percent more ambulatory care than do uninsured minorities, in both rural and urban areas. But even with insurance, strong racial differences persist.

Hospital Care

Despite the common perception that all disadvantaged persons can obtain hospital care from some charity facility, tremendous differentials in use of hospital care also exist by insurance status, residence, and race. The insured receive 90 percent more hospital care than do the uninsured (see Table 6). Differentials by insurance status are particularly marked in the South and in rural areas. In the South, insured persons receive three times as many days of hospital care annually as uninsured persons, regardless of race or ethnic background.

These hospital utilization differentials clearly demonstrate that the insured fare much better than the uninsured in obtaining health care services. Since those with insurance are likely to have basic coverage for hospitalization, the hospital utilization data provide a more accurate assessment of the role of insurance coverage in the use of health care services than do the ambulatory care differentials in the previous section.

These differentials remove any complacency about the accessibility of inpatient care. They reinforce similar findings by Wilensky and Berk (1982), who find that the insured poor use more hospital care than the uninsured poor. They find the biggest differences between those always uninsured and those on Medicaid all year. Those on Medicaid part of the year used fewer hospital services than those on Medicaid all year. The uninsured also used less hospital care than those privately insured. The analysis here extends these results to examine racial and regional differentials.

More disaggregated information is essential on the types of conditions for which the insured receive inpatient care and the uninsured do not. Standards for appropriate utilization of hospital services are still the subject of wide debate. Some of the differential between the

Table 6
Hospital Patient Days per 100 Persons under Age 65,
by Insurance Status, Residence, and Race, 1977

Insurance status, residence, and race	Uninsured	Insured	Ratio
Total	47	90	1.91*
South	35	104	2.97*
White	33	100	3.03*
Black and other	40†	119	2.98*
Non-South	56	84	1.50
White	51	81	1.59*
Black and other	89†	114	1.28
SMSA	50	86	1.72*
White	44	83	1.89*
Black and other	70†	106	1.51
Non-SMSA	42	99	2.36*
White	43	94	2.19*
Black and other	39†	175	4.49*

Source: Data from the U.S. Department of Health and Human Services, National Center for Health Services Research, National Medical Care Expenditure Survey.
* Indicates values for insured and uninsured are significantly different at the .05 level.
†Indicates relative standard error is equal to or greater than 30 percent.

insured and uninsured seen here may be the result of overutilization of hospital services by the insured. However, this is unlikely to explain the entire differential.

Some of the greater utilization of hospital care by the insured may represent self-selection. Those who expect to be hospitalized may obtain such coverage. Hospitalization may itself result in Medicaid coverage of some of the poor and near-poor. However, this should affect primarily those who are insured part of the year and uninsured the remainder of the year. Such partially insured persons are excluded from this analysis. These explanations are unlikely to account for a three-fold differential in use.

Some of the results by region and race are surprising. It is interesting to note that outside the South uninsured blacks receive more hospital days per 100 persons than insured whites. Insured blacks have the highest use. This may reflect greater health problems among blacks, or the tendency of blacks to receive care in public hospitals which have longer stays. Another unexpected result is high hospitalization among insured blacks in nonmetropolitan areas. This is one of the smallest population groups in the study and results, in this case, may simply be statistically unreliable.

Barriers to access to hospital services for the uninsured need to be explored. To what extent do hospitals require preadmission deposits for the uninsured? What are the consequences of such policies on access to care? Which hospitals serve the uninsured and the insured? Do the differences between metropolitan and nonmetropolitan areas reflect the role of teaching hospitals and public hospitals in caring for the uninsured in the inner city? Do the uninsured have to travel sizeable distances to obtain services? What are the health problems of the insured and uninsured, for what conditions are the insured hospitalized but not the uninsured, and what are the health consequences of lack of hospital care for the uninsured? To what extent do any or all of these factors influence the use of hospital care by the uninsured? Further exploration is certainly warranted.

Health Status and Use of Services

Lower utilization of ambulatory and inpatient care by the uninsured is not a reflection of lower need for health care services. Instead, as measured by self-assessment of health status, the uninsured tend to be somewhat sicker than the insured. Fifteen percent of the uninsured under age 65 rate their health as fair or poor, compared with 11 percent of the insured. Blacks and other minorities in the South systematically rate their health the worst. Of insured blacks and other minorities in the South, 19 percent assess their health as fair or poor, compared with 9 percent of insured whites outside the South.

One possible explanation of the higher rate of poor or fair health among the uninsured is that the lack of insurance is itself related to health status. Those who rate their health as poor or fair are more likely to be unable to work because of illness than those who rate their health good or excellent. Since insurance coverage in the United States is related to employment, those who are unemployed due to poor health are also likely to be without insurance. Under an employment-based insurance system, the working population enjoys both good health and insurance coverage, while those too ill to work suffer both lack of employment and lack of insurance.

The sick who are uninsured use medical care services less than their insured counterparts. Utilization of ambulatory services, adjusted for health status, shows that the insured in poor health see a physician 70 percent more often than the uninsured in poor health.

Physician visits per person under age 65 in fair or poor health average 6.9 among the insured, compared with 4.1 visits for the uninsured with similar health problems (Table 7). Blacks and other minorities with fair or poor health who are insured receive twice as much care as their uninsured counterparts.

Among the uninsured in poor or fair health, the differentials in physician visits by race and residence are especially noteworthy. Uninsured whites have greater access to physician services than do uninsured minorities. A southern white in fair or poor health sees a physician twice as often as a southern minority person in fair or poor health. The same relationship exists for utilization of physician services in metropolitan areas. However, the utilization differential between whites and minorities narrows in areas outside the South and in nonmetropolitan areas.

The number of physician visits by the uninsured versus the insured in fair or poor health warrants further examination. It is

Table 7
Physician Visits per Person under Age 65
in Fair or Poor Health per Year,
by Insurance Status, Residence, and Race, 1977

Insurance status, residence, and race	Uninsured	Insured	Ratio
Total	4.1	6.9	1.68*
South	3.8	6.1	1.61*
White	4.4	6.4	1.45*
Black and other	2.2†	5.0	2.27
Non-South	4.5	7.4	1.64*
White	4.6	7.6	1.65*
Black and other	3.5†	6.5	1.86
SMSA	4.1	7.2	1.76*
White	4.7	7.6	1.62*
Black and other	2.3†	5.9	2.57
Non-SMSA	4.2	6.3	1.50
White	4.3	6.4	1.49
Black and other	3.2†	5.4	1.69

Source: Data from the U.S. Department of Health and Human Services, National Center for Health Services Research, National Medical Care Expenditure Survey.
* Indicates values for insured and uninsured are significantly different at the .05 level.
† Indicates relative standard error is equal to or greater than 30 percent.

expected that the individual in fair or poor health would require frequent physician visits for diagnosis and treatment of the condition. The average of five to seven visits annually by the insured would appear to provide a reasonable level of physician contact. But for uninsured minorities in the South in fair or poor health, the average number of visits is 2 per year. This rate would provide no more than an initial visit and 1 follow-up visit, which might be insufficient to treat serious or complex illnesses. Thus, lower rates of physician visits could impair adequate treatment and follow-up to promote a rapid recovery.

Dental Care

Dental care, unlike hospital care and most physician services, is not covered under most insurance plans. Therefore, differentials in dental visits between the insured and uninsured are not meaningful. However, the NMCES data do show a striking contrast between dental visits by whites and minorities.

Whites obtain dental care twice as often as minorities, averaging 1.5 visits per year compared to 0.7 visits for minorities. Nonsouthern whites had two times the number of visits as nonsouthern minorities and over three times the number of visits as southern minorities. Rural minorities appear to have the least access to dental services.

The significant differential between access to dental services for minorities and whites warrants further examination. The extent to which this differential reflects differences in health practices and attitudes toward dental care or differences in availability and accessibility to dental care should be explored.

Usual Source of Care

The NMCES data confirm other studies that have found that disadvantaged groups are less likely to have a usual source of ambulatory care and more likely to receive their care from a hospital outpatient department or a clinic than from a physician's office. Table 8, for example, enumerates that 84 percent of the insured have a physician's office as their usual source of care compared with 67 percent of the uninsured. About 50 percent of uninsured blacks and other minorities have a physician's office as their usual source of care. While this percentage is quite low in comparison with other groups, it does not fit the stereotype that all minorities in urban areas receive the bulk of their care from public facilities or hospital outpatient departments.

Uninsured residents of nonmetropolitan areas are more likely to have a physician as a usual source of care than are residents of a metropolitan area. In nonmetropolitan areas, 73 percent of the uninsured have a physician as a usual source of care in contrast to only 63 percent of the uninsured in metropolitan areas. However, nonmetropolitan residents are still likely to have fewer physician visits than their metropolitan counterparts (see Table 5). The nonmetropolitan uninsured get more of their care from physicians but receive less total care. These differences in utilization among the uninsured undoubtedly reflect differences between metropolitan and nonmetropolitan areas in the availability of alternatives to physician care. Residents of metropolitan areas are more likely to have access to clinic and outpatient hospital services that can substitute for care in physicians' offices.

The metropolitan and nonmetropolitan differential for physicians as a usual source of care is markedly reduced among the insured. As seen in Table 8, 86 percent of insured nonmetropolitan residents

Table 8
Percent of Persons under Age 65 Whose Usual Source
of Care Is a Physician's Office, by Insurance Status,
Residence, and Race, 1977

Insurance status, residence, and race	Uninsured	Insured	Ratio
Total	67	84	1.25*
South	66	81	1.22*
White	70	82	1.16*
Black and other	53	76	1.41*
Non-South	68	85	1.25*
White	70	86	1.22*
Black and other	45	69	1.53*
SMSA	63	82	1.31*
White	66	84	1.27*
Black and other	49	71	1.43*
Non-SMSA	73	86	1.19*
White	76	87	1.15*
Black and other	52	79	1.53*

Source: Data from the U.S. Department of Health and Human Services, National Center for Health Services Research, National Medical Care Expenditure Survey.
* Indicates values for insured and uninsured are significantly different at the .05 level.

and 82 percent of insured metropolitan residents have a physician as a usual source of care. Insurance coverage significantly increases the proportion of minorities who have a physician's office as their usual source of care. Among the minority uninsured 49 percent of those living in metropolitan areas and 52 percent of those in non-metropolitan areas have a physician as a usual source of care. In contrast, for insured minorities, 71 percent in metropolitan areas and 79 percent outside of metropolitan areas have physicians as a usual source of care. This would suggest that Medicaid and private health insurance coverage enable a substantial number of minorities to obtain care in a physician's office.

Convenience of Care

When they are able to obtain care, the uninsured must travel longer distances than the insured to obtain it. As enumerated in Table 9, 25 percent of the uninsured travel 30 minutes or more to obtain care compared with 18 percent of the insured. Differentials

Table 9
Percent of Persons under Age 65 Traveling
More Than 29 Minutes to Receive Medical Care,
by Insurance Status, Residence, and Race, 1977

Insurance status, residence, and race	Uninsured	Insured	Ratio
Total	25	18	1.39*
South	29	21	1.39*
White	30	20	1.48*
Black and other	28	26	1.09
Non-South	21	16	1.29*
White	22	16	1.35*
Black and other	17	21	.81
SMSA	22	17	1.27*
White	21	16	1.32*
Black and other	24	24	1.00
Non-SMSA	29	20	1.46*
White	30	20	1.50*
Black and other	23	19	1.24

Source: Data from the U.S. Department of Health and Human Services, National Center for Health Services Research, National Medical Care Expenditure Survey.
* Indicates values for insured and uninsured are significantly different at the .05 level.

in travel time between the insured and uninsured are somewhat more marked in rural areas than in urban areas, but travel time is a problem for uninsured persons everywhere. These data suggest not only that the uninsured receive less care, but also that when they do obtain care they do so by searching over a longer distance for providers willing to see them. The effort involved in such a search for care may discourage the use of preventive services, resulting in the uninsured only seeking care for serious illness or in crises. This would help explain the lower utilization levels of the uninsured.

When the uninsured arrive at a care provider, they generally have to wait longer for care to be delivered. Regardless of residence, the waiting time for insured blacks and other minorities is longer than the waiting time experienced by uninsured whites. Waiting times are longer in the South. Uninsured southern minority persons experience the longest waiting times. The NMCES data show that they wait one-third longer than do insured southern whites (Department of Health and Human Services, 1982a).

Policy Implications

The utilization differentials between the insured and uninsured underscore the importance of financial barriers to health care. Lack of insurance coverage is the major barrier. It markedly affects the amount of both ambulatory and inpatient care received. Without insurance coverage, many individuals obviously do without care. Those able to obtain care incur substantial travel and waiting times.

Lack of insurance coverage has three major consequences: it contributes to unnecessary pain, suffering, disability, and even death among the uninsured; it places a financial burden on those uninsured who struggle to pay burdensome medical bills; and it places a financial strain on hospitals, physicians, and other health care providers who attempt to provide care to the uninsured.

Research is limited on both the health of the uninsured and the health consequences of having no insurance. Extensive data on utilization patterns by the uninsured disaggregated by residence and race are presented for virtually the first time in this report. But a number of recent studies have shown that medical care utilization has a dramatic impact on health. A recent Urban Institute report by Hadley (1982) explores the relation between medical care utilization and mortality rates. It contains persuasive evidence that utilization of medical care services leads to a marked reduction in mortality rates. A recent study by Grossman and Goldman (1981) at the

National Bureau of Economic Research has found that infant mortality rates have dropped significantly in communities served by federally funded community health centers. This growing body of evidence does provide considerable support to the importance of medical care utilization in assuring a healthy population—and at least indirectly provides a basis for concern that the lower medical care utilization of the uninsured contributes to unnecessary deaths and lowered health status.

Lack of insurance coverage also imposes serious financial burdens on those who try to make regular payments to retire enormous debts incurred in obtaining medical care. With the average cost of a hospital stay in the United States now in excess of $2,000, few individuals can afford to build payments for hospital care into their monthly living allowance (Department of Health and Human Services, 1982b). Yet, since the uninsured are more likely to be poor, the economic consequences of lack of insurance fall heaviest on those least able to bear the burden.

In addition to its consequences for the uninsured, lack of insurance also takes its toll on the health care system. One result is that the financial stability of hospitals and ambulatory care providers willing to provide charity care for those unable to pay is jeopardized. Health care providers serving the uninsured—particularly inner city community and teaching hospitals, county and municipal clinics, and community health centers—absorb much of the cost of this as charity care or a bad debt. Yet this burden is not evenly distributed among hospitals and other providers. A recent study by the Urban Institute found that one-seventh of a national sample of hospitals studied provided over 40 percent of the free care (Brazda, 1982).

Recent policy measures are likely to exacerbate this situation. The Omnibus Budget Reconciliation Act of 1981 reduced federal financial participation in Medicaid and curtailed eligibility under the Aid to Families with Dependent Children (AFDC) program. Actions by state governments in response to this legislation could swell the ranks of the uninsured poor by over 1 million people. Coupled with the highest rate of unemployment since the Great Depression and the loss of health insurance coverage frequently occurring with unemployment, the number of uninsured continues to rise. Undoubtedly the situation has worsened rather than improved since the NMCES study in 1977. Today, the access problems of the uninsured should be a pressing concern on the nation's health agenda.

For many of the uninsured, community health centers and migrant health centers have helped to fill the gap in access created by

the lack of insurance. This was especially important for those
ineligible for Medicaid. However, simultaneously with the cutbacks
in Medicaid, major reductions were made in these service delivery
programs. Overall funding was reduced by 25 percent in absolute
dollars, which may lead to 1.1 million fewer people being served
than the 6 million served in 1980. The National Health Service
Corps, while not as seriously affected now, will be substantially
reduced in future years since no new scholarships are being awarded
with commitments for service in underserved areas (Davis, 1981).

Financial strains on public hospitals and clinics supported by
state and local governments are leading to further curtailment of
services. Preadmission deposits, often sizeable in amount, impose
serious barriers for many of the uninsured seeking hospital care.
Teaching hospitals that have for years maintained an open-door
policy are reevaluating the fiscal viability of continuing such a
policy. In many areas, hospitals are beginning to transfer nonpaying
patients to public facilities, further expanding the charity load of
those facilities and reducing their ability to remain solvent (Brazda,
1982).

Public hospitals, traditionally the care provider of last resort, are
under new pressures to close or reduce services as local governments respond to shrinking revenues. Yet, shifting the responsibility
of public hospitals to community hospitals will not solve the problem of caring for the uninsured. Recent hearings have documented
the refusal of community hospitals to take uninsured patients, even
in emergency situations. This has led to documented cases of deaths
that could have been avoided with prompt medical attention (U.S.
Congress. House. Committee on Energy and Commerce, 1981).

Such disparities in access to care are unacceptable in a decent
and humane society. Several actions are required to assure progress
toward adequate access for all. Medicaid coverage should be expanded to provide basic insurance coverage for all low-income
individuals. The Medicaid programs in southern states have tended
to have very restrictive eligibility policies leaving many of the poor
uncovered (Department of Health and Human Services, 1982c).
Expanded coverage of the poor through Medicaid would improve
the scope of coverage in the South and could help to alleviate some
of the extreme utilization differentials between the South and non-
South. A minimum income standard set at some percentage of the
poverty level would be an important first step. In 1979, 23 states,
including most of the southern states, had income eligibility levels
for Medicaid below 55 percent of the poverty level. Texas, Alabama,
and Tennessee had the lowest standards in the nation—less than

$2,000 for a family of four. Coupled with implementation of a minimum income standard, Medicaid coverage should be broadened to include children and ultimately adults in two-parent families. Such steps would help assure access to care for the nation's poorest families.

Yet, the near-poor and working poor without insurance cannot be forgotten. Today, under Medicaid, only 29 states cover the medically needy to provide health coverage for those with large medical expenses. In effect, this catastrophe coverage provides some measure of protection to working families and is undoubtedly the source of care for many of the "sometimes insured." Coverage for the medically needy is currently very limited in the South; implementation of coverage for the medically needy would be another step toward reducing the disparities between the South and the rest of the country. Expansion of this coverage option is an important component of a positive health care agenda.

Finally, the extensiveness of unemployment in today's economy underscores the need to refine the link between employment and health insurance coverage. "Out of work" ought not to translate to "without health care services." Often, health needs are greatest during periods of stress related to unemployment (Brenner, 1973; Lee, 1979). Health insurance coverage should be extended through employer plans for a period following unemployment, and guaranteed through public coverage until reemployment. Employers should also be encouraged to provide comprehensive coverage, including prevention and primary care services, to all workers and their families.

These measures would help to provide protection and improved access to care for the 34 million or more Americans now without health care insurance. However, as the metropolitan and nonmetropolitan differentials among the insured demonstrate, financing alone is not enough to correct access differentials. Resources development must be coupled with improved financing in underserved areas to assure that needed providers are available. Continued funding and expansion of the community and migrant health center programs to assure physical access to services for residents of high poverty, medically underserved communities is an essential adjunct to broadened financing for low-income populations. Other important ways to provide expanded insurance coverage without perpetuating the cost inefficiencies of the existing system include: reform of Medicaid, Medicare, and private health insurance plans to encourage ambulatory care in cost-effective primary care programs; and experimentation with capitation payments to individual primary care centers, networks of centers, hospitals, or other major primary care providers for providing ambulatory and inpatient services to Medicaid beneficiaries.

This agenda of improved financing and resource development represents a positive strategy that can be employed to reduce major inequities in American health care. Today, some will argue that this agenda is too ambitious and costly and would instead opt for a more targeted and incremental approach. For example, instead of expanding Medicaid coverage, advocates of the incremental approach would favor renewed support to public hospitals and financial aid to hospitals serving large numbers of uninsured to mitigate the worst problems. These approaches are piecemeal, however, and do not address the fundamental problems identified in this paper. Such targeted approaches focus on protecting institutions serving the uninsured rather than protecting the uninsured themselves. Thus, they provide for the continued existence of a source of care for the uninsured seeking care, but do not provide comprehensive coverage to the uninsured to encourage early and preventive services. The poor and uninsured who do without care either because they do not live near an "aided facility" or do not know they could obtain free care from a hospital with a financial distress loan would still suffer inequitable health care differentials.

This paper demonstrates that lack of insurance makes a difference in health care utilization. Studies such as the recent work by Hadley (1982) point out the positive impact of medical care on mortality. Society ultimately bears the burden for care of the uninsured. The choice is between paying up front and directly covering the uninsured or indirectly paying for their care through subsidies to fiscally troubled health facilities, higher insurance premiums, and increased hospital costs to cover the cost of charity care and pay for the ill health caused by neglect and inadequate preventive and primary care. Thus, the best and most pragmatic approach is to provide health insurance coverage to the uninsured and to use targeted approaches to improve resource distribution and to remove remaining differentials. The inequities in health care in the United States described here will deepen unless a positive agenda is pursued.

References

Brazda, J., ed. 1982. Perspectives: Who Will Care for the Uninsured? (September 27) *Washington Report on Medicine and Health* 36 (38, Sept. 27): unpaged insert.

Brenner, H. 1973. *Mental Illness and the Economy.* Cambridge: Harvard University Press.

Davis, K. 1975. *National Health Insurance: Benefits, Costs, and Consequences.* Washington: Brookings Institution.

———. 1981. Reagan Administration Health Policy. (December). *Journal of Public Health Policy* 2(4):312–32.

———. 1982. Medicare Reconsidered. Paper presented at Duke University Medical Center Private Sector Conference on the Financial Support of Health Care of the Elderly and the Indigent, March 14–16.

Davis, K., and C. Schoen. 1978. *Health and the War on Poverty: A Ten Year Appraisal.* Washington: Brookings Institution.

Davis, K., M. Gold, and D. Makuc. 1981. Access to Health Care for the Poor: Does the Gap Remain? *Annual Review of Public Health* 2:159–82.

Department of Health and Human Services. 1982a. National Medical Care Expenditure Survey, 1977. Unpublished Statistics. Hyattsville, Md.: National Center for Health Services Research.

———. 1982b. *Health Care Financing Trends,* June. Baltimore: Health Care Financing Administration.

———. 1982c. *Medicare and Medicaid Data Book 1981.* Baltimore: Health Care Financing Administration.

———. 1982d. Usual Sources of Medical Care and Their Characteristics, Data Preview 12. Hyattsville, Md.: National Center for Health Services Research.

Grossman, M., and F. Goldman. 1981. The Responsiveness and Impacts of Public Health Policy: The Case of Community Health Centers. Paper presented at the 109th Annual Meeting of the American Public Health Association, Los Angeles, November.

Health Centers. Paper presented at the 109th Annual Meeting of the American Public Health Association, Los Angeles, November.

Hadley, J. 1982. *More Medical Care, Better Health?* Washington: Urban Institute.

Institute of Medicine. 1981. *Health Care in a Context of Civil Rights.* Washington: National Academy Press.

Kasper, J.A., D.C. Walden, and G.R. Wilensky. 1978. *Who Are the Uninsured?* National Medical Care Expenditures Survey Data Preview no. 1. Hyattsville, Md.: National Center for Health Services Research.

Lee, A.J. 1979. *Employment, Unemployment, and Health Insurance.* Cambridge, Mass.: Abt Books.

Rowland, D., and C. Gaus. 1983. Medicaid Eligibility and Benefits: Current Policies and Alternatives. In *New Approaches to the Medicaid Crisis*, ed. R. Blendon and T.W. Moloney. New York: Frost and Sullivan.

Taylor, A.K., and W.R. Lawson. 1981. Employer and Employee Expenditures for Private Health Insurance. National Medical Care Expenditures Survey Data Preview 7. Hyattsville, Md.: National Center for Health Services Research, June.

U.S. Congress. House. Committee on Energy and Commerce, U.S. House of Representatives. 1981. *Hearings on Medicaid Cutbacks on Infant Care.* Washington, 27 July.

Wilensky, G.R., and M.L. Berk. 1982. The Health Care of the Poor and the Role of Medicaid. *Health Affairs* 1(4):93–100.

Wilensky, G.R., and D.C. Walden. 1981. Minorities, Poverty, and the Uninsured. Paper presented at the 109th Meeting of the American Public Health Association, Los Angeles, November. Hyattsville Md.: National Center for Health Services Research.

Acknowledgments: This paper was prepared for the President's Commission for the Study of Ethical Problems in Medicine and Biomedical and Behavioral Research. We gratefully acknowledge the assistance of Susan Morgan and Kathryn Kelly of the commission staff, and reviewers for helpful comments. We also thank Gail Wilensky and Daniel C. Walden of the National Center for Health Services Research for supplying requested data and assisting in its interpretation, and Karen Pinkston and Mary Frances leMat of Social and Scientific Systems, Inc. for programming support.

Health Benefits: How the System Is Responding to AIDS

Staff of the National Health Law Program

Introduction

AIDS is not limited to select groups or to specific health problems: rather, AIDS affects all groups and challenges the entire health care system to respond.

This article updates our previous article on AIDS.[1] It will identify major health care problems that people with AIDS (PWAs) encounter and suggest solutions to these problems.

The Expanding AIDS Crisis

Since 1981, 74,447 cases of AIDS have been reported and 41,925 deaths have resulted from AIDS.[2] While homosexual and bisexual men account for most of these cases, recent figures show that the rate of increase among gay men is decreasing, while the incidence of AIDS among other groups is increasing.[3]

Perhaps the most significant change in groups contracting AIDS has been among IV drug users. While IV drug users have accounted for 19 percent of AIDS cases since 1981, they represent 24 percent of the reported cases since January 1, 1988.[4] In New York City, the

Staff of the National Health Law Program (NHELP), "Health Benefits: How the System Is Responding to AIDS," *Clearinghouse Review*, December 1988. Reprinted by Permission of the *Clearinghouse Review*.

number of IV drug users with AIDS is greater than the number of homosexual or bisexual men who have AIDS.[5] More than half of the women who have contracted AIDS have been IV drug users.[6]

AIDS cases among children (persons under age 13 at the time of contracting the disease) have also increased at an alarming rate. Most children are contracting AIDS *in utero*, suggesting that one or both of their parents may be IV drug users with AIDS.[7] The Centers for Disease Control (CDC) has reported 1,185 AIDS cases among children.[8]

Studies continue to confirm initial statistics indicating that minorities are disproportionately represented among PWAs. Blacks and Hispanics account for 41 percent of reported AIDS cases. This disparity is even worse among children; minorities account for over 75 percent of the reported AIDS cases in children.[9]

Publicly Funded Programs for People with AIDS

PWAs are able to obtain a variety of services with the assistance of federal,[10] state, and local programs. Unfortunately, these public programs have numerous and sometimes conflicting requirements and procedures that can obstruct access to care. Some programs lack sufficient funds to serve the increasing number of PWAs. Furthermore, people are frequently unaware of their eligibility for services.

Federal Programs

Medicare

Medicare currently covers less than 1 percent of total medical costs for PWAs and only one-half of 1 percent of all direct medical care expenditures.[11] Medicare eligibility is restricted to people who have worked a specific number of years and are either over 65 years of age or have met certain disability standards[12] for 24 months.[13] Because most PWAs die before the 24-month waiting period has expired, most never have access to the program.[14]

People who do qualify for Medicare quickly learn that many of the services they need are not covered. For example, nursing home care and home health services are extremely limited. Currently, coverage for prescriptions is limited to drugs administered in the hospital.[15] Beginning in 1991, however, Medicare will pay a portion of the cost of all prescription drugs after the patient pays a $600 deductible.[16] Notably, AIDS testing is covered by Medicare as a diagnostic service for symptomatic beneficiaries.

Medicare eligibility does not eliminate another barrier to care: eligible beneficiaries must pay for a significant portion of the services that Medicare does cover. In addition to Medicare premiums, beneficiaries must pay deductibles and 20 percent of the approved Medicare rate[17] (after 1990, limited to $1,350)[18] and any excess charges above the approved rate.

AIDS Drug Reimbursement Program

The AIDS Drug Reimbursement Program,[19] created by the federal government in 1987, is designed to help states cover the high cost of zidovudine (formerly called AZT) and other drugs found by the Food and Drug Administration to extend the lives of PWAs. Under the program, allocations are made available to states based on the number of PWAs in each state. The program is specifically limited to low-income, uninsured people who are ineligible for Medicaid or who are Medicaid recipients in states that do not cover zidovudine. It is unclear whether people with AIDS-Related Complex (ARC) may be eligible. States administer and establish income eligibility requirements for the program.[20]

The program is of limited duration. Initially set to expire on October 1, 1988, Congress has recently adopted a six-month reauthorization of the program, until April 1, 1989.[21] Individuals interested in the AIDS Drug Reimbursement Program must contact the appropriate state office.

Block Grants

Block grants under the Omnibus Budget Reconciliation Act of 1981 and related statutes allow states to fund programs for specified services, including alcohol, drug abuse, and mental health services: preventive health and health services; maternal and child health services; and community services programs.[22] Most of these grants can provide services to PWAs.[23] For example, because its Title V crippled children's program covers immunodeficiencies, Maryland uses crippled children's funds to cover costs of pediatric AIDS cases.[24] New Jersey uses its maternal and child health block grant to provide prenatal services, including AIDS testing, to women at risk. New Jersey also allocates block grant money to local organizations to provide case management to children with AIDS.[25]

Veterans' Benefits

Veterans and their families automatically qualify for veterans' benefits, including medical care.[26] Services provided may vary depending on individuals' particular circumstances (where and when they served) and whether they have a "service-connected" or "nonservice-connected" disability. Services may include hospital care, nursing home care, domiciliary care, medical treatment, and hospice care.[27]

Medicaid

Approximately 25 percent of all AIDS-related medical care costs are paid for by Medicaid. Nationwide, it is estimated that 40 percent of all PWAs receive some services paid for by Medicaid.[28] It has also been estimated that cumulative Medicaid costs for treating AIDS between 1986 and 1991 will be as low as $2 billion or as high as $47 billion, with an intermediate estimate falling at about $10 billion.[29] While Medicaid is clearly an important funding source for the provision of health care to PWAs, its complex eligibility rules and service coverage limitations—both of which vary from state to state—create many obstacles.

Medicaid Eligibility

States must provide Medicaid coverage to individuals who are categorically needy and may opt to cover additional groups referred to as the "optional categorically needy" and the "medically needy."[30] Categorically needy individuals include those who receive or who are "deemed" to be eligible for Aid to Families with Dependent Children (AFDC). By July 1, 1989, all states also will have to provide coverage to pregnant women and infants with incomes at or below 75 percent of the federal poverty level, and by July 1, 1990, coverage will be required for pregnant women with incomes below 100 percent of the poverty line.[31] Most states have already opted to cover pregnant women and infants up to the 100 percent limit. Meanwhile, all states have the option of covering pregnant women and infants with incomes up to 185 percent of the poverty line, and a number of states have made use of this option.[32] These recent expansions in Medicaid coverage are critical because they come at a time when the AIDS virus is affecting more low-income women and children.

Categorically, needy Medicaid recipients also include those aged, blind, or disabled persons who meet eligibility requirements for the Supplemental Security Income (SSI) program.[33] In 36 states, persons who are eligible for SSI automatically become eligible for

Medicaid.[34] Several so-called 209(b) states, however, apply eligibility rules in their Medicaid programs that are more restrictive than SSI's eligibility rules.[35] Nonetheless, in most states—assuming that income and resource criteria are met—it is the determination of disability under the SSI program that provides the avenue for Medicaid coverage for many PWAs. Essentially, SSI disability eligibility requires that the person be disabled and unable to work.

A claimant applying for SSI based on disability may receive up to three months' payments prior to the formal eligibility determination if there is a finding of "presumptive disability."[36] In February 1985, SSA added AIDS, as then defined by the CDC, to the impairment categories provided in SSI presumptive disability rules.[37] To qualify, an individual had to show that he or she suffered from an opportunistic AIDS infection, such as pneumonia or cancer. In February 1988, SSA issued a final rule, effective until December 31, 1989, adopting a revised, expanded CDC definition of AIDS, which includes dementia or wasting syndrome (emaciation) as manifestations of the disease in HIV-positive persons.[38]

The SSI regulatory changes in 1985 and 1988 should result in low-income PWAs receiving almost immediate SSI and Medicaid coverage. The preamble to the 1988 final rule states clearly that (1) confirmation of the AIDS "diagnosis will be by contact with a physician or some other medical or treating source such as a member of a hospital or clinic staff"; (2) "confirming contact may be made by telephone"; and (3) "presumptive disability may be found immediately upon confirmation of the diagnosis of AIDS ... and need not be delayed for the receipt of the actual medical reports or records."[39]

Individuals who would be eligible for AFDC or SSI but for the fact that they have excess income or resources may still be able to receive Medicaid coverage as "medically needy" recipients. Most states have adopted optional programs that allow applicants to receive Medicaid services if their incomes are below an established medically needy income level (MNIL) or after they "spend down" their income that exceeds the MNIL.[40] In many states, the spend down amount, and the time period in which a medically needy applicant must accomplish spend down, will be calculated on a six-month basis. States will not anticipate the expenditure of excess income during this time period. Consequently, Medicaid will not be available until the applicant has actually incurred (but not necessarily paid for) medical costs equal to his or her "excess" income. When making eligibility determinations for the medically needy program, the state Medicaid agency should follow the SSI definition of disability.[41] Given the high cost of AIDS treatment, the medically needy program will be the basis upon which many PWAs qualify for Medicaid.

Barriers to Medicaid Eligibility

Despite SSA's allowance of presumptive eligibility for PWAs, a number of barriers can preclude the receipt of Medicaid benefits. Obviously, immediate receipt of Medicaid benefits is dependent on the SSI presumptive eligibility process working smoothly. The SSA offices must ensure that applicants are able to apply for SSI with minimal administrative delay, that confirming diagnosis contacts are made quickly, and that state Medicaid offices are notified immediately of the SSI presumptive eligibility status so that the applicant can then get his or her Medicaid card.

The Medicaid process may be particularly formidable for PWAs living in 209(b) states (where SSI eligibility does not assure Medicaid eligibility) and for PWAs who have income and resources in excess of SSI eligibility standards (medically needy applicants). In these instances, persons must submit their applications to the state Medicaid agency, and delays can occur. The Medicaid Act, however, does provide protections against delay. According to the Act, all persons must be given the opportunity to apply for Medicaid "without delay,"[42] and assistance must be furnished with reasonable promptness.[43] Notably, eligibility of PWAs on the basis of disability must be determined within 60 days.[44]

Persons with AIDS-Related Complex (ARC) confront yet another eligibility barrier.[45] SSA has not extended automatic presumptive eligibility to persons with ARC. SSA's Program Operations Manual System (POMS) instruction on presumptive eligibility notes that, when diagnosing AIDS, it "must be confirmed that the individual has AIDS rather than AIDS-related complex."[46] Another POMS provision states:

> Those who do not meet the criteria [for identifying AIDS] but who have evidence of AIDS/ARC should not automatically be assumed to have an impairment which does not meet or equal the listings. Such individual claims must be assessed on a case-by-case basis. As with all medically determinable impairments, the assessment of severity must take into account signs, symptoms, and laboratory findings. Developments and assessment of activities of daily living may also be helpful in evaluating the severity of the impairment.[47]

*   *   *

Some people with ARC, therefore, may have to go through the full SSI disability determination process. These persons, however, should be able to apply separately for Medicaid and receive a determination no later than 60 days after application, even if their SSI applications are still pending.[48] Arguably, even if SSA determines that the applicant is not disabled, the state Medicaid agency could find that the applicant is disabled.[49]

Medicaid Services and Service Barriers

Services provided to PWAs under Medicaid programs are inadequate. Generally, state Medicaid plans are only required to cover inpatient hospital care, outpatient care, physician services, laboratory and X-ray services, skilled nursing services for those over 21, and home health care services for people eligible for skilled nursing services.[50]

States can also cover a number of optional services such as prescription drugs, intermediate care facility services, hospice care, case management, and private nursing.[51] There is substantial variation among the states with regard to the number and choice of optional Medicaid services they provide.

PWAs are also likely to be adversely affected by a state's limitation on the amount, duration, and scope of covered services. It is not uncommon for state Medicaid agencies to place numerical limits on hospital days, doctor visits, or prescription drugs. Some states may limit the overall dollar amount they will allow for a particular service or limit the kinds of services (e.g., prescription drugs or prosthetic devices) they will cover.[52]

Whatever the limitation, state Medicaid programs must be consistent with federal regulations requiring services to be sufficient in amount, duration, and scope to achieve their purpose to a reasonable extent. In addition, all "medically necessary" Medicaid services must be covered. Finally, states must not discriminate in the provision of service based on a person's diagnosis, type of illness, or condition.[53] If any of these provisions are violated, litigation can be filed. For example, indigent persons with AIDS or ARC have charged Parkland Hospital in Dallas with violating the Medicaid Act.[54] They argue that the hospital has targeted AIDS/ARC patients for a lower level of patient care and that it requires them to wait unreasonable lengths of time before receiving certain services, particularly drugs.

Medicaid amount, duration, and scope limitations come into play in the provision of costly zidovudine. Zidovudine prolongs life for certain people with AIDS/ARC and has been approved by the FDA. All states have opted to cover drugs as a Medicaid service. However, in three states—Alabama, Arkansas, and Colorado—zidovudine is not covered.[55] A legal challenge to a state's refusal to include zidovudine in its Medicaid program is viable. In *Mair v. Barton*, the state of Kansas was preliminarily enjoined from refusing to provide zidovudine for Medicaid recipients whose physicians prescribe the drug.[56]

Medicaid Provider Participation and Barriers to Service

Even when PWAs are determined to be eligible for Medicaid-covered services, they may still encounter difficulty finding a provider to render needed care. One hospital in Maryland, for example, will neither treat nor employ individuals testing positive for HIV.[57] Fully 35 percent of physicians surveyed in Sacramento, California, stated that they would not treat HIV-positive individuals.[58] A survey of state Medicaid directors by the National Governor's Association showed that half of the 38 directors have found providers resistant to treating PWAs.

Some states have tried to encourage providers to treat PWAs by increasing Medicaid reimbursement rates. For example, Florida doubled its Medicaid rate for skilled nursing facilities that accept PWAs; only 2 county facilities, however, have agreed to the terms of the program. Wisconsin established an independent Medicaid rate covering private room costs and certain supplies for PWAs who require nursing home care. New York pays enhanced Medicaid reimbursement rates to hospitals designated as treatment centers for PWAs. Services provided include housing, home health, and hospice care.[59]

In response to physicians' unwillingness to treat PWAs, authorities have found that physicians competent to treat PWAs are ethically obliged to do so.[60] Providers' concerns regarding the treatment of PWAs can be ameliorated—if not eliminated—by their taking precautions described by the CDC.[61] HHS and the Department of Labor have also listed precautions that employees should take to prevent the transmission of AIDS.[62]

Some case law suggests that sole providers of care in a community may be legally obligated to furnish treatment to patients in need.[63] If all of a community's providers of certain treatments for AIDS refuse to treat PWAs, they could be sued on such a theory.

Alternative Care as a Medicaid Service

Hospice and home- and community-based care often serve PWAs' needs better than inpatient care—and save money.[64]

The Consolidated Omnibus Budget Reconciliation Act of 1985 allows states to include hospice care as an optional Medicaid service.[65]

Currently, only a few states (e.g., Kentucky and Michigan) offer hospice services for palliative treatment as an alternative to hospital care.[66] To be eligible, the person who elects hospice care must be terminally ill and must waive his or her rights to other Medicaid services for treatment of his or her condition.

States can also provide home- and community-based care to PWAs if the state first obtains a "section 2176 waiver" from the federal government.[67] The waiver allows a state to limit recipients' freedom of choice of providers and to offer services in only certain geographic areas. Persons eligible for home- and community-based care under a waiver include those who would otherwise require hospital, skilled nursing, or intermediate facility care. In the Omnibus Budget Reconciliation Act of 1986, Congress authorized states to target waivers to groups of individuals at risk of institutionalized care, as defined by illness or diagnosis, e.g., AIDS or ARC.[68] Services available under such waivers include home-based narcotic and drug abuse treatment, case management,[69] private duty nursing, respite care, medical day care, personal care assistance services, and home-based hospice care.

There are some limitations on waivers. They cannot be used to provide home- and community-based services otherwise provided by the state Medicaid agency. They may not cover vocational or educational activities. Moreover, the federal application process for states to obtain waivers is rigid and requires ample time and staff to follow through on the application process.

In March 1987, New Jersey became the first state to offer home- and community-based care to persons with AIDS/ARC. Waiver services include individual care management, private duty nursing, medical day care, personal care services, home-based methadone treatment, psychotherapy, family therapy, and increased reimbursement for foster parents of children with AIDS/ARC.

Unfortunately, other states have been slow to follow New Jersey's lead. New Mexico has obtained waiver approval and orients its program toward individual case management in rural settings. Hawaii, Ohio, and South Carolina also have obtained waivers.[70] Illinois and North Carolina claim already to serve PWAs under existing waiver programs designed to aid the physically disabled.[71]

The recently enacted Medicare Catastrophic Coverage Act of 1988 offers an important new home- and community-based waiver option. States can extend waiver services to children under age five who, at birth, are infected with (or test positive for) AIDS, the AIDS virus, or drug dependency. These children also must be eligible for adoption or foster care assistance under Title IV-E. Services under the waiver must minimally include nursing care, respite care, physicians' services, prescribed drugs, medical devices and supplies, and transportation services. Services must be provided pursuant to a written plan of care. The provision became effective on July 1, 1988.[72]

State and Local Government Programs

Indigent Care Programs

All states except Kentucky and Tennessee have indigent health care programs.[73] The scope of services available under these programs, however, varies considerably. Moreover, PWAs have limited access to indigent care programs because most of these programs provide only limited outpatient care. However, over the past few years courts have expanded the scope of services available under indigent care programs. Several courts have required the provision of dental care to the medically indigent,[74] and an Idaho court recently ruled that the provision of "medical assistance" required county reimbursement for an indigent patient's private physician bills.[75] California, New Jersey, and New York do report treating large numbers of PWAs through their indigent care programs.[76]

Catastrophic Health Insurance Programs

Several states have created medical assistance programs for people with catastrophic illnesses.[77] Historically, such programs have been targeted at middle-income persons whose financial welfare is endangered by large medical bills. Most of these programs have eligibility criteria that utilize means tests and require cost-sharing. Coverage begins after medical expenses exceed a predetermined threshold or a certain percentage of an applicant's income and/or assets. With the high costs of AIDS treatment, PWAs can easily exceed such thresholds. Cost-sharing requirements may, of course, prove burdensome for many applicants.

Three states—Idaho, South Dakota, and Nevada—reimburse counties for catastrophic medical expenses that exceed a threshold amount. In Idaho, counties may establish their own eligibility criteria. Each county, however, pays premiums into a Catastrophic Health Expense Fund. The premiums are raised by a sales tax based on a per capita formula. All indigent hospitalization costs over $10,000 in a given year are reimbursed from the catastrophic fund. Oklahoma recently established a program that directly reimburses hospitals for catastrophic expenses that exceed 50 percent of the family's annual gross income.[78]

High-Risk Insurance Pools

Fifteen states have created high-risk insurance pools to cover the medically uninsurable—those unable to obtain insurance coverage due to preexisting medical conditions.[79] Persons with AIDS or ARC are considered uninsurable by the majority of insurance companies. PWAs will therefore benefit from risk pools, provided they can afford the premiums, which are generally 150–200 percent higher than normal private insurance rates. Wisconsin and Maine are the only states to operate a premium subsidy program for low-income persons.

Though such programs have succeeded in providing health coverage for a previously uninsurable population, the number of people enrolled has been substantially less than anticipated, and the programs' costs have been high.[80] There are no statistics on how many PWAs are enrolled in high-risk pools.

Most risk pools have a waiting period for preexisting conditions. However, services unrelated to the preexisting condition will be covered during the waiting period. Maine's new program has a more lenient waiting period of 90 days or $3,500, whichever comes first. Iowa, Indiana, Minnesota, Nebraska, and Oregon have placed PWAs on a presumptive eligibility list, thereby enabling them to avoid the customary waiting period.[81] By contrast, South Carolina considered implementing a high-risk pool that would exclude PWAs.[82]

Drug Programs

PWAs' inability to afford drugs can cause needless sickness, disability unemployment, and hospitalization. Nine states have prescription drug programs for low-income, disabled, or elderly residents.[83]

Eligibility criteria and the scope of drug coverage under these programs vary considerably. Eligibility requirements (including age restrictions) and copayments also can limit the ability of prescription drug programs to assist PWAs. In Maryland, for example, the income eligibility cutoff is $5,100/year for one person; the comparable limit in New Jersey is $13,250. Illinois, Rhode Island, and Maine pay for only certain categories of drugs used for chronic illnesses. Most states include copayments ranging from $1/prescription in Maryland to 50 percent of the drug cost in Connecticut. The New York program requires copayments ranging from $3 to $15, depending on the cost of the drug. In Illinois, beneficiaries pay an $80 annual fee to receive free drugs for the entire year.[84]

Special State and Local Programs for PWAs

States and localities are taking steps to combat AIDS by targeting affected groups. Children with AIDS are beginning to receive particular attention. The physical complications of AIDS infections in children are often more severe than in adults because the child's immune system has never had an opportunity to develop. Thus, children often need aggressive, acute medical care from the onset of the disease. Florida and Maryland have created state programs for children infected with HIV.[85] In New Jersey, the Children's Hospital AIDS program in Newark has cared for children in both inpatient and outpatient care settings since 1984.

Programs are also being implemented for IV drug users with AIDS. For instance, Massachusetts has established a comprehensive ambulatory-inpatient care unit that can serve the special medical needs of drug users and the homeless. In New Jersey, the state finances an outreach program providing IV drug users coupons for a free visit to a public health clinic for medical screening and counseling.

Private Health Insurance Coverage

Seventy percent of Americans are covered by private health insurance through their employers.[86] However, insurance companies, alarmed by the costs of AIDS, are using a variety of methods to avoid providing coverage and/or claims payments to people with AIDS or ARC or people suspected of having these conditions.[87]

Uninsured persons with AIDS or ARC are deemed "uninsurable" by the vast majority of private insurers. Thus, they will have difficulty qualifying for private insurance. There are, however, a few avenues that can be explored. If the person can get a job with a company that employs large groups of people, he or she may be able to avoid a showing of individual insurability. Some Blue Cross/ Blue Shield insurers have periods of open enrollment when they will insure persons who can pay the premium regardless of individual insurability.[88] Absent these paths, however, private insurance coverage is unlikely.

Problems obtaining insurance are not limited to persons diagnosed with AIDS/ARC. Some insurance companies are suspected of denying coverage to certain persons, regardless of their health status. This includes persons who live in designated zip code areas with a high concentration of people whose lifestyle may make them a potentially high risk. Companies have also been suspected of denying policies to people who live with someone of the same gender or of using investigative companies to determine an applicant's lifestyle.[89] In at least one case, *National Gay Rights Advocates v. Great Republic Life Insurance Co.*,[90] plaintiffs have charged an insurance company with targeting single males who worked in "suspected" vocations, such as floral, fashion, and interior design. They claim such actions violate the state civil rights act.

Most insurance policies are regulated by state law.[91] Therefore, state insurance laws may provide a remedy against these practices. For example, if an individual suspects that AIDS-related questions on an application for insurance are unfair, he or she should contact the state department of insurance to determine whether the questions have been approved. Additionally, state unfair trade practices acts and public accommodations laws may be helpful. Section 504 of the Rehabilitation Act, discussed later in this article, may provide another remedy for aggrieved employees.

Another method used to deny health policies is to require a test for the HIV antibody. It was recently estimated that 50 percent of health and life insurers test applicants for the antibody.[92] Ninety-one percent of insurers indicated in a recent survey that they reject applicants with AIDS- or HIV-positive tests.[93]

Some states have responded to this practice by prohibiting AIDS testing. For example, Washington, D.C., prohibits testing for AIDS or suppressed immune systems for health, life, or disability insurance. Massachusetts and New York do not allow testing for the AIDS antibody for individual health insurance. Oregon requires insurers to obtain written consent from applicants taking the AIDS antibody test and to inform applicants of the use of the test, its purpose, and of who might see test results.

These laws may offer only temporary relief from the problem. They are under heavy attack from the insurance industry and, in some cases, have been invalidated or temporarily barred.[94] In response to the Washington, D.C., law, many insurers have refused to write new policies in the city.[95] Congress, through its control over D.C. appropriations, is now pressuring the city council to repeal this law.

On yet another front, some insurers are attempting to avoid reimbursement to PWAs, even though the health insurance policy is valid. Known techniques include cancelling the policy or refusing to pay—citing a preexisting condition, fraud, or the experimental nature of treatments.[96] One company, Circle K, recently took yet another approach when it announced to its 8,000 employees that, for new employees, the company health plan would no longer cover

AIDS unless it was contracted from a blood transfusion.[97] The company quickly abandoned this plan after considerable negative publicity.

Some insurers are refusing to continue or to convert a person's policy after employment.[98] The COBRA Continuation Provision of the federal Consolidated Omnibus Budget Reconciliation Act now requires employers to continue health insurance for former employees for 18 months, regardless of preexisting conditions.[99] State continuation laws may also provide a remedy.[100]

Discrimination Against PWAs

HIV-positive individuals and people with AIDS or ARC encounter discrimination in the receipt of health care. A legal services office recently handled a case challenging the actions of a Medicare-participating hospital. A client was diagnosed as having AIDS upon his admission to the hospital. During his inpatient stay, nurses often cracked open his door and called in to him to learn of his condition, but would not enter the room. Hospital staff would not bathe him, and he was not allowed to shower. Bloody linens were not removed from his room. His emergency bedside signal was left unanswered for as long as eight hours. A pamphlet was left at his bedside that described homosexuality as a sinful practice.[101] Increasingly, such activities are being challenged in litigation based on antidiscrimination laws.

Federal Antidiscrimination Provisions

Section 504 of the Rehabilitation Act

Section 504 prohibits discrimination by all federal and federally funded agencies. It is thus applicable to hospitals and nursing facilities that receive federal money, as well as to state Medicaid agencies.

According to section 504, "otherwise qualified handicapped individuals" may not be denied the benefits of or excluded from a "program or activity" that receives federal financial assistance. Handicapped persons include those who have a physical or mental impairment that substantially limits one or more major life activities, those who have a record of such an impairment, or those who are regarded as having such an impairment.[102]

In an October 1988 memorandum, the Justice Department ruled that PWAs and persons infected with HIV were protected by the

Rehabilitation Act. The decision overruled a June 1986 conclusion that such persons were not covered by section 504. The October memorandum cited recent legislative and judicial decisions that, in effect, had rejected the earlier position.[103]

In *School Board of Nassau County v. Arline*, the Supreme Court affirmed a Ninth Circuit decision holding that an infectious disease, tuberculosis, is a handicap within section 504.[104] The court noted that "allowing discrimination based on the contagious effects of a physical impairment would be inconsistent with the basic purpose of section 504, which is to ensure that handicapped individuals are not denied jobs or other benefits because of the prejudiced attitudes or ignorance of others."[105] Although the court expressly noted that it was not ruling on the question of AIDS,[106] the broad language of the decision is most certainly helpful.

Lower federal court decisions since *Arline* expressly find that AIDS is a handicapping condition within the Rehabilitation Act.[107] Most recently, a federal district court in *Doe v. Centinela Hospital* held that persons infected with HIV but asymptomatic for AIDS were entitled to protection under section 504 if they were "otherwise qualified" to participate in the activity from which they had been excluded. In this case an HIV-infected person alleged that he had been discharged from a hospital residential and day rehabilitation program because staffers feared that they would contract AIDS. The court cited *Arline* to support its conclusion that "discrimination based solely on fear of contagion is discrimination based on a handicap when the impairment has that effect on others."[108]

Meanwhile, Congress took note of *Arline* in an amendment to the Civil Rights Restoration Act of 1988, which became effective in March 1988. The amendment notes that the protection of section 504 does not extend to individuals who, by reason of a currently contagious infection, pose a "direct threat" to the health or safety of other individuals or to individuals who are unable to perform the duties of the job.[109] According to members of Congress, the amendment does nothing more than clarify the existing requirements of section 504 and incorporate the standards set by the Supreme Court in *Arline*.[110] Although referring almost solely to AIDS in the employment setting, the amendment applies to all federal agencies and recipients of federal funds.[111]

Hill-Burton Act

Hospitals and nursing homes with Hill-Burton community service obligations must make services available without discrimination on any basis "unrelated to an individual's need for the service or the availability of the needed service in the facility."[112] A recent lawsuit filed by the ACLU challenges a public hospital bed quota limitation for PWAs, on the basis that a bed quota violates the Hill-Burton Act.[113]

Antidumping Provisions

If a PWA arrives at a hospital and is in need of emergency treatment, the hospital will be required to admit the person pursuant to the anti-patient-dumping provisions of the Consolidated Omnibus Budget Reconciliation Act of 1985 (and some state emergency care laws).[114] The COBRA provision requires hospitals at least to treat and stabilize persons in need of emergency care before discharge or transfer to other facilities. If the hospital is not equipped to handle the patient's emergency needs, the duty to treat may encompass the duty to transfer the patient to an institution where essential treatment methods are available. Hospitals and physicians may be subject to severe sanctions and civil liability if they violate these antidumping provisions.

State Antidiscrimination Laws

Florida is the first state to bar discrimination specifically against PWAs and those infected with HIV.[115] Forty-four states and the District of Columbia have passed statutes prohibiting the private sector from discriminating against the handicapped.[116] Five other states prohibit state agencies and recipients of state funds from discriminating against the handicapped in employment.[117] Only the state of Delaware has not passed a prohibition on discrimination against the handicapped.

Under many state and local discrimination laws, AIDS- or HIV-positive status will be interpreted as a handicap or disability. The statutory language and judicial interpretations of differing state statutes vary considerably. Thus, remedies and procedural requirements will differ from state to state. It is critical to examine the precise wording of the law in your particular state. Several statutes that on their face protect only the disabled have been interpreted by the courts or state agencies to prohibit discrimination on the basis of perceived disability as well.[118] Though some statutes explicitly exclude "infectious" or "communicable" diseases, such exceptions were drafted to protect co-workers from being infected in the work place. Given how AIDS is transmitted, these exceptions should not apply to AIDS.[119]

Relief is available through private rights of action or administrative hearings.[120] Most states allow damage awards as well as injunctive relief.[121]

State courts have ruled favorably upon the issue of whether AIDS is a handicap under state law. The Florida Commission on Human Relations, for example, ruled in *Shuttleworth v. Broward County Office of Budget & Management Policies*[122] that an employee who was fired because he had AIDS was a victim of unlawful handicap discrimination.[123] In September 1987, sixteen nursing homes in Minnesota were charged with discrimination against PWAs by the State Department of Human Rights.[124] Delaware's attorney general ordered one of the state's largest pediatric institutions to rescind a controversial policy of not treating PWAs, stating that the hospital's policy violated the state's public accommodation/antidiscrimination policy.[125]

State privacy and civil rights laws also may be applicable to local government activities and may protect PWAs from discrimination. Public hospitals may be required to treat all who seek care as a condition of their subsidies, and tax-exempt nonprofit hospitals may risk their state tax-exempt status if they deny access to PWAs in need of hospital care.

Several cities, such as Austin, Los Angeles, San Francisco, Sacramento, Oakland, Berkeley, Hayward, Riverside, West Hollywood, New York, and Philadelphia, have enacted legislation specifically designed to prohibit AIDS-related discrimination. A number of California counties also have adopted measures to bar discrimination against people with AIDS-related disorders. In light of the broad relief that is sometimes available, many plaintiffs may be encouraged to rely upon these local ordinances.

Conclusion

The AIDS epidemic is creating a tremendous strain on the public and private health care system. It is clear that problems regarding PWAs need more than temporary solutions. While the societal problem of how to deal with the AIDS crisis will not be solved overnight, this article has sought to illustrate how legal services attorneys can help their clients obtain access to care that they might not otherwise receive.[126]

NOTES

1. Perkins & Boyle, *AIDS and Poverty: Dual Barriers to Health Care*, 19 CLEARINGHOUSE REV. 1283 (Mar. 1986).

2. CENTERS FOR DISEASE CONTROL, AIDS WEEKLY SURVEILLANCE REPORT (Sept. 26, 1988). Statistics are available from the CDC by telephone. (404) 330-3020.

3. *See* D. Weber, *AIDS Infects Million Worldwide*, 2 HEALTHWEEK 20 (June 20, 1988) (suggesting part of decline may be due to AIDS education efforts); CENTERS FOR DISEASE CONTROL, *supra* note 2.

4. CENTERS FOR DISEASE CONTROL. *supra* note 2.

5. *New York Reports Shifts in AIDS Patients, N.Y. Times*, Apr. 19, 1988, at 40, col. 1.

6. CENTERS FOR DISEASE CONTROL, *supra* note 2; Weber, *supra* note 3, at 21.

7. Citizens Committee of New York. The Invisible Emergency. Children and AIDS in New York (Apr. 1987) (available from National Health Law Program, Los Angeles).

8. CENTERS FOR DISEASE CONTROL, *supra* note 2. The presence of IV drug abuse, along with the poverty status of many of the children's families, make the effort to cope with AIDS difficult. "Boarder babies," infants thought to have AIDS, are sometimes left at hospitals because their parents are not able to care for them. These abandoned children are difficult to place in foster care homes and, consequently, represent an inappropriate financial and staff drain on the hospitals that board them. National Comm'n to Prevent Child Mortality, Report on Perinatal AIDS 7 (1987).

9. CENTERS FOR DISEASE CONTROL, *supra* note 2. *See also* Friedman, *The AIDS Epidemic Among Blacks and Hispanics*, 65 MILBANK Q. 455 (1987).

10. In addition to the programs discussed *infra.* numerous other federal programs can assist PWAs. For instance, migrant health centers can provide primary health services to migratory agricultural workers, seasonal agricultural workers, and family members who are PWAs or who have AIDS-related conditions. *See* 42 U.S.C. §254B (1988 Supp.). Similarly, community health centers can provide primary care to PWAs who live in areas that have a shortage of health services or a population lacking health services. 42 U.S.C. §254C (1988 Supp.); 53 Fed. Reg. 11345, 11346 (Apr. 6, 1988). (Community and migrant health center grant applications "must include a description of the needs of special population groups for whom the centers are the primary care providers, such as the homeless, AIDS patients and substance abusers.")

11. Roper, *From the Health Care Financing Administration*, 258 J. AM. MED ASS'N 3489 (Dec. 25, 1987); Laudicina. *States Move Ahead to Pay for Costs Related to AIDS*. 29 THE INTERNIST 10, 14 (Aug. 1988).

12. To determine disability, SSA looks at the person's ability to work in a "substantial gainful activity." If the person is not working, the impairment must be recognized as a disability by SSA. SSA has described the symptoms that must be documented for an individual to be considered disabled with AIDS. *See* 42 U.S.C. §416 and the Medicaid eligibility section in this article.

13. 42 U.S.C. §426. Proposals have been made to eliminate the 24-month waiting requirement.

14. M. Rowe & C. Ryan, AIDS: A Public Health Challenge 6–26 (Oct. 1987) (available from Intergovernmental Health Policy Project, Washington, D.C.).

15. 42 U.S.C. §1395x(y); 42 U.S.C. §1395x(m); 42 U.S.C. §1395x(s); 42 U.S.C. §1395(d).

16. Medicare Catastrophic Coverage Act, Pub. L. No. 100–360, §201 (July 1, 1988).

17. 42 U.S.C. §1395(e).

18. Medicare Catastrophic Coverage Act, Pub. L. No. 100–360. §202 (July 1, 1988).

19. 52 Fed. Reg. 30255 (Aug. 13, 1987).

20. *Id.*

21. *Elsewhere on Capitol Hill,* 42 MED. & HEALTH 3 (Oct. 10, 1988).

22. *See* 47 Fed. Reg. 29472 (July 6, 1982); 52 Fed. Reg. 37957 (Oct. 13, 1987). *See also* 42 U.S.C. §§300w–330y *et seq.;* 42 U.S.C. §§701 *et seq.;* 42 U.S.C. §§8621 *et seq.;* 42 U.S.C. §§9901 *et seq.;* 31 U.S.C. §1243.

23. Conversation between Robert Raymond, HHS, and Amy Leizman, National Health Law Program (July 19, 1988).

24. M. Rowe & C. Ryan, *supra* note 14, at 6–27.

25. *Id.*

26. 38 U.S.C. §§610 *et seq.*

27. *Id.*

28. Roper, *supra* note 11.

29. A. Pascal, The Cost of Treating AIDS Under Medicaid: 1986–1991 (May 1987) (available from the Rand Corp., Santa Monica, Cal.). *See also* Andrulis, *State Medicaid Policies and Hospital Care for AIDS Patients,* 5 HEALTH AFFAIRS 110 (Winter 1987).

30. 42 U.S.C. §1396a(a)(10) (1988 Supp.). *See generally* NATIONAL HEALTH LAW PROGRAM, AN ADVOCATE'S GUIDE TO THE MEDICAID PROGRAM (June 1985) (Clearinghouse No. 40,200).

31. 42 U.S.C. §§1396a(a)(10)(A)(i), (ii) and 42 U.S.C. §1396a(1), as amended by section 302 of the Medicare Catastrophic Coverage Act of 1988, Pub. L. No. 100–360 (July 1, 1988).

32. 42 U.S.C. §1396a(1).

33. 42 U.S.C. §1396a(a)(10)(A)(i).

34. In five of these states (Idaho, Oregon, Kansas, Arkansas, and Nevada), the state Medicaid office makes the eligibility determination but uses SSI eligibility rules.

35. These states include Connecticut, Hawaii, Minnesota, North Carolina, Virginia, North Dakota, Missouri, Indiana, Ohio, Illinois, New Hampshire, Nebraska, and Oklahoma.

36. 42 U.S.C. §1383(a)(4)(B).

37. 50 Fed. Reg. 5573 (Feb. 11, 1985). *See* 20 C.F.R. §416.934.

38. 53 Fed. Reg. 3739 (Feb. 9, 1988). SSA, in its final rule, notes that it is adopting the CDC definition as of September 1, 1987, and that future CDC revisions will not automatically affect SSA presumptive disability determinations.

39. *Id.* at 3740.

40. All *but* the following states have medically needy spend down programs: Alabama, Arkansas, Colorado, Delaware, Idaho, Indiana, Missouri, Nevada, New Mexico, South Carolina, South Dakota, and Wyoming. The Texas and Georgia programs only cover pregnant women and children. Ohio, Missouri, and Indiana, while not having a medically needy program, provide spend down eligibility for elderly, blind, and disabled persons as part of their 209(b) obligation. However, in these states the disability definition can be more restrictive than SSI's definition.

41. 42 C.F.R. §435.540.

42. 42 C.F.R. §435.906.

43. 42 U.S.C. §1396a(a)(8).

44. 42 C.F.R. §435.911. HHS has proposed regulations that would extend the determination time to 90 days. 52 Fed. Reg. 47414 (Dec. 14, 1987). *See also* Alexander v. Hill. 549 F. Supp. 1355 (W.D.N.C.), *amended in part,* 553 F. Supp. 1261 (W.D.N.C. 1982), *aff d.* 707 F.2d 780 (4th Cir.). *cert. denied sub nom.* Syria v. Alexander, 464 U.S. 874 (1983); Rousseau v. Murray, No. 84–0213S (D.R.I. Oct. 1, 1984).

45. ARC is the disease's milder form wherein exposure to the AIDS virus causes, among other things, swollen glands and a reduced ability to fight off disease.

46. POMS, DI 11055.240.D (Transmittal No. 6, SSA Pub. No. 68–0411000) (Sept. 1987).

47. POMS, DI 24525.015 (Transmittal No. 10, SSA Pub. No. 68–0424500) (Sept. 1987).

48. *See e.g., Alexander,* 549 F. Supp. 1355 (W.D.N.C. 1982); *Murray,* No. 84–02135 (D.R.I. Oct. 1, 1984).

49. HHS's position is that a state Medicaid office could not find an applicant disabled if SSI has determined that he or she is not disabled. *See* 52 Fed. Reg. 47414 (Dec. 14, 1987) (preamble). *See also* Fratone v. New Jersey Dep't of Human Servs., No. 87–2569 (D.N.J. Feb. 2, 1988). Several decisions, however, do not agree with the HHS position. *See* Rousseau v. Bordeleau, 625 F. Supp. 355 (D.R.I. 1985): Armstrong v. Norman, No. 86–889–B (S.D. Iowa May 24, 1988): Mullins v. Kenley, 639 F. Supp. 1252 (W.D. Va. 1986). *aff d in part and remanded in an unpublished opinion sub nom.* Mullins v. Lukhard, No. 86–3595 (4th Cir. Apr. 10, 1987).

50. 42 U.S.C. §§1396a(a)(10)(A), 1396d(a).

51. *Id.*

52. States have successfully defended against challenges to numerical limits on services. *See* Dorn, Parks, & Schwartz, *Maximizing Coverage for Medicaid Clients.* 20 CLEARINGHOUSE REV. 411 (Summer 1986).

53. *Id.*

54. Dallas Gay Alliance v. Dallas County Hosp. Dist., No. 88–6346 (N.D. Tex. May 20, 1988).

55. Laudicina, *supra* note 11, at 13.

56. Mair v. Barton, Medicare & Medicaid Guide (CCH) 36.697 (D. Kan. July 27, 1987) (preliminary injunction). In issuing the injunction order, the court looked to Medicaid's regulatory prohibition on denying the "amount, duration and scope of a required service to an otherwise eligible recipient solely because of the diagnosis, type of illness or condition." The parties thereafter entered into a stipulated settlement wherein the state Medicaid agency agreed to cover the drug. *See also* Weaver v. Reagan, No. 87–4314–CV–C–5 (W.D. Mo. Sept. 29, 1988), wherein the State of Missouri agreed to provide AZT under its Medicaid coverage, but not to those who failed to meet FDA criteria for the use of AZT. The district court ruled for the plaintiff AIDS patients based on their having established that AZT is "medically necessary" treatment.

57. CENTERS FOR DISEASE CONTROL, AIDS WEEKLY SURVEILLANCE REPORT 18 (July 4, 1988).

58. *Id.*

59. M. Rowe & C. Ryan, *supra* note 14, at 6–8–11.

60. American Medical Ass'n Council on Ethical & Judicial Affairs, Ethical Issues Involved in the Growing AIDS Crisis (1987). *See also* Emanuel, *Do Physicians Have an Obligation to Treat Patients with AIDS?*, 318 NEW ENG. J. MED. 1686 (June 23, 1988).

61. *See* 36 MORBIDITY & MORTALITY WEEKLY REPORT 37 (Nov. 15, 1985) (published by the Centers for Disease Control). According to the Occupational Safety and Health Act, employers must provide a safe and healthy working environment. Employees may not be disciplined for refusing to work in a situation that they reasonably believe creates a significant risk of injury. 29 U.S.C. §651 (1985). Whether workers will raise OSHA as a vehicle to avoid working with PWAs and whether they can successfully defend that position in court are open questions. *See generally* Thigpen v. Executive Comm. of the Baptist Convention. 114 Ga. App. 839. 152 S.E.2d 920 (1960) (nurse's aide not cautioned on how to avoid staph infection).

62. 52 Fed. Reg. 41818 (Oct. 30, 1987).

63. *See e.g.*, Leach v. Drummond Medical Group, 144 Cal. App. 3d 362, 192 Cal. Rptr. 650 (1985); Payton v. Weaver, 131 Cal. App. 3d 38, 182 Cal. Rptr. 225 (1982).

64. For example, the State of New Jersey, which has implemented a home- and community-based care program for PWAs, estimates that the program will save $3,948 per capita. Prior to implementation of the waiver, hospitals in the state estimated 25 percent of their patients with AIDS could be discharged to a lower level of care. Laudicina, *Financing for AIDS Care*, 11 J. of AMBULATORY CARE MANAGEMENT 55 (May 1988).

65. Pub. L. No. 99–272, §9505 (Apr. 7, 1986) (amending 42 U.S.C. §1396d). The Omnibus Budget Reconciliation Act of 1987 (OBRA 87) offers expanded hospice services to Medicaid recipients. Pub. L. No. 100–203, §4114 (adding 42 U.S.C. §11396d(o)(1)(B) effective December 22, 1987). Prior to the amendment, a hospice contracting with Medicaid or Medicare would have to assure HHS that total days of inpatient care provided recipients would not be more than 20 percent of the total days during which the recipients' election to receive hospice services was in effect. OBRA 87 provides that, for Medicaid services, a hospice can exclude days of inpatient care provided to PWAs from the 20-percent inpatient day limit.

66. Memorandum from Marlin W. Johnston, Commissioner, Texas Dep't of Human Servs., Implementation of Texas Hospice Program (Nov. 25, 1987).

67. Section 2176 of the Omnibus Budget Reconciliation Act of 1981 (codified as 42 U.S.C. §1396n).

68. Omnibus Budget Reconciliation Act of 1986, §9411. Pub. L. No. 99–509 (Oct. 21, 1986) (amending 42 U.S.C. §1396n(c)(1)).

69. Case management services can also be offered separately through a waiver or as an optional Medicaid service. The state of Washington has sought approval to offer case management to PWAs.

70. Conversation between Alice Litwimowicz, HCFA, and Jane Perkins, National Health Law Program (Oct. 12, 1988).

71. *Id.*

72. The Medicare Catastrophic Coverage Act of 1988, Pub. L. No. 100–360, §411(k)(17) (July 1, 1988) (to be codified as 42 U.S.C. §1396n(e)).

73. Dowell, *State and Local Government Legal Responsibilities to Provide Medical Care for the Poor*, J. OF LAW & HEALTH (forthcoming fall 1988). Programs are administered by the state or county, or jointly by the state and county, sometimes as part of general assistance programs.

74. *See e.g.*, Pickerell v. Stanislaus County Bd. of Supervisors, No. 222813 (Stanislaus County, Cal., Super. Ct. Mar. 14, 1988); Noble v. Placer County Bd. of Supervisors, No. 81031 (Placer County, Cal., Super. Ct. Mar. 16, 1988).

75. Saxtom v. Gem County, 113 Idaho 929, 750 P.2d 950 (1988).

76. Laudicina, *supra* note 11, at 14.

77. The following states have programs: California, Idaho, Nevada, New Hampshire, New York, Oklahoma, Rhode Island, and South Dakota. Alaska, Maine, and Minnesota have abandoned their catastrophic programs.

78. Dowell, National Health Law Program Conference on Increasing Access for the Medically Indigent (Washington, D.C., June 2–3, 1988) (available from National Health Law Program, Los Angeles).

79. These states are: Connecticut, Florida, Illinois, Indiana, Iowa, Maine, Massachusetts, Montana, Nebraska, New Mexico, North Dakota, Oregon, Tennessee, Washington, and Wisconsin.

80. Drinkwater, *Costs Impact of AIDS on Health and Life Insurance*, EMPLOYEE BENEFITS PRAC., June 1988, at 2.

81. Laudicina, *supra* note 11, at 15.

82. S.C. S.B. 499 (introduced Apr. 30, 1987).

83. Connecticut, Delaware, Illinois, Maine, Maryland, New Jersey, New York, Pennsylvania, and Rhode Island.

84. Dowell, National Health Law Program Conference on Increasing Access for the Medically Indigent (Washington, D.C., June 2–3, 1988).

85. The Florida legislature has also appropriated funds to Jackson Memorial Medical Center in Miami to develop an AIDS patient care network in Dade County; in addition, funds have been appropriated for patient care among five other counties with the highest incidences of AIDS. M. Rowe & C. Ryan, *supra* note 14, at 6-24. *See also* CENTERS FOR DISEASE CONTROL, AIDS WEEKLY SURVEILLANCE REPORT 15 (Jan. 4, 1988) (San Francisco has leased a hospital from the U.S. Army to provide treatment to PWAs beginning January 1989).

86. Law & Emsminger, *Negotiating Physicians' Fees: Individual Patients or Society?* (A Case Study in Federalism), 61 N.Y.U.L. REV. 1 (1986).

87. Address by Benjamin Schatz, Insurance Discrimination, Health Treatment Rights: HIV and AIDS Conference (Chicago, Ill., May 19–21, 1988).

88. Scherzer, *Insurance and AIDS-Related Issues*, in AIDS PRACTICE MANUAL: A LEGAL AND EDUCATIONAL GUIDE VIII-2 (1988).

89. *Gay Legal Organization Fights AIDS Insurance Bias*, N.Y. Native, May 19, 1986, at 12.

90. National Gay Rights Advocates v. Great Republic Life Ins., No. 857323 (San Francisco Super. Ct. filed May 5, 1986). A motion to dismiss the case has been denied.

91. Some companies that self-insure are exempt from state insurance laws. However, self-insured plans must meet IRS standards for tax-exempt status. The IRS has already said that one such company, Circle K, will not lose federal tax exemption if it excludes AIDS. *See* note 97, *intra.*

92. Drinkwater, *supra* note 80, at 3.

93. *Id.*

94. *Id.* (New York invalidated its regulation, with an appeal expected: Massachusetts temporarily blocked its legislation: attempts are being made to repeal the Washington, D.C., law). *See also* Howard, *N.Y. Outlaws Proposed AIDS Test*, MED BENEFITS. June 15, 1988, at 2.

95. Drinkwater, *supra* note 80, at 3.

96. Schatz, *supra* note 87.

97. Health Daily, Aug. 9, 1988, at 1.

98. Drinkwater, *supra* note 80, at 3.

99. 26 U.S.C. §162(k); 29 U.S.C. §§1002, 1161–1168.

100. *See* Perkins & Waxman, *The COBRA Continuation Option: Questions and Answers*, 21 CLEARINGHOUSE REV. 1315 (Apr. 1988).

101. Conversation between Darcy Norville, Evergreen Legal Services, and Jane Perkins, National Health Law Program (Aug 12, 1988). In a controversial decision that would have most certainly seen litigation grow even more, the President's Commission on AIDS recommended that antidiscrimination laws be extended to the private sector. The Administration, at that time, decided to leave this matter to the states.

102. 29 U.S.C. §§701 *et seq.*; 45 C.F.R. §83.3(j). For a more extensive discussion of section 504, see Dorn, Dowell, & Perkins, *Anti-Discrimination Provisions and Health Care Access: New Slants on Old Approaches*, 20 CLEARINGHOUSE REV. 438 (Summer 1986).

103. *Compare* Ostrow & Cimons, *AIDS Covered Under Anti-Bias Law, U.S. Rules,* L.A. Times, Oct. 7, 1988, at 1, col. 4 (reporting that AIDS is covered under section 504), *with* U.S. Dep't of Justice, Memorandum for Ronald Robertson, General Counsel, Department of HHS (June 20, 1986) (AIDS is not protected by section 504).

104. School Bd. of Nassau County v. Arline, 107 S. Ct. 1123 (1987).

105. *Id.* at 1129.

106. *Id.* at 1128 n. 7.

107. *See e.g.,* Chalk v. United States Dist. Court, 832 F.2d 1158 (9th Cir. 1987). ("Although handicapped because of AIDS, appellant [teacher] is otherwise qualified to perform his job within the meaning of section 504 of the Rehabilitation Act of 1973."). Thomas v. Atascadero Unified School Dist., 662 F. Supp. 376, 381 (C.D. Cal. 1987) (plaintiff teacher with AIDS was a handicapped person protected by section 504); Local 1812, Am. Fed. of Gov't Employees v. United States Dep't of State, 662 F. Supp. 50, 54 (D.D.C. 1987); Ray v. School Dist. of DeSota County, 666 F. Supp. 1525 (M.D. Fla. 1987).

108. Doe v. Centinela Hosp., 57 U.S.L.W. 2034 (C.D. Cal. June 30, 1988) (No. CV 87–2514 PAR).

109. Pub. L. No. 100–259, §9, 102 Stat. 31–32 (Mar. 22, 1988); 134 CONG. REC. H587–88 (Mar. 2, 1988).

110. *See e.g.,* 134 CONG. REC. S772 (Feb. 16, 1988) (statement of Sen. Inouye); 134 CONG. REC. S1738–40 (Mar. 2 1988) (statements of Sen. Kennedy, Sen. Weicker, and Sen. Harkin).

111. *See e.g.,* 134 CONG. REC. S30322-25 (Sept. 20, 1988).

112. 42 C.F.R. §124.601.

113. Conversation with Nan Hunter and Ben Sidran, American Civil Liberties Union (Aug. 17, 1988).

114. COBRA, Pub. L. No. 99–272, §9121 (Apr. 17, 1986) (adding 42 U.S.C. §1395dd); Dowell, *Indigent Access to Hospital Emergency Room Services,* 18 CLEARINGHOUSE REV. 483 (Oct. 1984).

115. HEALTH MANAGER'S UPDATE, July 13, 1988, at 4.

116. *AIDS Discrimination,* 15 FLA. ST. U.L. REV. 221, 268 (1987).

117. *Handicap Discrimination,* 40 ARK. L. REV. 261, 269 (1986).

118. *See generally,* AIDS PRACTICE MANUAL: A LEGAL AND EDUCATIONAL GUIDE at IV-2 (1988) (available from National Gay Rights Advocates or National Lawyers Guild AIDS Network, New York). *But see* Elstein v. State Div. of Human Rights, 57 U.S.L.W. 212 (N.Y. Sup. Ct., Onondaga County, Aug. 18, 1988) (physician not liable under state antidiscrimination law for refusing to treat a PWA).

119. AIDS PRACTICE MANUAL: A LEGAL AND EDUCATIONAL GUIDE (1988), *supra* note 118.

120. *Handicap Discrimination, supra* note 117, at 317 & n.277.

121. *Id.* at 317 & n.279.

122. Shuttleworth v. Broward County Office of Budget & Management Policies, No. 54 U.S.L.W. (Fla. Comm'n on Human Relations Dec. 11, 1985).

123. *See also* Chadbourne v. Raytheon (Cal. Super. Ct. Feb. 1987) (reported in 86 Daily Labor Reports (BNA) A-1 (Feb. 13, 1987)); Cronan v. New England Tel. Co., (settled Sept. 1986) (reported in 179 Daily Labor Reports (BNA) A-4 (Sept. 16, 1986)); Racine Educ. Ass'n v. Racine Unified School Dist., (Equal Rights Div., Wis. Dep't of Indus., Labor, & Human Relations, 1986) (reported in 98 Daily Labor Reports (BNA) E-1 (May 21, 1986)).

124. Taravella, *Settlement Near in AIDS Discrimination Lawsuit,* 17 MOD. HEALTHCARE 70 (Nov. 20, 1987).

125. *Delaware Hospital Ordered to Treat AIDS Patients,* AM. MED. NEWS, July 29, 1988, at 6.

126. *See* Byrd, *A Solitary Path: Representing People with AIDS,* Texas Legal Services Center ALERT, June 1988, at 8; Senak, *When Your Client Has AIDS,* 74 A.B.A.J. 76 (July 1, 1988).

AIDS and the Future of Hospital Care

Jesse Green, Ph.D.

AIDS APPEARED ON THE health care horizon ten years ago, suddenly and without warning. Although the entirely new and phenomenally complex disease did not even have a name, hospitals immediately became involved in its diagnosis and treatment, as well as in research. A whole new field of therapeutics had to be invented to deal with its myriad manifestations. Whole hospital wards became AIDS units. AIDS teams were formed. Physicians learned about a new disease from scratch. Thousands of nurses, residents, social workers, technicians, dieticians, and orderlies dealt with personal fears and—in the vast majority of cases—overcame them and kept on working.

Ten years later, New York City's hospitals are still at the forefront of the provision and development of AIDS treatment. They too have responded, by and large, by doing their job—providing care and treatment to those with AIDS. As Bruce Vladeck, president of the United Hospital Fund, has said, "We need to begin by taking note of the extraordinary response of this city's hospital community ... to the extraordinary challenges with which the epidemic has confronted it."[1]

The impact of AIDS on New York City hospitals is far out of

Jesse Green, Ph.D., "AIDS and the Future of Hospital Care," *The Crisis in AIDS Care: A Call to Action*, Working Group of the Citizens Commission on AIDS, March 1989, 3–14. Reprinted by Permission of the Citizens Commission on AIDS for New York City and Northern New Jersey.

proportion to its impact on any other city. Presently, the AIDS census in New York City's hospitals grows by more than *1 bed every day*. There are more AIDS patients hospitalized every day at Bellevue Hospital in New York City than in the entire city of San Francisco. New York City hospitals admit more than 4 times as many AIDS patients and devote more than 8 times as many beds to AIDS treatment as San Francisco hospitals. And while San Francisco's one public hospital has an AIDS caseload composed almost entirely (97 percent) of gay men, New York City's 11 public hospitals have an AIDS caseload that is more than two-thirds IV drug users—individuals with a host of special problems including homelessness, histories of poor health and poor nutrition, responsibilities for young children without other caretakers, lack of insurance, poor access to primary care physicians, and detoxification needs.

As a result of AIDS and other health care crises, New York City's hospitals are stretched to the breaking point. Occupancy levels are dangerously high; emergency rooms are backed up; staffing shortages are critical; revenues are not covering costs. New York may be the only American city with fewer hospital beds than it needs and this gap is likely to widen significantly. The result will be a serious loss of access to hospital care for all New Yorkers and a constant state of crisis in these facilities. Despite the danger, there is no sign that major efforts are underway to find systemwide solutions.

New York City's Hospitals at the Breaking Point

New York City's hospitals are operating at occupancy levels higher than at any time in recent history and higher than in any other city in the country. The average hospital occupancy rate in the United States is 60 percent. In many parts of the country, hospitals aggressively attract patients through marketing efforts. In New York City, by contrast, most hospitals have occupancy rates above 90 percent and many exceed 100 percent.

Like any service delivery system, hospitals require a buffer between average occupancy level and maximum capacity in order to deal with peak times and with crises. There are large daily fluctuations in hospital census totals due primarily to the ebb and flow of unscheduled admissions. If the average day brings a hospital to 90–100 percent of capacity, what happens on a busy day? On a very busy day? What happens during a catastrophe, such as an explosion, a plane crash, a riot, or a terrorist incident? How can the system cope with the outbreak of another epidemic illness, such as Legionnaire's disease, a virulent strain of flu, or something else that we can't even predict?

In a report entitled *New York City's Hospital Occupancy Crisis: Caring for a Changing Patient Population,* the Bigel Institute and the United Hospital Fund describe the factors that created the current crisis. During the early 1980s, hospital utilization in New York City declined, reaching a ten-year low in 1986. A similar trend occurred throughout the United States. Forecasters and planners expected the trend to continue, but instead it reversed dramatically, with hospital occupancy levels soaring from 82 percent to above 90 percent. According to the report, "the annual cycle of winter highs and summer lows disappeared, replaced by relentless increases in utilization."[2]

A number of factors combined to cause the occupancy crisis: planned downsizing of the hospital plant in New York City, resulting in a 9 percent decrease in beds; additional bed reductions due to staff shortages and the need to isolate some patients; increased demand for services among New York City's growing population of the poor; dramatic increases in the use of emergency rooms as points of entry; and the large numbers of newborns requiring very long hospital stays. City hospitals may well have been able to absorb these shocks were it not for the simultaneous pressure placed on acute services by three interrelated epidemics: psychiatric disorders, substance abuse, and AIDS. Although AIDS has actually contributed the smallest share of bed need to date, it is by far the fastest-growing epidemic and its full impact is yet to be felt.

Along with the occupancy crisis, New York City hospitals face a severe financial crunch. The 1988 deficit for New York City hospitals is estimated to be $120 million.[3] Hospitals anticipate an additional $169 million loss statewide ($100 million in New York City) as a result of recent changes in Medicare payment policy for patients whose hospitalizations are much longer than expected. A large reduction is also expected in Medicare payments to teaching hospitals, where many New York City AIDS patients are hospitalized. In addition, Governor Mario Cuomo has announced substantial cuts in Medicaid. Coupled with the large budget deficits at both the federal and state levels, these cutbacks create pressure to reduce rather than expand health care resources.

Current Bed Needs in New York City

In its most recent survey (September 1988) of New York City hospitals, the Greater New York Hospital Association found that 1,679 beds—more than 6 percent of the City's total medical/surgical beds—were occupied by patients with confirmed AIDS or suspected AIDS. This is up sharply from 1,071 in March, 1987 when the survey was first conducted. In February 1989, the New York City AIDS Task Force reported 1,800 beds used for HIV illness and AIDS.

Why does New York City have so many AIDS patients in the hospital? First, because the epidemic has hit the region hard. One in 4 U.S. AIDS cases has occurred in New York City. There have been more AIDS cases reported here than in the next 4 highest-incidence cities (San Francisco, Los Angeles, Houston, and Newark) combined. If the City Department of Health's estimate of 200,000 New Yorkers infected with HIV is accurate, it is *4 times higher* than similar estimates for San Francisco. And, if the estimate is accurate, 90 percent of those infected in New York City have not yet developed AIDS.

In addition, AIDS patients typically require hospitalization for acute illness twice between diagnosis and death. A majority of the hospital admissions occur within 6 months of diagnosis and lengths of stay vary greatly. Some AIDS-related hospitalizations (about 10 percent) are for just 1 day. More than one-third are for one week or less. But a significant number of hospitalizations last a very long time, skewing the average stay to just under 20 days. In particular, long stays characterize the 1 in 5 hospital admissions for AIDS that end in the patient's death.

Comparisons of utilization data across cities indicate that AIDS patients in New York City are hospitalized about as often as in San Francisco but for longer periods of time. This difference is due in part to the greater availability of subacute services in San Francisco and to the extensive support by a network of volunteers. Other likely reasons include differences in patient mix, and the fact that IV drug users (IVDUs) have a more complex set of medical problems.

Some observers have suggested that a relatively large subgroup of the 1,800 AIDS and HIV patients currently hospitalized can be cared for outside the hospital in order to ease the strain on services and possibly reduce the cost of care. However, there is little hard evidence that many hospitalized AIDS patients do not actually need acute care. Although there has been little systematic study of the question, some estimates do exist for New York City. These range from a low of 5 percent, based on alternate level of care days, to highs of about 20 percent[4] or 25 percent.[5] Even the State's projections assume only a 10 percent reduction in bed need when alternate care settings become available. And a national survey of public hospitals found that 10 percent of hospitalized AIDS patients do not need acute care. Thus, it appears that subacute services, even if they could be made available quickly, would reduce by a relatively small degree the need for acute care beds.

Further, it is not clear that alternatives to hospitalization for AIDS patients actually save money. Comparing the average cost of a day in the hospital with a day in long-term care, for example, oversimplifies the cost tradeoffs involved. The hospitalization costs for an AIDS patient who is ready to be discharged is less per day than for the typical and sicker hospital patient, whereas once admitted to long-term care that patient is likely to generate higher costs than the average patient in a hospital. There are also costs involved in creating alternative beds and in coordinating the efficient transfer of patients to alternative sites (case management). And we cannot guarantee that additional beds outside the hospital will be used exclusively as substitutes for hospital days.

Forecasts of Hospital Bed Needs for AIDS in New York City

Projections of future bed needs have been made separately by the New York City AIDS Task Force and the New York State Department of Health (see table). The State's projections are somewhat lower because they are based on *reported* HIV-related hospitalizations whereas the City AIDS Task Force adjusted to account for substantial underreporting.

Either of these projections suggest a citywide acute care crisis of major proportions by 1991. Even the lowest estimate shows that an additional 1,100 beds will be needed. By 1993, 2,100 more AIDS beds will be called for. If these projections are accurate and if other factors stay constant, all of New York City's hospitals could be operating above 100 percent capacity. Clearly this could create serious access problems for any New Yorker seeking hospital care. And if other problems, including drug abuse, homelessness, psychiatric disorders and nursing shortages worsen as well, the strain on hospital care in New York City in the next decade will be almost unimaginable.

Projections of Aids-related Hospital Beds
Needed in New York City

End of year	NY State DOH*	NYC AIDS Task Force**
1989	2,071	2,420
90	2,477	3,020
91	2,909	***2,940
92	3,351	3,470
93	3,792	4,020

Sources:
* B. Pasley and P. Vernon, "Health Care Resource Requirements for AIDS Patients in New York State: Acute Care 1987-1994." Paper presented at the American Public Health Association Annual Meeting, Boston, MA. November 14, 1988. The authors applied the official New York State bed need methodology to New York City.
** New York City AIDS Task Force, presentation of Needs Assessment Work Group, February 22, 1989.
*** The task force's methodology involves a downward adjustment beginning in 1991 for the addition of nonhospital options to the system.

How Accurate Are the Projections?

Both state and city forecasts of hospital bed need depend on the so-called linear extrapolation method to project future need from past trends. The method makes two critical assumptions: (1) the rate at which AIDS incidence has been growing will continue at a constant rate; and (2) the average length of a hospital stay by AIDS patients will continue to decline.

The assumption that AIDS cases will grow at a constant rate may be unsound because HIV did not spread at a constant rate. The best epidemiologic data available shows that among gay men in San Francisco the spread of infection took place very rapidly about 4 or 5 years ago and slowed substantially after that.[6] There is evidence of a similar history among New York City IVDUs.[7] If the pattern does prove to be similar, the State's projections—which show the incidence of AIDS levelling off among gay men but growing sharply among IVDUs—will be inaccurate. Further, our ability to estimate the rate of infection in other populations, such as female partners of IVDUs, other heterosexuals, and infants, is even more imprecise.

The second questionable assumption is that the average length of hospital stay by AIDS patients will continue to drop. This is based solely on data from 1983 through 1986, when average length of stay decreased, and ignores a more recent upward trend in New York

City (from 19.2 days in 1986 to 19.7 days in 1987). Nationally, the length of stay for AIDS cases has increased from 19 days to 20.29 days.[8] The state's estimate also fails to take into account the trend toward increasing proportions of AIDS cases among IVDUs, whose lengths of stay in the hospital are generally longer than average. Finally, the state assumes that lengths of stay will decline 10 percent when alternate facilities are available and the New York City AIDS Task Force has said that subacute facilities may lower average length of stay to 16 days by 1991, but, as the studies cited earlier suggest, these may be optimistic assessments.

Given the high degree of uncertainty surrounding the projections, the only thing that can be forecast with confidence is that estimates will change. This past year the New York City Commissioner of Health changed the City's best estimate of HIV-infected gay men in New York City from about 200,000 to between 60,000 and 90,000. An expert panel has reviewed the new estimates and found them justifiable. Recent data about seroprevalence among gay men, IVDUs, infants and women, which *have not been incorporated* into the projections, will also need to be considered. Although fluctuations in data often make policymakers feel they are aiming at a moving target, it obviously remains critical to plan on the basis of the best available information and then revise when necessary.

Why Poor Neighborhoods and Public Hospitals Bear a Heavy Burden

Because of its link to drug abuse, AIDS has become especially prevalent in the poorest neighborhoods, among a population with very limited resources and very few medical services. Staten Island, for example, has barely been affected at all while certain Manhattan, Bronx, and Brooklyn neighborhoods have been devastated. Ernest Drucker of Montefiore Medical Center has estimated that 10 to 20 percent of young men (17–34 years old) in the South Bronx are seropositive.[9] The impact of this level of infection (and future disease) on an impoverished neighborhood is immense. And if 20 percent of sexually active young men are infected, the implications for the young women in the South Bronx and their babies are equally ominous.

In poor neighborhoods the local hospital emergency room (ER) often provides the only available access to a physician. A systemic problem that transcends the AIDS epidemic is highlighted here: Like other residents of impoverished neighborhoods, HIV-infected patients make inappropriate use of the ER simply because no other health care is available. For the same reason, a disproportionate share of AIDS patients is being handled by public Health and Hospitals Corporation hospitals, which account for 16 percent of New York City medical/surgical beds but 36 percent of the AIDS census. The New York City Strategic Plan for AIDS cites the readjustment of this share between public and voluntary hospitals as one of the City's most important AIDS policy objectives. Realistically, however, this cannot be achieved without a major change in the way the poor receive their health care. And in any event, the redistribution of patients will not solve the need for more beds.

Current Plans and Programs to Meet the Acute Care Needs of PWAs

The state has sent out mixed signals in response to the hospital crisis in general and specifically to AIDS-related hospital needs. Some state initiatives have helped hospitals cope with AIDS, most notably the supplemental reimbursement for AIDS care that is provided through the Designated AIDS Center program, and the adoption of AIDS-specific Diagnosis Related Groups (DRG), which are unique to New York State. (DRGs are rates of reimbursement established for various illnesses based on typical resource requirements.) The Designated AIDS Center program was modeled on San Francisco General Hospital's combination of a dedicated unit, an interdisciplinary team, case management, and community-based alternative care. The program has since evolved to fit the realities of New York State's health care environment and has developed standards of care that are constantly monitored. The New York State Department of Health has announced a goal to provide 60 percent of AIDS hospital beds through Designated Centers. So far, however, there are only 14 centers statewide, 9 of which are in New York City. None of the city's public hospitals has become a center.

The City has long recognized the need for additional beds but has little power to create them. The State, which does have the power, has had a more restrained response to anticipated need. Early in the crisis, Dr. David Axelrod, the state health commissioner, announced that the AIDS epidemic could not be used to allow New York City to enlarge its hospital system. Since the state has labored for 10 years to contract that system, a reluctance to see its effort reversed is natural. As a result, even when state health planners began to project expanded needs as a consequence of AIDS, the hope was that most of this capacity would be created by shorter stays among non-AIDS patients. The thinking here was that implementing an all-payor DRG system in New York State would reduce lengths of stay across the board thus freeing up many beds. Unfortunately, the opposite has occurred. The average length-of-stay has increased in the State since DRGs were implemented.[10]

The state's recently released five-year plan continues to acknowledge the huge increase in AIDS cases and the need for new beds. Given the ongoing interest in downsizing hospitals, however, it is safe to anticipate that the State will attempt to reallocate existing beds rather than add new ones. A number of revealing actions in this direction have already been taken. First, the New York State Department of Health has issued emergency regulations to allow for the temporary certification of 500 "mothballed" beds in New York City. But the fate of these 500 beds remains much in doubt. To date only about 10 percent have actually been brought on line, with the others apparently stymied by staffing shortages. There are also some beds in the under construction.

Second, the state has begun to look at Veterans Administration (VA) hospitals around the city, which have relatively low occupancy levels. The New York State Department of Health recently drafted a memo instructing hospitals to check on the veteran status of inpatients and, where feasible, to transfer veterans to VA hospitals. The VA has responded by demanding Medicaid funds to handle the extra cases. The outcome of this struggle is unclear. However, if the state is successful, the federal share of the burden would increase somewhat.

Third, the state will continue and perhaps step up its efforts to reduce hospital utilization through regulatory and reimbursement mechanisms; such a reduction was the major purpose of the all-payor DRG system. Undoubtedly, hospitals will also continue to be pressured to discharge patients sooner, to perform more surgery on an outpatient basis, and to reduce or delay admissions for discretionary procedures.

Finally, a certain number of beds can be effectively returned to service by providing *more staff*. About 4 percent of New York City's medical/surgical beds are out of service due to a critical shortage of nurses and other health care workers.[11] Despite the demand, some hospitals have had to reduce admission levels because of the acute shortages. In addition, recent regulations have reduced the long hours interns and residents work, a measure which was designed to enhance quality of care but which also reduces available staff in the hospital.

The shortage of health care workers has its roots in some fundamental demographic and societal changes.[12] Solving the problem will require major initiatives including economic incentives, redefinition of functions, and scholarship programs. It may also require an overhaul of the city educational system in order to increase the number and quality of high school graduates.

The State faces some very tough choices. Given the great uncertainty about future resource needs, it must decide whether to stay the course on downsizing New York City's hospital system or accept the need to change in response to recent ominous trends. Any decision is a gamble because we don't know for sure whether the upward trends in utilization are an aberration or a reflection of protracted need in New York City. Faced with such uncertainty, there will be a strong temptation to take a wait-and-see approach. Given the lead time required to increase the capacity of New York City's health care system, however, this would be unwise. Instead, the state should intervene now to assure that adequate hospital beds are available to meet projected need.

Hospitals in New Jersey

New York's hospital crisis may appear to overshadow the problem in New Jersey where there is no comparable bed shortage. However, AIDS has created a serious strain on New Jersey's hospital system.

In New Jersey, where inner-city hospitals in Newark, Paterson, and Jersey City provide services to a disproportionate number of AIDS patients, AIDS has added a layer of unexpected cost. According to the *Community AIDS Needs Assessment*, 72 percent of these cases are found in the five most densely populated counties—Essex, Hudson, Bergen, Passaic, and Union—though Middlesex and Monmouth counties are now reporting well over 200 cases each.[13] The New Jersey Hospital Association has stated that some inner-city hospitals regularly have a daily census of over 50 patients with AIDS, in addition to the hundreds of outpatients who are also receiving care.[14]

This problem is compounded by the fact that roughly 80 percent of these AIDS patients are indigent drug users and their sexual partners. These patients generally do not enter the health care system until they are too sick to be placed in units with ordinary levels of nursing care and they often require more hours of nursing care than the average medical-surgical patients. Care for these indigent AIDS patients not only requires extra financial resources but also affects the recruitment and retention of practitioners and health care workers who are already in short supply. In addition, absent equitable reimbursement mechanisms, a lack of long-term health care facilities and other support services, and the care needs of these indigent patients limit the ability of these hospitals to provide adequate services to other patients.

The "all-payer system" for hospital reimbursement in New Jersey has effectively reduced the "dumping" of patients, that is, referring them to other hospitals. In this system, the New Jersey Department of Health administers an Uncompensated Care Trust Fund that is financed by a uniform, statewide add-on to all hospital bills. Public and private hospitals are reimbursed for care provided to all patients regardless of their ability to pay. Nevertheless, AIDS-specific dumping, characterized by subtle discrimination practices and inappropriate referrals, does occur. Moreover, the Trust Fund does not cover the cost of physician's fees or the costs of subacute care.

Therefore, hospitals in Hudson and Essex counties are still struggling with the extraordinarily high cost of treatment. And although the "all-payer system" will be continued at least until 1990, it is possible that the rising costs of hospital uncompensated care (linked to an increase in AIDS-related care) may lead the legislature to replace it with a system that provides less certain access to hospital care.

Regulatory changes which place enormous burdens on the hospitals have already been instituted. For example, hospitals are now required to document a patient's financial status and to prove indigent status; they are required to provide social services that include efforts to insure that the patient has applied to Medicaid and that every effort has been made to obtain payment from the patient for any amount that is deemed appropriate. These procedures are burdensome for inner-city hospitals. Although it is ultimately to the advantage of the hospitals to help their patients obtain access to Medicaid, more often than not these hospitals cannot provide the required documentation because the patients being served are frequently impoverished, homeless, and difficult to locate.

Although New Jersey has no AIDS-specific diagnosis-related groups (DRGs), the Department of Health has approved a surcharge of $600 per AIDS admission. However, these rates of reimbursement still do not take into account the particular characteristics of HIV-infected persons. Because the system operates on the basis of prospective hospital payments that are determined by a patient's admitting diagnosis (increased by $600), they cannot take into account variables resulting from the clinical course of HIV infection. Some hospital officials claim that DRG rates of reimbursement are $150–$300 less than the actual costs per day incurred by a PWA. The episodic nature of HIV-infection requires more specific DRGs that accurately reflect the nature of the illness and the population being served. More specifically, DRGs, as they now exist, underestimate the cost of caring for HIV-infected individuals who are IV drug users, often homeless, and without recourse to any significant network of community support services.

The financial impact of AIDS on urban hospitals in New Jersey is exacerbated by the relative lack of long-term care facilities for persons with AIDS (see following article "Long-term Care, A Long-term Commitment"). There are currently many patients in the system who meet normal discharge criteria but remain in acute care settings simply because there are no subacute facilities available.

Although there are currently a significant number of beds available in residential health care facilities (boarding homes with a minor nursing component), many of these institutions are reluctant to admit HIV-positive individuals. Moreover, there are no reimbursement mechanisms that adequately fund these facilities.

The financial burden resulting from uncompensated care, linked to the increase in costs of AIDS-related care, combined with a reduction in Federal Medicare participation in the program, and the lack of long-term facilities, have created a cash-flow problem for hospitals that is expected to worsen as more individuals become hospitalized with HIV-related illnesses.

NOTES

1. B. Vladeck, United Hospital Fund, "Social Morbidity and the Transformation of New York's Hospital System," *President's Letter* (July 1988): 1.

2. L. P. Myers, B. Spitz, B. C. Vladeck et al., *New York City's Hospital Occupancy Crisis: Caring for a Changing Patient Population*, Bigel Institute for Health Policy, United Hospital Fund (August 1988).

3. K. Raske, "AIDS Takes Its Toll on New York Hospitals," *Health Week*, 27 December, 1988.

4. B. Pasley and P. Vernon, "Health Care Resource Requirements for AIDS Patients in New York State: Acute Care 1987–1994," Paper presented at the

American Public Health Association Annual Meeting, Boston, MA. 14 November, 1988.

5. Nassau-Suffolk Health Systems Agency, "Plan for a Comprehensive Response to HIV Infection and Related Diseases in Nassau and Suffolk Counties," Executive Summary (November 1988).

6. W. Winkelstein, M. Samuel, N. S. Padian et al., "The San Francisco Men's Health Study: III. Reduction in Human Immunodeficiency Virus Transmission among Homosexual/Bisexual Men, 1982–86," *American Journal of Public Health* 76 (1987): 685–689.

7. D. C. Des Jarlais, S. R. Friedman, D. M. Novick et al., "HIV-1 Infection among Intravenous Drug Users in Manhattan, New York City, 1988–1989," *Journal of the American Medical Association* 261 (1989): 1008–1012.

8. D. P. Andrulis et al., "Medical Care for AIDS Patients in U.S. Hospitals: 1987 Preliminary Report," *Medical Benefits* 5 (1988): 2–3.

9. E. Drucker and S. H. Vermund, "Estimating Prevalence of Human Immunodeficiency Virus Infection in Urban Areas with High Rates of Intravenous Drug Abuse: A Model of the Bronx in 1987," *American Journal of Epidemiology* (in press).

10. New York Business Group on Health, Inc., "Experience with DRGs in NYS," *NYBGH Newsletter* 8, no. 6: 1, 8.

11. New York State Department of Health, Bureau of Health Facility Planning, *Recent Trends in New York City Hospital Utilization* (January 1988).

12. New York State Department of Health, New York State Labor–Health Industry Task Force on Health Personnel, *Report to the Commissioner of Health* (Draft: January 1988).

13. The *Community AIDS Needs Assessment* was prepared by the New Jersey Community AIDS Partnership Advisory Commitee of the Community Foundation of New Jersey, January 1989.

14. New Jersey Hospital Association Statement on AIDS presented to The Assembly Health and Human Resources Committee of the New Jersey State Legislature, 9 February 1989.

Long-term Care:
A Long-term Commitment

Jesse Green, Ph.D.

> Long-term care concerns the details of the life and death of people in this country ... long-term care is not about placements, cases, and target groups but about people, their families, their communities, and their lives.
>
> (Kane and Kane, 1987)[1]

> "We pray our way in and we pray our way out."
>
> (Plight of the Home Care Workers, 1988)[2]

A PERSON WITH AIDS (PWA) suffers from a chronic illness characterized by progressive deterioration of the immune system, likely neurological impairment including dementia, a bewildering variety of opportunistic infections, and malignancies. From the time AIDS diagnosis occurs, generally after an individual has a significant bout of illness, median survival is about one year.[3] However, new therapies are rapidly improving survival rates,[4] leading to growing need for long-term, chronic care. When they are not hospitalized, AIDS patients often remain fairly ill with a number of medical problems.[5] These problems can be met by a range of services that can be delivered at home (if there is a suitable home) or in nonacute facilities.

It is easy to misunderstand long-term care, since even the language we use to describe it is murky. The phrase "long-term care,"

Jesse Green, Ph.D., "Long-term Care: A Long-term Commitment," *The Crisis in AIDS Care: A Call to Action*, Working Group of the Citizens Commission on AIDS, March 1989, 17–30.

with its emphasis on duration, tells us little. "Nursing home" is a misleading term, since most facilities have few nurses and are not much like home. Nor do any of the technical terms, such as "skilled nursing facility (SNF)," "intermediate care facility (ICF)," "health-related facility (HRF)," or even "home care" tell us much.

Though the demographic characteristics of AIDS patients (mostly young, mostly male, often minority) are 180 degrees opposite from the usual recipients of long-term care (mostly elderly females over 75 years of age), there are some striking similarities in long-term care needs.[6] Most such care (whether in the patient's home or in an organized facility) emphasizes assistance with the basics of daily life, including eating, cleaning, cooking, and going to the bathroom. Symptoms such as fatigue, weight loss, diarrhea, fever, shortness of breath, and difficulties with mental functioning often make it difficult to perform these tasks. Many people with AIDS, like many of the elderly, receive help from friends, relatives, or neighbors and never enter the health care system at all. Others are cared for by specially trained paraprofessionals.

Another dimension of long-term care reflects the development of sophisticated medical technology over the past decade. Many patients can now receive relatively intensive medical services at home, including 24-hour nursing care, intravenous therapy, and oxygen therapy,[7] thus avoiding hospitalization while receiving the care they need. AIDS patients and the elderly also both have medical needs, such as nutritional support, guidance in taking medication, and monitoring that can be provided outside the hospital environment.

PWAs entering long-term care must choose between two basic philosophies of care: rehabilitative and palliative.[8] Unlike rehabilitative care, which involves active treatment to restore strength and functional capacity, palliative or hospicelike care emphasizes the relief of pain, physical discomfort, and mental anguish. If palliative care is elected, the goal of therapy is only to "provide relief from pain, depression, agitation, or psychosis."[9] For PWAs, who are generally young men or women in the prime of life, the desire to continue living is very strong. Therefore it is very difficult for young people to embrace the hospice philosophy. Many PWAs also hold out great hope that one of the many avenues of research underway will lead to a breakthrough, and so they don't want to "give up." The choice between rehabilitative and palliative care is therefore only appropriate as part of a spectrum of choices.[10] No patient or care partner should ever be pressured into opting for hospice, a decision that involves a human being's most basic rights.

Whatever long-term care services PWAs select are generally provided by home care attendants or nursing home aides. A study of home care services in Los Angeles found that the average PWA used nearly 50 hours of attendant services for every hour of professional nursing.[11]

How Are AIDS Patients Receiving Long-term Care Now?

The three basic approaches to long-term care are care in the home, care in residential health care facilities, mainly nursing homes, and supported housing, although day care and adult foster care also need to be developed as part of the family of available services. Despite the demand, and despite some exemplary models, most of the need for long-term care is *not being met*. The table gives an indication of just how great the gap is between need and availability in long-term care services in New York City.

Without even considering future projections, the state's estimates of the current need for nursing home beds (600) exceeds what is now available by 474 beds. The state's estimate of 1,370 PWAs currently needing home care exceeds by nearly 1,000 the number being served by formal programs. While 1,280 PWAs need supported housing now, only 66 units are actually provided (about 5 percent of

LONG-TERM CARE FOR PERSONS WITH AIDS IN NEW YORK CITY: NEED VS. ACTUAL SERVICES

	Nursing home beds*	Supported housing units*	Home care average daily clients**
Currently provided:	126	66	400
Projected need:			
End of 1989	600	1,280	1,370
1990	740	1,590	1,638
1991	910	1,930	1,922
1992	1,060	2,280	2,219
1993	1,220	2,640	2,517

Sources:
*Projections are from the New York City AIDS Task Force.
**Projections are based on *AIDS: New York's Response* (The 5-year Interagency Plan).

need). Some long-term care needs are currently being met by hospitals because of the lack of alternatives. At a time when overcrowding has reached critical levels in New York City, any unnecessary use of beds is a serious problem. Some of the gaps in formal care are also being met informally by friends, relatives, neighbors, and other volunteers. By the end of 1993, the situation will be worse: to meet expected needs we must increase the availability of nursing home beds tenfold, housing units fortyfold, and home care services sixfold.

Services that are available to PWAs today come from a handful of sources. Only 2 of New York City's 147 nursing homes—Coler Memorial and Goldwater hospitals, which are part of the City's Health and Hospitals Corporation—currently have beds for PWAs. With a total of 52 dedicated skilled nursing facility beds, this is by far the largest such undertaking in the country. At Coler, 89 percent of the PWAs are male, 43 percent are black, and 32 percent are Hispanic. More than 80 percent have a history of intravenous drug use.

The Coler/Goldwater experience in providing long-term care services to AIDS patients since 1985 was recently described in the first published account of nursing home services to PWAs.[12] The authors address the issues of which patients are most appropriate for placement in a long-term care facility; the special training and staffing that are required to care for these patients; and the differences between caring for AIDS patients and other chronic care patients.

A 1-day survey of 17 PWAs at Coler illustrates the broad range of care needs that a residential health care facility is asked to meet. The survey found 5 patients requiring isolation, 4 on tube feeding, 5 with herpes simplex, 5 with disseminated mycobacteria, 4 with pulmonary tuberculous, 4 with *pneumocystis* pneumonia, 1 with Kaposi's sarcoma, 1 with meningitis, 1 with disseminated candidiasis, 2 with toxoplasmosis, 2 with cryptococcoses, and 2 with cytomegalovirus. Fifteen of the 17 patients suffered from some form of dementia, 7 were on psychotropic drugs, 9 were receiving psychiatric treatment, and 12 were being treated by neurology.[13] Clearly, service demands go beyond what is available in most nursing homes.

In New Jersey, as in New York City, long-term care has been the most difficult part of the continuum of care to establish.[14] Several programs and/or facilities designed to address this need are in various stages of planning.

The Wanaque Convalescent Center in Wanaque, New Jersey, will provide 120 skilled nursing beds for PWAs in the near future. Ten to

21 beds are currently being occupied by PWAs and the remainder will slowly be filled at a rate of about 8 beds per month. When the plan was first announced in April 1988, it was challenged by local residents and officials from Wanaque as well as from neighboring Bloomingdale, Pompton Lakes, and Ringwood.[15] However, the challenges failed. The facility is being reimbursed (through Medicaid) at a rate of approximately $350 per day, about 3 times the normal skilled nursing home rate, and almost twice the normal rate for "heavy duty" rehabilitative skilled nursing. However, at the end of April 1989 there will be an audit. If the rate of reimbursement is found to be too high, it will be cut to reflect more costs more accurately.

Other attempts to place PWAs in nursing homes have not been successful. Plans for a Newark nursing home run by Continental Affiliates of Englewood Cliffs were dropped because of opposition from both the mayor's office and the city council.[16]

The Department of Health is also attempting to encourage non-profit and private entities to provide residences for people with AIDS. The Jersey City Medical Center in Jersey City has already announced its intention to open a 40-bed subacute facility for Hudson County residents within its current building. While the medical center does not preclude taking AIDS patients from outside Hudson County, the emphasis will be on taking care of local need, with priority going to the medical center's patients.[17] This project was initiated jointly by the hospital and a private firm, Stopwatch, headed by former state health commissioner Dr. J. Richard Goldstein. Anthony Cucci, the Jersey City mayor, supports the plan. The project has received a certificate of approval from the New Jersey Department of Health and is ready to be implemented.

Five hospitals in Newark including University Hospital, United Hospitals, St. Michael's Hospital, Beth Israel Hospital, and Columbus Hospital, have formed a consortium to create a series of facilities for PWAs. The first step is intended to be a subacute facility located in or near one of the hospitals. Also on the drawing board are outpatient clinics, congregate and scatter-site housing, and respite and hospice facilities.

The facilities will be managed by a new incorporated entity under the direction of Marc Lory, current chair of the consortium and vice-president and CEO of University Hospital in Newark. It is intended to serve all Newark, and it apparently has the backing of the Newark city government, which includes the mayor and the city council. Discussions have begun with the New Jersey Department of Health, which is being supportive but as yet nonspecific in discussions of licensing and funding. No discussions have taken place with Medicaid officials.

Although the programs mentioned above are beginning to provide long-term care in New Jersey, the number of PWAs in need of long-term care continues to rise at an alarming rate. Many more programs and facilities will have to be designed to address this need.

Home care to PWAs in New York City is primarily provided by the Visiting Nurse Service (VNS), which has a contract with New York City's Human Resources Administration (HRA) to serve Medicaid patients. As of December 1988, the caseload of Medicaid clients with AIDS was 367. The VNS/HRA AIDS Home Care Program provides a wide range of services, including home attendants, home health aides, rehabilitation therapists, and nursing visits. The program is designed to accommodate the level of service to fluctuations in a client's condition. Some patients with private insurance also receive services from HRA/VNS but many insurance policies either fail to cover or severely limit coverage for home care.

In addition to VNS, a number of certified home health agencies (CHHA) provide some home care services to PWAs, although not in large volume. One CHHA serving Manhattan, Brooklyn, and Queens provided services to 19 cases in 1987. Another CHHA in New York City provided services to 54 cases in 1988.

The issue of how to care for PWAs who lack appropriate housing is a controversial one. In projecting future needs, the state's methodology prioritizes the lowest level of care, meaning that if home care is possible, the patient is assigned to home care even if there is no home. In so doing, the state makes the assumption that housing for homeless PWAs will be provided so that they can be served by home care. In practice, however, nursing home construction seems likely to proceed more rapidly than the development of housing for PWAs. Currently, the AIDS Resource Center's Bailey House with 44 beds and about 22 scatter-site apartments in New York City provide the only available supported housing units. As a result, the state may end up placing homeless PWAs projected to be served by home care in nursing home beds instead. This could double or triple the volume of such beds anticipated by the state's plan and deny PWAs access to more appropriate care through supported housing.

Hospices represent a final long-term care option. The Ritter Scheuer Hospital in New York City has been providing care to PWAs since 1986. As of January 1988 the hospice had served 62 PWAs whose average stay lasted 35 days. Unlike the traditional mix of hospice care which (according to federal reimbursement rules) consists of

80 percent home care and 20 percent institutional care, Ritter Scheuer found the AIDS hospice care was 91 percent institutional care and only 9 percent home care.[18]

Home and Community-Based Services Waiver in New Jersey

Beginning in March 1987, New Jersey received a federal waiver from Medicaid regulations that permitted the Department of Human Services to provide, in addition to the usual Medicaid services, community-based case management, skilled nursing in the home, personal health care assistance in the home, medical day care, provision of drug use treatment in the home, residential placement for treatment, and increased reimbursement for family-based foster care. The program is available to persons who have diagnoses of AIDS or advanced ARC, who have a maximum monthly income of about $1,050, and who are qualified for nursing home level of care under Medicaid principles as well as for HIV-infected children up to the age of 2. It is a 3-year waiver program with 350 slots in year 1, 650 in year 2, and 1,000 in year 3. All these slots have not been filled. As of March 17, 1989, there were 349 participants in the program; 713 persons had participated in the program to that date.

Although the home- and community-based waiver program can potentially provide badly needed care to PWAs in their homes, there are several problems. (1) The program has had difficulty recruiting and training personnel, primarily nurses and home health aides; the program has resisted efforts, thus far, to provide enhanced reimbursement for these services. (2) Many of the individuals who could benefit from the program cannot participate because they have no housing. The services can only be provided in a home. (3) The program requires that a participant who receives private duty nursing also have a primary care giver who lives with the patient (private duty nursing is provided for a maximum of 16 hours per day). Some potential recipients of services are ineligible for this reason. (4) Many individuals who are IV drug users are difficult to locate and follow because they have no permanent housing. (5) Although the program has made some significant improvements to expedite the process to determine eligibility, some hospital personnel and program officials are still concerned about the excessive paperwork required to establish eligibility.

The components of the home- and community-based services

waiver can help individuals with AIDS remain in their communities for a longer period of time. Because the goal of the program is both compassionate and pragmatic (hospital care is much more expensive), the Department of Human Services should conduct a formal evaluation of the program. This evaluation would help to identify and resolve programmatic problems, and might be a guide to other states considering the waiver.

The Quality of Long-term Care

As we began to write this section, *The New York Times* reported that a sad chapter in New York State history ended with the payment of the last $1.4 million installment by Bernard Bergman's estate of the fines he incurred in the nursing home scandals that were first reported 15 years ago.[19] The article was an important reminder of how bad things can get but also a recognition of how far we have come. The same article pointed out that federal auditors recently found the quality of New York State's nursing homes better than that of most other states. Still, as we gear up to construct hundreds of nursing home beds for PWAs, many of whom are very poor and politically powerless, we must remember the lessons of the Bergman era and build in the standards and enforcement mechanisms that will assure excellence.

The difference between good- and poor-quality nursing home care is based on many factors, both tangible and intangible. The physical environment should be comfortable, unrestricted, and pleasant.[20] Access to a physician is vitally important for all nursing home patients but perhaps especially for PWAs. Yet as Linda Aiken states, "physicians participate very little in nursing home care."[21] According to her research, only 8.3 percent of all doctors make any nursing home visits at all and those who do average only 1.5 hours per month.

Even access to a nurse can be a problem since most skilled nursing facilities (SNFs) lack 24-hour-a-day RN coverage. The average SNF has a ratio of 1 nurse to 49 patients, which amounts to 15 minutes of nursing care per patient per day.[22] Misuse and overuse of medications remain serious problems in nursing homes.[23] Overuse of psychoactive drugs for behavior control, the use of inappropriate drugs, and the administration of medicines by inadequately trained nurses' aides are the most commonly noted problems.[24] Since PWAs often have multiple prescriptions, some for new, experimental drugs, the need to monitor this component of care is crucial. It should also be stressed that in any nursing home (or home care) program that is not exclusively a hospice, PWAs must have access to clinical trials and experimental therapies.

Careful monitoring of quality is also important in providing home care. In our haste to discharge AIDS patients from the hospital we must be careful not to swing too far in the direction of "quicker and sicker."[25,26] A thorough clinical assessment should be part of any decision to discharge a patient to home care. With 60,000 New Yorkers receiving care at home,[27] it is difficult to monitor or regulate quality of care, but the establishment of AIDS-specific standards, surveillance, and follow-up of complaints are a minimal part of any effort to expand home care.

New York State's Initiative for AIDS Nursing Homes

In July 1988, New York State issued new regulations intended to "encourage development of high quality services and facilities for PWAs who need institutional alternatives to the hospital."[28] These may be skilled nursing facility beds or less intensive health-related facility beds and can be part of an existing facility or a separate AIDS nursing home.

The regulations specify that enhanced reimbursement rates will be available for care of persons with AIDS, ARC, or other symptomatic HIV illnesses. The enhanced reimbursement is quite generous, since it first assigns PWAs to a high-paying Resource Utilization Group (RUG) and then *adds* to that payment a sum equal to the amount paid for the average nursing home patient. Thus payment is 2 or 3 times the average rate. This approach appears to be attracting nursing home operators. Terence Cardinal Cooke Health Care Center will soon open an AIDS HRF on the Upper East Side of Manhattan. The Village Nursing Home, Bronx-Lebanon Hospital, Samaritan House, and Brookdale Institute have reportedly applied to license nursing home beds for PWAs.[29]

In addition, capital financing is being developed. The State of New York Mortgage Association will insure bonds to raise $8.5 million to construct a 5-story nursing home in New York City. Shearson Lehman Hutton is managing the issue, and the New York State Medical Care Fair Financing Agency (MCFFA) is issuing the bonds. The MCFFA is also trying to add 800 to 1,000 beds by raising $80 to $100 million through tax-exempt bonds.[30]

The National Council of Health Facilities Finance Authority has called New York State's efforts to obtain capital financing for AIDS exemplary, but New York's efforts have been frustrated by federal intransigence, specifically the refusal to raise the $150 million ceiling on tax-exempt debt, which precludes many of New York City's teaching hospitals from financing needed AIDS nonacute care. The federal government has also refused to allow the state to pool the bond issues for 12 AIDS facilities. Presently, HUD approves mortgages one by one, which creates unconscionable delays.[31]

In the field of home care, the state has developed enhanced Medicaid reimbursement rates (30 percent above average) for CHHAs providing home nursing to PWAs. But there is no special rate for attendants' visits, which are reimbursed on an hourly basis and make up the vast majority of AIDS care. The suggestion that higher reimbursement rates be paid to home care workers for visiting AIDS patients has received no city or state response. Whether or not differential wages (a kind of combat pay) for AIDS care is supported, the broader issue of low wages for home care workers needs to be addressed. Ninety-three percent of these workers are black women, and their average salary does not even raise them above the poverty line. Every day these women care for 60,000 disabled New Yorkers, often under extremely difficult circumstances, yet they are among the most undervalued workers in our society. Not surprisingly, turnover is very high; a job in a fast-food restaurant often pays more and is more dependable.

With the emphasis now being placed on the need for home care for PWAs, we must remember the burdens that fall on workers who cannot earn enough to make ends meet in their own homes. A statement by David Gould of the United Hospital Fund made the point very well: "We can no longer call for and design a system of high quality home care services and ground it on a foundation of minimum wages, marginal benefits and dead-end jobs."[32]

Will Providing Long-term Care Be Cost Effective?

On the surface, long-term care saves money. One day in a nursing home costs $100, while a single day of hospitalization costs $800. In fact, though, studies of care for the elderly have shown that long-term care fails to decrease costs significantly and sometimes actually increases them. Similar findings have resulted when nursing home services were substituted for hospital services, and when home care services were substituted for either nursing home or hospital services.[33,34,35] After reviewing a number of such studies W. G. Weissert concluded that long-term care is "a complement not a substitute" for hospitalization[36] because it is very difficult to channel services only to those currently receiving acute care. Inevitably, people in the community with unmet needs also find their way to the new services.[37] Studies have also found that hospitalized patients ready for discharge incur costs much below the average for hospital care. Such patients use only about 24 percent to 30 percent of average daily hospital resources.[38]

Though a substantial body of research indicates that long-term care does not reduce hospital use or lower costs, the belief that it would do so for AIDS patients has long been almost an article of faith. Probably the major reason for this has been the shorter lengths of stay in San Francisco hospitals, where community care is more prevalent. But as A. E. Benjamin points out, "It is one thing to show that San Francisco has more AIDS community care and shorter hospital stays but quite another to demonstrate empirically that there is a cause and effect relationship."[39] Moreover, though there may initially have been more out-of-hospital AIDS care in San Francisco than in New York City,[40] it is not clear that this remains true today. In 1988, New York City served considerably more AIDS patients in nursing home beds than San Francisco. In home care, San Francisco had an average daily census of 80 clients in 1988; New York City's HRA/VNS program served more than 300 per day.[41] And the Shanti project's 48 supported housing units in San Francisco are fewer than the 66 units of the AIDS Resource Center in New York City. But as New York City moves ahead of San Francisco in providing long-term care for AIDS patients we should not expect hospital stays and costs to drop to anything like San Francisco levels.

Both the city and state are depending on the notion that providing long-term care to PWAs will substantially reduce the per-patient use of the hospital and thereby decrease costs. Though there may be such an effect on a small scale, it is not something we can depend on in our planning.

What Should Be Done?

On any given day, 186,000 New Yorkers are served by long-term care programs of one kind or another. But the existing system has absolutely no slack. Nursing homes in New York are full. Waiting lists are long. The availability of supported housing is minimal. Formal home care programs do not meet current needs, let alone needs projected for the future. And even if there were no AIDS epidemic, projected growth in the elderly population would create a need for 11,000 new long-term care slots in the next few years.[42]

PWAs are not an easy client population to serve. Few have private insurance. Care needs are complex. Many have a history of IV drug use. Some, despite their illness, continue to use and engage in drug trafficking. To a nursing home operator or a home care administrator with a clientele consisting mainly of elderly women, the prospect of adding all these difficulties to their daily list of problems may be a considerable deterrent. Even the promise of increased reimbursement for nursing home care to PWAs has only brought in nursing home operators like the archdiocese and some hospitals that are already familiar with AIDS. Most existing nursing home operators have decided not to open their doors to PWAs, even at reimbursement rates 2 to 3 times average rates.

To generate the needed home care capacity will require financial investment, but dollars alone are not sufficient. Leadership and innovation are also needed. For example, to provide home care to PWAs, home care workers will need more support—not just financial, but also added security from escorts, better supervision, and help with management of the case. To increase availability of nursing home care for PWAs, government regulations should be made flexible, with an eye toward encouraging participation and innovation while setting high standards of quality. Construction of long-term care facilities which had been planned primarily for the elderly should be expedited if we are to avoid a crisis in home care analogous to the one we are experiencing in acute care today.

Nursing home operators and home care agencies should do their share, but they must be provided with technical assistance to handle the special problems of this population. They also need to be assured that the state and city are making a long-term commitment and will not lose interest in the issue after the beds are built. New York has accomplished a great deal in long-term care over the years. We came through the nursing home scandals and greatly improved industry standards. We have led the nation in the provision of home care services to the elderly. We now have an opportunity to set an example for the nation in providing home care to PWAs.

NOTES

1. R. L. Kane and R. A. Kane, *Long-Term Care: Principles, Programs and Policies* (New York: Springer Publishing Co., 1987).

2. New York City Office of the President of the Borough of Manhattan, *Plight of the Home Care Worker: Report of the Manhattan Borough President's Hearing on April 29, 1987* (New York: January 1988).

3. R. Rothenberg, M. Woelfel, R. Stoneburner et al., "Survival with Acquired Immunodeficiency Syndrome: Experience with 5833 Cases in New York City," *The New England Journal of Medicine* 317 (1987): 1297–1302.

4. T. Creagh-Kirk, P. Doi, E. Andrews et al., "Survival Experience Among Patients with AIDS Receiving Zidovudine," *Journal of the American Medical Association* 260 (1988): 3009–3015.

5. D. Werdegar and J. Amory, *AIDS in San Francisco: Status Report for Fiscal Year 1987-88 and Projections of Service Needs and Costs for 1988–93* (San Francisco: San Francisco Department of Public Health, 22 April, 1988).

6. A. E. Benjamin, "Long-term Care and AIDS: Perspective from Experience with the Elderly," *Milbank Quarterly* 67 (1989).

7. J. Fuller and G. Gordon, "Home Health Care Takes on a New Role," *Business and Health* (November 1988): 34–35.

8. N. Rango, "Nursing Home Care for Persons with AIDs," in David E. Rogers and Eli Ginzberg, eds., *The AIDS Patient: An Action Agenda* (Boulder and London: Westview Press, 1988), 35–41.

9. Ibid.

10. New York City Interagency Task Force on AIDS, *New York City Strategic Plan for AIDS* (New York: New York City Department of Health, May 1988).

11. J. Little, S. Daley, A. Long, and H. Fortson, *AIDS Home Health, Attendant or Hospice Care Pilot Study—April 1, 1986 to May 31, 1987* (Los Angeles, CA: AIDS Project Los Angeles [prepared for the Office of AIDS, California Department of Health Services], January 1988).

12. N. Afzal and A. Wyatt, "Long Term Care of AIDS Patients," *Quality Review Bulletin* 15 (1989): 20–25.

13. New York City Interagency Task Force on AIDS, *New York City Strategic Plan for AIDS* (New York: New York City Department of Health, May 1988).

14. Richard Conviser, Stephen Young, "Providing and Funding a Continuum of Care for People with AIDS: An Update" (Prepared for the Public Health Plenary Session, Southern Health Association and Virginia Public Health Association Meetings, Richmond, 5 May 1988).

15. "Wanaque Says It Has Legal Grounds to Bar AIDS Care at Nursing Home," *The (Newark) Star-Ledger*, 7 April 1988.

16. "40-Bed AIDS Facility Planned in New Jersey," *The (Newark) Star-Ledger*, 11 April 1988.

17. Ibid.

18. W. Bulkin, L. Brown, D. Fraioli et al., "Hospice Care of the Intravenous Drug User AIDS Patient in a Skilled Nurse Facility," *Journal of Acquired Immune Deficiency Syndrome* 1 (1988): 375–380.

19. S. Roberts, "Bergman Legacy: $1,376,032 Check and 110 Auditors," *The New York Times*, 13 February 1989, B1.

20. N. Rango, "Nursing Home Care in the United States," *The New England Journal of Medicine* 307 (1982): 883–889.

21. L. H. Aiken, M. D. Mezey, J. E. Lynaugh, and C. R. Buck, Jr., "Teaching Nursing Homes: Prospects for Improving Long-Term Care," *Journal of the American Geriatrics Society* 33 (1985): 196–201.

22. Ibid.

23. Kane and Kane, *Long-Term Care*.

24. M. Beers, J. Avron, S. B. Soumerai et al., "Psychoactive Medication Used in Intermediate-Care Facility Residents," *Journal of the American Medical Association* 260 (1988): 3016–3020.

25. A. M. Smith, "Alternatives in AIDS Homecare," *AIDS Patient Care* 1 (1987): 28–32.

26. Benjamin, "Long-term Care and AIDS."

27. United Hospital Fund, Home Care in New York City, Providers, Payors and Clients.

28. New York State Department of Health, Memo #88–63, and New York State Code of Rules and Regulations, Amendments to Subpart 86-2 of Title 10.

29. Greater New York Hospital Association, *Status of Plans for Long-Term Care Beds for AIDS* (1988).

30. J. Nemes, "Agency to Insure Bonds for AIDS Facilities," *Modern Healthcare* 46 (23 December 1988).

31. S. P. Palm, "Bond Pool Would Help Build AIDS Facilities," *Modern Healthcare* 56 (24 June 1988).

32. New York City Office of the President of the Borough of Manhattan, *Plight of the Home Care Worker: Report of the Manhattan Borough President's Hearing on April 29, 1987* (New York, January 1988).

33. S. C. Hedrick and T. S. Inui, "The Effectiveness and Cost of Home Care: An Information Synthesis," *HSR: Health Services Research* 20 (1986): 852–880.

34. C. J. Newschaffer, "The Future Demand for RNs in Home Care: An Examination of Issues and Projections," in U.S. Department of Health and Human Services, *Secretary's Commission on Nursing: Support Studies & Background Information*, Volume II (III-1 to III-5) (Washington, DC: U.S. Government Printing Office, December 1988).

35. W. G. Weissert, C. M. Cready, and Pawelak, "The Past and Future of Home- and Community-based Long-term Care," *The Milbank Quarterly* 66 (1988): 309–389.

36. W. G. Weissert, "Seven Reasons Why It Is so Difficult to Make Community-Based Long-Term Care Cost-Effective," *Health Services Research* 20 (1985): 423–433.

37. P. Kemper, R. Applebaum, and M. Harrigan, "Community Care Demonstrations: What Have We Learned?" *Health Care Financing Review* 8 (1987): 87–100.

38. A. Hochstein, "Treating Long-Stay Patients in Acute Hospital Beds: An Economic Diagnosis," *The Gerontologist* 25 (1985): 161–165.

39. Benjamin, "Long-term Care and AIDS."

40. P. S. Arno and R. G. Hughes, "Local Policy Responses to the AIDS Epidemic: New York and San Francisco," *NY State Journal of Medicine* 87 (May 1987): 264–272.

41. "AIDS in San Francisco: Status Report for Fiscal Year 1987-88," HRA/VNS Homecare data (Unpublished, 1988).

42. New York State Department of Health, Office of Health Systems Management, *New York State Long Term Care Need Methodology* (Draft: November 1988).

Testimony of David Barr
of the Lambda Legal Defense
and Education Fund
at the NYS Legislature
Hearings on Primary
Health Care and AIDS

I AM HERE TODAY in both my capacity as staff attorney at Lambda Legal Defense Fund and as a person who is HIV seropositive. Rather than talk about statistics regarding AIDS and the increased burden on our health delivery systems over the next five years, I will discuss some of my personal experiences with being HIV positive, and how having a primary care physician has been essential in maintaining my well-being.

I work on AIDS policy issues at a nonprofit organization that focuses on lesbian and gay rights legal advocacy. Needless to say, I am able to be open about my sero-status without fear of employment discrimination. I have a health insurance plan that, so far, has covered the costs of my HIV-related treatments without opposition. I have a supportive partner of fourteen years and a strong support system of family and friends that have made it easier for me to cope with living with the fatal potential of this disease. I have utilized the latest research findings in treatment to forestall the development of illness. Most important, I have a good working relationship with my physician, who has a large AIDS practice here in Manhattan. In some ways, you might say that I am the state of the art in HIV patients.

I tested HIV positive last February at an anonymous test site run

"Testimony of David Barr," of Lambda Legal Defense and Education Fund Testimony at the New York State Legislature Hearings on Primary Health Care and AIDS, December 19, 1989. Reprinted by Permission of David Barr.

by the NYC Department of Health. It was the first time I had ever taken the test. After receiving my results, I soon realized that knowing that I was positive was an empty piece of information without knowing the status of my immune system. I made my first appointment with my doctor. In addition to a complete blood work-up which would, among other things, determine what my T-cell count was, I was fully examined, a medical history was taken, and then we sat for about an hour and discussed the various options open to me for treatment. My doctor explained what markers he thought indicated progression of HIV disease and at which point in that progression that he felt treatment was advised. We discussed opportunistic infections related to HIV and what signs I should look for onset of such infections. We also discussed ways to remain calm and how not to jump to conclusions every time I coughed or noticed a black and blue mark on my leg. This, and subsequent conversations with my doctor have been an essential part of my treatment.

My first T-cell test showed a T4 count of 385 (a normal count averages 1000). I had not developed any symptoms of illness and agreed with my doctor that no treatment was indicated at that time. I continued to have my status monitored every three months. Each time I tested, there was a drop in my T4 count. When my count reached 230 in July, my doctor and I again discussed treatment options. I first went on Bactrim as prophylaxis against PCP. Fortunately, unlike 60 percent of people with HIV infection, I have been able to tolerate Bactrim without any allergic reactions. I then began to take AZT. I was worried about initial side effects and suggested to my doctor that instead of starting at the full dose I was to take (600 mg. daily), I would start taking the drug slowly and gradually increase my dosage. I did this and found it to be a useful way to begin AZT treatment. I experienced none of the nausea, achiness, agitation, or irritability that many of my friends suffered for the initial six weeks of treatment. I am now also taking a high dose of acyclovir (2000 mg. daily) as prophylaxis against cytomegalovirus and naltrexone as an immunomodulator. My T4 count is back up to 385 and climbing. I have still not experienced any symptoms of illness.

Each decision regarding treatment is a painstaking one. It is confusing to begin taking several different drugs, some of which may be highly toxic, without ever having been sick from this infection. My doctor plays an essential role in helping me to shape my treatment plan. Because HIV affects one systemically, a primary-care physician is crucial to care. My doctor has to be able to determine the status of my immune system using a totally inefficient set of markers, determine if the rash I have is related to HIV, the drugs I am taking, or something completely unrelated to AIDS, ascertain if I am developing anemia or other problems related to AZT, be able to diagnose CMV retinitis, MAI, thrush, Kaposi's sarcoma, tuberculosis, toxoplasmosis, PCP, meningitis, HIV-related dementia, etc., and be able to reassure me when I get frantic about living and possibly dying with all this.

I contrast my experience with a call I received recently. The social worker of a Latina woman in the Bronx who had recently tested HIV positive called to tell me about her client. The woman had tested positive and was fortunate enough to know that she should follow up with a T-cell test. A Medicaid recipient, she went to the clinic at the public hospital in her neighborhood. A blood test was done. Every two weeks she returned to the hospital and was told that her test results had not been received. She speaks little English. Finally, after waiting ten weeks, she returned to the hospital with a social worker who speaks Spanish. They waited for three hours only to have the doctor tell her that again her test results were not available and that she should return in two weeks. The doctor then said that since she was HIV-positive, she should start taking 1500 mg. of AZT every day, wrote out a prescription, and left.

Unfortunately, I do not believe that this case is an isolated incident and I cannot blame the doctor (at least wholly), given the conditions he or she is forced to work under. The state of AIDS care, of health care generally, for me and for this woman is a completely different one. She is living in a Third World country and I am not even though we live in the same city. I may live through this epidemic, she will not. It is no accident that poor people, that women, that people of color, die faster from AIDS than us white, middle-class gay men. We have access to doctors and information, and treatment. The poor do not. If I did not have a physician to oversee my case and work with me toward treatment, I would be sick today. The development of a health care system based on a primary physician model is essential in the fight against AIDS. So many AIDS deaths are now unnecessary. Unless the state acts to provide care and treatment immediately, then it is the state—and not lack of medical knowledge—which is responsible for these deaths.

Recent events in Eastern Europe highlight the power of people to effect change in their society. Their need for recognition of political freedoms is no more important or essential than our need for recognition of economic freedom. The United States is the only country in the industrialized world other than South Africa which does not guarantee health care to its people. The time has come to recognize that not only must we all have the right to speak freely, but we must also have the right to eat, to have shelter, and to have a doctor when we are sick.

HIV AND THE ISSUES OF PREVENTION

Introduction

No ISSUE SURROUNDING AIDS has had more attention than the issue of the public health threat of the HIV virus. More than any other aspect of the epidemic, the issue of the transmission of the disease has been given great social prominence over issues of medical need or of discrimination against those who are HIV-affected. What is often forgotten is that the issues of "transmission" of the virus are really a part of a larger issue—the issues of "prevention" of disease.

"HIV and the Issues of Prevention" is about two things. This section deals first with the debate about HIV-antibody testing and its historical, ethical, and legal limitations. There is continuing controversy over screening for the HIV virus and this debate inevitably ends up with questions of the ethical and constitutional issues of the treatment of persons and the social and political jeopardy of stigmatization. "HIV and the Issues of Prevention" expands upon the issue of the prevention of transmission to include discussion of the prevention of the onset of disease and the complications that medical advances create for HIV-antibody testing policies.

Late into the epidemic, biomedical science has given us a fairly reliable test for HIV antibodies so that we have been able to clear our blood supply and to test individuals for the antibodies, given sufficient reason to do so. And it has given us drugs like AZT and aerosolized pentamidine, which essentially stave off some of the infections that constitute the disease of AIDS. But, as the articles in this section make clear, the information from tests about HIV status, whether for the prevention of transmission or for early medical intervention, are only as good as the social and political policies that make actual interventions possible.

After 10 years, some issues about HIV transmission, testing, and public health restrictions are becoming clearer, and there is increasingly a consensus against any mass screening of the HIV-affected. But the issue of mandatory testing or incentives for testing for the HIV virus continues to come up quite often. It is still the case, however, that the public health community advises against involuntary or coercive testing for the HIV antibodies. Yet, as biomedical progress is made in testing for the HIV virus (so far we have the Elisa and Western Blot, as well as the polymerase chain-reaction technique [PCR]), it is all too easy not to have to think about the social/political or even psychological consequences of a positive test to the patient.

It is instructive to review the history of epidemics and see what, if anything, we can learn from the public health strategies that were used in the past. As Allan Brandt of Harvard suggests in "AIDS in Historical Perspective: Four Lessons from the History of Sexually Transmitted Diseases," the first apparently commonsensical move in reviewing our public health policies, particularly as they pertain to transmission of disease, is to look for models of epidemics that have some analogies with the HIV epidemic. The second, more important move, however, is to see how the HIV epidemic is *different* from other epidemics. Once both analyses are in place, it is possible to learn from history.[1]

History has no simple truths. The history of epidemics is no exception. The highly political and social nature of disease makes political the very interpretation we are attempting. HIV, like syphilis, is "socially constructed." Its apparent danger in transmission, its meaning, its assumed "carriers" are all a part of cultural assumptions about society, its weaknesses, its morality, its "enemies."

Our notion of public health as that set of broad protective strategies of "containment" of infectious and contagious disease grew out of the social hygiene movement in America initiated in direct response to syphilis. The belief that there could be a "public" hygiene emerged out of the threat of venereal disease at the end of the nineteenth century. The social hygiene movement had a number of goals: control of syphilis and gonorrhea; education of the public about these diseases; the direct protection of women and children from infection. Its advances were a mixed blessing. On the one hand, quite a lot of technical expertise was developed in which the medical profession became proficient in detecting disease. But the same development of expertise involved a great leap in medical authority whereby the medical profession became a state officialdom overseeing what, before that time, had been the province of individuals.

There were always the assumptions of class difference at the core of the new public health policies, since the most visible (but not the most common—a great proportion of middle-class men had syphilis but this remained largely unacknowledged) transmitters of venereal disease were the poor. The same medical association that called for increased surveillance of likely contagious groups— immigrants, prostitutes, the poor-in-general—also quite often themselves refused to treat patients with venereal disease, feeling that such work was beneath them as physicians. This kind of double standard was operative at other social levels and constituted part of the enormous complexity of the social response to the epidemic. Such hypocrisy shows the difficulties people, even experts, have in dealing evenly with public health emergencies.

Issues of public health bring into relief our unreflective tendencies to blame the victim and to imbue the victims of contagious disease with our assumptions about their likelihood of endangering the commonwealth. A public health emergency—a medical event occurring in the public domain, either from some environmental factor or from the facts of contagion—brings out a response whereby the public, including its experts, mentally assigns or conceptualizes a "barrier" between the healthy and the unhealthy. Naturally, the assignment of such a barrier between the healthy and the unhealthy is not a purely scientific assignment but one that carries with it the value assumptions of the assigner. These value assumptions are operative in a time of nonemergency as part of the social/political landscape of the culture. The social configuration of syphilis was its association with sexuality and with the breakdown of the family. And today, persistent fears of the destitute, of the drug user, and of "sexual deviance" form the core of the assumptions about the HIV epidemic.

It should not surprise us, then, that historically those who underwent restrictions by public health authorities did so not because they were the primary transmitters of the disease but because they were easy to control and were thought, erroneously, to be the center of infection. During World War I, Congress passed a bill that allowed anyone suspected of having venereal disease to be detained and incarcerated by public health authorities. More than 20,000 women were held in camps because they were thought to be spreaders of disease. The bill had no apparent impact on rates of infection.

As Brandt, and the other authors in this section make clear, compulsory public health measures are usually counterproductive—they drive underground the very people they wish to contact.

Allan Brandt makes a forceful claim in "AIDS in Historical Perspective" that fear of disease will powerfully influence medical approaches and public health response to HIV. Because of that tragic fact, neither education nor public health policies are likely to work. Brandt's point is not to darken the horizon of response to the epidemic. Rather, it is intended to require us to evaluate the social and political obstacles that pervade the American landscape of AIDS response. A political landscape very much like what Dr. Brandt had predicted it would be when he wrote the article. We must, then, take up the issues of prevention of the transmission of the HIV virus with a dogged scrutiny of our own assumptions about human nature and about social, cultural, and political standards. And we must do so with as much allegiance as possible to the individual's rights to respect and autonomy and with equal fidelity to the voices of the communities most affected by the epidemic.

As Ronald Bayer, Carol Levine, and Susan Wolf suggest in "HIV Antibody Screening: An Ethical Framework for Evaluating Proposed Programs," principles *do* exist for the analysis of screening programs for the HIV epidemic that allow us to act without the cloud of political and cultural bias. These principles are ethical assumptions at the heart of medicine, research, and public health and reflect this culture's commitment to the rights of the individual and the prudent limitations of the individual in the face of harm they or their actions may cause. While the Bayer et al. article stresses the ethical issues involved in the use of the HIV-antibody test for mass screening of infection, it is important to note that the ethical obligations they point to are also embodied in recent developments in American constitutional law. The ethical and legal restraints on the public sector reflect the last 50 years of civil rights legislation in America.

Bayer, Levine, and Wolf do an extensive treatment of the issue of screening for HIV antibodies. The proposals that they make have now essentially been integrated into public health law in New York State as the state has developed a response to the HIV epidemic. The article should be closely read, for it provides a very specific set of guidelines for the use of the HIV-antibody test on individuals. These guidelines include the importance of informed consent, the obligation to give those tested the results of their test, the requirements of pre- and post-test counseling for the HIV-antibody test, and the strictures of confidentiality. Also discussed in the piece are screening procedures in special settings which are already implemented (as in states requiring screening in premarital testing; the U.S. armed services; and the Job Corps) or are at issue: clinical and residential settings, employment, insurance. The authors go into some detail over the issue of HIV-antibody testing for health insurance and are forceful in their disapproval of its use to decrease financial burden for insurers.

The authors join with the Centers for Disease Control in not recommending the compulsory testing of individuals in any setting except the screening of the anonymous blood supply, of donors for artificial insemination, and organ donations. The authors end the article with an emphasis upon voluntary testing and a call for strict enforcement of anti-discrimination law for the HIV affected, stressing that "the greatest hope for stopping the spread of HIV infection lies in the voluntary cooperation of those at higher risk."[2]

In "The Ethics of Screening for Early Intervention in HIV Disease," Carol Levine and Ronald Bayer broaden their analysis of the issue of testing and look at the need for strict ethical judgment with respect to the HIV-antibody test in its possible use for early medical treatment for the HIV-affected. Their analysis is very detailed and worthy of careful scrutiny. Recently, some public health officials, as well as some community groups, have suggested that knowing one's HIV status places one in a more optimal situation for treatment merely by the fact that some recently developed drugs can stop or slow down the replication of the virus or stave off some opportunistic infections. Levine and Bayer recommend caution and ask the reader to carefully weigh the costs and the benefits of a decision to be tested for the HIV antibodies to the virus.

The authors spend the first part of their article outlining the medical evidence in favor of early intervention in the HIV virus. They are quick to point out that the combined ELISA HIV antibody test and Western Blot are not accurate in identifying seropositive individuals. And what accuracy there is with adults cannot be applied to infants. (For a short treatment of the specific problems of HIV-antibody testing for perinatal transmission [transmission from mother to fetus], see the introduction to Section Five, as well as the Anatos and Marte article in Section Five of this book.)

As they review the therapeutic offerings for seropositive individuals, Levine and Bayer find little that is not still experimental, outrageously expensive, and extremely care-intensive. Published evidence that zidovudine (AZT) inhibits viral replication is scant. Aerosolized pentamidine does inhibit a recurrence of *pneumocystis carinii* pneumonia but not the other infections associated with the disease.

The authors end their analysis by providing seven conclusions derived from an ethical consideration of HIV-antibody screening for early intervention. In their conclusion they stress that the next phase of the epidemic will be marked by medical improvements and new challenges to the ethical principles that must govern medicine and public health. Only by an abiding and vigilant respect for persons and their privacy, coupled with a public shouldering of our obligations to the sick, can we assure that the cautious medical optimism now reigning will develop sound and ethical policy.

We end this section with a speech by Dr. June Osborn, the Chair of the National Commission on AIDS, which she gave at the Fifth International Conference on AIDS. In "Prevention: Can We Mobilize What Has Been Learned?" Dr. Osborn is expansive in her view of the epidemic, which was at the time *only* eight years old. We are asked to look at prevention as an effort of scientists and of communities; of biomedical science and of caretaking; of political science and politics; of strict statistical advance and the ability to know the faces behind the numbers. She challenges us to understand that the split between science, particularly biomedical science and social policy, between medical advance and medical economics is one that grossly impedes our utilizing what we know about the HIV epidemic. But, more than anything else, this piece is an ethical meditation on health expertise, health care, and the *will* to compassion.

NOTES

1. Brandt has done an extensive history of the social hygiene movement that grew out of the venereal disease epidemics in America in the 1890s. See *No Magic Bullet, A Social History of Venereal Disease in the United States since 1880.* (Oxford University Press, 1985, rev. ed. 1987).

2. A new antidiscrimination bill is currently before Congress. The Americans with Disabilities Act includes those affected with the HIV virus. It is likely that it will pass.

AIDS in Historical Perspective: Four Lessons from the History of Sexually Transmitted Diseases

Allan M. Brandt, Ph.D.

Introduction

It has become abundantly clear in the first six years of the AIDS (acquired immunodeficiency syndrome) epidemic that there will be no simple answer to this health crisis. The obstacles to establishing effective public health policies are considerable. AIDS is a new disease with a unique set of public health problems. The medical, social, and political aspects of the disease present American society and the world community with an awesome task.

The United States has relatively little recent experience dealing with health crises. Since the introduction of antibiotics during World War II, health priorities shifted to chronic, systemic diseases. We had come to believe that the problem of infectious, epidemic disease had passed—a topic of concern only to the developing world and historians.

In this respect, it is not surprising that in these first years of the epidemic there has been a desire to look for historical models as a means of dealing with the AIDS epidemic. Many have pointed to past and contemporary public health approaches to sexually transmitted diseases (STDs) as important precedents for the fight against

Allan M. Brandt, Ph.D., "AIDS in Historical Perspective: Four Lessons from the History of Sexually Transmitted Diseases," *American Journal of Public Health* 78, no. 4 (1988): 367–371. Reprinted by Permission of the Author and the *American Journal of Public Health.*

AIDS.[1] And indeed, there are significant similarities between AIDS and other sexually transmitted infections which go beyond the mere fact of sexual transmission. Syphilis, for example, also may have severe pathological effects. In the first half of the twentieth century, it was both greatly feared and highly stigmatized. In light of these analogues, the social history of efforts to control syphilis and other STDs may serve to inform our assessments of the current epidemic.

But history holds no simple truths. AIDS is not syphilis; our responses to the current epidemic will be shaped by contemporary science, politics, and culture. Yet the history of disease does offer an important set of perspectives on current proposals and strategies. Moreover, history points to the range of variables that will need to be addressed if we are to create effective and just policies.

In these early years of the AIDS epidemic, there has been a tendency to use analogy as a means of devising policy. It makes sense to draw upon past policies and institutional arrangements to address the problems posed by the current crisis. But we need to be sophisticated in drawing analogues; to recognize not only how AIDS is like past epidemics, but the precise ways in which it is different. This article draws four "lessons" from the social history of sexually transmitted disease in the United States and assesses their relevance for the current epidemic.

Lesson #1—Fear of Disease Will Powerfully Influence Medical Approaches and Public Health Policy

The last years of the nineteenth century and first of the twentieth witnessed considerable fear of sexually transmitted infection, not unlike that which we are experiencing today. A series of important discoveries about the pathology of syphilis and gonorrhea had revealed a range of alarming pathological consequences from debility, insanity, and paralysis, to sterility and blindness. In this age of antibiotics, it is easy to forget the fear and dread that syphilis invoked in the past.

Among the reasons that syphilis was so greatly feared was the assumption that it could be casually transmitted. Doctors at the turn of the twentieth century catalogued the various modes of transmission: pens, pencils, toothbrushes, towels and bedding, and medical procedures were all identified as potential means of communication.[2] As one woman explained in an anonymous essay in 1912:

At first it was unbelievable. I knew of the disease only through newspaper advertisements [for patent medicines]. I had understood that it was the result of sin and that it originated and was contracted only in the underworld of the city. I felt sure that my friend was mistaken in diagnosis when he exclaimed, "Another tragedy of the public drinking cup!" I eagerly met his remark with the assurance that I did not use public drinking cups, that I had used my own cup for years. He led me to review my summer. After recalling a number of times when my thirst had forced me to go to the public fountain, I came at last to realize that what he had told me was true.[3]

The doctor, of course, had diagnosed syphilis. One indication of how seriously these casual modes of transmission were taken is the fact that the US Navy removed doorknobs from its battleships during World War I, claiming that they had become a source of infection for many of its sailors. We now know, of course, that syphilis cannot be contracted in these ways. This poses a difficult historical problem: Why did physicians believe that they could be?

Theories of casual transmission reflected deep cultural fears about disease and sexuality in the early twentieth century. In these approaches to venereal disease, concerns about hygiene, contamination, and contagion were expressed, anxieties that reflected a great deal about the contemporary society and culture. Venereal disease was viewed as a threat to the entire late Victorian social and sexual system, which placed great value on discipline, restraint, and homogeneity. The sexual code of that era held that sex would receive social sanction only in marriage. But the concerns about venereal disease and casual transmission also reflected a pervasive fear of the urban masses, the growth of the cities, and the changing nature of familial relationships.[4]

Today, persistent fears about casual transmission of AIDS reflect a somewhat different, yet no less significant, social configuration. First, AIDS is strongly associated with behaviors which have been traditionally considered deviant. This is true for both homosexuality and intravenous drug use. After a generation of growing social tolerance for homosexuality, the epidemic has generated new fears and heightened old hostilities. Just as syphilis created a disease-oriented xenophobia in the early twentieth century, AIDS has today generated a new homophobia. AIDS has recast anxiety about contamination in a new light. Among certain social critics, AIDS is seen as "proof" of a certain moral order.

Second, fears are fanned because we live in an era in which the authority of scientific expertise has eroded. This may well be an aspect of a broader decline in the legitimacy of social institutions, but it is clearly seen in the areas of science and medicine. Despite significant evidence that HIV (human immunodeficiency virus) is not casually transmitted, medical and public health experts have been unable to provide the categorical reassurances that the public would like. But without such guarantees, public fear has remained high. In part, this reflects a misunderstanding of the nature of science and its inherent uncertainty. While physicians and public health officials have experience tolerating such uncertainty, the public requires better education in order to effectively evaluate risks.[5,6]

Third, as a culture, we Americans are relatively unsophisticated in our assessments of relative risk. How are we to evaluate the risks of AIDS? *How shall social policy be constructed around what are small or unknown risks?* The ostracism of HIV-infected children from their schools in certain locales, the refusal of some physicians to treat AIDS patients, job and housing discrimination against those infected (and those suspected of being infected) all reveal the pervasive fears surrounding the epidemic. Clearly, then, one public health goal must be to address these fears. Addressing such fears means understanding their etiology. They originate in the particular social meaning of AIDS—its "social construction." We will not be able to effectively mitigate these concerns until we understand their deeper meaning. The response to AIDS will be fundamentally shaped by these fears; therefore, we need to develop techniques to assist individuals to distinguish irrational fears of AIDS from realistic and legitimate concerns. In this respect, many have focused on the need for more education.

Lesson #2—Education Will Not Control the AIDS Epidemic

Early in the twentieth century, physicians, public health officials, and social reformers concerned about the problem of syphilis and gonorrhea called for a major educational campaign.[7] They cogently argued that the tide of infection could not be stemmed until the public had adequate knowledge about these diseases, their mode of transmission, and the means of prevention. They called for an end to "the conspiracy of silence"—the Victorian code of sexual ethics—that considered all discussion of sexuality and disease in respectable society inappropriate. Physicians had contributed to this state of affairs by hiding diagnoses from their patients and families, and upholding what came to be known as the "medical secret." One physician described the nature of the conventions surrounding sexually transmitted diseases:

> Medical men are walking with eyes wide open along the edge of despair so treacherous and so pitiless that the wonder can only be that they have failed to warn the world away. Not a signboard! Not a caution spoken above a whisper! All mystery and seclusion. . . . As a result of this studied propriety, a world more full of venereal infection than any other pestilence.[8]

Prince Morrow, the leader of the social hygiene movement, the antivenereal disease campaign, concluded, "Social sentiment holds that it is a greater violation of the properties of life publicly to mention venereal disease than privately to contract it."[9]

During this period, the press remained reticent on the subject of sexually transmitted infections, refusing to print accounts of their effects. Reporters employed euphemisms such as "rare blood disorder" when forced to include a reference to a venereal infection. Nevertheless, magazines and newspapers did accept advertisements for venereal nostrums and quacks. In 1912, the US Post Office confiscated copies of birth control advocate Margaret Sanger's *What Every Girl Should Know* because it considered the references to syphilis and gonorrhea "obscene" under the provisions of the Comstock law.[4]

Enlightened physicians vigorously called for an end to this hypocrisy. "We are dealing with the solution of a problem," explained Dr. Egbert Grandin, "where ignorance is *not* bliss but is misfortune, and where, therefore, it is folly not to be wise."[10] Social reformers viewed education and publicity as a panacea; forthright education would end the problem of sexually transmitted infection. If parents failed to perform their social responsibilities and inform their children, then the schools should include sex education. By 1919, the U.S. Public Health Service endorsed sex education in the schools, noting, "As in many instances the school must take up the burden neglected by others."[11] By 1922, almost half of all secondary schools offered some instruction in sex hygiene.

Educational programs devised by the social hygienists emphasized fear of infection. Prince Morrow, for example, called fear "the protective genius of the human body." Another physician explained, "The sexual instinct is imperative and will only listen to fear." Margaret Cleaves, a leading social hygienist, argued, "There should be taught such disgust and dread of these conditions that naught would induce the seeking of a polluted source for the sake of gratifying a controllable desire."[12]

In this sense, educational efforts may have actually contributed to the pervasive fears of infection, to the stigma associated with the diseases, and to the discrimination against its victims. Indeed, educational materials produced throughout the first decades of the twentieth century emphasized the inherent dangers of all sexual activity, especially disease and unwanted pregnancy. In this respect, such educational programs, rather than being termed sex education were actually antisex education. Pamphlets and films repeatedly emphasized the "loathsome" and disfiguring aspects of sexually transmitted disease; the most drastic pathological consequences (insanity, paralysis, blindness, and death); as well as the disastrous impact on personal relations.

This orientation toward sex education reached its apogee during World War I, when American soldiers were told, *"A German bullet is cleaner than a whore."* Despite their threatening quality, these educational programs did not have the desired effect of reducing the rates of infection. And indeed, sexual mores in the twentieth century have responded to a number of social and cultural forces more powerful than the fear of disease.

There are, nonetheless, some precedents for successful educational campaigns. During World War II, the military initiated a massive educational campaign against sexually transmitted disease. But unlike prior efforts, it reminded soldiers that disease could be prevented through the use of condoms, which were widely distributed. The military program recognized that sexual behaviors could be modified but that calls for outright abstinence were likely to fail. Given the need for an efficient and healthy army, officials maintained a pragmatic posture that separated morals from the essential task of prevention. As one medical officer explained, "It is difficult to make the sex act unpopular."[13]

Today, calls for better education are frequently offered as the best hope for controlling the AIDS epidemic. But this will only be true if some resolution is reached concerning the specific content and nature of such educational efforts. The limited effectiveness of education that merely encourages fear is well-documented. Moreover, AIDS education requires a forthright confrontation of aspects of human sexuality that are typically avoided. To be effective, AIDS education must be explicit, focused, and appropriately targeted to a range of at-risk social groups. As the history of sexually transmitted diseases makes clear, we need to study the nature of behavior and disease. If education is to have a positive impact, we need to be far more sophisticated, creative, and bold in devising and implementing programs.

Education is not a panacea for the AIDS epidemic, just as education did not solve the problem of other sexually transmitted diseases earlier in the twentieth century. It is one critical aspect of a fully articulated program. As this historical vignette makes clear, we need to be far more explicit about what we mean when we say "education." Certainly education about AIDS is an important element of any public health approach to the crisis, but we need to substantively evaluate a range of educational programs and their impact on behavior for populations with a variety of needs.

Because the impact of education is unclear and the dangers of the epidemic are perceived as great (see lesson #1), there has been considerable interest in compulsory public health measures as a primary means of controlling AIDS.

Lesson #3—Compulsory Public Health Measures Will Not Control the Epidemic

Given the considerable fear that the epidemic has generated and its obvious dangers, demands have been voiced for the implementation of compulsory public health interventions. (The history of efforts to control syphilis during the twentieth century indicates the limits of compulsory measures which range from required premarital testing to quarantine of infected individuals.)

Next to programs for compulsory vaccination, compulsory programs for premarital syphilis serologies are probably the most widely known of all compulsory public health measures in the twentieth century United States. (The development of effective laboratory diagnostic measures stands as a signal contribution in the history of the control of sexually transmitted diseases.) With the development of the Wassermann test in 1906, there was a generally reliable way of detecting the presence of syphilis. The achievement of such a test offered a new series of public health potentials. No longer would diagnosis depend on strictly clinical criteria. Diagnosis among the asymptomatic was now possible, as was the ability to test the effectiveness of treatments. *The availability of the test led to the development of programs for compulsory testing.*

Significantly, calls for compulsory screening for syphilis predated the Wassermann exam. Beginning in the last years of the nineteenth century, several states began to mandate premarital medical examinations to assure that sexually transmitted infections were not communicated in marriage. But without a definitive test, *such examinations were of limited use.* With a laboratory test, however, calls were voiced for requiring premarital blood tests. In 1935, Connecticut became the first state to mandate premarital serologies of all prospective brides and grooms. The rationale for premarital screening was clear. If every individual about to be married were tested, and, if found to be infected, treated, the transmission of infection to marital partners and offspring would be halted. The legislation was vigorously supported by the public health establishment, organized women's groups, magazines, and the news media. Many clinicians, however, argued against the legislation, suggesting that diagnosis should not rely exclusively on laboratory findings which were, in some instances, incorrect. N.A. Nelson of the Massachusetts Department of Public Health explained, "Today, it is becoming the fashion to support, by law, the too common notion that the laboratory is infallible."[14] Despite such objections, by the end of World War II, virtually all the states had enacted provisions mandating premarital serologies.

Legislation is currently pending in 35 state legislatures that would require premarital HIV serologies. The rationale for such programs is often the historical precedent of syphilis screening. The logic seems intuitively correct: We screen for syphilis. AIDS is a far more serious disease, we should therefore screen for AIDS. In this respect it is worth reviewing the effectiveness of premarital syphilis screening as well as those factors that distinguish syphilis from AIDS.

Mandatory premarital serologies never proved to be a particularly effective mechanism for finding new cases of syphilis. First, physicians and public health officials recognized that there was a *significant rate of false positive tests,* which occurred because of technical inadequacies of the tests themselves or as a result of biological phenomena (such as other infections). As the concepts of sensitivity (the test's performance among those with the disease) and specificity (the test's performance among those free of infections) came to be more fully understood in the 1930s, the oversensitivity of tests like the Wassermann was revealed. *As many as 25 percent of individuals determined to be infected with syphilis by the Wassermann test were actually free of infection; nevertheless, these individuals often underwent toxic treatment with arsenical drugs, assuming the tests were correct.* Beyond this, individuals with false positive tests often suffered the social repercussions of being infected: deep stigma and disrupted relationships. As many physicians pointed out, a positive serology did not always mean that an individual could transmit the disease. Because the tests tended to be mandated for a population at relatively low risk of infection, their accuracy was further compromised. Some individuals reportedly avoided the test altogether.[15]

Many of the difficulties associated with the high numbers of false positives were alleviated as new, more specific tests were developed in the 1940s and 1950s, but the central problem remained. Premarital syphilis serologies failed to identify a significant percentage of the infected population. In 1978, for example, premarital screening accounted for only 1.27 per cent of all national tests found to be positive for syphilis. The costs of these programs were estimated at $80 million annually.[16] Another study in California projected the costs per case found through premarital screening to be $240,000.[17] Moreover, premarital screening for syphilis continued to find a significant number of false positives. *As these studies indicated, the benefits of screening programs are dependent on the prevalence of the disease in the population being screened.* In this respect, it seems unlikely that premarital screening effectively served the function of preventing infections within marriage that its advocates assumed it would. These data led a number of states to repeal mandatory premarital serologies in the early 1980s.

Compulsory premarital syphilis serologies thus offer a dubious precedent for required HIV screening. The point, of course, is *not* that the test is inaccurate. ELISA (enzyme-linked immunosorbent assay) testing coupled with the Western Blot *can be* quite reliable, but only when applied to populations that are likely to have been infected. Screening of low-prevalence populations, like premarital couples, is unlikely to have any significant impact on the course of the epidemic. *Not only will such programs find relatively few new cases, they will also reveal large numbers of false positives. A recent study concluded that a national mandatory premarital screening program would find approximately 1,200 new cases of HIV infection, one-tenth of 1 percent of those currently infected. But it would also incorrectly identify as many as 380 individuals— actually free of infection—as infected, even with supplementary Western Blot tests. Such a program would also falsely reassure as many as 120 individuals with false negative results.*[18] Moreover, the inability to treat and render noninfectious those individuals who are found to be infected severely limits the potential benefits of such mandatory measures. With syphilis serologies, *the rationale of the program was to treat infected individuals.*

This, of course, is *not* to argue that testing has no role in an effective AIDS public health campaign. During the late 1930s, a massive voluntary testing campaign heightened consciousness of syphilis in Chicago, bringing thousands of new cases into treatment. AIDS testing, conducted voluntarily and confidentially, targeted to individuals who have specific risk factors for infection, may have significant public health benefits. Compulsory screening, however, could merely discourage infected individuals from being tested. This makes clear the need to enact legislation guaranteeing the confidentiality of those who volunteer to be tested and prohibiting discrimination against HIV-infected individuals.

As a mandatory measure, premarital screening is a relatively modest proposal. During the course of the twentieth century, more radical and intrusive compulsory measures to control STDs, such as quarantine, have also been attempted. These, too, have failed. During World War I, as hysteria about the impact of STDs rose, Congress passed legislation to support the quarantine of prostitutes suspected of spreading disease. The Act held that anyone suspected of harboring a venereal infection could be detained and incarcerated until determined to be noninfectious. During the course of the war, more than 20,000 women were held in camps because they were suspected of being "spreaders" of venereal disease.

The program had no apparent impact on rates of infection, which actually climbed substantially during the war. In sexually transmitted infections, the reservoir of infection is relatively high, modes of transmission are specific, and infected individuals may be healthy. In the case of AIDS, where there is no medical intervention to render individuals noninfectious, quarantine is totally impractical because it would require lifelong incarceration of the infected.

Compulsory measures often generate critics because such policies may infringe on basic civil liberties. From an ethical and legal viewpoint, the first question that must be asked about any potential policy intervention is: Is it likely to work? Only if there is clear evidence to suggest the program would be effective does it make sense to evaluate the civil liberties implications. Then it is possible to evaluate the constitutional question: Is the public health benefit to be derived worthy of the possible costs in civil liberties? Is the proposed compulsory program the least restrictive of the range of potential measures available to achieve the public good?[19]

In this respect, it is worth noting that compulsory measures may actually be counterproductive. First, they require substantial resources that could be more effectively allocated. Second, they have often had the effect of driving the very individuals that the program hopes to reach farther away from public health institutions. Ineffective draconian measures would serve only to augment the AIDS crisis. Nevertheless, despite the fact that such programs offer no benefits, they may have substantial political and cultural appeal (see lesson #1).

Because compulsory measures are controversial and unlikely to control the epidemic, there is considerable hope that we will soon have a "magic bullet"—a biomedical "fix" to free us of the hazards of AIDS.

Lesson #4—The Development of Effective Treatments and Vaccines Will Not Immediately or Easily End the AIDS Epidemic

As the history of efforts to control other sexually transmitted diseases makes clear, effective treatment has not always led to control. In 1909, German Nobel laureate Paul Ehrlich discovered Salvarsan (arsphenamine), an arsenic compound which killed the spirochete, the organism which causes syphilis. Salvarsan was the first effective chemotherapeutic agent for a specific disease. Ehrlich called Salvarsan a "magic bullet," a drug that would seek out and destroy its mark.[20] He claimed that modern medicine would seek the discovery of a series of such drugs to eliminate the microorganisms which cause disease. Although Salvarsan was an effective treatment, it was toxic and difficult to administer. Patients required a painful regimen of injections, sometimes for as long as two years.

Unlike the arsphenamines, penicillin was truly a wonder drug. In early 1943, Dr. John F. Mahoney of the US Public Health Service found that penicillin was effective in treating rabbits infected with syphilis. After repeating his experiments with human subjects, his findings were announced and the massive production of penicillin began.[21]

With a single shot, the scourge of syphilis could be avoided. Incidence fell from a high of 72 cases per 100,000 in 1943 to about 4 per 100,000 in 1956.[22] In 1949, Mahoney wrote, "As a result of antibiotic therapy, gonorrhea has almost passed from the scene as an important clinical and public entity."[23] An article in the *American Journal of Syphilis* in 1951 asked, "Are Venereal Diseases Disappearing?" Although the article concluded that it was too soon to know, by 1955 the *Journal* itself had disappeared. *The Journal of Social Hygiene*, for half a century the leading publication on social dimensions of the problem, also ceased publication. As rates reached all time lows, it appeared that venereal diseases would join the ranks of other infectious diseases that had come under the control of modern medicine.

Although there is no question that the nature and meaning of syphilis and gonorrhea underwent a fundamental change with the introduction of antibiotic therapy, the decline of venereal diseases proved short-lived. Rates of infection began to climb in the early 1960s. By the late 1950s much of the machinery, especially procedures for public education, case-finding, tracing and diagnosis had been severely reduced.[1]

In 1987, the Centers for Disease Control (CDC) reported an increase in cases of primary and secondary syphilis. The estimated annual rate per 100,000 population rose from 10.9 to 13.3 cases, the largest increases in 10 years. These figures are particularly striking in that they come in the midst of the AIDS epidemic which many have assumed has led to a substantial decline in sexual encounters. Moreover, after an 8-year decline, rates of congenital syphilis have also reportedly risen since 1983. The CDC concluded that individuals with a history of sexually transmitted infection are at increased risk for infection with the AIDS virus.[24]

Despite the effectiveness of penicillin as a cure for syphilis, the disease has persisted. The issue, therefore, is not merely the development of effective treatments but the *process* by which they are deployed; the means by which they move from laboratory to full allocation to those affected. Effective treatments without adequate education, counseling, and funding may not reach those who most need them. Even "magic bullets" need to be effectively delivered. Obviously effective treatments should be a priority in a multifaceted approach to AIDS and will ultimately be an important component in its control; but even a magic bullet will not quickly or completely solve the problem.

No doubt new and more effective treatments for AIDS will be developed in the years ahead, but their deployment will raise a series of complex issues ranging from human subject research to actual allocation. And while effective treatments may help to control further infection, as they do for syphilis and gonorrhea, treatments which prolong the life of AIDS patients may have little or no impact on the rates of transmission of the virus, which occurs principally among individuals who have no symptoms of disease.

This suggests certain fundamental flaws in the biomedical model of disease. Diseases are complex bio-ecological problems that may be mitigated only by addressing a range of scientific, social, and political considerations. No single intervention—even an effective vaccine—will adequately address the complexities of the AIDS epidemic.

Conclusions

As these historical lessons make clear, in the context of fear surrounding the epidemic (lesson #1), the principal proposals for eradicating AIDS (lessons #2–4) are unlikely to be effective, at least in the immediate future. These lessons should not imply, however, that nothing will work; they make evident that no single avenue is likely to lead to success. Moreover, they suggest that in considering any intervention we will require sophisticated research to understand its potential impact on the epidemic. While education, testing, and biomedical research all offer some hope, in each instance we will need to fully consider their particular effectiveness as measures to control disease.

Simple answers based upon historical precedents are unlikely to alleviate the AIDs crisis. History does, however, point to a range of variables which influence disease, and those factors which require attention if it is to be effectively addressed. Any successful approach to the epidemic will require a full recognition of the important social, cultural, and biological aspects of AIDS. A public health priority will be to lead in the process of discerning those programs likely to have a beneficial impact from those with considerable political and cultural appeal, but unlikely to positively affect the course of the epidemic. Only in this way will we be able to devise effective and humane public policies.

NOTES

1. Cutler J.C., Arnold R.C.: Venereal disease control by health departments in the past: Lessons for the present. Am J Public Health 1988; 78:372–376.

2. Bulkey L.D.: Syphilis of the Innocent. New York: Bailey and Fairchild, 1894.

3. Anon: What one woman has had to bear. Forum 1912; 68:451–454.

4. Brandt A.M.: No Magic Bullet: A Social History of Venereal Disease in the United States since 1880. New York: Oxford University Press, 1985, rev. ed. 1987.

5. Eisenberg L.E.: The genesis of fear: AIDS and public's response to science. Law, Med Health Care 1986; 14:243–249.

6. Becker M.H., Joseph J.G.: AIDS and behavioral change to reduce risk: A review. Am. J. Public Health 1988; 78:394–410.

7. Yankauer A.: AIDS and Public Health. (editorial) Am J Public Health 1988; 78:364–366.

8. Willson R.N.: The relation of the medical profession to the social evil. JAMA 1906; 47:32.

9. Morrow P.A.: Publicity as a factor in venereal prophylaxis. JAMA 1906; 47:1246.

10. Grandin E.: Should the Great Body of the General Public Be Enlightened? Charities and Commons, February 24, 1906.

11. US Public Health Service: The Problem of Sex Education in the Schools. Washington, DC, 1919; p 9.

12. Cleaves M.: Transactions of the American Society for Social and Moral Prophylaxis 1910; 3:31.

13. Pappas J.P.: The venereal problem in the US Army. Milit Surg August 1943; 93:182.

14. Nelson N.A.: Marriage and the laboratory. Am J Syphilis 1939; 23:289.

15. Kolmer J.A.: The problem of falsely doubtful and positive reactions in the serology of syphilis. Am J Public Health 1944; 34:510–526.

16. Felman Y.: Repeal of mandated premarital tests for syphilis: A survey of state health officers. Am J Public Health 1981; 71:155–159.

17. Haskell R. J.: A cost benefit analysis of California's mandatory premarital screening program for syphilis. West J Med 1984; 141:538–541.

18. Cleary P.D., Barry M. J., Mayer K.H., Brandt A.M., Gostin L., Fineberg H.V.: Compulsory premarital screening for the human immunodeficiency virus. JAMA 1987; 258:1757–1762.

19. Gostin L., Curran W.: The Limits of Compulsion in Controlling AIDS. Hastings Center Report 1986; 16(suppl):24–29.

20. Marquardt M.: Paul Ehrlich. New York: Henry Schuman, 1951.

21. Dowling H.: Fighting Infection. Cambridge: Harvard University Press, 1977.

22. Brown W.J., Donohue J.F., Axnick N.W., Blount J.H., Jones O.G., Ewen N.J.: Syphilis and Other Venereal Diseases. Cambridge: Harvard University Press (APHA), 1970.

23. Mahoney J.F.: The effect of antibiotics on the concepts and practices of public health. In: Galdston I. (ed): The Impact of Antibiotics on Medicine and Society. New York: 1958; 98–120.

24. USPHS, Centers for Disease Control: MMWR 1987; 36:393.

HIV Antibody Screening:
An Ethical Framework for
Evaluating Proposed Programs

Ronald Bayer, Ph.D., Carol Levine, M.A., and Susan M. Wolf, J.D.

October 1986

THE ACQUIRED IMMUNODEFICIENCY SYNDROME (AIDS) poses a compelling ethical challenge to medicine, science, public health, the legal system, and our political democracy. This report focuses on one aspect of that challenge: the use of blood tests to identify individuals who have been infected with the retrovirus human immunodeficiency virus (HIV). In this article we follow the terminology recently proposed by the International Committee on the Taxonomy of Viruses; that is, we use the term *human immunodeficiency virus*. This replaces the more cumbersome dual terminology of human T-cell lymphotropic virus type III/lymphadenopathy-associated virus (HTLV-III/LAV).

The issue is urgent: The tests are already in use and plans to implement them much more broadly are being proposed.[1] The issue is also complex: At stake is a potential conflict between the community's interests in stopping the spread of a devastating disease and in preserving important values of individual liberty and equal rights.

Screening may seem to be a minor intrusion in the face of a deadly disease; yet even such an ostensibly limited intervention can have dramatic and deleterious consequences for individuals. Such

Ronald Bayer, Ph.D., Carol Levine, M.A., Susan M. Wolf, J.D., "HIV Antibody Screening: An Ethical Framework for Evaluating Proposed Programs," *Journal of the American Medical Association* 256, no. 13 (October 3, 1986): 1768–1774. Copyright © 1986 American Medical Association. Reprinted by Permission of the Authors and the *Journal of the American Medical Association*.

intrusions must, therefore, be warranted by the potential public health benefits.

It is important to reaffirm our society's commitment to promoting the health of its citizens, but public health efforts undertaken with a beneficent intent have sometimes had the opposite effect. An example is mandatory screening for sickle cell trait among blacks in the 1970s, which resulted in misinformation, stigmatization, and discrimination.[2]

This report is addressed to all those considering the introduction of screening and testing programs, including employers, public health officials, legislators, health care providers, and insurers, as well as those who would be screened and whose interests would be affected. We have adopted prevailing usage and define "screening" as the application of the HIV antibody tests to populations and "testing" as the application of that procedure to individuals on a case-by-case basis.[3] Using this distinction, blood donations tested for HIV antibodies are screened; people who go to an alternative test site for the same procedure are tested.

We believe that in each situation in which screening is considered, the proposed program should be subjected to ethical analysis. This report provides a framework for that task. Ethical evaluation is necessary but not sufficient for decision making; it should be performed in conjunction with other types of evaluation, such as legal and economic analyses, before screening is instituted.* In addition, those who consider screening should consult with members of affected populations, since these individuals are best able to identify the potential hazards of proposed programs.

This document argues at various points in favor of moral obligations without advocating legal coercion. In a society that recognizes individual privacy and liberty, law and ethics are often distinct spheres. Not all moral obligations should be translated into law.

---

*Important to consider will be pertinent constitutional provisions, laws, and legal precedent on the federal, state, and local levels, such as the Fourteenth Amendment to the US Constitution, the Federal Vocational Rehabilitation Act of 1973, 29 USC 794, state statutes such as California Health and Safety Code Chapter 1, 11 §199 20 et seq, city ordinances such as the San Francisco Police Code Article 38, and judicial decisions such as *Codero vs Coughlin*, No. 84, Civ 728 (SD NY 1984); *District 27 Community School Board vs Board of Education*, 130 Misc 2d 398, 502 NYS2d 325 (NY Sup 1986); *South Florida Blood Service, Inc vs Rasmussen*. 467 S2d 798 (Fla App 1985); and *La Rocca vs Dalsheim*, 120 Misc 2d 697, 467 NYS2d 302 (NY Sup 1983). This list is by no means exhaustive, and the specifics of any screening or testing proposal will dictate the legal research required.

AIDS: Status Today

As of June 1986 about 73 percent of the 21,517 cases of AIDS have occurred among homosexual or bisexual men, some of whom were intravenous drug users; 17 percent were heterosexual intravenous drug users; 1.6 percent were people who had received contaminated blood transfusions; 0.8 percent were hemophiliacs who had received contaminated units of factor VIII, a plasma blood product; and 1 percent were heterosexual partners of persons at increased risk for AIDS. The remainder are people without a known risk factor, primarily recent immigrants from Haiti or people who died before complete case histories could be taken.[4]

The reported cases of AIDS represent what is commonly called the tip of the iceberg. Using the Centers for Disease Control's projections of ten cases of AIDS-related complex (ARC) (not a reportable condition) for every case of AIDS, the concealed portion includes an estimated 210,000 cases of ARC, many more cases of minor illness, and up to 1.5 million people who have been infected with the virus but who show no clinical signs of disease.[4,5]

Because HIV is a retrovirus whose genome becomes permanently integrated into its host's genetic material, all people infected can be presumed to be infected for life. Experts disagree on how many infected individuals will go on to develop disease. Early estimates of 5 to 10 percent were optimistic. Some now suggest that as many as 45 percent will develop AIDS or ARC within 5 years. How many will do so over more extended periods of time is at present not known. However, it must now also be assumed that all infected individuals can transmit the virus to others because the naturally produced antibodies do not completely neutralize the virus.[6] Although the virus has been isolated in nearly all body fluids, it is most concentrated in blood.[7]

The human immunodeficiency virus is transmitted through intimate sexual contact and blood, and not through air, water, or other vectors. Its transmission can be stopped at present only by behavioral change, through avoiding intimate sexual contact with an infected person and the use of contaminated needles and syringes. Risk can be reduced through "safer" or "protected" sex practices (such as the use of condoms and the avoidance of receptive intercourse).[8] Infection with HIV affects individuals differently, with the factors leading to greater susceptibility to infection or illness still unknown. The latency period (the time between infection and onset of symptoms) is highly variable but in some individuals may be years. When HIV infection culminates in AIDS, it is ultimately fatal.

From a civil liberties perspective, HIV infection has so far predominantly affected groups that are already at risk of social and economic discrimination. Many of the behaviors implicated are expressions of sexual orientation and occur in private settings, and information about individuals with AIDS or at risk of AIDS can be used in ways that have no legitimate public health purpose and can be detrimental to their interests.

Screening for HIV Antibodies

The test now being used to detect the presence of antibodies elicited by HIV viral antigens is an enzyme-linked immunosorbent assay—the ELISA (or EIA) test. Because the ELISA test was developed to protect the blood supply, the cutoff between reactive and nonreactive values was set very low to capture all true-positives. The price of such sensitivity is a loss of specificity. In high-risk populations there will be comparatively few false-positives. In low-risk populations, however, as many as 90 percent of the small number of initially reactive results will be false-positives. To distinguish true-positives, it is necessary to repeat the ELISA and to use an independent, supplemental test such as the Western Blot.[9]

In addition to the false-positives, there may be false-negatives; that is, the tests may fail to detect antibodies, or there may be none, even though the person is infected. The problem of false-negatives is only partly a characteristic of the test; it also reflects the latency period (on rare occasions as long as 6 months) between infection with the HIV virus and the development of antibodies.

Despite these problems, the ELISA test has served its initial purpose—screening blood donations—satisfactorily. The antibody test also enables clinicians to monitor the infection status of their patients. It may be useful in establishing risk to the patient when immunosuppressive therapy is contemplated. It may provide epidemiologists with baseline data for the conduct of longitudinal studies of the natural history of AIDS. Finally, it may provide many individuals with data useful in supporting their voluntary modification of sexual, drug-using, and reproductive behavior.

The current screening method (a repeated ELISA plus a supplemental test) compares favorably in terms of accuracy to other

screening methods used in medical practice, all of
limitations. Concern about the possible misuses
not be confused with challengers to the accura

Principles and Prerequisites for
Evaluating a Screening Program

To evaluate the ethical acceptability of a proposed screening program, we *recommend an analysis based on seven prerequisites.*
The prerequisites are based on the principle of respect for persons,
the harm principle, beneficence, and justice. These 4 widely accepted ethical principles are derived from secular, religious, and
constitutional traditions and are commonly applied to medicine,
research, and public health.[10,11]

Principles

1. *Respect for persons* requires that individuals be treated as
autonomous agents who have the right to control their own destinies. Respect for persons requires that persons be given the opportunity to decide what will or will not happen to them. The right to
privacy and the requirement of informed consent flow from this
principle. A corollary—requiring persons with diminished autonomy
to be given special protections—may also apply to some populations such as children and prisoners.

2. The *harm* principle permits limitations on an individual's liberty to pursue personal goals and choices when others will be
harmed by those activities.

3. *Beneficence* requires that we act on behalf of the interests and
welfare of others. The obligations of beneficence apply to actions
affecting both individuals and the community. Potential risks must
be weighed against potential benefits and the actions with the most
favorable risk-to-benefit ratio adopted. The justification for public
health authority derives from both the harm principle and beneficence.

4. *Justice* requires that the benefits and burdens of particular
actions be distributed fairly. It also prohibits invidious discrimination.

These ethical principles may sometimes conflict. For example,
the principle of beneficence and the harm principle may outweigh
the need to obtain consent in some situations, but they never
outweigh the obligation to treat persons with respect for their
intrinsic worth and dignity.

rerequisites for Screening

he following seven prerequisites constitute the threshold requirements for ethical acceptability, but as we will discuss later, they do not cover all the ethical problems that may arise.

1. *The purpose of the screening must be ethically acceptable.* There is at present one acceptable purpose for screening: to stop the spread of AIDS. This purpose draws on the principle of beneficence—our duty to protect the welfare of those who might become infected with HIV. The use of medical tests and the public health power of the state is justifiable to protect the health of the community. However, to use these resources merely to express social disapproval of sexual orientation or drug use violates the principles of justice and respect for persons. If a therapy or vaccine becomes available, screening may be justified to benefit those at risk.

2. *The means to be used in the screening program and the intended use of the information must be appropriate for accomplishing the purpose.* If a screening program is intended to stop the spread of HIV infection, but designed in a way that precludes achieving that end, it is unjustifiable. It would involve an invasion of privacy without any public health benefit. For example, screening all food handlers is not justifiable, since there is no evidence that the disease is spread through food.

3. *High-quality laboratory services must be used.* Given the importance of interpreting not just one but a series of tests to arrive at a confirmed positive result, the availability of highly qualified technicians and laboratory services is essential. Beneficence requires that persons not be subjected to any risk—whether social, psychological, or medical—if the information about them to be generated in screening does not meet the current standard levels of accuracy. The need for confirmatory testing applies to both low- and high-risk populations.

4. *Individuals must be notified that screening will take place.* Respect for persons requires that individuals be notified that they are or may be the subjects of screening. In some cases individuals may choose not to participate in the activity for which screening is required (for example, they may choose not to donate blood or semen). In other cases, they may not have that option, but they should, nevertheless, be notified to protect their autonomy; they should also be made aware that highly sensitive data about them will be generated, with the associated psychological burdens and risks of breaches of confidentiality. Physicians who contemplate

testing an individual on the basis of membership in a risk group should notify the person and should seek consent. This prerequisite does not preclude the use, without notification, of blood or other samples unlinked to personal identifiers in Institutional Review Board-approved research.

5. *Individuals who are screened have a right to be informed about the results.* There is no ethical justification for withholding test results. Certainly that information may be profoundly disturbing—not just to the individual but to the health care provider who has to convey it—but both respect for persons and beneficence support notification.

The converse—whether individuals have a "right not to know"—is a disputed question. We believe that persons who are screened and whose seropositivity is confirmed have a moral obligation to learn that information; that is, we reject the "right not to know" in this case.[12]

The most important potential benefit of the knowledge of a positive test result to an individual is the motivation to change behavior that puts others at risk. A person at low risk (for example, a blood donor who has no knowledge of a sexual partner's drug abuse) had no reason to suspect that he or she is infected and, therefore, has no reason to change behavior. To protect others, that person must know the fact of potential infectiousness.

This conclusion is generally accepted; the major controversy concerns the right of individuals at high risk not to know. The claim is made that as long as such an individual acts as though he or she were seropositive and avoids high-risk behavior, there is no need for knowledge of seropositivity. Moreover, the argument continues, such information may be so psychologically devastating that the individual will suffer greatly without any benefits to himself or herself or additional benefits to others.

We acknowledge the potential burden of such information. We also recognize that there is insufficient evidence to determine whether notification will in fact motivate behavioral change or whether it will lead to enormous distress with no compensating benefits. However, there are two problems with the arguments in favor of a "right not to know." First, they underestimate the power of denial and the difficulty of sustaining behavioral change in the absence of specific information. Second, there is no way to discern in advance who of the infected people will modify their behavior without notification and who will not, much less who will be consistent in these changes.

Therefore, we conclude that given the disastrous consequences of HIV infection and the imperative of the harm principle, those who are infected have an obligation to know their antibody status, to inform their sexual partners, and to modify their behavior. We urge immediate research into both the positive and negative consequences of notification.

6. *Sensitive and supportive counseling programs must be available before and after screening to interpret the results, whether they are positive or negative.* Individuals should be counseled about the test before screening, told the significance of both positive and negative results, and informed about the availability of future counseling. A confirmed positive test result should not be conveyed by letter. It should be provided by personal contact in the context of, or with referral to, competent counseling services. Referral to a person's private physician may not be adequate, since many physicians in general practice, particularly those in low-incidence areas, have little experience with interpreting HIV antibody test results.

7. *The confidentiality of screened individuals must be protected.* Respect for the privacy of those who undergo therapeutic and diagnostic procedures demands that the results of such procedures be kept confidential. In the case of HIV antibody testing, where the inadvertent or unwarranted disclosure of positive test results could have disastrous social consequences for individuals, the importance of preserving confidentiality is especially critical.

However, there are a few circumstances in which public health reasons could provide a justification for the breach of confidentiality. For example, if it were known that a seropositive individual had recently donated blood, notifying the blood collection agency would be appropriate on grounds of benefiting blood recipients. However, that agency would then have the obligation to protect the confidentiality of the information received.

Appropriate legislation or administrative regulations should be designed to protect the confidentiality of antibody test results. Whenever disclosure is to occur, individuals must be informed that a breach of confidentiality will take place and why it is necessary. Under no circumstances should test results be used in ways that bear no relationship to legitimate public health concerns.

Mass Screening and Screening in Special Settings: Applying the Ethical Prerequisites

Using the framework we have established in the previous section, we now turn to the specific application of the principles and prerequisites to the current policy debates.

Should Universal Mandatory Screening Be Undertaken?

Universal mandatory screening can be justified on the basis of beneficence when a therapeutic intervention is available or when an infectious state puts others at risk merely by casual contact. However, neither is the case with AIDS. Thus, there is no demonstrable public health benefit that justifies universal mandatory screening, given the invasion of privacy involved.

At the most extreme, advocates of universal mandatory screening suggest it be a prelude to isolation.[13] This would entail a sweeping deprivation of civil and human rights—the segregation of a million or more people for life on the assumption that they will behave in ways that spread disease. Such a drastic measure cannot be justified, particularly when less intrusive measures are available. Isolation would probably increase the incidence of disease because those who were segregated would become a closed community, with the prospect of repeated reinfection.

Others justify mandatory screening less drastically. They see it as a way of making each individual learn his or her antibody status, hoping it will prompt behavioral change. However, long-term behavioral modification is a complex process that is less likely to be achieved under circumstances of coercion, where long-term follow-up and support are nearly impossible to provide on a mass scale. Even in this case, universal mandatory screening would require the creation of an enormous and costly apparatus. Since screening would have to be periodically repeated, it would be necessary to trace each individual's whereabouts to preclude avoidance of the test. Even were such screening feasible, it would require an extraordinary and repeated intrusion into the privacy of all Americans for little probable benefit. Therefore, on grounds of beneficence, it would be unacceptable.

Should Mandatory Screening Be Implemented in Special Settings?

There are limited circumstances in which mandatory screening is appropriate—only where it can be shown, under stringent standards of scientific evidence, to reduce certain dangers. The mandatory screening of all blood donations has aroused virtually no opposition because everyone has an interest in a blood supply that is free of HIV. For similar reasons there should be routine screening of semen donors for artificial insemination and organ donations for transplant purposes under conditions consistent with our ethical prerequisites.[14] In blood, semen, or live organ donations, individuals can avoid screening by avoiding the activity; these activities may be desired but are not central to a person's life plans.

Screening all applicants for marriage licenses presents quite a different situation. Marriage, unlike donating blood, is central to an individual's freedoms. The likelihood of detecting a significant number of true-positives, a goal that might be defended on grounds of beneficence, is exceedingly small in relation to the economic costs and ethical dangers of invasions of privacy and potential curbs on individual liberties in instituting a screening program. Those at risk for contracting AIDS are not likely to be the ones applying for marriage licenses. Moreover, neither sex nor childbearing is dependent on marriage in our society.

The state has an interest in stopping the spread of AIDS, but any bar to marriage for a seropositive individual would pose serious legal and ethical problems. Seropositive heterosexuals, like gay men in long-term relationships, can practice "safer sex" and take their antibody status into account in making childbearing plans. Individuals who are at high risk, or who are concerned about their own or their partner's antibody status, may voluntarily take the test before marriage, with appropriate counseling.

General workplace screening is unjustifiable under our ethical prerequisites because the usefulness of such screening for the protection of others is unsupported by epidemiologic or clinical evidence.[15] In some cases the protection of the public health is the stated purpose for workplace screening, while the underlying reason is the desire to avoid the economic burden of providing health care benefits for people who might become ill with AIDS. The economic costs of AIDS are a matter of serious concern and ought to be addressed directly so that equitable mechanisms for sharing the burden can be developed. However, to disguise these concerns as matters of public health serves neither purpose well.

But are there circumstances that fall between the extremes of blood screening and general employment screening where mandatory screening might be ethically acceptable?

Employment Settings

Since casual contact is not a route of transmission of HIV, the only employment settings in which mandatory screening might be justified are, first, health care involving the open wounds of others and, second, prostitution. Careful investigation of the potential of HIV transmission from infected workers and professionals to patients indicates no evidence of such transmission when standard infection control precautions are taken.[16] Since the risks are, therefore, only theoretical, there are no grounds at present for instituting routine screening of health care workers, including dentists. Prudence, however, dictates that health care personnel at high risk for AIDS, whether or not they know their antibody status, take all precautions when they come into a situation where contact might pose a hazard to others.

A strong public health argument can be made for screening prostitutes. First, male and female prostitutes may have significant rates of seropositivity, either because of drug use, because of a greater risk of infection due to their large numbers of sexual contacts, or because of high-risk sexual practices in which they may engage. Second, seropositive prostitutes can potentially infect large numbers of people. Because the great majority of infected persons in this country are male, and because male-to-male transmission of HIV is most common, it is likely that male prostitutes constitute a greater threat to their clients than do female prostitutes at this time. Finally, prostitutes' motivation to practice "safer sex" or to stop prostitution may be questionable; even if they are so motivated, the pressures to maintain their current behavioral patterns are probably considerable.

As a practical matter, however, only where prostitutes are licensed and subject to periodic health examinations could such screening, when used in conjunction with license revocation, interrupt the transmission of HIV without creating enormous problems. Nevada has recently introduced such screening.[17] Where prostitution is illegal, screening can occur only as an adjunct to arrest. Those prostitutes who are seropositive would have to be threatened with rearrest and perhaps isolation if they continued to engage in prostitution. Effective and consistent enforcement would raise difficult logistical and legal questions.

These practical difficulties, and the moral issues raised by singling out one group for a regimen of screening, arrest, and isolation, warrant immediate attention. Although moving incrementally is morally permissible, targeting a specific population requires particular justification to prevent invidious discrimination. There is an urgent need for educating prostitutes and their clients. It is also important to examine possible ways to reduce the spread of HIV that take account of the social realities of prostitution.

Since the only ethical justification for workplace screening is based on beneficence—reducing the risk of infection to others—the Department of Defense's routine screening of all recruits and active duty personnel is troubling. Communal living does not result in the transmission of HIV. The Department of Defense publicly justifies its policy with the claim that each member of the armed services is a potential blood donor and that in a battlefield emergency there would be no time to screen blood.[18] However, it is not at all clear that soldier-to-soldier battlefield transfusions are in fact standard practice today. Moreover, the rejection of seropositive recruits cannot be justified on such grounds if seropositive active duty personnel are not also being discharged. Even if all seropositive individuals were discharged, one-time screening would not suffice to protect the military donor pool over time. Given the social costs associated with repeated screening, it would be more appropriate to ensure alternatives to battlefield soldier-to-soldier transfusion.

More plausible is the justification that screening identifies those whose compromised immune system might lead to adverse reactions to live-virus vaccines routinely given to recruits. But even this paternalistic justification is weak. The HIV tests are not the only way to identify these individuals.

As in general employment screening, other factors may be concealed under the guise of public health: the military's policies against homosexuality and drug use, relations with foreign governments concerned about the exportation of AIDS by American servicemen, and the desire to avoid the economic burden of AIDS. Here, too, we urge direct discussion of these concerns, not masking them as purported public health issues.

Clinical and Residential Settings

Because hepatitis B is far more infectious than HIV, it is widely accepted that those institutional precautions currently in place to prevent infection by hepatitis B are sufficient to protect against infection by HIV.[15] Since the routine screening of hospital admissions for hepatitis B is not deemed necessary, neither is the routine mandatory screening of all hospital admissions for HIV infection.

The only clinical setting in which routine hepatitis B screening occurs is in dialysis centers. Yet here the Centers for Disease Control has argued against routine antibody screening for HIV because of the potential breaches of confidentiality, although it does not object to dialysis on separate machines for those with clinically diagnosed AIDS.[19] Epidemiologic evidence has provided no evidence thus far of transmission of HIV infection in dialysis centers. However, given the frequent occurrence of blood spills in such centers, we believe that the routine screening of dialysis patients for HIV and the adoption of especially careful precautions for those who are seropositive require further consideration. Such screening, however, should never be used to deny dialysis.

In other settings, such as mental hospitals and residential homes for retarded people, routine screening might be considered because of the possibility of sexual contacts among residents or patients. Especially in those settings where sexual segregation is practiced, homosexual contact—voluntary and involuntary—is known to occur. Given the reduced competence and diminished autonomy that characterize residents of mental hospitals and homes for retarded people, it might be appropriate to consider screening residents and patients in such settings as a way of protecting those who are uninfected from possible HIV infection. However, the need to provide extra supervision for those who are seropositive does not warrant isolation, stigmatization, or the deprivation of services.

The screening of infants born to mothers at high risk, prior to foster care or adoption placement, raises unique problems.[20] The purpose of antibody testing under these circumstances would not be to stop the spread of AIDS or to benefit the child. The purpose would be to provide potential foster and adoptive parents with information that would undoubtedly play a role in their decision to care for the child. But for that purpose the test results may be inconclusive. Some babies born to seropositive mothers may be seropositive at birth but not viremic and may lose the antibodies in the first year of life.[21]

A seropositive child may be difficult, if not impossible, to place in foster or adoptive homes, even though the child may never develop illness. Isolation and stigmatization would almost inevitably follow. The tension is between the potential harm to such children and the interests of the prospective foster and adoptive parents in obtaining this information. The issues require further study.[22]

Finally, screening in prisons has been discussed. Since there are substantial numbers of intravenous drug users in prisons, and since homosexual activity, including instances of homosexual rape, is

known to occur, proponents of screening argue that it is the obligation of the state to protect inmates from possible infection. Those
who oppose such screening point out that the identification of
seropositive prisoners might well place them in imminent danger of
violence from other inmates. To prevent such violence, and to
protect other inmates from infection, isolation has been suggested
by proponents of prison screening. The logical consequence of such
a proposal would be the creation of a separate prison system. The
logistical problems posed by such an effort would be staggering.
Furthermore, segregating those who are seropositive without measures to educate and protect them from repeated infection would
only increase the likelihood of disease.

In prison and in clinical and residential settings, a question ought
to be asked of all proposals for mandatory screening. Are there
alternative measures less intrusive than screening that could provide the necessary protections? If there are alternative measures,
then screening cannot be justified.

In fact there are alternatives to screening in prisons. The state
could reduce the risk of forcible spread of HIV infection by seeking
to reduce the incidence of prison rape. Finally, the spread of HIV
infection in prison would also be reduced by providing condoms
and education regarding the risks of drug use and high-risk sexual
behaviors.

Screening and Insurance

Health Insurance

As a society we have determined that, with the exception of the
very poor and the elderly, health insurance will be available through
the private sector, largely through the workplace. The acquired
immunodeficiency syndrome has provided the occasion to reexamine elements of that system, including exclusions for preexisting
conditions and reliance on experience rather than community rating.[23]

The sole purpose for which screening would be instituted by
health insurance carriers would be either to deny coverage or to
increase sharply premiums for those who are seropositive ("White
paper: The acquired immunodeficiency syndrome & HTLV-III antibody testing," mimeograph. American Council of Life Insurance,
Health Insurance Association of America, February 1986.). Persons
who apply for insurance as individuals, rather than as members of
groups, are particularly vulnerable, but there are dangers for persons covered by group plans as well. Employers who are self-
insured may seek to dismiss employees, penalize them, or refuse to

hire applicants who could increase the costs of health care coverage. In any case, given the proportion of the population that would be involved, screening for group health insurance would be, in essence, universal mandatory screening, and the arguments presented against that policy apply here as well.

Although we recognize that this view is controversial, we believe that state regulatory agencies should not permit those who provide group or individual health insurance coverage to exclude those who are at increased risk for any illness, including AIDS. A denial of health insurance would ultimately create overwhelming burdens for the public and private hospitals that would be forced to provide uncompensated care to the uninsured. From a societal perspective, the central issue is whether the cost of health care for AIDS patients and others at high risk for illness will be broadly distributed or borne by those who become sick, and by their friends and families, reducing them to dependency on the welfare system. The moral issue is one of justice.

Life Insurance

The moral problems posed by life insurance are more difficult to evaluate since it is not as basic a need as is health insurance. The social purpose of life insurance is to provide protection for dependents in the event of death, although individuals may purchase life insurance for other purposes as well. Those at increased risk for a broad range of medical conditions face barriers to life insurance either through formal exclusion or prohibitive premium rates, especially when insurance is purchased individually rather than through a group.

Insurance carriers fear that those who know that they are at risk for AIDS will seek large amounts of life insurance coverage, thus potentially endangering a company's solvency and its ability to pay other claims. Consequently, insurers seek to protect the interests of their other policyholders and stockholders by screening applicants in high-risk categories for HIV antibodies.

Despite such fears, there is no solid information yet on the potential impact of AIDS on insurance companies' solvency or on future premium rates. Moreover, there is a substantial risk to individuals who are screened; the information produced may be accessible to employers and others with no legitimate public health interest. Those who are denied life insurance coverage may also be denied loans, mortgages, and other forms of credit.

In determining public policy, state regulatory agencies must entertain the full range of issues beyond narrow actuarial considerations. If screening is ultimately permitted by state regulatory agencies for life insurance, these agencies should also explore innovative arrangements to provide appropriate coverage to seropositive individuals and should mandate strict confidentiality requirements as well.

Alternatives to Screening: The Promise of Voluntarism

We believe that those at high risk for developing AIDS have a moral obligation to take all possible steps to prevent harm to others, including taking the antibody test. This moral obligation should not, however, be translated into legal coercion. Mandating universal screening, as we have explained, would violate norms of beneficence and respect for persons and might drive the HIV infection underground, thus subverting public health goals.

Where voluntary testing programs are instituted, they should follow the relevant ethical prerequisites set out earlier: that is, high-quality laboratory and data services must be used; individuals who are tested must be informed about the results; sensitive and supportive counseling programs must be available before and after testing to interpret the results, whether positive or negative; and the confidentiality of tested individuals must be protected, In addition, voluntary testing should involve full disclosure of risks and benefits and informed consent.

Some have rejected the moral obligation to take the test, arguing that all members of high-risk groups should simply act as if they are antibody positive. They cite dramatic changes in sexual behavior (as measured by a reduction in sexually transmitted diseases in homosexual men in San Francisco and New York) in populations that include men who have not taken the test.

If such advice were sufficient to motivate radical alterations in sexual conduct and in childbearing plans among the diverse populations involved, it might not be necessary to encourage the use of the antibody test. There is no conclusive evidence on either side, but there is reason to doubt that advice alone provides sufficient motivation.[24] Given the risks associated with AIDS and the uncertainty about what will in fact modify high-risk behavior, there is a strong community interest in encouraging voluntary testing. Public health authorities and clinicians should encourage the use of such tests, to be taken anonymously or with strict confidentiality protections.

In addition, there is a moral obligation for antibody-positive individuals to notify their sexual partners, especially when their partners have no reason to suspect that they have had contact with an individual at risk for HIV infection. Counselors have a professional duty to encourage such notification.

We recognize that sexual contact tracing by public health officials might be considered the next logical step because some individuals may refuse to notify their sexual partners directly. This is an issue that needs further discussion, to consider both whether this is an appropriate strategy at this time and what kinds of protection would be needed. Sexual contact tracing might be justified in low-risk groups and low-incidence areas, for example, but not in other settings.[25]

Women who are at high risk should be encouraged to undergo testing as they consider the prospect of childbearing.[26] In the case of positive results, pregnant women should be fully informed about the risks to themselves and their fetuses (which is high but not inevitable) so that they can make informed decisions about whether to terminate the pregnancy. However, encouragement should not be coercive.

Because of the uncertainty and anxiety that surround the issue of confidentiality, antibody testing has been undertaken under conditions of anonymity in many cities at alternative test sites. In these settings individuals do not provide their names, they are counseled about the test, and if they decide to take it, they are given a number. It is up to the tested individual to request the results and to obtain further counseling. Anonymous testing thus offers the greatest protection for the confidentiality of test results. As a result, testing under such circumstances has been recommended as the single most effective way of encouraging the voluntary use of the test. There are, however, drawbacks to such testing. It may preclude appropriate counseling and follow-up and make long-term epidemiologic studies in the tested populations difficult or impossible. In the short run, anonymous testing may be the only effective strategy for both privacy and public health reasons. Ultimately, if it were possible to construct stringent confidentiality protections, anonymous testing with its obvious limitations might be replaced.

The most serious threat to the widespread use of voluntary testing comes from proposals or already enacted regulations that require reporting the names of those who are antibody positive to state public health officials. The arguments for such reporting are like those that are used to justify the mandatory reporting of AIDS itself—now universally required in the United States—as well as other venereal diseases and infectious conditions. It has been asserted that epidemiologic study, sexual contact tracing, and future therapeutic interventions all require mandatory reporting by private physicians as well as all health care facilities.

In fact mandatory reporting by name rather than code may deter rather than encourage voluntary testing. The knowledge that names will be given to public health authorities, even when those authorities affirm their commitment to confidentiality, is not conducive to voluntary testing. Some have even suggested that mandatory reporting may encourage anonymous sexual activity, so that individuals could not be named as sexual partners if contact tracing were implemented.

Testing should be widely available, not only in alternative test sites, but also in clinics established for the treatment of sexually transmitted diseases, drug treatment facilities, and prenatal clinics. Information in these settings should describe the services available in alternative test sites under conditions of anonymity as well.

Moreover, under the principle of justice, voluntary testing should be publicly funded. Many individuals at high risk, especially those who are intravenous drug users, do not have the resources to pay the cost of testing. The cost of widely available testing programs will be substantial, especially when the requisite services of counselors are considered. But to the extent that significant public health benefits might be achieved, these costs should not be a barrier to the creation of testing centers throughout the United States. Furthermore, since the primary purpose of testing is the protection of other individuals, including potential offspring, the burden of paying for testing ought to be borne by the public.

Summary

We believe that the greatest hope for stopping the spread of HIV infection lies in the voluntary cooperation of those at higher risk—their willingness to undergo testing and to alter their personal behavior and goals in the interests of the community. But we can expect this voluntary cooperation—in some cases, sacrifice—only if the legitimate interests of these groups and individuals in being protected from discrimination are heeded by legislators, professionals, and the public. Yet voluntary testing is not enough. We must proceed with vigorous research and educational efforts to eliminate both the scourge of AIDS and the social havoc that has accompanied it.

NOTES

1. Additional recommendations to reduce sexual and drug abuse-related transmissions of human T-lymphotropic virus type III/lymphadenopathy-associated virus. *MMWRR* 1986;35:152–155.

2. Murray RF Jr, Chamberlain M, Fletcher J, et al: Special considerations for minority participation in prenatal diagnosis. *JAMA* 1980;243:1254–1256.

3. Last JM: *Dictionary of Epidemiology.* New York, Oxford University Press, 1982, pp 32–33.

4. Public Health Service plan for the prevention and control of AIDS and the AIDS virus. Read before the Coolfront Planning Conference, Berkeley Springs, WVa, June 4–6, 1986.

5. Curran JW, Morgan WM: Acquired immunodeficiency syndrome: The beginning, the present, and the future, in Cole HM, Lundberg GD (eds): *AIDS From the Beginning.* Chicago, American Medical Association, 1986, p 23.

6. Landesman SH, Ginzburg HM, Weiss SH: The AIDS epidemic. *N Engl J Med* 1981;253:221–225.

7. An evalutation of acquired immunodeficiency syndrome (AIDS) reported in health-care personnel—United States. *MMWR* 1983;32:358–360.

8. Prevention of acquired immune deficiency syndrome (AIDS): Report of inter-agency recommendations. *MMWR* 1983;32:101–104.

9. Weiss SH, Goedart JJ, Sarngadharan MG, et al: Screening test for HTLV-III (AIDS agent) antibodies: Specificity, sensitivity, and applications. *JAMA* 1985;253:221–225.

10. National Commission for the Protection of Human Subjects of Biomedical and Behavioral Research: *The Belmont Report: Ethical Principles and Guidelines for the Protections of Human Subjects of Research,* publication (OS) 78–0013. US Dept of Health, Education, and Welfare, 1978.

11. Beauchamp TL, Childress JF: *Principles of Biomedical Ethics.* New York, Oxford University Press, 1979, pp 97–126.

12. Provisional public health service interagency recommendations for screening donated blood and plasma for antibody to the virus causing acquired immunodeficiency syndrome. *MMWR* 1985;34:1–5.

13. Grutsch J, Robertson AD: The coming of AIDS: It didn't start with homosexuals and it won't end with them. *Am Spectator* 1986;19:12–15.

14. Testing donors of organs, tissues, and semen for antibody to human T-lymphotropic virus type-III/lymphadenopathy-associated virus. *MMWR* 1985;34:294.

15. Recommendations for preventing transmission of infection with human T-lymphotropic virus type III/lymphadenopathy-associated virus in the workplace. *MMWR* 1985;34:681–686, 691–695.

16. Update: Evaluation of human T-lymphotropic virus type III/lymphadenopathy-associated virus infection in health-care personnel—United States. *MMWR* 1985;34:575–578.

17. Prostitute to undergo HTLV-III testing. *Am Med News* 1986;29:30.

18. Norman C: Military AIDS testing offers research bonus. *Science* 1986;232:818–820.

19. Favero MS: Recommended precautions for patients undergoing hemodialysis who have AIDS or non-A, non-B hepatitis. *Infection Control* 1985;6:301–305.

20. Education and foster care of children infected with human T-lymphotropic virus type III/lymphadenopathy-associated virus. *MMWR* 1985;34:517–521.

21. Marion RW, Wiznia AA, Hutcheon RG, et al: Human T cell lymphotropic virus type III (HTLV-III) embryopathy: A new dysmorphic syndrome associated with intrauterine HTLV-III infections. *AJDC* 1986;140:638–640.

22. Acquired immunodeficiency syndrome in correctional facilities: A report of the National Institute of Justice and the American Correctional Association. *MMWR* 1986;35:195–199.

23. Oppenheimer GM, Padgug RA: AIDS: The risk to insurers, the threat to equity. *Hastings Cent Rep* 1986;16:18–22.

24. Stevens CE, Taylor PE, Zang EA, et al: Human T-cell lymphotropic virus type III infection in a cohort of homosexual men in New York City. *JAMA* 1986;255:2167–2172.

25. Mills M, Wofsey CB, Mills J: Special report: The acquired immunodeficiency syndrome. *N Engl J Med* 1986;314:931–936.

26. Recommendations for assisting in the prevention of perinatal transmission of HTLV-III/LAV and acquired immunodeficiency syndrome. *MMWR* 1985;34:721–726, 731–732.

The Ethics of Screening for Early Intervention in HIV Disease

Carol Levine, M.A. and
Ronald Bayer, Ph.D.

THE TREATMENT OF AIDS and HIV infection has entered a new, more hopeful era, marked by incremental advances in therapy rather than heralded by a single dramatic breakthrough. For those ill with AIDS itself, the prognosis remains grim. But many clinicians, public health officials, patients, and AIDS activists are now convinced that early treatment of asymptomatic HIV infection is beneficial in preventing or delaying the onset of illness.

The voices supporting this view are many and varied. Drs. Robert R. Redfield and Donald S. Burke, of the Walter Reed Army Institute of Research in Washington, D.C., were early advocates of HIV-antibody testing for prompt diagnosis of HIV infection. In a recent summary, they stated: "Prompt diagnosis of HIV infection enables the patient to receive optimal medical care from the earliest moments of the disease. Such care can often prevent complications from developing or getting unnecessarily out of hand."[1]

From a community-based perspective, Project Inform, a San Francisco information and advocacy group, gives its constituents this remarkably similar "Basic Message":

Get tested, anonymously.
If positive, consider antiviral treatment.

Carol Levine, M.A.; Ronald Bayer, Ph.D., "The Ethics of Screening for Early Intervention in HIV Disease," *American Journal of Public Health*, December 1989, vol. 79, no. 12, pp. 1661–1667. Reprinted by Permission of the Authors and the *American Journal of Public Health*.

Monitor T4 cells quarterly, charting the trend.
If the trend of T4 cells is downward or falls consistently below
500, consider both antiviral therapy and immune-boosting
therapy.
If the trend of T4 cells falls below 200, consider prophylactic (preventive) treatment against pneumocystis (aerosol or oral forms).[2]

After a review of available evidence, the United States Public
Health Service has issued the same advice.[3] The San Francisco
AIDS Foundation has launched a campaign to encourage everyone
at risk to be tested voluntarily in order to take advantage of early
medical intervention.[4] Dr. Anthony S. Fauci, director of the National
Institute of Allergy and Infectious Diseases, has said that there is
"no question" that it is now medically advantageous to know one's
HIV status.[5] In the most sweeping recommendation, Drs. Frank S.
Rhame and Dennis G. Maki recommended HIV testing "to all U.S.
adults under the age of 60 regardless of their reported risk history."[6]

Testing patients with symptoms suggestive of HIV disease under
conditions of informed consent as part of a diagnostic workup
has never posed ethical problems. However, when HIV-antibody
testing became available in 1985, there were no clinical grounds
for testing asymptomatic individuals, although there were public
health reasons to encourage testing. Substantial changes in therapeutic prospects and the anticipation of even greater advances
to come have fundamentally altered the context of the discussion about HIV-antibody testing. Because of these changes it is
critical at this point to reconsider the ethics of screening for HIV
infection.[7]

It is precisely when medicine's capacity to enhance patient welfare appears to be increasing that there is a danger that important
ethical concerns can be overridden or disregarded. This is especially so in the case of AIDS—a disease that will continue to exact
an enormous toll in human suffering for the foreseeable future and
that continues to have a social and cultural impact far beyond the
numbers of people affected.

In this article we discuss the ethical aspects of screening and
testing to detect asymptomatic HIV-infected individuals for clinical
purposes. Adopting customary usage, we define "screening" as the
application of the HIV-antibody tests to populations and "testing" as
the application of that procedure to individuals on a case-by-case
basis.[8] It is important to distinguish among the many potential
justifications for screening such as prevention of transmission, infection control, epidemiological surveillance, and medical care. We

believe that all justifications for screening should be evaluated independently and should not be masked by the language of potential therapeutic benefit to the individual.

The Evidence for Early Intervention

Earlier, more accurate identification of seropositive individuals would ideally make it possible to offer them the benefits of: (a) inhibition of viral replication or improvement of immunological status; (b) better management of symptoms or prevention of the onset of opportunistic infections; (c) better general health care.

Identification of True Seropositives

The combined ELISA HIV-antibody test and the supplementary Western Blot provide a high but not absolute level of accuracy in identifying seropositive individuals. Indeterminate Western Blots occur in a small percentage of samples that are repeatedly reactive on ELISA tests, making necessary further testing for viral culture.[9] Recent evidence has indicated that antibody response may be delayed, in some cases as long as 35 months, in some unknown proportion of infected individuals, leading to false negative results.[10]

The level of accuracy that can be obtained with adults does not yet apply to infants. Infants born to infected mothers have maternal HIV antibodies, which may indicate true infection or which may disappear up to 15 or 16 months after birth. Recent studies indicate that from 20 to 50 percent of infants with HIV antibodies are truly infected, a decrease from earlier estimates.[11] Dr. Stephen C. Joseph reported during the Kenneth D. Blackfan Lecture in June 1989 that the most recent evidence from New York City shows a 29 percent transmission rate from infected mother to fetus.

New techniques for the direct identification of viral infection have been reported, primarily the polymerase chain-reaction technique (PCR).[12] This technique can detect the presence of HIV provirus DNA sequences as long as 6 months prior to seroconversion from negative to positive on a Western Blot. PCR may be of assistance in clarifying the meaning of indeterminate Western Blots, but it is still highly experimental, expensive, and difficult to perform except under specialized laboratory conditions. Limited studies with infants show promise; in one study of seven infants positive results proved reliable (the babies later developed AIDS or symptoms of HIV infection), but negative results are much less reliable and may miss as many as 60 percent of infected infants.[13] PCR is not, and may never be, useful as a mass screening tool.

An enhanced ability to detect truly infected individuals is relevant because of the potential to provide early therapeutic benefit. At this juncture infected adults but not infected infants can be reliably identified.

Inhibition of Viral Replication

The published evidence on early intervention to inhibit viral replication is scant. A group led by Frank de Wolf and Jan Mulder of the University of Amsterdam reported in February 1988 on the treatment of 18 asymptomatic men with long-standing HIV infection with low doses of zidovudine (AZT), either alone or in combination with acyclovir. They found that zidovudine has "an inhibitory effect on viral replication ... in blood and (in 1 subject) the central nervous system."[14] Later that year they reported that only 2 of 24 healthy seropositive men treated with AZT needed blood transfusions, compared with 20 to 50 percent of patients with AIDS. Furthermore, the side effects of zidovudine in asymptomatic patients were "mild, transient, and infrequent."[15] In a study presented at the Fifth International Conference on AIDS in June 1989, the Amsterdam group reported that "even with early zidovudine treatment and considerable suppression of HIV-Ag production disease progression can still occur."[16]

Several studies of asymptomatic, HIV-positive persons are underway at the National Institutes of Health and in the United Kingdom and France.[17] The largest NIH study is a Phase III, placebo-controlled study consisting of two doses of AZT. This trial, which began recruiting subjects in 1987, is a 3-year study; it originally expected to enroll 1,562 subjects, but that number has been increased to 3,000. Recruitment for this trial has been slow. Many potential subjects, convinced that the drug is effective, are unwilling to enter a placebo-controlled trial.[18] Other, smaller NIH studies are also underway, involving zidovudine as well as other drugs.

So far there is no solid evidence that early treatment inhibits viral replication or improves immune status. However, there are persuasive theoretical arguments and promising initial reports that may, in time, be substantiated. In his review of the development of early intervention strategies against HIV infection, Dani Bolognesi concluded on a hopeful note. Nevertheless he cautioned that "the emerging picture is far from clear.... One can [however] begin to visualize certain lines of investigation to pursue" for more definitive answers.[19]

Prevention of Opportunistic Infections

Clearly the symptoms of the opportunistic infection associated with AIDS are better managed today than in earlier years. The most dramatic difference is in the management of *Pneumocystis carinii pneumonia*, the most common infection and the one most often associated with early death. Sulfa-based drugs are used to prevent recurrences. Many patients have allergic reactions to this class of drugs, however.

Aerosolized pentamidine had been widely used to prevent the recurrence of *Pneumocystis*, even before the FDA approved its use under a Treatment IND for this purpose. The FDA also approved the drug for patients with 200 or fewer T4 helper cells per cubic millimeter, who are at high risk for developing PCP.[20] The Public Health Service recommendations on primary prophylaxis (for individuals who have not had an episode of *Pneumocystis*) are largely based on extrapolations from evidence from trials of secondary prophylaxis.

Improved General Health Status

A clear benefit of early identification of HIV infection is the opportunity to test for other diseases, such as tuberculosis and syphilis, and to institute appropriate prophylaxis or therapies. Moreover, many persons who learn they are HIV-positive are motivated to engage in healthier lifestyles, changing their diets, exercising more, and reducing cigarette, alcohol, and drug use. There are no studies to support the belief that these changes affect the progression of HIV disease, but many people who have altered their lifestyles report an enhanced feeling of control over their lives and higher energy levels.

Potential Benefits and Risks

Since HIV becomes part of the individual's genetic material, only a therapy that eliminated the virus from DNA or that permanently inhibited viral expression could be considered a cure. At best, early therapeutic intervention at this point can offer an individual longer disease-free intervals, a better quality of life through symptom management, and the hope that the longer one lives the greater the likelihood that even better therapies will be available. These are substantial benefits.

As is the case in adults, there is no proven therapy for asymptomatic HIV infection in newborns. However, knowing that an infant is potentially infected may make possible the aggressive treatment of infections that might otherwise be treated routinely. The more vigilant medical monitoring of such infants could prove especially beneficial since the majority of them are from poor and minority backgrounds and thus vulnerable to many other ailments that are common in economically deprived areas. Moreover, special vigilance can act as a counterbalance to some of the more general problems of health care in poor communities, including access and the lack of a single primary caregiver who can follow the infant's progress.

Providing patients or their guardians with such medically relevant information enhances autonomy. However, the uncertain nature of the information about possible infection can also create situations in which healthy, uninfected infants are subjected to aggressive and potentially risky interventions. In addition, there is no assurance that identified infants will actually receive special attention; according to the New York City Human Rights Commission, some mothers have encountered difficulties in obtaining health care for HIV-infected babies.

Innovative therapies currently available carry substantial risks. Early intervention in HIV infection is not analogous to a short course of penicillin to treat syphilis. All the drugs that are believed to have an anti-viral effect also have toxicities. These may be mild or moderate in low doses; long-term toxicities are unknown. Furthermore, some viral strains are already becoming resistant to drugs.[21] With so little scientific evidence to substantiate the therapeutic claims put forward as justification for the early identification of HIV-infected but asymptomatic individuals, in most instances such interventions should be considered experimental.

The method of administration may also be a burden. Drugs may have to be taken orally every few hours or intravenously. Over time this regimen can become onerous to a healthy person. Presumably any regimen that was effective would have to be continued for an indefinite period. The asymptomatic person may also find the psychological burdens of becoming a "patient" restrictive. All the regimens will require frequent monitoring by physicians or nurses as well as accurate self-reporting by the patient. Administration of some therapies to newborns may require hospitalization, intravenous infusions, and the attendant medical and psychological risks.

There are also potential, well-documented social risks to being identified as HIV-positive. These include the risks of loss of health insurance (especially significant to a person entering a lengthy regimen of expensive treatment); loss of job or housing, and isolation from friends and relatives who may reject the individual known to be infected. Maintaining confidentiality about HIV status is difficult enough for a healthy person; it is much harder for a healthy person undergoing regular medical treatment.

Treatments will be costly. For example, if zidovudine were to be administered to an asymptomatic patient at half or full dosage currently prescribed for AIDS patients, the annual costs would be between $4,891 and $10,382.[22] Aerosolized pentamidine costs about $1,500 to $2,500 annually, plus the costs of the nebulizer and office visits.[23] Monitoring of T-cell counts, recommended at six-month intervals, costs $150. On the other hand, there would be savings in hospital costs for patients who did not get *Pneumocystis*. However, patients would still be vulnerable to other opportunistic infections requiring hospitalization. Furthermore, treatment for asymptomatic patients during the next few years will primarily involve experimental interventions or drugs, which are not covered by most private insurance companies or Medicaid programs. Many policies also do not fully reimburse the costs of drugs or treatment given in outpatient settings.

Finally, seropositive patients may have a very difficult time locating physicians willing to treat them. Few community physicians will care for AIDS patients, and there are even fewer willing to undertake still unproven therapeutic regimens for asymptomatic HIV-infected persons.

In sum, the benefit-risk calculus is not clear-cut. Treatment for asymptomatic HIV infection is as yet unproven, costly, and with significant potential risks. But AIDS is still ultimately a fatal disease, and early intervention offers both the potential of prolonging life and the psychological benefit of giving individuals a sense of control over their destinies. Given such uncertainty, patients, in consultation with their physicians, will weigh the various elements differently. Some will choose an aggressive, all-out approach; others will select certain treatments and not others; and some may prefer to watch and wait.

Justifications for and Limits of Screening for Early Intervention

In our ethical analysis, we draw on the principles of respect for persons, the harm principle, beneficence, and justice. As we have stated elsewhere, these four widely accepted ethical principles are derived from secular, religious, and constitutional traditions and are commonly applied to medicine, research, and public health.

Respect for persons requires that individuals be treated as autonomous agents who have the right to control their own destinies. Respect for persons requires that persons be given the opportunity to decide what will or will not happen to them. The right to privacy and the requirement of informed consent flow from this principle. A corollary—requiring persons with diminished autonomy to be given special protections—may also apply to some populations such as children and prisoners.

The *harm* principle permits limitations on an individual's liberty to pursue personal goals and choices when others will be harmed by those activities.

Beneficence requires that we act on behalf of the interests and welfare of others. The obligations of beneficence apply to actions affecting both individuals and the community. Potential risks must be weighed against potential benefits and the actions with the most favorable risk-to-benefit ratio adopted. The justification for public health authority derives from both the harm principle and beneficence.

Justice requires that the benefits and burdens of particular actions be distributed fairly. It also prohibits invidious discrimination.

These ethical principles may sometimes conflict. For example, the principle of beneficence and the harm principle may outweigh the need to obtain consent in some situations, but they never outweigh the obligation to treat persons with respect for their intrinsic worth and dignity.

Considering both benefits and risks, and drawing on the ethical principles of autonomy, beneficence, and justice, we reach several conclusions:

1. *There are now clinical and ethical grounds for establishing voluntary anonymous or confidential screening programs in settings where individuals who may have been infected with HIV are treated.*

Defining the populations for whom such routinely offered screening would represent a benefit will not be simple. Certainly those who report a history of high-risk sexual or drug-using behavior could benefit from early identification. On the other hand, some investigators have observed that self-reported behavior may fail to identify all those at increased risk for HIV infection.[24] Therefore, it will be necessary to recommend HIV testing to persons seen in clinical settings, such as STD clinics, where the level of HIV infection is high, and to others, for example, pregnant women, in geographic areas where there is an elevated level of infection.

Private physicians should discuss HIV testing with their patients and recommend it to those whose sexual or drug-using history reveals risk behaviors and those who are not sure about their past risks. Recommending testing to all adults, regardless of their history, as suggested by Rhame and Maki, would result in a massive diversion of resources with few benefits.

Adolescents who may be at high risk of HIV infection should also be offered counseling and testing. Adolescents at highest risk because of sexual or drug-using behavior are often alienated from their families. Ideally parents or another family member or trusted adult should be involved in the decision, both to provide emotional support for the adolescent and to facilitate therapeutic follow-up.

2. *Testing of competent adults for clinical purposes should be based on explicit informed consent.*

As the clinical justification for offering HIV testing increases, there will inevitably be a trend toward incorporating testing into the standard panel of "routine" tests. We use the term "routine" to mean that physicians should as a matter of good medical practice and beneficence initiate discussions about HIV antibody testing with their patients.[25] We reject any use of "routine" that involves testing first and talking about it later.[26] HIV testing should not be performed under the conditions of general or presumed consent that governs many other, but not all, medical tests. Presumed consent is an unwritten contract by which the patient, by supplying urine or allowing blood to be drawn, agrees to the routine testing of these materials. If the tests for HIV antibodies were not blood tests, but procedures that involved patient cooperation such as tests for colorectal cancer or mammograms, there would be no question that specific consent would be required.

HIV infection is not like other clinical conditions, even those that are potentially lethal. It carries not only great psychological burdens but the possibility of severe stigma and discrimination, including rejection or avoidance by health care workers and poor-quality treatment.

The consent procedure preceding testing should carefully define the benefits and risks of testing. An honest appraisal of the situation enhances patient autonomy. When the possible benefits of testing are inflated, when the limited therapeutic possibilities are exaggerated, the difficulty of enrolling in clinical trials understated, or the fact that such trials may be placebo-controlled omitted from the discussion, the patient's right to an informed choice is undermined.

Some mothers, because of illness or drug addiction, may be unable to make decisions on testing for their children. Many others are competent to do so, however. Competence is not a single standard; the determination in this case should focus on the specific question of decision-making for children, and not on other issues such as competence to make financial decisions or even decisions about the woman's own health care. Mothers' consent for testing is critical since their involvement in monitoring the health status of their children will be especially important. In addition, newborn screening will also carry significant psychological and social consequences for mothers identified as infected. For some infants, who have no parent present or competent to give consent, there are significant barriers to testing, treatment, and enrollment in experimental protocols. These questions are beyond the scope of this article but should be addressed by policymakers to find ways to both protect vulnerable infants and offer them whatever benefits exist for their conditions.

Individuals with diminished capacity to consent—those with mental illness or retardation, for example—should be considered on a case-by-case basis, with the involvement of guardians or other representatives. Here too the absence of a guardian may result in the denial of some kinds of care because of concern about the individual's competence to consent. Those with diminished capacity to consent should not be denied the benefits of potential therapeutic intervention. Procedures should be established to review individual cases of guardians' refusal to permit testing, or the absence of a guardian to give consent.

In the case of adolescents clinicians will have to determine, again on a case-by-case basis, if an adolescent is mature enough to make the decision about testing, either alone or in consultation with a responsible adult. If so, parental consent ought not be required, even though it is clearly desirable. The notification of parents should be determined on a case-by-case basis, weighing the crucial role that they may be called upon to play in their children's health care against the possibility that they may harm the adolescent. There is no cure or effective treatment for HIV infection. Since long-term follow-up is required, with significant medical interventions, parental involvement is more essential than in STDs. In addition, nearly all teenagers will be unable to pay for treatment on their own.

3. *There is no justification for mandatory screening on the grounds of therapeutic benefit.*

Competent Adults. Mandatory, that is legally required or institutionally enforced, screening for early intervention for competent adults would be a major departure from the accepted standards of medical practice. In our legal and ethical systems, competent adults have the ultimate decision-making authority over their medical care. Despite the well-documented clinical benefits of screening for other potentially fatal diseases—breast cancer, for example—screening programs are entirely voluntary. Changing this standard because of the infectious and stigmatized nature of HIV disease would be a grave mistake.

The few situations in which mandatory screening for individual benefit occur, for example, screening for lead toxicity in the workplace, are narrowly construed and result in beneficial responses, such as offering affected persons different jobs without loss of salary or benefits. Even premarital syphilis screening, which many states have in recent years rescinded on grounds of cost-effectiveness, has as its primary goal the prevention of transmission, not the treatment of an affected individual. While many types of mandatory screening, such as drug screening in some narrowly defined employment settings, may be constitutional, their stated justification is the prevention of harm to others.[27] Proposals for mandatory HIV screening on clinical grounds do not fall into this category.

Because of the limitations of screening based on well-defined patient characteristics or community prevalence rates, the Centers for Disease Control recommended in 1988 that all pregnant women be "routinely" screened for hepatitis B surface antigen in order to initiate the available prophylactic treatment.[28] Such a universal, quasi-mandatory approach to screening pregnant women cannot be justified in the case of HIV.

If there were an intervention that both benefited an infected person and also prevented transmission by rendering him or her noninfectious, mandatory screening might be considered and might be justified on the basis of the harm principle. But even in that entirely hypothetical situation, the likelihood of public health benefit would have to be weighed against the possible side effects and the intrusive and long-term nature of the intervention. Since HIV is transmitted through behavior that can be modified, clinical intervention is not the only possible means of controlling the spread of infection.

Even those who acknowledge that mandatory screening is not justified for purposes of prevention, transmission, or therapeutic benefit might argue that the three purposes, when combined, may indeed create a justification. We reject such a claim. These three weak arguments do not make a strong one. It is ethically unacceptable to require or encourage testing on grounds of potential therapeutic advantage when in fact the purpose of screening is entirely different.

Newborns. The case of newborns presents a more complex situation. Infants cannot consent for themselves, and society has an obligation to assure that they are not deprived of potentially life-saving therapeutic benefits. Nevertheless, the welfare of children is assumed in general to be most effectively protected by deferring to parents. While respect for persons is usually considered to be a principle affecting individuals, family autonomy has a long legal and moral tradition as well.

Unlike the situation with competent adults, there are mandatory or quasi-mandatory newborn screening programs in place for a few conditions. Screening for phenylketonuria (PKU), for example, is mandated in most states. In the case of PKU, there is a definitive test to identify the rare infant with the genetic enzyme deficiency that prevents the metabolization of phenylalanine. There is a well-established therapeutic regimen—a diet low in phenylalanine—that is highly effective in preventing retardation. It must be initiated early in infancy and continued until the child is 5 or older.

But even here there is controversy. Ruth Faden and others have argued that "there are cogent moral arguments against requirements of parental consent for PKU screening" and "compelling moral arguments against a policy of honoring parental refusals of PKU screening."[29] However, George Annas has asserted that *voluntary* screening for PKU can be equally effective and that the focus should be on improving the consent process and not on those few parents who withhold consent.[30]

In 1987, a National Institutes of Health consensus conference concluded that states should mandate the routine offering of sickle cell disease screening to newborns.[31] Sickle cell screening programs had been championed in the early 1970s but were beset by problems caused by the resulting stigmatization of those identified, the confusion between sickle cell disease and trait, and the absence of therapeutic interventions. The NIH consensus conference reviewed new evidence that prophylactic penicillin treatment of affected newborns prevented serious episodes of disease, and in some cases, death. Despite the clear potential benefits, the conference report called upon states to "mandate the availability of these services while permitting parental refusal." According to Dr. Marilyn Gastin of the National Institutes of Health, at present about twenty states are implementing, or planning to implement, sickle cell newborn screening programs. Some of these allow parental refusal; many do not provide any mechanism to inform parents about their right to refuse.

Unlike the cases of PKU and sickle cell screening, however, there is at present no definitive screening test to identify the HIV-infected infant, no proven therapy, and no proven benefits to early intervention. There are also strong arguments *against* mandatory HIV screening at present. Mandatory screening of all newborns would entail the coercive identification of infected mothers, since the HIV antibodies in the infant reveal infection in the mother. These women are typically from minority communities. Often they are poor and have a history of drug use. They are particularly subject to attempts to override their parental rights. Unless specifically demonstrated to be unable to act in their child's best interests, mothers at high risk for HIV infection should have the power to exercise the rights accorded to other parents, including the right to refuse HIV testing for their infants.

Only when a definitive test that accurately identifies HIV-infected infants becomes available and when a treatment has been demonstrated to be safe and effective in prolonging life and improving its quality for the child will overriding parental refusal for HIV testing be ethically defensible on the basis of the harm principle. This position conforms to the conclusion of the President's Commission for the Study of Ethical Problems in Medicine and Biomedical and Behavioral Research that "programs requiring the performance of low-risk, minimally invasive procedures may be justified if voluntary testing would fail to prevent an avoidable, serious injury to people—such as children—who are unable to protect themselves."[32]

4. *Mandatory named reporting of those diagnosed with HIV infection is unnecessary for clinical purposes and may be counterproductive.*

The potential benefits that can follow from the early identification of infection has led some officials to reconsider their earlier opposition to the reporting by name of individuals with HIV infection to public health registries.[33] Such reporting, they have asserted, would permit careful follow-up and counseling regarding the importance of early clinical intervention and would facilitate partner notification to provide the same benefits to individuals reached through public health programs. In the first years of the AIDS epidemic the issue of reporting was the source of bitter controversy, especially in states with relatively low levels of HIV infection.[34] When the Institute of Medicine of the National Academy of Sciences considered the question in 1988 it declared that "although some arguments for mandatory reporting have merit ... the costs far outweigh the benefits, especially if mandatory reporting discourages individuals from seeking voluntary testing."[35]

Now that the prospects for early clinical intervention are emerging and more people at risk are voluntarily seeking testing, it is especially critical to avoid public health measures that may foster anxiety about breaches of confidentiality. That is true regardless of the exemplary record of state health departments in maintaining the confidentiality of the records of those reported with AIDS and other diseases. To assure the proper counseling of HIV-infected individuals about the possibilities of early clinical intervention, it would be wiser to launch aggressive education campaigns targeted at both physicians and those at risk of infection. Partner notification is not dependent on named reporting. Counselors working with HIV-infected people should stress the importance of partner notification for clinical and public health reasons, and programs should be in place to assist in notification when the infected individual is unwilling or unable to do it personally.

5. *High-quality laboratory services must be used.* Beneficence requires that persons not be subjected to any risk—whether social, psychological, or medical—if the information about them to be generated in screening does not meet the current standard levels of accuracy. According to Lawrence Miike, testifying before the House subcommittee in October 1987, studies by the Office of Technology Assessment have found extremely wide variability in laboratory performance. High-quality laboratory services will be essential not only for HIV antibody testing but also for T-cell monitoring, and as consideration is given to wider reliance on PCR techniques.

6. *HIV-infected individuals should be protected against discrimination.*

Fear of the discriminatory consequences of being labeled as HIV-infected continues to affect decisions regarding the willingness to be tested for clinical purposes.[36] Despite some advances of the past two years in providing statutory protections against the unconsented disclosure of HIV status, and in protecting the civil rights of infected individuals, patients must be informed that whatever benefits may currently flow from the early identification of HIV infection may be compromised by violations of confidentiality and acts of discrimination. This underscores the importance of the protection of the rights of HIV-infected persons, which should be enacted in federal law, as recommended by the Presidential Commission on the HIV Epidemic.

7. *Screening programs to identify asymptomatic individuals for clinical purposes which do not at the same time plan for appropriate follow-up services fail to meet the ethical standards of justice or beneficence.*

The demands of justice go beyond a prohibition of discrimination. They require a systematic and full-scale commitment to planning for and providing the medical and social services that will be required to meet the needs of HIV-infected individuals.

With over 100,000 cases of CDC-defined AIDS reported so far, one-third of them in the New York City-northern New Jersey region, the health care systems in heavily affected areas have been severely strained. Providing experimental and therapeutic regimens as well as careful monitoring for the estimated 1.5 million asymptomatic individuals with HIV infection will require a dramatic expansion of services.[37] If the majority of asymptomatic seropositive people were treated on the basis of the current Public Health Service recommendations, costs would run into the billions of dollars.

The need for such a commitment has been recognized by the Public Health Service as well as by some public health officials who are now pressing for more aggressive programs to identify individuals infected with HIV. Thus Dr. Stephen C. Joseph, Commissioner of Health for New York City, has stated, "[The] shift toward a disease control public health approach must be accompanied by ensured availability of needed clinical and social services."[33] But more than assertions will be necessary. The next phase of the epidemic will require a major infusion of public resources and a willingness to mobilize and organize the services that will so clearly be necessary.

Following the principles of justice and beneficence, the economic barriers that could restrict access to therapeutic agents that may retard the progress of HIV infection must be eliminated. This is an especially critical issue since so many of the infected are poor, uninsured, underinsured, and medically underserved. Only a last-minute intervention by Congress assured that individuals clinically eligible for zidovudine would continue to get it regardless of their ability to pay. But the willingness of the federal government to continue to fund such special AIDS-specific programs is not at all certain.

In its report on genetic screening and counseling the President's Commission for the Study of Ethical Problems in Medicine and Biomedical and Behavioral Research declared, "Screening programs should not be undertaken unless accurate results will be produced and a full range of pre-screening and follow-up services are available."[38] That conclusion applies with equal force to screening for HIV infection. It is not ethically defensible to encourage individuals to undergo HIV testing for clinical purposes unless they will have access to available therapies regardless of ability to pay.

Some public health officials who acknowledge the critical shortage of affordable services nevertheless have objected to this conclusion. They have argued that only when individuals are identified through testing and begin to demand access to services will the resources be made available. Whatever the validity of such claims—and there is reason to doubt that the demands of the poor and disenfranchised would have such a desired impact in this case any more than they have had in the case of drug treatment and primary care—they are irrelevant from the perspective of this analysis. To encourage HIV testing for clinical benefit without informing individuals without insurance and primary health care that the necessary follow-up clinical services are virtually inaccessible would represent a breach of the principles that govern the process of informed consent. As Dr. June Osborn, dean of the University of Michigan School of Public Health declared at the Fifth International Conference on AIDS, "We must not use the cruelly false lure of access to inaccessible care to justify abandoning principles we have learned so dearly about the fundamental importance of confidentiality and human rights."

The challenge posed by AIDS is not unique: It simply underscores dramatically and urgently the importance of addressing the systemic failures of the American health care system, noted by every major organization and institution that has studied this question. Resolution of these problems is integral to any ethically justified clinical program of screening for HIV infection.

Conclusions

When HIV-antibody testing first became available in mid-1985, its primary function was to prevent the spread of infection through the screening of blood, and, in conjunction with counseling, to foster behavior change. Out of the many sharp debates that surrounded the test at that time a broad alliance of clinicians, public health officials, political leaders, and AIDS activists forged a consensus that stressed the importance of specific informed consent for testing and the protection of the confidentiality of the test results. That consensus emerged in the context of relative therapeutic impotence.

Now that the clinical options for those with HIV infection have improved, and in light of the prospects for further advances, that consensus will be subject to challenge. The next phase of the HIV epidemic will thus be marked by improvements in therapies and by profound challenges to the ethical principles that should govern the practice of medicine and public health. Only if careful consideration is given to the rights of individuals, to respect for their privacy, and to society's obligations to provide the needed clinical and social services will it be possible to assure that the cautious optimism that is now medically justified will be translated into policies that are ethically justified.

NOTES

1. Redfield RR, and Burke DS: HIV infection: The clinical picture. Sci Am, October 1988:90.

2. PI Perspective, April, 1988:7.

3. U. S. Public Health Service: Guidelines for prophylaxis against Pneumocystis carinii pneumonia for persons infected with Human Immunodeficiency Virus disease. Morbidity and Mortality Report, 38(supp. #5), June 16, 1989.

4. Wall Street Journal, April 21, 1989.

5. New York Times, April 24, 1989.

6. Rhame FS, Maki DG: The case for wider use of testing for HIV infection. N Engl J Med 1989;320 (19):1248–1254.

7. Bayer R, Levine C, and Wold S. HIV antibody screening: An ethical framework for evaluating proposed programs. JAMA 1986; 256:1768–1774.

8. Last JM: Dictionary of Epidemiology. New York, Oxford University Press, 1982; 32–33.

9. The Consortium for Retrovirus Serology Standardization: Serological diagnosis of human immunodeficiency virus infection by Western blot testing, JAMA 1988;260:674–679.

10. Imagawa DT, Lee MH, Wolinsky SM, et al.: Human Immunodeficiency Virus Type 1 infection in homosexual man who remain seronegative for prolonged periods. N Engl J Med 1989; 320:1458–1462.

11. European Collaborative Study, Mother-to-child transmission of HIV infection. Lancet, November 5, 1988;1039–1043.

12. Hart C, Spira T, Moore J et al.: Direct detection of HIV RNA expression in seropositive subjects. Lancet, August 20, 1988;418–421.

13. Rogers, MF, Ou, C-Y, Rayfield, M, et al.: Use of the polymerase chain reaction for early detection of the proviral sequences of Human Immunodeficiency Virus in infants born to seropositive mothers. N Engl J Med 1989; 320: 1649–1654.

14. de Wolf F, Gouldsmit J, deGan J et al.: Effect of zidovudine on serum human immunodeficiency virus antigen levels in symptom-free subjects. Lancet, February 20, 1988;373–376.

15. Reported in Campbell D.: AIDS: Patient power puts research on trial. New Scientist, November 12, 1988;27.

16. Lange J, Mulder J, de Wolf F, et al.: Disease progression despite antigen decline during zidovudine treatment of asymptomatic HIV-infected subjects: Need for placebo-controlled trials. Abstracts of the V International Conference on AIDS, 1989:M.B.P. 352, p. 280.

17. Zidovudine in symptomless HIV infection, Lancet, February 25, 1989;415–416.

18. New York Times, December 19, 1988:1, 46.

19. Bolognesi DP: Prospects for prevention of an early intervention against HIV. JAMA 1989;261(2):3007–3013.

20. 'Treatment IND' for aerosolized pentamidine. JAMA 1989; 261:1398.

21. Larder BA, Darby G, Richman DD: HIV with reduced sensitivity to zidovudine (AZT) isolated during prolonged therapy. Science 243 (4899): 1731–1734.

22. Citizens Commission on AIDS, "The Crisis in AIDS Care: A Call to Action," New York, March 1989.

23. State of New York Department of Health news release dated June 15, 1989.

24. Landesman S, Minkoff H, Holman S, McCalla S, and Siijin O: Serosurvey of human immunodeficiency virus infection in parturients: implications for human immunodeficiency virus testing programs of pregnant women. JAMA 1987;258:2701–2703. Krasinski K, Borkowsky W, Bebenroth D, Moore T: Failure of voluntary testing for human immunodeficiency virus to identify infected parturient women in a high-risk population. N Engl J Med 1988;318:185.

25. American Medical Association: HIV blood test counseling: AMA physician guidelines. 1988.

26. Sherer R: Physician use of the HIV antibody test: The need for consent, counseling, confidentiality, and caution. JAMA 1988;259:264–265.

27. For an analysis of other screening issues, see Annas GJ: Crack, symbolism, and the Constitution. Hastings Center Report 1989;19(3):35–37.

28. Prevention of perinatal transmission of hepatitis B virus: Prenatal screening of all pregnant women for hepatitis B surface antigen. Morbidity and Mortality Weekly Report 1988;37:341–346.

29. Faden R, Holtzman N, and Chwalow A: Parental rights, child welfare, and public health: The case of PKU screening. Am J Public Health 1982;72:1396–1400.

30. Annas GJ: Mandatory PKU screening: The other side of the looking glass. Am J Public Health, 1982;72:1401–1403.

31. Newborn screening for sickle cell disease and other hemoglobinopathies. NIH Consensus Conference. JAMA 1987; 258: 1205–1209.

32. President's Commission for the Study of Ethical Problems in Medicine and Biomedical and Behavioral Research, Screening and Counseling for Genetic Conditions, Washington DC: 1983.

33. Joseph SJ: Premarital AIDS testing: Public policy abandoned at the altar. Editorial, JAMA 1987;261:3456.

34. Bayer, R: Private Acts, Social Consequences: The Politics of Public Health. New York: Basic Books, 1989, 101–136.

35. Institute of Medicine, National Academy of Sciences: Confronting AIDS: Update 1988. Washington, DC:National Academy Press, 1988;11.

36. Report of the Presidential Commission on the Human Immunodeficiency Virus Epidemic, Washington DC: June, 1988;74.

37. Arno, PS, Shenson, D, and Franks, P: The economic and social impact of early intervention in HIV disease. J Am Med Assn, in press.

38. President's Commission for the Study of Ethical Problems in Medicine and Biomedical and Behavioral Research, Summing Up;25.

Prevention: Can We Mobilize What Has Been Learned?

June E. Osborn, M.D.

EIGHT YEARS AGO THIS week in June 1980, the first reports of AIDS appeared. Sometimes that seems like only yesterday, but in many ways it feels like an eternity, for the time when there was a world without HIV epidemic has almost escaped the memory of those caught in its path or deeply committed to its conquest. For 8 years awful realities of the epidemic and its ferocious pandemic potential have crowded into our awareness, and it is difficult to keep in mind what a brief instant that is in the annals of human endeavor.

The epidemic monster has taken a sad toll already in many countries, and it has darkened the entire globe with its frightening shadow, making us uneasily aware of our vulnerablility; but even where its tracks are still fresh, the loving compassion of individuals and the innovative care mobilized by communities in many lands has reminded us also of our power to overcome disaster if we keep in mind that our strength comes from solidarity as members of one human family.

During those 8 long epidemic years scientists and clinicians have made significant advances in ways to care for persons with AIDS even as they have had too struggle to cope with escalating numbers of chronically ill young adults and children. It is not for lack of trying that we still seem to be far short of a cure for HIV disease—

June E. Osborn, M.D., "Prevention: Can We Mobilize What Has Been Learned?" Paper read at the V International AIDS Conference, Montreal, Canada, June 8, 1988, President's Commission on AIDS. Reprinted by Permission of the Author.

rather it is because of the complexity of retrovirus biology and the subtlety of the virus-host relationship that definitive biomedical solutions continue to prove elusive. Nevertheless, a genuine cure is not in sight and a universal vaccine remains troublesome and problematic. Because of those realities, it is important that we take special note of the productive research and experience that has transpired beyond the laboratory, for there is a great deal we *can* do.

Keeping pace with the rapid advance of science has been a growing awareness that intellectual understanding is an esoteric luxury if it cannot be put to use. For instance:

- We know more and more about how to extend life and enhance its quality for persons already caught in the monster's path. And yet discrimination threatens so ominously that many do not dare seek to learn their HIV-infection status. For them such progress remains an abstraction rather than a merciful regime.
- We know what we need to know to interrupt further spread of the virus, for it is sharply limited in its available modes of transmission. Even more wonderfully, those lessons seem to pertain to other human retroviruses, which share epidemiologic properties with HIV-1, meaning that what we can teach about *avoidance* of risk behavior may have broad utility for primary prevention. And yet we sometimes become befuddled by the arguments of pseudo-moralists. They shout their concerns that in giving names to widespread risk behaviors we might seem to condone. But look what horrors we condone if we acquiesce with silence.
- We can reach ready scientific agreement that the epidemic of illicit drug use carries crucial keys to the future scope of our epidemic problems—yet we tolerate rigid laws governing needle access and in some places even prohibit public information about effective antiviral cleansing of injection apparatus, despite the absence of available treatment options for addicted persons caught in the path of HIV.

All these examples lead to a compelling question for those of us at the interface between biomedical science, health care, and public health—can we really mobilize what we learn?

The epidemic does not lend itself to tidy disciplinary dissection but rather slashes across all facets of science and society—and our effective responses must do so as well. With that in mind, there are several kinds of prevention I want to discuss: there is need to prevent illness, to the extent possible, in people already infected by HIV. When illness does intervene, there is a need to provide care, and particularly to prevent disarray in health care systems that would threaten the quality of available medical attention. And of course there is a compelling need to keep the numbers from increasing, so we must prevent further spread of the virus.

These kinds of prevention are fairly obvious, and new data offer hope in each arena. But it is also important to discuss two other facets of the epidemic where we have learned useful lessons. As the numbers grow we must prevent disruption of the infrastucture of public health and health care. And since our tasks are made vastly more difficult by pervasive fear and discrimination that plagues our efforts, prevention of such ignorant and ugly social reactions would help greatly in every other aspect of our endeavors.

I will try to deal briefly, in sequence, with these several preventive goals.

First let me turn to prevention of specific illness in persons with HIV disease. New data presented this week have advanced the ways in which clinical care can defer illness and extend longevity through a combination of innovations in prophylaxis and therapy of persons with HIV disease. Where its cost and side effects have not proved to be prohibitive, Zidovudine has provided a merciful reprieve for many persons with AIDS, and clinical investigators have made progress in finding ways to mitigate its toxicity. Studies are underway to achieve further attenuation of toxicity through combination antiviral therapies, and recent efforts have been diversified to include more complex biological approaches, combining antiviral and immunomodulatory components in treatment regimens. Such sophistication reflects an elegance of scientific understanding and reminds skeptics not to be too gloomy in their predictions, for the only excuse for hopelessness is helplessness, and we are far from helpless in this struggle.

In a different vein, more has been learned to retard or diminish the onslaught of opportunistic infections that form the most lethal cornerstone of the AIDS definition. The deadliness of *pneumocystis carinii* has been partially foiled by several prophylactic strategies that hold promise. Aerosolized Pentamidine is to become more available for such use, and studies reported here offer hope of less costly prophylaxis with other drugs in the near future. To use these strategies, of course, we must have ways to make contact with infected persons, to provide them with care, and to follow their immunologic status so that we will be in a position to anticipate trouble. Those are not easy tasks, and they will require resources and planning. We already fall short of present standards of care in some areas, however, because of lack of resources, and we must not use the cruelly false lure of inaccessible care to justify abandoning principles we have learned so dearly about the fundamental importance of confidentiality and human rights.

Extensive studies are now underway to intervene even earlier in the pathogenetic progression of HIV, using antiviral drugs in an attempt to delay the onset of immunodeficiency itself. I am very concerned that AZT is now used frequently—sometimes even carelessly—in the context of accidental exposure of health care personnel, on the unvalidated assumption that early therapy will interrupt establishment of viral infection. We should be worried about this for we have now seen that HIV may become resistant to Zidovudine. It has only happened in a few instances thus far, but the role of that drug in the treatment of AIDS is unique, and we must be alert to prevent the tragic loss of its therapeutic efficacy for persons with AIDS. *Severe* workplace exposure is a serious and legitimate concern, but there is a great difference between indiscriminate use and systematic assessment of degree of risk in deciding how to proceed. It makes good sense to establish standards in this context and to collect and document as much experiential data as we can during such use.

I have even greater concern about development of resistance should a policy encourage treatment of asymptomatic HIV-infected individuals. We are still learning about the range of HIV manifestations and we do not yet know how to predict for an *individual* the likely duration of symptom-free infection. Therefore assessment of chemoprophylactic effect is intrinsically difficult—and we must be sure the measured gain in duration of well-being is worth the distinct risk of losing our *only* therapeutic weapon for persons who are ill.

In the context of health care delivery there is a different kind of preventive action to be taken. As numbers of persons with HIV disease grow, we must anticipate institutional and personnel needs and plan to assure their adequacy. If we fail to do so, our elegant clinical advances and scientific knowledge will be of little use to the persons who need them most. In particular, reliance on high-technology hospitals not only exaggerates costs but also fails to optimize the quality of life of persons with chronic illness. The need for a continuum of care options is already evident, and as Zidovudine and other attenuating therapies extend life expectancy still further, the need will grow greater.

How to prevent further spread of HIV is the facet of the epidemic that has occasioned the stormiest debates. Uniform consensus about transmission mechanisms points to specific sexual and drug-using behaviors that are ordinarily beyond the realm of public discourse, and yet it is those very matters that must be discussed in order to be amended in the interest of decreasing risk. Despite the clarity of need for behavioral research and interventions, we continue to cripple ourselves with specious quarrels about appropriateness of language—and rather than addressing the need for more knowledge about sexual behavior, we try to finesse our ignorance by relying solely on technology in a vacuum of social understanding.

There are some successful exceptions to that generalization. For instance, we have reiterated since 1983 the message that the chief protection of the blood supply in developed countries with well-established blood banking systems lies in self-deferral by persons who recognize themselves to be at behavioral risk. Antibody screening gains its full protective potential because of this behavioral layer of safeguard. The emergence of HIV-2 and HTLV-1 as potential threats to the blood supply can be met in part by the same caveats concerning self-deferral. I do not want to minimize the important contribution made by screening tests, but rather to underscore the point that we must use *all* facets of our knowledge and insight in order to maximize our preventive capabilities.

Other public health uses of antibody testing and screening in the interest of prevention are more problematic. In general there is an inverse correlation between perceived risk of discrimination and public health usefulness of programs, and in all contexts the value of the test is secondary to the value of associated counseling about its meaning and implications for personal health and risk avoidance through behavior modification.

Fear of discrimination is powerful as a detractor from the usefulness of testing and counseling—and when coercion is an element, as in mass screening programs intermittently proposed by frightened politicians, antibody testing becomes exorbitantly costly and counterproductive, in both human and economic terms.

Conversely, the effectiveness of education as a means of reducing spread has been documented by a number of specific and useful studies. Most encouragingly, data continue to accumulate showing that modification of high-risk sexual practices in defined gay communities has markedly decreased the spread of HIV within those communities. The reduction in risk behavior has not been total, nor has the rate of spread dropped to zero, and concerns about recidivism are valid. However, they do not negate the hopeful message—

rather they indicate the need to search further for strategies to reinforce and sustain changed behavior.

The success thus far achieved is dramatic and encouraging, for these are, after all, difficult and relatively untrammeled areas of behavioral research. Some caveats are necessary, however. There is a remarkably frequent tendency to accept those successes as total victories—I have been astonished to hear people conclude from these focal studies that the perils are over for gay men and that we can therefore shift our preventive efforts elsewhere. Clearly that is not true, for the large majority of gay men do not live in open communities and have not had access to such clearly crafted messages, and I worry about the naivete of such a facile declaration of triumph at the very outset of a long and difficult campaign.

What I think we really learned from those studies is that education *can* be effective, especially when it is *community-based*, sustained, and conducted in the language of its intended listeners, rather than in terms chosen to mollify civic censors. And persons whose risk behavior is closeted from fear of discrimination and censure will be the *last*, not the first, to participate and learn. I think we must assume that great numbers of men with a covert same-sex orientation and/or bisexual behavior *remain* at high risk and that new—probably different—educational strategies will surely be needed to reach them. Furthermore we must not be lulled by successes in *mature* cohorts into the comfortable assumption that they pertain to other age groups, for to do so is to risk missing whole new generations of children and adolescents whose lifestyle choices are still under consideration.

I have used studies from gay communities to illustrate what is involved in making AIDS information usable—but other examples can be brought forward as well. In the important arena of heterosexual spread, there are data to suggest that condoms can decrease risk of HIV transmission during vaginal intercourse very substantially—by an order of magnitude or more—and yet advocacy of condom usage has had equivocal support in many countries. Indeed, in some places where *women* are urged to help implement condom usage, laws remain on the books that would brand them as prostitutes were they found to be carrying condoms.

Furthermore cultural sensitivity is paramount in all aspects of AIDS education, and nowhere more than in this context. It has become evident that there are several cultures in which male domination of sexual relationship is such that the mere suggestion by a woman that condoms be used may provoke a beating or even threaten the integrity of the partnership—with social and economic ramifications that are far more immediate and disastrous than the abstract fear of HIV. We have much to learn about such matters, and indeed about sexual behavior in general, before we can really *use* some of the fundamental facts we have learned about preventing sexual transmission of HIV.

In a different area, the potential of shared drug-injection apparatus as a source of sudden trouble has been dramatically underscored by the evolving tragedy in Thailand in the past year and a half. That experience evokes dismal echoes of Edinburgh and New York and leaves one deeply apprehensive about the rest of the world, for illicit drug use is also pandemic and is out of control at present. We now know to our sorrow that sharing of so-called works is an alarmingly efficient vehicle of HIV spread, that intravenous cocaine is even more threatening than intravenous heroin, and that even injection isn't necessary to perpetuate HIV spread in the context of "crack" cocaine because of the currency of sex-for-drugs that closes the loop of HIV transmission. Those facts are awesome, but can we use them?

Yes—but only if we develop the social and political will to do so. Needle-exchange programs, for instance, have been implemented in a number of European countries with apparently positive results. In no instance has evaluation found drug use to be increased by such programs, and while the data are mixed about effectiveness in preventing HIV spread, some studies are positive and most indicate that many drug users respond eagerly to the implicit offer of access to care. Even such simple efforts as instruction in the use of bleach as an antiviral measure combined with AIDS information seem to have had salutory effects. It should startle us into remembering that in many countries—and particularly my own—persons addicted to drugs had been abandoned as lost souls. We had written them off as criminals, and have been forgetting to offer them hope.

Needle-exchange programs or bleach interventions must *not* be discussed as *solutions*, I agree, for that is nihilistic. They are short-term strategies to buy time. But that time is precious, for it is all the time some addicted persons will have. Where drug treatment is readily available, it may prove problematic or even counterproductive to test or implement such stop-gap measures—but where it is *not* available, failure to use what we know condemns us all to a merciless and cruel extension of the HIV epidemic.

Vaccines are the traditional means of preventing viral infection, and while the topics of vaccine research and development have been dealt with earlier, I want to note briefly that vaccine deployment and utilization will be critical factors in preparing for a time when a promising vaccine might be available The assumption that such a vaccine could be put directly to use is worrisomely simplistic. In some countries—again, the U.S. may be the most striking example—problems of litigiousness and feared corporate liability for potential adverse vaccine effects must be dealt with in advance. Thorny problems of design of vaccine trials, informed consent of subjects, choice of target groups, and assessment of vaccine efficacy in low-risk populations crowd the agenda of vaccine utilization planners. Delicate issues arise if higher-risk populations are sought in nations other than those where the vaccines are being developed. Happily, efforts are underway to address these problems, both under the aegis of the global program on AIDS of the World Health Organization and in other forums.

As noted earlier, two other kinds of prevention are important: One involves preventing serious distortion of the infrastructure of public health by the ebb and flow of epidemic crises. In this context let me return briefly to the impending situation in which specific chemoprophylaxis might be advocated to delay the advent of illness in HIV-infected persons, for such a capability—while welcome—will aggravate problems already apparent in competing public health programs that have suffered because of the urgency of AIDS activities. For instance, tenuously funded sexually-transmitted-disease control programs have sometimes, quixotically, been compromised by AIDS initiatives and find themselves losing in direct competition for funding. Dr. N'Galy documented the explosive increases in tuberculosis in parts of Africa in conjunction with HIV that will surely bring new stresses to bear.

If HIV chemoprophylaxis were to be recommended without advance planning, distortions of ongoing public health programs would almost surely follow, and in areas of the world where total resources available for health care are extremely limited, even such basic activities as childhood immunization or maternal and child health might collapse under the pressure to expand access to costly HIV diagnosis, treatment, and continuing care. We must use what we know about public health administration and management in order to plan and to prevent inequity and chaos.

Finally, we must prevent fear, for that is the great hidden distractor that saps our collective strength and diverts human energies that could arise from compassion. In a world full of fearsome things, HIV should *not* be high on the list, for risk behavior can be avoided. That is the one bit of truly good news in this awful epidemic, and we should pause to celebrate it, for it might not have been that way. One could not have said the same had the new microbial pathogen

spread like measles or polio or influenza. That gives us the historically lucky opportunity to respond to an awful epidemic with *both*
knowledge and compassion.

But still we face public fear, and it is remarkable to note how
disabling that fear has been to our collective efforts. General education must be our preventive strategy—perhaps by now it would be
more accurate to call it a "curative" strategy, for the fear is deep-
seated and advanced in many societies. I cringe when I hear people
in the U.S. say that we have already "done" education, for in
proportion to the need we have only just begun. Given the stakes,
we must reflect on how much would be "enough." Certainly if we
were intent on marketing a commercial product for profit we would
not consider efforts to date even vaguely adequate—and what we
want to sell here is nothing less than critical to our children's safety
and future, for HIV is here to stay and its *avoidance* must become
second nature to us all.

The task of educating the public is not easy, for it flies in the face
of grandmothers' common sense that anything so deadly should be
so difficult to transmit. It gets tangled, too, with the anxious whimsy
of the late twentieth century. After all, there are far more people
well-read in science fiction than in science, and calm reassurance
that modes of transmission are well-understood sounds like foolish
overconfidence to those more accustomed to the unpredictability of
the genetic oddities that crowd paperback book shelves. There are
also those who do not want to hear what we say—some who barely
acknowledge their risk to themselves from covert behavior but who
sense that it would be convenient to have mosquitoes to blame if
the worst were to happen.

All that says is that we must try harder, for defeatism is no more
useful in this war against the AIDS monster than it is in any other
war.

My comments about fear pertain with special poignancy to health
care workers. Sometimes, because of fear, there has been a tendency to try to evade the AIDS epidemic—to avoid caring for
persons with AIDS or to assert that it surely "won't happen here."
But HIV infection has seeded every country on the globe and HIV
illness will expand much further before it ebbs, even if all our
primary preventive efforts were to succeed. There are much greater
risks than HIV in the health care workplace, not the least of which
is to forget the humane commitment that brought us to the privilege
of being health care workers and professionals in the first place. It
is reasonable to be alert, to exercise sensible precautions and to
exercise prudence in the health care workplace—but panic is un-

reasonable and abandonment of the obligation to care for sick people because of personal fear is intolerable.

There is a very special reason to improve public understanding and that is to unleash the power of compassion. I am of the opinion that there are no two more incompatible human emotions than personal fear and compassion, and we are in great need of the latter as the epidemic grows.

On Tuesday David Roy spoke about humanity with a passion that was thrilling. He said that *humanity* is where many wonderful things are, but that, sadly, humanity is not *always* where human beings are. He drew our attention to the unforgettable image of a lone Chinese student stopping a column of tanks, and he let us know that our challenges were equally desperate but that the same power could be unleashed in their behalf. He reminded us that bars depicted in graphs were the condensation of populations, that populations were collections of loving, suffering individuals, and that if we could only learn to gaze closely enough into the faces of those individuals, we would see ourselves.

He touched on a related point that I would like to underscore: We must learn to value and celebrate our diversity if we are to gain the full benefit of human creativity. The wonder of biology lies in its infinite variety, and there is nowhere better than an international gathering of committed people to remind ourselves that we in the human family are marvelous manifestations of that diversity. We will enhance the strength and boldness of our stride if we learn to cherish heterogeneity instead of fighting against it.

So we have two charges: to learn to gaze long enough at others that we can see ourselves, and yet to value the details that make each of us unique. They are compatible—indeed, inseparable—goals, and if we achieve them, we will unleash a power that can stop tanks and despair and discrimination and HIV. If we collect what we have learned and find how to mobilize it, the net gain for our human communities will reach far beyond the conquest of AIDS.

HIV and the Political Crisis of the Private

Introduction

THE PRECEDING SECTION DEALT with the ethical and social issues of the prevention of the HIV virus and of the medical condition of AIDS. It treated the transmission issues as ones relating the individual to the public space we all share and to the inherent right we all have to be left alone. Respect for the individual forms the core of ethical social policy. And it is the essence of democratic government to protect individuals as a matter of course from violations of their intimacy, of their relations to their bodies, to their emotional connections to partners and to community.

This chapter expands on the right to privacy. It demonstrates how the HIV epidemic highlights the current cultural tensions surrounding homosexuality, drug use, and reproductive rights. It also addresses the paradoxes of the protection of privacy by showing that the emphasis upon the right to privacy often serves to exacerbate invisibility and disenfranchisement—a political isolation for the individual only remedied through very strict and rigorous constitutional protection.

Before addressing the *right* to privacy, it is important to have a way of understanding how American law and philosophy have understood what privacy is. Democracy differs from other forms of government because it makes the individual the sole end of government. Government has no reason for being except to protect the individual.

According to John Locke, one of the most influential Englishmen for our American Constitution, and later to John Stuart Mill, government serves the exclusive purpose of allowing individuals to coordinate their varying interests. Government's function is to allow for ordered liberty. And ordered liberty basically translates into being free to pursue one's interests, as long as those interests do not conflict with the interest of another individual.

When we ask what an "individual" is, or what makes up the realm of privacy, things get complicated. This is because the English view and the view of early American law were views that embodied a male definition of the individual and that tied the realm of the "private" exclusively to the existence of the family. We have, of course, developed a much more complicated view of the person and of the state since our English forefathers and we have progressed in our legal precedents to the point where the basic human rights to the pursuit of happiness are not so uniformly wedded to male and familial concerns. It is now generally accepted and a development of our constitutional law that the realm of the private is one that includes the control an individual has over their body, as well as affectional and emotional preference. And that "individuals" cannot be viewed solely by their function in human reproduction and familial unity. The rationale for democratic government continues to be that it is essentially the common arm that allows each of us to be "left alone." In that sense, government is negative and defines no positive rights.

This brief reminder about democracy gives us a way in which to situate what is currently controversial in the HIV epidemic about privacy in the questions of drug use, the moral and, now, legal proscriptions against homosexuality, as well as some issues of reproductive rights. As each of the articles reiterate in their own way, what is at stake in the questions of privacy is not only the rights of individuals but the preeminence that right has in our form of government.

Today, the debates about privacy and individualism are often focused on the right to the exercise of privacy itself. Many argue that democracy is dedicated to the protection of the individual but that an *equal* corollary of this protection is the protection of the "moral climate" of everyday life. In this last sense, civil libertarians confront conservatives who feel that what is at stake constitutionally is the preservation of a way of life that is perceived to be dictated by nature and exemplified in the "majority." Nowhere is this more evident than in the rights of minorities as they relate to prevailing moral opinions about sexuality and reproduction.

What is most at issue in the HIV epidemic is the question of the equal protection individuals deserve in their privacy. And this debate is about basic civil liberties like sexual preference, reproductive privacy, medical confidentiality, and drug use, as well as about the limits of majoritarian rule.

If the protection of privacy were the only issue, the issues of HIV affection would be largely constitutional issues. Unfortunately, the issue of privacy is even more complicated than what has been briefly outlined. What the foregoing assumes is that the public–private distinction is one that is always beneficial. What it doesn't address sufficiently is the generic problem of privacy itself.

The government's violation of the privacy of the individual is not the only transgression of the individuals' rights. Privacy is also abused when democracy begins to degenerate into majoritarian politics. Being left alone by government might, in fact, be a *terrible* fate. Due to the arbitrariness of nature or of the economic sphere, or due to a social climate that sets up prejudice against an individual because of his/her classification in a group, individual differences must not only be protected in the private sphere of "being left alone." They must also be addressed by the state. This is the origin of civil and human rights law and affirmative action policy. People cannot be left alone by government if, in being left alone, they are at the mercy of other individuals, socially or economically. Their relative disadvantage must be redressed.

"HIV and the Political Crisis of the Private" begins with the opinion of the Supreme Court in Bowers v. Hardwick. The Supreme Court decision concerned Hardwick, a Georgia man engaged in homosexual intimacy at the time of a police search of his home. Georgia law prohibits sodomy—any kind of contact between the sexual organs of one partner and the oral or anal region of the body of the other partner. The Georgia prohibition was challenged by Hardwick and his partner, as well as by a married couple who maintained that the Georgia law also restricted their rights to sexual intimacy. In *upholding* the Georgia sodomy law, the Supreme Court rendered a judgment that has implications not only for privacy as it relates to sexuality but also to abortion and any other intimate act that does not relate to family, procreation, marriage.

Whether the act of sodomy is a right covered under the notion of fundamental rights depends upon two interpretations of fundamental rights. One interpretation maintains that sodomy is a private act and is intimately related to the right to be "left alone." The second interpretation views fundamental liberties to be ones that are "deeply rooted in this Nation's history and tradition." The Justices, in overturning the Court of Appeals which supported the Hardwick petition, maintain that "no connection between family, marriage, or procreation on the one hand and homosexual activity on the other, has been demonstrated, either by the Court of Appeals or by respondent."

Justice Blackmun, in his dissenting opinion, argues that sodomy is a part of the basic right to be left alone. Sexual preference is attached to a person's fundamental identity. As a "sexual intimacy," it is a "sensitive, key relationship for human existence, central to family life, community welfare, and the development of human personality."

Dan Beauchamp ("Morality and the Health of the Body Politic") takes up the question of the relation between the state and morality. Beauchamp also greatly regrets the Supreme Court decision in Bowers v. Hardwick and asks the question at the basis of constitutional guarantees: "Who is worthy of such guarantees and what is the basis upon which we decide? Does a culture have the right to enforce a morality?"

Embracing the view that the state must institute a moral code may be one way in which to eliminate democracy altogether. During a public health emergency like the HIV epidemic, the value of the protection of privacy for setting up trust and candor cannot be overemphasized. "How healthy is the enforcement of a morality for the body politic?" Beauchamp's article highlights the purely ethical basis of our constitutional rights and questions the ethical practical bases of "legal moralism." In outlining the necessity of a viable social pluralism, Beauchamp makes clear the social and public health importance of the protection of the moral *minority*.

The right to privacy has the constitutional weight that it does because it is considered an innate moral principle of human interaction. Hence, the right to privacy is not only expressed politically but also in institutions which must deal with the private information that each of us has which makes us vulnerable to other human beings. One of the major institutions in which privacy and its respect are paramount is the medical institution. Here privacy is expressed in the laws of medical confidentiality between physician and patient, laws that have been accepted for millennia and that form the basis for state laws of medical practice. With the advent of the HIV epidemic the issue of medical confidentiality has become problematic as some physicians feel they cannot adhere to rules of strict confidentiality because of the public health threat of HIV. They argue that medical confidentiality impedes knowledge of transmission and does not sufficiently take into account third party vulnerability, like the possibility of transmission to a partner or spouse. Medical confidentiality and the public right to know form the poles of this debate.

In "Medical Confidentiality: An Intransigent and Absolute Obligation," Dr. Michael Kottow argues vigorously against any new limitation on medical confidentiality. Offered as an express protection of privacy when initiating the doctor-patient relationship, the promise of confidentiality cannot be withdrawn after the fact without violations of fairness to the patient. Medical confidentiality is unconditional. And Dr. Kottow argues that without such protection of privacy medicine would be impossible to practice.

The reproductive decisions associated with the HIV epidemic are contained in the Anastos and Marte article in Section Two. It is important in this context, however, to reiterate some of the constitutional issues that emerge for women, particularly as these issues relate to the intersection of reproductive choice, pediatric AIDS, and the neglect of women by the health care system.

It is, of course, women's roles as mothers that enormously complicate what legal protection they have as individuals. This is particularly true in the current climate which gives preference to children over mothers. A further complicating factor is the current social attitude toward low-income minority women—that they are somehow less responsible about personal and public health concerns that they, through this self-neglect, endanger their unborn children. Within the structure of our bifurcated health care system, these attitudes get played out with official, if tacit, sanction. Low-income women (who are the women who are largely affected by the epidemic) depend upon public agencies for prenatal, contraceptive, and medical care. Because these agencies are also state agencies and because they are vastly overutilized, low-income women have severely limited access to medical care for themselves and for their children. These limitations change the time frame for reproductive decisions and, as is the case in New York where one routinely waits for 3 months for a prenatal appointment, makes the state a de facto decision-maker. These differences are continued in the power differences and value difference that occur in the extent to which women's *right* to refuse to be tested for the HIV virus is balanced against the health official's assumptions that this choice is not hers alone, given the possible HIV status of her fetus. The issue of consent to testing dovetails here with the issue of the woman's right to confidentiality if she is seropositive—a confidentiality that many health officials feel they cannot honor given the existence of the fetus.

The preeminent status of women-as-mothers makes their constitutional right to birthing choice and their ethical right to medical confidentiality *conditional* rights—rights conditioned upon the status of the potential child. This ambiguity in legal and ethical obligation is increased further for the low-income woman who, due to her dependence upon the state, must deal with health experts who see themselves as practitioners ethically bound to protect their patient's autonomy as well as instruments of social policy aimed at birth control.

Race and class differences stratify the medical promise that experimental drugs hold for women and their children. They also have a direct bearing upon fundamental rights. On the other hand, pregnant women are encouraged to be tested for the HIV virus with the threat of perinatal transmission but equally with the offer of experimental drugs for the newborn. The true extent to which their infants may be helped by these early interventions is heatedly debated. Some maintain that AZT may be very dangerous to a new immune system and point to the less-than-two-year experimental research period for adult subjects. Others point to the need for wide dissemination of AZT as the most promising therapeutic intervention. However the debate concludes, assurances of unalloyed blessing or unalloyed tragedy with respect to early intervention fall inevitably on uninformed ears unless health experts take quite seriously their obligation to educate women to the true benefits and the true consequences of treatments for their newborns. Nowhere is informed consent more meaningful than in experimental regimens targeted to groups of people likely to serve as subjects for medical advance.

Nowhere is the crisis of the private and the real test of democracy more visible than in the areas of drug use, reproductive rights, and, importantly, homosexuality. The public or civic execution of rights puts a great burden on privacy—it makes the individual have to choose between constitutional rights and anonymity. The standard predicament is that of the homosexual who gets beat up because he is gay. ("Gay-bashing" has increased fourfold since the epidemic began.) If the gay man goes to the police he must tell them that he was beaten because he is gay or perceived to be gay. The police may be unsympathetic. Worse, the news may get back to his landlord, his employer, his family. More often than not, gay individuals choose to live with the violence of their personal lives rather than try to exercise their rights to protection. In the HIV epidemic, the choices are even harsher—the choice between one's rights and one's access to resources like housing, public accommodation, even health care.

One of the components of the crisis of the private is this burden of invisibility: for the invisibly disabled (HIV-antibody-positive; the intravenous drug user); for the homosexual; for the woman who is pregnant. All are invisible minorities who have civil rights just like everyone else; but, unlike the minorities of race, disability, religion, they can't execute those rights without untold consequences. In order to procure or secure those rights they must become visible in a climate that protects their behavior, in effect, *only as long as they keep it private* (invisible). "Invisible Minorities, Civic Rights Democracy: Three Arguments for Gay Rights" takes up the constitutional challenge that invisible minorities offer to the functioning of democracy.

At the core of the Supreme Court decision in Bowers v. Hardwick is the question of the role of the family and its relation to democracy. Some argue that the family is the preeminent goal of life and that democracy, in its protection of the individual, is protecting that individual for his or her right to procreate. With the overidentification of government with the goals of family, a new danger emerges. The problem is not so much that government will intrude on the private to such an extent that the distinction between the public and the private vanishes but, rather, that the government will define itself with a private goal and require citizens to uphold it. Such a position by the state is synonymous with making the protection of the family a national goal. At the extreme of the privacy debate, then, is the notion that the protection of the family is the national goal in a democracy and that the "private" constitutes the *terminus* of that nationalism.

The "private," once the sacrosanct basis of English and American law, is being construed as the enemy of tradition, of family, of nation. This issue should make us all pause to rethink the emergence of the general invasions of privacy exemplified by drug testing, abortion proscription, fetal rights, and proscriptions against homosexuality.

The final article in this section deals directly with law. David Schulman, the supervising attorney in the AIDS/HIV Discrimination Unit of the Los Angeles City Attorney's Office, addresses himself to the discriminatory impact of the epidemic. In this article we are able to see the arguments for civil rights that come out of our form of government, as well as the function of discrimination as it emerges against those who are affected by the HIV epidemic. One particularly important aspect of this article is the way in which it develops the social basis of prejudice and its treatment of cases of AIDS discrimination as they come within the purview of California state and Los Angeles city law. One uncommon issue is the question of AIDS euthanasia and the law. Shulman offers a profound analysis of this issue. Individual control over one's own death and the interest of the state in allowing or disallowing such control forms a natural end to our discussions of the right to privacy in all of its everyday constitutional, social, and personal expressions.

SUPREME COURT OF THE UNITED STATES

Syllabus

BOWERS, ATTORNEY GENERAL OF GEORGIA
v. HARDWICK ET AL.

CERTIORARI TO THE UNITED STATES COURT OF APPEALS FOR
THE ELEVENTH CIRCUIT

No. 85-140. Argued March 31, 1986—Decided June 30, 1986

After being charged with violating the Georgia statute criminalizing
sodomy by committing that act with another adult male in the bedroom
of his home, respondent Hardwick (respondent) brought suit in Federal
District Court, challenging the constitutionality of the statute insofar as
it criminalized consensual sodomy. The court granted the defendants'
motion to dismiss for failure to state a claim. The Court of Appeals
reversed and remanded, holding that the Georgia statute violated respondent's fundamental rights.

Held: The Georgia statue is constitutional. Pp. 3–9.

(a) The Constitution does not confer a fundamental right upon homosexuals to engage in sodomy. None of the fundamental rights announced
in this Court's prior cases involving family relationships, marriage, or
procreation bear any resemblance to the right asserted in this case. And
any claim that those cases stand for the proposition that any kind of
private sexual conduct between consenting adults is constitutionally
insulated from state proscription is unsupportable. Pp. 3–4.

(b) Against a background in which many States have criminalized
sodomy and still do, to claim that a right to engage in such conduct is
"deeply rooted in this Nation's history and tradition" or "implicit in the
concept of ordered liberty" is, at best, facetious. Pp. 4–8.

(c) There should be great resistance to expand the reach of the Due
Process Clauses to cover new fundamental rights. Otherwise, the Judiciary necessarily would take upon itself further authority to govern the
country without constitutional authority. The claimed right in this case
falls far short of overcoming this resistance. P. 8.

(d) The fact that homosexual conduct occurs in the privacy of the
home does not affect the result. *Stanley v. Georgia,* 394 U. S. 557,
distinguished. Pp. 8–9.

"Opinion, Supreme Court of the United States July, 1986, Bowers v. Hardwick."

(e) Sodomy laws should not be invalidated on the asserted basis that majority belief that sodomy is immoral is an inadequate rationale to support the laws. P. 9.

760 F. 2d 1202, reversed.

WHITE, J., delivered the opinion of the Court, in which BURGER, C. J., and POWELL, REHNQUIST, and O'CONNOR, JJ., joined. BURGER, C. J., and POWELL, J., filed concurring opinions. BLACKMUN, J., filed a dissenting opinion, in which BRENNAN, MARSHALL, and STEVENS, JJ., joined. STEVENS, J., filed a dissenting opinion, in which BRENNAN and MARSHALL, JJ., joined.

JUSTICE WHITE delivered the opinion of the Court.

In August 1982, respondent was charged with violating the Georgia statute criminalizing sodomy[1] by committing that act with another adult male in the bedroom of respondent's home. After a preliminary hearing, the District Attorney decided not to present the matter to the grand jury unless further evidence developed.

Respondent then brought suit in the Federal District Court, challenging the constitutionality of the statute insofar as it criminalized consensual sodomy.[2] He asserted that he was a practicing homosexual, that the Georgia sodomy statute, as administered by the defendants, placed him in imminent danger of arrest, and that the statute for several reasons violates the Federal Constitution. The District Court granted the defendants' motion to dismiss for failure to state a claim, relying on *Doe* v. *Commonwealth's Attorney for the City of Richmond*, 403 F. Supp. 1199 (ED Va. 1975), which this Court summarily affirmed, 425 U. S. 901 (1976).

A divided panel of the Court of Appeals for the Eleventh Circuit reversed. 760 F. 2d 1202 (1985). The court first held that, because *Doe* was distinguishable and in any event had been undermined by later decisions, our summary affirmance in that case did not require affirmance of the District Court. Relying on our decisions in *Griswold* v. *Connecticut*, 381 U. S. 479 (1965), *Eisenstadt* v. *Baird*, 405 U. S. 438 (1972), *Stanley* v. *Georgia*, 394 U. S. 557 (1969), and *Roe* v. *Wade*, 410 U. S. 113 (1973), the court went on to hold that the Georgia statute violated respondent's fundamental rights because his homosexual activity is a private and intimate association that is beyond the reach of state regulation by reason of the Ninth Amendment and the Due Process Clause of the Fourteenth Amendment. The case was remanded for trial, at which, to prevail, the State would have to prove that the statute is supported by a compelling interest and is the most narrowly drawn means of achieving that end.

Because other Courts of Appeals have arrived at judgments contrary to that of the Eleventh Circuit in this case,[3] we granted the State's petition for certiorari questioning the holding that its sodomy statute violates the fundamental rights of homosexuals. We agree with the State that the Court of Appeals erred, and hence reverse its judgment.[4]

This case does not require a judgment on whether laws against sodomy between consenting adults in general, or between homosexuals in particular, are wise or desirable. It raises no question about the right or propriety of state legislative decisions to repeal their laws that criminalize homosexual sodomy, or of state court decisions invalidating those laws on state constitutional grounds. The issue presented is whether the Federal Constitution confers a fundamental right upon homosexuals to engage in sodomy and hence invalidates the laws of the many States that still make such conduct illegal and have done so for a very long time. The case also calls for some judgment about the limits of the Court's role in carrying out its constitutional mandate.

We first register our disagreement with the Court of Appeals and with respondent that the Court's prior cases have construed the Constitution to confer a right of privacy that extends to homosexual sodomy and for all intents and purposes have decided this case. The reach of this line of cases was sketched in *Carey* v. *Population Services International*, 431 U. S. 678, 685 (1977). *Pierce* v. *Society of Sisters*, 268 U. S. 510 (1925), and *Meyer* v. *Nebraska*, 262 U. S. 390 (1923), were described as dealing with child rearing and education; *Prince* v. *Massachusetts*, 321 U. S. 158 (1944), with family relationships; *Skinner* v. *Oklahoma ex rel. Williamson*, 316 U. S. 535 (1942), with procreation; *Loving* v. *Virginia*, 388 U. S. 1 (1967), with marriage; *Griswold* v. *Connecticut, supra*, and *Eisenstadt* v. *Baird, supra*, with contraception; and *Roe* v. *Wade*, 410 U. S. 113 (1973), with abortion. The latter three cases were interpreted as construing the Due Process Clause of the Fourteenth Amendment to confer a fundamental individual right to decide whether or not to beget or bear a child. *Carey* v. *Population Services International, supra*, at 688–689.

Accepting the decisions in these cases and the above description of them, we think it evident that none of the rights announced in those cases bears any resemblance to the claimed constitutional right of homosexuals to engage in acts of sodomy that is asserted in this case. No connection between family, marriage, or procreation on the one hand and homosexual activity on the other has been demonstrated, either by the Court of Appeals or by respondent.

Moreover, any claim that these cases nevertheless stand for the proposition that any kind of private sexual conduct between consenting adults is constitutionally insulated from state proscription is unsupportable. Indeed, the Court's opinion in *Carey* twice asserted that the privacy right, which the *Griswold* line of cases found to be one of the protections provided by the Due Process Clause, did not reach so far. 431 U. S., at 688, n. 5, 694, n. 17.

Precedent aside, however, respondent would have us announce, as the Court of Appeals did, a fundamental right to engage in homosexual sodomy. This we are quite unwilling to do. It is true that despite the language of the Due Process Clauses of the Fifth and Fourteenth Amendments, which appears to focus only on the processes by which life, liberty, or property is taken, the cases are legion in which those Clauses have been interpreted to have substantive content, subsuming rights that to a great extent are immune from federal or state regulation or proscription. Among such cases are those recognizing rights that have little or no textual support in the constitutional language. *Myers*, *Prince*, and *Pierce* fall in this category, as do the privacy cases from *Griswold* to *Carey*.

Striving to assure itself and the public that announcing rights not readily indentifiable in the Constitution's text involves much more than the imposition of the Justices' own choice of values on the States and the Federal Government, the Court has sought to identify the nature of the rights qualifying for heightened judicial protection. In *Palko* v. *Connecticut*, 302 U. S. 319, 325, 326 (1937), it was said that this category includes those fundamental liberties that are "implicit in the concept of ordered liberty," such that "neither liberty nor justice would exist if [they] were sacrificed." A different description of fundamental liberties appeared in *Moore* v. *East Cleveland*, 431 U. S. 494, 503 (1977) (opinion of POWELL, J.), where they are characterized as those liberties that are "deeply rooted in this Nation's history and tradition." *Id.*, at 503 (POWELL, J.). See also *Griswold* v. *Connecticut*, 381 U. S., at 506.

It is obvious to us that neither of those formulations would extend a fundamental right to homosexuals to engage in acts of consensual sodomy. Proscriptions against that conduct have ancient roots. See generally, Survey on the Constitutional Right to Privacy in the Context of Homosexual Activity, 40 Miami U. L. Rev. 521, 525 (1986). Sodomy was a criminal offense at common law and was forbidden by the laws of the original thirteen States when they ratified the Bill of Rights.[5] In 1868, when the Fourteenth Amendment was ratified, all but 5 of the 37 States in the Union had criminal sodomy laws.[6] In fact, until 1961,[7] all 50 States outlawed sodomy, and today, 24 States and the District of Columbia continue to provide criminal penalties for sodomy performed in private and between consenting adults. Survey, Miami U. L. Rev., *supra*, at 524, n. 9. Against this background, to claim that a right to engage in such conduct is "deeply rooted in this Nation's history and tradition" or "implicit in the concept of ordered liberty" is, at best, facetious.

Nor are we inclined to take a more expansive view of our authority to discover new fundamental rights imbedded in the Due Process Clause. The Court is most vulnerable and comes nearest to illegitimacy when it deals with judge-made constitutional law having little or no cognizable roots in the language or design of the Constitution. That this is so was painfully demonstrated by the face-off between the Executive and the Court in the 1930's, which resulted in the repudiation of much of the substantive gloss that the Court had placed on the Due Process Clause of the Fifth and Fourteenth Amendments. There should be, therefore, great resistance to expand the substantive reach of those Clauses, particularly if it requires redefining the category of rights deemed to be fundamental. Otherwise, the Judiciary necessarily takes to itself further authority to govern the country without express constitutional authority. The claimed right pressed on us today falls far short of overcoming this resistance.

Respondent, however, asserts that the result should be different where the homosexual conduct occurs in the privacy of the home. He relies on *Stanley* v. *Georgia*, 394 U. S. 557 (1969), where the Court held that the First Amendment prevents conviction for possessing and reading obscene material in the privacy of his home: "If the First Amendment means anything, it means that a State has no business telling a man, sitting alone in his house, what books he may read or what films he may watch." *Id.*, at 565.

Stanley did protect conduct that would not have been protected outside the home, and it partially prevented the enforcement of state obscenity laws; but the decision was firmly grounded in the First Amendment. The right pressed upon us here has no similar support in the text of the Constitution, and it does not qualify for recognition under the prevailing principles for construing the Fourteenth Amendment. Its limits are also difficult to discern. Plainly enough, otherwise illegal conduct is not always immunized whenever it occurs in the home. Victimless crimes, such as the possession and use of illegal drugs do not escape the law where they are committed at home. *Stanley* itself recognized that its holding offered no protection for the possession in the home of drugs, firearms, or stolen goods. *Id.*, at 568, n. 11. And if respondent's submission is limited to the voluntary sexual conduct between consenting adults, it would be difficult, except by fiat, to limit the claimed right to homosexual conduct while leaving exposed to prosecution adultery, incest, and other sexual crimes even though they are committed in the home. We are unwilling to start down that road.

Even if the conduct at issue here is not fundamental right, respondent asserts that there must be a rational basis for the law and that there is none in this case other than the presumed belief of a majority of the electorate in Georgia that homosexual sodomy is immoral and unacceptable. This is said to be an inadequate rationale to support the law. The law, however, is constantly based on notions of morality, and if all laws representing essentially moral choices are to be invalidated under the Due Process Clause, the courts will be very busy indeed. Even respondent makes no such claim, but insists that majority sentiments about the morality of homosexuality should be declared inadequate. We do not agree, and are unpersuaded that the sodomy laws of some 25 States should be invalidated on this basis.[8]

Accordingly, the judgment of the Court of Appeals is

Reversed.

NOTES

1. Ga. Code Ann. § 16–6–2 (1984) provides, in pertinent part, as follows: "(a) A person commits the offense of sodomy when he performs or submits to any sexual act involving the sex organs of one person and the mouth or anus of another. . . .

"(b) A person convicted of the offense of sodomy shall be punished by imprisonment for not less than one nor more than 20 years. . . ."

2. John and Mary Doe were also plaintiffs in the action. They alleged that they wished to engage in sexual activity proscribed by § 16–6–2 in the privacy of their home, App. 3, and that they had been "chilled and deterred" from engaging in such activity by both the existence of the statute and Hardwick's arrest. *Id.*, at 5. The District Court held, however, that because they had neither sustained, nor were in immediate danger of sustaining, any direct injury from the enforcement of the statute, they did not have proper standing to maintain the action. *Id.*, at 18. The Court of Appeals affirmed the District Court's judgment dismissing the Does' claim for lack of standing, 760 F. 2d 1202, 1206–1207 (1985), and the Does do not challenge that holding in this Court.

The only claim properly before the Court, therefore, is Hardwick's challenge to the Georgia statute as applied to consensual homosexual sodomy. We express no opinion on the constitutionality of the Georgia statute as applied to other acts of sodomy.

3. See *Baker* v. *Wade*, 769 F. 2d 289, reh'g denied, 774 F. 2d 1285 (CA5 1985) en banc). *Dronenburg* v. *Zech*, 239 U. S. App. D. C. 229, 741 F. 2d 1388, reh'g denied, 241 U. S. App. D. C. 262, 746 F. 2d 1579 (1984).

4. The State also submits that the Court of Appeals erred in holding that the District Court was not obligated to follow our summary affirmance in *Doe*. We need not resolve this dispute, for we prefer to give plenary consideration to the merits of this case rather than rely on our earlier action in *Doe*. See *Usery* v. *Turner Elkhorn Mining Co.*, 428 U. S. 1, 14 (1976); *Massachusetts Board of Retirement* v. *Murgia*, 427 U. S. 307, 309, n. 1 (1976); *Edelman* v. *Jordan*, 415 U. S. 651, 671 (1974). Cf. *Hicks* v. *Miranda*, 422 U.S. 332, 344 (1972).

5. Criminal sodomy laws in effect in 1791:

Connecticut: Public Statute Laws of the State of Connecticut, 1808, Title LXVI, Ch. 1, § 2(rev. 1672).

Delaware: 1 Laws of the State of Delaware, 1797, ch. 22, § 5 (passed 1719).

Georgia had no criminal sodomy statute until 1816, but sodomy was a crime at common law, and the General Assembly adopted the Common Law of England as the law of Georgia in 1784. The First Laws of the State of Georgia, pt. 1 (1981).

Maryland had no criminal sodomy statute in 1791. Maryland's Declaration of Rights, passed in 1776, however, stated that "the inhabitants of Maryland are entitled to the common law of England," and sodomy was a crime at common law. 4 Sources and Documents of United States Constitutions 372 (W. Swindler ed. 1975).

Massachusetts: Acts and Laws passed by the General Court of Massachusetts, ch. 14, Act of March 3, 1785.

New Hampshire passed its first sodomy statute in 1718. Acts and Laws of New Hampshire 1680–1726, p. 141 (1978).

Sodomy was a crime at common law in New Jersey at the time of the ratification of the Bill of Rights. The State enacted its first criminal sodomy law five years later. Acts of the Twentieth General Assembly, March 18, 1796, Ch. DC, § 7, p. 93.

New York: Laws of New York, ch. 21, p. 391 (passed 1787).

At the time of ratification of the Bill of Rights, North Carolina had adopted the English statute of Henry III outlawing sodomy. See Collection of the Statutes of the Parliament of England in Force in the State of North Carolina 314 (1792).

Pennsylvania: Laws of the Fourteenth General Assembly of the Commonwealth of Pennsylvania, ch. CLIV, § 2, p. 293 (passed 1790).

Rhode Island passed its first sodomy law in 1662. The Earliest Acts and

Laws of the Colony of Rhode Island and Providence Plantations 1647–1719 142 (1977).

South Carolina: Public Laws of the State of South Carolina, p. 49 (1790).

At the time of the ratification of the Bill of Rights, Virginia had no specific statute outlawing sodomy, but had adopted the English common law. 9 Hening's Laws of Virginia, ch. 5, § 6, p. 127 (1821) (passed 1776).

6. Criminal sodomy statutes in effect in 1868:

Alabama: Ala. Code, § 3604 (1867).

Arizona (Terr.): Howell Code, ch. 10, § 48(1865).

Arkansas: Ark. Stat., ch. 51, Art. IV, § 5 (1858).

California: 1 Cal. Gen. Laws, ch. 99 § 48 (1865).

Colorado (Terr.): Colo. Rev. Stat., ch. 22, §§ 45, 46 (1868).

Connecticut: Conn. Gen. Stat., Tit. 122, ch. 7 § 124 (1866).

Delaware: Del. Code Ann., Tit. 20, ch. 131, § 7 (1852).

Florida: Acts and Resolutions, ch. 8 § 17 (1868).

Georgia: Ga. Code §§ 4286, 4287, 4290 (1867).

Kingdom of Hawaii: Hawaii Penal Code, ch. 13, § 11 (1868).

Illinois: Ill. Rev. Stat., div. 5, §§ 49, 50 (1845).

Kansas: Kan. (Terr.) Stat., ch. 53, § 7 (1855).

Kentucky: 1 Ky. Rev. Stat., ch. 28, Art. IV, § 11 (1860).

Louisiana: La. Rev. Stat., Crimes and Offences, § 5 (1856).

Maine: Me. Rev. Stat., tit. XII, ch. 160, § 4 (1847).

Maryland: 1 Md. Code, Art. 30, § 201 (1860).

Massachusetts: Mass. Gen. Laws, ch. 165, § 18 (1860).

Michigan: Mich. Rev. Stat., Tit. 30, ch. 158, § 16 (1846).

Minnesota: Minn. Stat., ch. 96, § 13 (1859).

Mississippi: Miss. Rev. Code, ch. 64, Art. 238, § LII, art. 238 (1857).

Missouri: 1 Mo. Rev. Stat., ch. 50, Art. VIII, § 7 (1856).

Montana (Terr.): Mont. Laws, Criminal Practice Acts, ch. IV, § 44 (1864).

Nebraska (Terr.): Neb. Rev. Stat., Crim. Code, ch. 4, § 47 (1866).

Nevada (Terr.): Nev. Comp. Laws, ch. 28, § 45 (1862).

New Hampshire: N. H. Rev. Laws, Act. of June 19, 1812, § 5 (1815).

New Jersey: N. J. Rev. Stat., Tit. 8, ch. 1, § 9 (1847).

New York: 3 N. Y. Rev. Stat., pt. 4, ch. 1, tit. 5, art. 3, § 20 (1858).

North Carolina: N. C. Rev. Code, ch. 34, § 6 (1854).

Oregon: Laws of Ore., Crimes—Against Morality, etc., ch. 7, § 655 (1874).

Pennsylvania: Act of March 31, 1860, § 32, Pub. Law 392, in 1 Digest of Statute Law of Pa. 1700–1903 1011 (Purdon 1905).

Rhode Island: R. I. Gen. Stat., ch. 232, § 12 (1872).

South Carolina: Act of 1712, in 2 Stat. at Large of S. C. 1682–1716, p. 493 (1837).

Tennessee: Tenn. Code, ch. 8, Art. 1, § 4843 (1858).

Texas: Tex. Rev. Stat., Penal Code, tit. 10, ch. 5, Art. 342 (1887) (passed 1860).

Vermont: Laws of the State of Vermont (1779).

Virginia: Va. Code, ch. 149, § 12 (1868).

West Virginia: W. Va. Code, ch. 149, § 12 (1860).
Wisconsin (Terr.): Wis. Stat., § (1839).

7. In 1961, Illinois adopted the American Law Institute's Model Penal Code, which decriminalized adult, consensual, private, sexual conduct. Criminal Code of 1961, §§ 11–2, 11–3, 1961 Ill. Laws 1985, 2006 (codified as amended at Ill. Rev. Stat., ch. 38, ¶¶ 11–2, 11–3 (1983) (repealed 1984).
See American Law Institute, Model Penal Code § 213.2 (Proposed Official Draft 1962).

8. Respondent does not defend the judgment below based on the Ninth Amendment, the Equal Protection Clause or the Eighth Amendment.

CHIEF JUSTICE BURGER, concurring.

I join the Court's opinion, but I write separately to underscore my view that in constitutional terms there is no such thing as a fundamental right to commit homosexual sodomy.

As the Court notes, *ante* at 5, the proscriptions against sodomy have very "ancient roots." Decisions of individuals relating to homosexual conduct have been subject to state intervention throughout the history of Western Civilization. Condemnation of those practices is firmly rooted in Judeao-Christian moral and ethical standards. Homosexual sodomy was a capital crime under Roman law. See Code Theod. 9.7.6; Code Just. 9.9.31. See also D. Bailey, Homosexuality in the Western Christian Tradition 70–81 (1975). During the English Reformation when powers of the ecclesiastical courts were transferred to the King's Courts, the first English statute criminalizing sodomy was passed. 25 Hen. VIII, c. 6. Blackstone described "the infamous crime against nature" as an offense of "deeper malignity" than rape, an heinous act "the very mention of which is a disgrace to human nature," and "a crime not fit to be named." Blackstone's Commentaries *215. The common law of England, including its prohibition of sodomy, became the received law of Georgia and the other Colonies. In 1816 the Georgia Legislature passed the statute at issue here, and that statute has been continuously in force in one form or another since that time. To hold that the act of homosexual sodomy is somehow protected as a fundamental right would be to cast aside millennia of moral teaching.

This is essentially not a question of personal "preferences" but rather that of the legislative authority of the State. I find nothing in the Constitution depriving a State of the power to enact the statute challenged here.

JUSTICE BLACKMUN, with whom JUSTICE BRENNAN, JUSTICE MARSHALL, and JUSTICE STEVENS join, dissenting.

I

In its haste to reverse the Court of Appeals and hold that the Constitution does not "confe[r] a fundamental right upon homosexuals to engage in sodomy," *ante*, at 3, the Court relegates the actual statute being challenged to a footnote and ignores the procedural posture of the case before it. A fair reading of the statute and of the complaint clearly reveals that the majority has distorted the question this case presents.

First, the Court's almost obsessive focus on homosexual activity is particularly hard to justify in light of the broad language Georgia has used. Unlike the Court, the Georgia Legislature has not proceeded on the assumption that homosexuals are so different from other citizens that their lives may be controlled in a way that would not be tolerated if it limited the choices of those other citizens. Cf. *ante*, at 2, n. 2. Rather, Georgia has provided that "[a] person commits the offense of sodomy when he performs or submits to any sexual act involving the sex organs of one person and the mouth or anus of another." Ga. Code Ann. § 16–62(a). The sex or status of the persons who engage in the act is irrelevant as a matter of state law. In fact, to the extent I can discern a legislative purpose for Georgia's 1968 enactment of § 16–6–2, that purpose seems to have been to broaden the coverage of the law to reach heterosexual as well as homosexual activity.[1] I therefore see no basis for the Court's decision to treat this case as an "as applied" challenge to § 16–6–2, see *ante*, at 2, n. 2, or for Georgia's attempt, both in its brief and at oral argument, to defend § 16–6–2 solely on the grounds that it prohibits homosexual activity. Michael Hardwick's standing may rest in significant part on Georgia's apparent willingness to enforce against homosexuals a law it seems not to have any desire to enforce against heterosexuals. See Tr. of Oral Arg. 4–5; cf. *Hardwick* v. *Bowers*, 760 F. 2d 1202, 1205–1206 (CA11 1985). But his claim that § 16–6–2 involves an unconstitutional intrusion into his privacy and his right of intimate association does not depend in any way on his sexual orientation.

Second, I disagree with the Court's refusal to consider whether § 16–6–2 runs afoul of the Eighth or Ninth Amendments or the Equal Protection Clause of the Fourteenth Amendment. *Ante*, at 9, n. 8. Respondent's complaint expressly invoked the Ninth Amendment, see App. 6, and he relied heavily before this Court on *Griswold* v.

Connecticut, 381 U. S. 479, 484 (1965), which identifies that Amendment as one of the specific constitutional provisions giving "life and substance" to our understanding of privacy. See Brief for Respondent 10–12; Tr. of Oral Arg. 33. More importantly, the procedural posture of the case requires that we affirm the Court of Appeals' judgment if there is *any* ground on which respondent may be entitled to relief. This case is before us on petitioner's motion to dismiss for failure to state a claim, Fed. Rule Civ. Proc. 12(b)(6). See App. 17. It is a well settled principle of law that "a complaint should not be dismissed merely because a plaintiff's allegations do not support the particular legal theory he advances, for the court is under a duty to examine the complaint to determine if the allegations provide for relief on any possible theory." *Bramlet* v. *Wilson*, 495 F. 2d 714, 716 (CA8 1974); see *Parr* v. *Great Lakes Express Co.*, 484 F. 2d 767, 773 (CA7 1973); *Due* v. *Tallahasee Theatres Inc.*, 333 F. 2d 630, 631 (CA5 1964); *United States* v. *Howell*, 318 F. 2d 162, 166 (CA9 1963); 5 C. Wright & A. Miller, Federal Practice and Procedure: Civil, § 1357, pp. 601–602 (1969); see also *Conley* v. *Gibson*, 355 U. S. 41, 45–46 (1957). Thus, even if respondent did not advance claims based on the Eighth or Ninth Amendments, or on the Equal Protection Clause, his complaint should not be dismissed if any of those provisions could entitle him to relief. I need not reach either the Eighth Amendment or the Equal Protection Clause issues because I believe that Hardwick has stated a cognizable claim that § 16–6–2 interferes with constitutionally protected interests in privacy and freedom of intimate association. But neither the Eighth Amendment nor the Equal Protection Clause is so clearly irrelevant that a claim resting on either provision should be peremptorily dismissed.[2] The Court's cramped reading of the issue before it makes for a short opinion, but it does little to make for a persuasive one.

II

"Our cases long have recognized that the Constitution embodies a promise that a certain private sphere of individual liberty will be kept largely beyond the reach of government." *Thornburgh* v. *American Coll. of Obst. & Gyn.*,—U. S.—,— (1986) (slip op. 23). In construing the right to privacy, the Court has proceeded along two somewhat distinct, albeit complementary, lines. First, it has recognized a privacy interest with reference to certain *decisions* that are properly for the individual to make. *E.g.*, *Roe* v. *Wade*, 410 U. S. 113 (1973); *Pierce* v. *Society of Sisters*, 268 U. S. 510 (1925). Second, it has recognized a privacy interest with reference to certain *places* without regard for the particular activities in which the individuals who occupy them are engaged. *E.g., United States* v. *Karo,* 468 U.S. 705 (1984); *Payton* v. *New York,* 445 U. S. 573 (1980); *Rios* v. *United States,* 364 U. S. 253 (1960). The case before us implicates both the decisional and the spatial aspects of the right to privacy.

A

The Court concludes today that none of our prior cases dealing with various decisions that individuals are entitled to make free of governmental interference "bears any resemblance to the claimed constitutional right of homosexuals to engage in acts of sodomy that is asserted in this case." *Ante,* at 4. While it is true that these cases may be characterized by their connection to protection of the family, see *Roberts* v. *United States Jaycees,* 468 U. S. 609, 619 (1984), the Court's conclusion that they extend no further than this boundary ignores the warning in *Moore* v. *East Cleveland,* 431 U. S. 494, 501 (1977) (plurality opinion), against "clos[ing] our eyes to the basic reasons why certain rights associated with the family have been accorded shelter under the Fourteenth Amendment's Due Process Clause." We protect those rights not because they contribute, in some direct and material way, to the general public welfare, but because they form so central a part of an individual's life. "[T]he concept of privacy embodies the 'moral fact that a person belongs to himself and not others nor to society as a whole.'" *Thornburgh* v. *American Coll. of Obst. & Gyn.,* — U. S., at —, n. 5 (STEVENS, J., concurring) (slip op. 6, n. 5), quoting Fried, Correspondence, 6 Phil. & Pub. Affairs 288–289 (1977). And so we protect the decision whether to marry precisely because marriage "is an association that promotes a way of life, not causes; a harmony in living, not political faiths; a bilateral loyalty, not commercial or social projects." *Griswold* v. *Connecticut,* 381 U. S., at 486. We protect the decision whether to have a child because parenthood alters so dramatically an individual's self-definition, not because of demographic considerations or the Bible's command to be fruitful and multiply. Cf. *Thornburgh* v. *American Coll. of Obst. & Gyn., supra,* at —, n. 6 (STEVENS, J., concurring) (slip op. 6, n. 6). And we protect the family because it contributes so powerfully to the happiness of individuals, not because of a preference for stereotypical households. Cf. *Moore* v. *East Cleveland,* 431 U. S., at 500–506 (plurality opinion). The Court recognized in *Roberts,* 468 U. S., at 619, that the "ability independently to define one's identity that is central to any concept of liberty" cannot truly be exercised in a vacuum; we all depend on the "emotional enrichment of close ties with others." *Ibid.*

Only the most willful blindness could obscure the fact that sexual intimacy is "a sensitive, key relationship of human existence, central to family life, community welfare, and the development of human personality," *Paris Adult Theatre I* v. *Slayton*, 413 U. S. 49, 63 (1973); see also *Carey* v. *Population Services International*, 431 U. S. 678, 685 (1977). The fact that individuals define themselves in a significant way through their intimate sexual relationships with others suggests, in a Nation as diverse as ours, that there may be many "right" ways of conducting those relationships, and that much of the richness of a relationship will come from the freedom an individual has to *choose* the form and nature of these intensely personal bonds. See Karst, The Freedom of Intimate Association, 89 Yale L. J. 624, 637 (1980); cf. *Eisenstadt* v. *Baird*, 405 U. S. 438, 453 (1972); *Roe* v. *Wade*, 410 U. S., at 153.

In a variety of circumstances we have recognized that a necessary corollary of giving individuals freedom to choose how to conduct their lives is acceptance of the fact that different individuals will make different choices. For example, in holding that the clearly important state interest in public education should give way to a competing claim by the Amish to the effect that extended formal schooling threatened their way of life, the Court declared: "There can be no assumption that today's majority is 'right' and the Amish and others like them are 'wrong.' A way of life that is odd or even erratic but interferes with no rights or interests of others is not to be condemned because it is different." *Wisconsin* v. *Yoder*, 406 U. S. 205, 223–224 (1972). The Court claims that its decision today merely refuses to recognize a fundamental right to engage in homosexual sodomy; what the Court really has refused to recognize is the fundamental interest all individuals have in controlling the nature of their intimate associations with others.

B

The behavior for which Hardwick faces prosecution occurred in his own home, a place to which the Fourth Amendment attaches special significance. The Court's treatment of this aspect of the case is symptomatic of its overall refusal to consider the broad principles that have informed our treatment of privacy in specific cases. Just as the right to privacy is more than the mere aggregation of a number of entitlements to engage in specific behavior, so too, protecting the physical integrity of the home is more than merely a means of protecting specific activities that often take place there.

Even when our understanding of the contours of the right to privacy depends on "reference to a 'place,'" *Katz* v. *United States*, 389 U. S., at 361 (Harlan, J., concurring), "the essence of a Fourth Amendment violation is 'not the breaking of [a person's] doors, and the rummaging of his drawers,' but rather is 'the invasion of his indefeasible right of personal security, personal liberty and private property.'" *California* v. *Ciraolo*,—U.S.—,—(1986) (POWELL, J., dissenting) (slip op. 11), quoting *Boyd* v. *United States*, 116 U. S. 616, 630 (1886).

The Court's interpretation of the pivotal case of *Stanley* v. *Georgia*, 394 U. S. 557 (1969), is entirely unconvincing. *Stanley* held that Georgia's undoubted power to punish the public distribution of constitutionally unprotected, obscene material did not permit the State to punish the private possession of such material. According to the majority here, *Stanley* relied entirely on the First Amendment, and thus, it is claimed, sheds no light on cases not involving printed materials. *Ante*, at 8. But that is not what *Stanley* said. Rather, the *Stanley* Court anchored its holding in the Fourth Amendment's special protection for the individual in his home:

> "'The makers of our Constitution undertook to secure conditions favorable to the pursuit of happiness. They recognized the significance of man's spiritual nature, of his feelings and of his intellect. They knew that only a part of the pain, pleasure and satisfactions of life are to be found in material things. They sought to protect Americans in their beliefs, their thoughts, their emotions and their sensations.'

> "These are the rights that appellant is asserting in the case before us. He is asserting the right to read or observe what he pleases—the right to satisfy his intellectual and emotional needs in the privacy of his own home." *Id.*, at 564–565, quoting *Olmstead* v. *United States*, 277 U. S., at 478 (Brandeis, J., dissenting).

The central place that *Stanley* gives Justice Brandeis' dissent in *Olmstead*, a case raising *no* First Amendment claim, shows that *Stanley* rested as much on the Court's understanding of the Fourth Amendment as it did on the First. Indeed, in *Paris Adult Theatre I* v. *Slaton*, 413 U. S. 49 (1973), the Court suggested that reliance on the Fourth Amendment not only supported the Court's outcome in *Stanley* but actually was *necessary* to it: "If obscene material unprotected by the First Amendment in itself carried with it a 'penumbra' of constitutionally protected privacy, this Court would not have found it necessary to decide *Stanley* on the narrow basis of the 'privacy of the home,' which was hardly more than a reaffirmation that 'a man's home is his castle.'" *Id.*, at 66. "The right of the people to be secure in their ... houses," expressly guaranteed by the Fourth Amendment, is perhaps the most "textual" of the various constitutional provisions that inform our understanding of the right to privacy, and thus I cannot agree with the Court's statement that "[t]he right pressed upon us here has no ... support in the text of the Constitution," *ante*, at 8. Indeed, the right of an individual to conduct intimate relationships in the intimacy of his or her own home seems to me to be the heart of the Constitution's protection of privacy.

III

The Court's failure to comprehend the magnitude of the liberty interests at stake in this case leads it to slight the question whether petitioner, on behalf of the State, has justified Georgia's infringement on these interests. I believe that neither of the two general justifications for § 16–6–2 that petitioner has advanced warrants dismissing respondent's challenge for failure to state a claim.

First, petitioner asserts that the acts made criminal by the statute may have serious adverse consequences for "the general public health and welfare," such as spreading communicable diseases or fostering other criminal activity. Brief for Petitioner 37. Inasmuch as this case was dismissed by the District Court on the pleadings, it is not surprising that the record before us is barren of any evidence to support petitioner's claim.[3] In light of the state of the record, I see no justification for the Court's attempt to equate the private, consensual sexual activity at issue here with the "possession in the home of drugs, firearms, or stolen goods," *ante*, at 9, to which *Stanley* refused to extend its protection. 394 U. S., at 568, n. 11. None of the behavior so mentioned in *Stanley* can properly be viewed as "[v]ictimless," *ante*, at 9: drugs and weapons are inherently dangerous, see, *e.g.*, *McLaughlin* v. *United States*,—U.S.—(1986), and for property to be "stolen," someone must have been wrongfully deprived of it. Nothing in the record before the Court provides any justification for finding the activity forbidden by § 16–6–2 to be physically dangerous, either to the persons engaged in it or to others.[4]

The core of petitioner's defense of § 16–6–2, however, is that respondent and others who engage in the conduct prohibited by § 16–6–2 interfere with Georgia's exercise of the " 'right of the Nation and of the States to maintain a decent society,'" *Paris Adult Theater I* v. *Slaton,* 413 U. S., at 59–60, quoting *Jacobellis* v. *Ohio,* 378 U. S. 184, 199 (1964) (Warren, C. J., dissenting). Essentially, petitioner argues, and the Court agrees, that the fact that the acts described in § 16–6–2 "for hundreds of years, if not thousands, have been uniformly condemned as immoral" is a sufficient reason to permit a State to ban them today. Brief for Petitioner 19; see *ante,* at 3, 5–8, 9.

I cannot agree that either the length of time a majority has held its convictions or the passions with which it defends them can withdraw legislation from this Court's scrutiny. See, *e.g., Roe* v. *Wade,* 410 U. S. 113 (1973); *Loving* v. *Virginia,* 388 U. S. 1 (1967); *Brown* v. *Board of Education,* 347 U. S. 483 (1954).[5] As Justice Jackson wrote so eloquently for the Court in *West Virginia Board of Education* v. *Barnette,* 319 U. S. 624, 641–642 (1943), "we apply the limitations of the Constitution with no fear that freedom to be intellectually and spiritually diverse or even contrary will disintegrate the social organization.... [F]reedom to differ is not limited to things that do not matter much. That would be a mere shadow of freedom. The test of its substance is the right to differ as to things that touch the heart of the existing order." See also Karst, 89 Yale L. J., at 627. It is precisely because the issue raised by this case touches the heart of what makes individuals what they are that we should be especially sensitive to the rights of those whose choices upset the majority.

The assertion that "traditional Judeo-Christian values proscribe" the conduct involved, Brief for Petitioner 20, cannot provide an adequate justification for § 16–6–2. That certain, but by no means all, religious groups condemn the behavior at issue gives the State no license to impose their judgments on the entire citizenry. The legitimacy of secular legislation depends instead on whether the State can advance some justification for its law beyond its conformity to religious doctrine. See, *e. g., McGowan* v. *Maryland,* 366 U. S. 420, 429–453 (1961); *Stone* v. *Graham,* 449 U. S. 39 (1980). Thus, far from buttressing his case, petitioner's invocation of Leviticus, Romans, St. Thomas Aquinas, and sodomy's heretical status during the Middle Ages undermines his suggestion that § 16–6–2 represents a legitimate use of secular coercive power.[6] A State can no more punish private behavior because of religious intolerance than it can punish such behavior because of racial animus. "The Constitution cannot control such prejudices, but neither can it tolerate them. Private biases may be outside the reach of the law, but the law cannot, directly or indirectly, give them effect." *Palmore* v. *Sidoti,*

466 U. S. 429, 433 (1984). No matter how uncomfortable a certain group may make the majority of this Court, we have held that "[m]ere public intolerance or animosity cannot constitutionally justify the deprivation of a person's physical liberty." *O'Connor* v. *Donaldson*, 422 U. S. 563, 575 (1975). See also *City of Cleburne* v. *Cleburne Living Center,* — U. S. — (1985); *U. S. Dept. of Agriculture* v. *Moreno*, 413 U. S. 528, 534 (1973).

Nor can § 16–6–2 be justified as a "morally neutral" exercise of Georgia's power to "protect the public environment," *Paris Adult Theatre I*, 413 U. S., at 68–69. Certainly, some private behavior can affect the fabric of society as a whole. Reasonable people may differ about whether particular sexual acts are moral or immoral, but "we have ample evidence for believing that people will not abandon morality, will not think any better of murder, cruelty and dishonesty, merely because some private sexual practice which they abominate is not punished by the law." H. L. A. Hart, Immorality and Treason, reprinted in The Law as Literature 220, 225 (L. Blom-Cooper ed. 1961). Petitioner and the Court fail to see the difference between laws that protect public sensibilities and those that enforce private morality. Statutes banning public sexual activity are entirely consistent with protecting the individual's liberty interest in decisions concerning sexual relations: the same recognition that those decisions are intensely private which justifies protecting them from governmental interference can justify protecting individuals from unwilling exposure to the sexual activities of others. But the mere fact that intimate behavior may be punished when it takes place in public cannot dictate how States can regulate intimate behavior that occurs in intimate places. *See Paris Adult Theatre I*, *supra*, at 66, n. 13 ("marital intercourse on a street corner or a theater stage" can be forbidden despite the constitutional protection identified in *Griswold* v. *Connecticut*, 381 U. S. 479 (1965)).[7]

This case involves no real interference with the rights of others, for the mere knowledge that other individuals do not adhere to one's value system cannot be a legally cognizable interest, cf. *Diamond* v. *Charles*,— U. S. —, — (1986) (slip op. 10–11), let alone an interest that can justify invading the houses, hearts, and minds of citizens who choose to live their lives differently.

IV

It took but three years for the Court to see the error in its analysis in *Minersville School District* v. *Gobitis*, 310 U. S. 586 (1940), and to recognize that the threat to national cohesion posed by a refusal to salute the flag was vastly outweighed by the threat to those same values posed by compelling such a salute. See *West Virginia Board of Education* v. *Barnette*, 319 U. S. 624 (1943). I can only hope that here, too, the Court soon will reconsider its analysis and conclude that depriving individuals of the right to choose for themselves how to conduct their intimate relationships poses a far greater threat to the values most deeply rooted in our Nation's history than tolerance of nonconformity could ever do. Because I think the Court today betrays those values, I dissent.

NOTES

1. Until 1968, Georgia defined sodomy as "the carnal knowledge and connection against the order of nature, by man with man, or in the same unnatural manner with woman." Ga. Crim. Code § 26–5901 (1933 In *Thompson* v. *Aldredge*, 187 Ga. 467, 200 S. E. 799 (1939), the Georgia Supreme Court held that § 26–5901 did not prohibit lesbian activity. And in *Riley* v. *Garrett*, 219 Ga. 345, 133 S. E. 2d 367 (1963), the Georgia Supreme Court held that § 26–5901 did not prohibit heterosexual cunnilingus. Georgia passed the act-specific statute currently in force "perhaps in response to the restrictive court decisions such as *Riley*," Note The Crimes Against Nature, 16 J. Pub. L. 159, 167, n. 47 (1967).

2. In *Robinson* v. *California*, 370 U. S. 660 (1962), the Court held that the Eighth Amendment barred convicting a defendant due to his "status" as a narcotics addict, since that condition was "apparently an illness which may be contracted innocently or involuntarily." *Id.*, at 667. In *Powell* v. *Texas*, 392 U. S. 514 (1968), where the Court refused to extend *Robinson* to punishment of public drunkenness by a chronic alcoholic, one of the factors relied on by JUSTICE MARSHALL, in writing the plurality opinion, was that Texas had not "attempted to regulate appellant's behavior in the privacy of his own home." *Id.*, at 532. JUSTICE WHITE wrote separately:
"Analysis of this difficult case is not advanced by preoccupation with the label 'condition.' In *Robinson* the Court dealt with 'a statute which makes the "status" of narcotic addition a criminal offense....' 370 U. S., at 666. By precluding criminal conviction for such a 'status' the Court was dealing with a condition brought about by acts remote in time from the application of the criminal sanctions contemplated, a condition which was relatively permanent in duration, and a condition of great magnitude and significance in terms of human behavior and values.... If it were necessary to distinguish between 'acts' and 'conditions' for purposes of the Eighth Amendment, I would adhere to the concept of 'condition' implicit in the opinion in *Robinson.* ... The proper subject of inquiry is whether volitional acts brought about the 'condition' and whether those acts are sufficiently proximate to the 'condition' for it to be permissible to impose penal sanctions on the 'condition.' " *Id.*, at 550–551, n. 2.

Despite historical views of homosexuality, it is no longer viewed by mental health professionals as a "disease" or disorder. See Brief for American Psychological Association and American Public Health Association as *Amici Curiae* 8–11. But, obviously, neither is it simply a matter of deliberate personal election. Homosexual orientation may well form part of the very fiber of an individual's personality. Consequently, under JUSTICE WHITE's analysis in *Powell*, the Eighth Amendment may pose a constitutional barrier to sending an individual to prison for acting on that attraction regardless of the circumstances. An individual's ability to make constitutionally protected "decisions concerning sexual relations," *Carey* v. *Population Services International*, 431 U. S. 678, 711 (1977) (POWELL, J., concurring in part and concurring in the judgment), is rendered empty indeed if he or she is given no real choice but a life without any physical intimacy.

With respect to the Equal Protection Clause's applicability to §16–6–2, I note that Georgia's exclusive stress before this Court on its interest in prosecuting homosexual activity despite the gender-neutral terms of the statute may raise serious questions of discriminatory enforcement, questions that cannot be disposed of before this Court on a motion to dismiss. See *Yick Wo* v. *Hopkins*, 118 U. S. 356, 373–374 (1886). The legislature having decided that the sex of the participants is irrelevant to the legality of the acts, I do not see why the State can defend § 16–6–2 on the ground that individuals singled out for prosecution are of the same sex as their partners. Thus, under the circumstances of this case, a claim under the Equal Protection Clause may well be available without having to reach the more controversial question whether homosexuals are a suspect class. See, *e.g.*, *Rowland* v. *Mad River Local School District*,— U. S. —, —(1985) BRENNAN, J., dissenting from denial of certiorari); Note, The Constitutional Status of Sexual Orientation: Homosexuality as a Suspect Classification, 98 Harv. L. Rev. 1285 (1985).

3. Even if a court faced with a challenge to § 16–6–2 were to apply simple rational-basis scrutiny to the statute, Georgia would be required to show an actual connection between the forbidden acts and the ill effects it seeks to prevent. The connection between the acts prohibited by § 16–6–2 and the harms identified by petitioner in his brief before this Court is a subject of hot dispute, hardly amenable to dismissal under Federal Rule of Civil Procedure 12(b)(6). Compare, *e. g.*, Brief for Petitioner 36–37 and Brief for David Robinson, Jr., as *Amicus Curiae* 23–28, on the one hand, with *People* v. *Onofre*, 51 N. Y. 2d 476, 489, 415 N. E. 2d 936, 941 (1980); Brief for the Attorney General of the State of New York, joined by the Attorney General of the State of California, as *Amici Curiae* 11–14; and Brief for the American Psychological Association and American Public Health Association as *Amici Curiae* 19–27, on the other.

4. Although I do not think it necessary to decide today issues that are not even remotely before us, it does seem to me that a court could find simple, analytically sound distinctions between certain private, consensual sexual

conduct, on the one hand, and adultery and incest (the only two vaguely specific "sexual crimes" to which the majority points, *ante*, at 9), on the other. For example, marriage, in addition to its spiritual aspects, is a civil contract that entitles the contracting parties to a variety of governmentally provided benefits. A State might define the contractual commitment necessary to become eligible for these benefits to include a commitment of fidelity and then punish individuals for breaching that contract. Moreover, a State might conclude that adultery is likely to injure third persons, in particular, spouses and children of persons who engage in extramarital affairs. With respect to incest, a court might well agree with respondent that the nature of familial relationships renders true consent to incestuous activity sufficiently problematical that a blanket prohibition of such activity is warranted. See Tr. of Oral Arg. 21–22. Notably, the Court makes no effort to explain why it has chosen to group private, consensual homosexual activity with adultery and incest rather than with private, consensual heterosexual activity by unmarried persons or, indeed, with oral or anal sex within marriage.

5. The parallel between *Loving* and this case is almost uncanny. There, too, the State relied on a religious justification for its law. Compare 388 U. S., at 3 (quoting trial court's statement that "Almighty God created the races white, black, yellow, malay and red, and he placed them on separate continents. . . . The fact that he separated the races shows that he did not intend for the races to mix"), with Brief for Petitioner 20–21 (relying on the Old and New Testaments and the writings of St. Thomas Aquinas to show that "traditional Judeo-Christian values proscribe such conduct."). There, too, defenders of the challenged statute relied heavily on the fact that when the Fourteenth Amendment was ratified, most of the States had similar prohibitions. Compare Brief for Appellee in *Loving* v. *Virginia*, O. T. 1966, No. 395, pp. 28–29, with *ante*, at 5–7 and n. 6. There, too, at the time the case came before the Court, many of the States still had criminal statutes concerning the conduct at issue. Compare 388 U. S., at 6, n. 5 (noting that 16 States still outlawed interracial marriage), with *ante*, 6–7 (noting that 24 States and the District of Columbia have sodomy statutes). Yet the Court held, not only that the individious racism of Virginia's law violated the Equal Protection Clause, see 388 U. S., at 7–12, but also that the law deprived the Lovings of due process by denying them the "freedom of choice to marry" that had "'long been recognized as one of the vital personal rights essential to the orderly pursuit of happiness by free men." *Id.*, at 12.

6. The theological nature of the origin of Anglo-American antisodomy statutes is patent. It was not until 1533 that sodomy was made a secular offense in England. 25 Hen. VIII, cap. 6. Until that time, the offense was, in Sir James Stephen's words, "merely ecclesiastical." 2 J. Stephen, A History of the Criminal Law of England 430 (1883). Pollock and Maitland similarly observed that "[t]he crime against nature. . . . was so closely connected with heresy that the vulgar had but one name for both." 2 F. Pollock & F.

Maitland, The History of English Law 554 (1895). The transfer of jurisdiction over prosecutions for sodomy to the secular courts seems primarily due to the alteration of ecclesiastical jurisdiction attendant on England's break with the Roman Catholic Church, rather than to any new understanding of the sovereign's interest in preventing or punishing the behavior involved. Cf. E. Coke, The Third Part of the Institutes of the Laws of England, ch. 10 (4th ed. 1797).

7. At oral argument a suggestion appeared that, while the Fourth Amendment's special protection of the home might prevent the State from enforcing § 16–6–2 against individuals who engage in consensual sexual activity there, that protection would not make the statute invalid. See Tr. of Oral Arg. 10–11. The suggestion misses the point entirely. If the law is not invalid, then the police can *invade the home to enforce it, provided, of course, that they obtain a determination of probable cause from a neutral magistrate. One of the reasons for the Court's holding in Griswold* v. *Connecticut*, 381 U. S. 479 (1965), was precisely the possibility, and repugnancy, of permitting searches to obtain evidence regarding the use of contraceptives. *Id.*, at 485–486. Permitting the kinds of searches that might be necessary to obtain evidence of the sexual activity banned by § 16–6–2 seems no less intrusive, or repugnant. Cf *Winston* v. *Lee*, — U. S. —(1985); *Mary Beth G.* v. *City of Chicago*, 723 F. 2d 1263, 1274 (CA7 1983).

Morality and the Health of the Body Politic

Dan E. Beauchamp

THE ACQUIRED IMMUNODEFICIENCY SYNDROME (AIDS) is clearly a public health threat. The view that it is also a threat to the majority's values is a form of legal moralism.[1] Like public health, legal moralism relies on the use of law and regulation to promote community aims. But legal moralism restricts liberty as a defense against a moral rather than a physical harm. It uses law to protect the majority's morality from the deviant group.

The classic defense of moralism is found in James F. Stephen's *Liberty, Equality, Fraternity*, published in 1873,[2] a rebuttal to John Stuart Mill's essay "On Liberty."[3] Stephen argued that the majority in any society is a moral majority. In the moralist's view a principal function of the criminal law and public policy should be to enforce the norms of that shared morality, punishing whatever is "offensive, degrading, vicious, sinful, corrupt, or otherwise immoral."[4]

In recent times this view has been most forcefully stated by Lord Patrick Devlin in his critique of the 1957 British Wolfenden Report—the Report of the Committee on Homosexual Offences and Prostitution —which recommended removing criminal sanctions for private homosexual conduct between consenting adults. Devlin said: "What makes a society of any sort is community of ideas, not only political ideas but also ideas about the way its members should behave and

Dan E. Beauchamp, "Morality and the Health of the Body Politic," *Hastings Center Report*, December 1986, pp. 30–36. Reprinted by Permission of the Author and the *Hastings Center Report*.

govern their lives; these latter ideas are its moral.... [W]ithout shared ideas on politics, morals and ethics no society can exist.... For society is not something that is kept together physically; it is held by the invisible bonds of common thought."[5] Moralism binds the community tightly within a narrow and precise morality. Moralism seeks to purify the community, dividing the citizenry into the wheat and the chaff. (My discussion of "loose-boundedness" and "tight-boundedness" in culture and politics is drawn from Richard Merelman, *Making Something of Ourselves* [Berkeley: University of California Press, 1984]. However, I depart from Merelman's notion of loosely bounded societies in which a sense of group attachment and limits has vanished. I use the term "loosely bounded" to mean restrictions that, while less all-encompassing and restrictive than the restrictions of tightly bounded groups, nevertheless limit autonomy and liberty to promote a shared and common good.)

Opposition to moralism is sometimes expressed as: "Law has no business restricting private conduct." But it is using law to restrict private conduct in order to promote a private morality that is the crux of the problem.

The most powerful objections to moralism lie in disputing two claims often made on its behalf. According to the first thesis, if a common morality is shared by a majority, this alone is sufficient justification to include it in the criminal law.[6] The second thesis is that because a common morality holds a society together, legal moralism is justified on the grounds of self-preservation. But to opponents of legal moralism, serious restrictions on liberty cannot rest solely on appeals to tradition, even when backed by majority approval. Furthermore, there is no evidence that violations of the majority's moral norms, like homosexuality, threaten the existence of society.

The most potent challenge to legal moralism is its frequent collision with a more widely shared value—public health. Restrictions on liberty to promote the public health—paternalism—are today more widely accepted than legal moralism. The trend seems to be, at least over the long run, toward rejecting tightly bounded moral codes in favor of loosely bounded restrictions that promote the public health as a common good. By permitting the majority the right to enforce legally its traditional prejudices, particularly in the sexual realm, the health and safety of the public can be directly threatened.

AIDS mainly strikes two groups—gay men and intravenous drug users—who under normal circumstances are shunned by the larger society. According to the Centers for Disease Control (CDC), the number of cases of heterosexual transmission is rising, but the percentage of all cases due to heterosexual transmission remains very low, roughly 1 percent, and shows no sign of change.

Our best weapon against AIDS would be a public health policy resting on the right to be different in fundamental choices and the democratic community as "one body" in matters of the common health. This new policy would mean the right of every individual to fundamental autonomy, as in abortion and sexual orientation, while viewing health and safety as a common good whose protection (through restrictions on liberty) promotes community and the common health. The public health policy would reject moralism as a threat to the right of each individual, including gays, to fundamental autonomy and also a threat to the common health.

AIDS, at least in developed countries, does not seem to behave like a typical infectious disease, which spreads rapidly or easily. Until a vaccine is developed, AIDS will resemble drunk driving or cigarette smoking more than diphtheria or malaria; that is, mortality will rise to a high and stubborn level, which will prove very difficult to reduce. And, as in drunk driving, we will be strongly tempted to use the criminal law to punish the offender rather than to explore the roots of the disease, because the roots of the problem lie in American practices generally.

AIDS policy must begin with a realistic admission that, given the poor prospects for developing a vaccine in the immediate future, there is little hope for elimination of the disease. We can only hope to control the rate of increase among high-risk groups, and to prevent the spread into other groups. By how much we can't say for sure, but reducing the incidence of AIDS by one-half seems an almost utopian goal. Hence, neither quarantine nor isolation can be the principal path to conquering AIDS. Education is our only hope for prevention, and here we confront the barrier of societal practices regarding homosexuality.

The Public Health Service guidelines to reduce the risk of contracting or transmitting AIDS stress eliminating sex with strangers and anal intercourse, and urge the use of condoms at all times.[7] Gay groups have strongly criticized these guidelines, because their global character seems to imply that the main sexual activities of gay men are, by definition, risky. Discouraging anal intercourse, sex with strangers, or almost any sexual activity that is stimulating with those suspected of being exposed to the HIV virus, does seem unrealistic. In many states and localities the publication of such guidelines might provide grounds for criminal charges. Sodomy statutes and other laws against homosexuality serve as a powerful brake on the most potent weapon we have against AIDS—the use of a vigorous public education campaign.

Societal discrimination against gay people slows up the battle against AIDS in two ways. It threatens their health directly, and it impedes changes in gay sexual practices that heighten the risk of AIDS.

The laws against homosexuality in about half the states, as well as containing social prejudice, prevent public health agencies from developing and aggressively carrying out frank and open sex education campaigns for safer homosexual sex, as well as frustrating prompt medical attention as a part of an overall prevention strategy. We already have ample evidence that this will occur. In the case of the federal government's recent solicitation for "Innovative Projects for AIDS Risk Reduction," the federal government requires that a program review panel, the majority of whom are not the members of at-risk groups, should review program materials to determine that the general public is not offended by sexually explicit material.[8] Federal officials obviously became jittery that successful applicants might draw the ire of opposed groups and even lawsuits, based on state sodomy statutes.

Many might conclude that, because some media and some locales permit rather extensive and public discussion of gay sexuality, these statutes are not a serious problem. While some media carry rather explicit information about "safe sex," the details of such practices are not widely publicized. It is very difficult in many areas in the U.S. to assure that these data are widely disseminated and that homosexuals can freely debate and discuss critical changes in their practices. Where openness is the rule, evidence seems to show a dramatic decline in at-risk sex.

The sodomy statutes also contribute to the poor health of many gays by discouraging their seeking prompt medical advice and treatment for many sexually transmitted diseases (STDs). The high rate of STDs among homosexual males may increase the risk that those who become infected will develop symptoms or become full-blown AIDS cases. The same might well be true for gay men using drugs of various kinds to increase sexual stimulation. Antisodomy statutes and fear of prosecution or exposure discourage prompt medical attention and limit opportunities for communicating clear advice about safer sexual practices. Indeed, the antisodomy statutes may encourage prejudice among the medical community toward homosexual patients.

The antisodomy statutes and other restrictions on gay men may also make it more likely that the sexual practices of some such individuals remain high-risk for venereal disease and AIDS. If the sexual practices of many gay men are to change, and if homosexual sex is to occur in the context of more stable relationships, the larger society will have to permit permanent forms of gay association and civil liberties that encourage such stable relationships. While societal discrimination is not the whole story behind gay liberation, gay sexual practices may have been shaped in part by societal pressures and laws forcing gay men to associate secretly in bars and bathhouses out of view of the majority community, while at the same time proscribing gay association by cohabitation and marriage. Gay people cannot now marry and are denied many other legal and social privileges of straights. The freedoms to live where one wants and with whom one wants; to make contracts; and to obtain employment in a normal manner are likely linked in subtle ways to encouraging enduring relationships, which lower the risk of exposure to STDs.

Success in the battle against AIDS depends on replacing old images of the tightly bound community based on sodomy statutes—"us" and "them"—with a more complex public health policy that combines the right to be different with the view that in matters of the common health and safety we are "one body" with a common good. This complex vision, combining equality and community, rests on a double movement; the health of the body politic depends on mutual trust and a willingness to accept the burdens of a citizenship; these burdens are accepted because a narrow moralism is rejected and all are equal partners in the body politic, free to pursue their own ultimate ends.

Therefore, health education against AIDS should involve far more than disseminating explicit sex education materials. Health education means building and strengthening both equality and community, challenging traditional superstitions and defending the legitimate rights of homosexuals. Health officials should actively—albeit prudently—seek the repeal of state laws proscribing homosexuality as major barriers to this public education, laws whose continued existence threatens the public health. Public health groups should also support efforts to broaden the civil liberties of gay people and eliminate laws that permit employers, landlords, the military, or commercial establishments to discriminate in employment, housing, insurance, or military service.

While public health and the rights to citizenship are a cornerstone in any community, removing centuries of prejudice and discrimination dictates caution and political prudence. The prejudices against homosexuality are deep-seated and not likely to give way easily.

Of course, the moralist sees laws against homosexuality as ordained by God and tradition. In this view, laws forbidding sodomy among males and females or partners of the same sex are a vital bulwark against AIDS. If homosexuality were to decline sharply, the number of AIDS cases would fall in turn. Guidelines for safe sex are, accordingly, guidelines for safe sodomy and are, as such, patently repugnant.

Similarly the moralist is reluctant to distribute sterile needles to intravenous drug users as a strategy to stop the spread of AIDS. Drug use, to the moralist, is not just a health problem; it is a vice.

There are many parallels between AIDS and abortion. In Roe v. Wade, legal abortion was justified not on grounds of privacy alone (equality) but also on public health grounds (the common good); Justice Blackmun justified his decision in significant part because legal abortions were much safer for the mother than pregnancy and illegal abortions.[9] Securing the right to abortion strengthened the public health by removing the barriers to safe abortions.

Understandably, health officials might want to avoid another issue as contentious as abortion. But it is unlikely that they will be able to do so. The same groups that object, in the name of religion, to abortion, to sex education, and to teenage contraception also object to eliminating the sodomy laws and to expanding the right of privacy in matters of sex, as well as strengthening the rights of homosexuals to decent medical care, to employment, housing, and military service. Public health cannot ignore the blunt truth that society's restrictions on sexual freedom are a fundamental public health issue. Legal moralism has always been concerned at its core with sexual practices believed to hold together and strengthen the traditional family unit.

This is not to say that the majority has no legitimate interest in regulating gay sexual practices on the grounds of morality. Many of these practices may give deep offense to members of the community, much as many features of heterosexual practices placed on public display are offensive. The public peace surely demands reasonable regulation of public sexual practices. The majority seems especially fearful regarding the relation of homosexuals and the young, despite the evidence that sexual molestation seems largely a crime of heterosexual males. Yet prudence seems to indicate that with repeal of sodomy statutes, statutes against child abuse need to be strengthened where necessary.

Moralists believe that certain forms of behavior must be observed if society's central orders—religion, work, family, and relations between the sexes—are to be upheld. Honor to parents, devotion to family, chastity, hard work, and the fear of God are in themselves valuable and should be preserved. But religious morality often becomes a triumph of form over substance. Like those who demythologize superstitions and myths in the Bible, replacing these with the timeless ethic of love and community, the health official must seek to transcend a traditional morality and focus debate on the link between the common good and the equal rights of our fellow citizens who are gay.

In the case of the Bible, John Boswell's exhaustive study of the issue of homosexuality suggests that Sodom was destroyed not because of the abomination of homosexuality, but because the Sodomites refused hospitality to strangers.[10] In fact, homosexuality is explicitly forbidden in only one place in the Old Testament and there for reasons of ritual impurity (like the eating of pork), and not as a fundamental sin.

In the New Testament, Jesus did not mention homosexuality at all; and his ministry to prostitutes, thieves, beggars, and the poor constituted a scandal to the moralists of his time. In fact, Jesus' reference to the story of Sodom's fall in Matthew 10:14 refers to the Sodomites' lack of hospitality: "Whosoever shall not receive you, nor hear your words, when ye depart out of that house or city, shake off the dust of your feet. Verily I say unto you, it shall be more tolerable for the land of Sodom and Gomorrah in the day of judgment, than for that city." Jesus' attack on religious moralism and his elevation of a gospel of love and community were the principal reasons for his being put to death.

Even Paul, who had some harsh things to say about homosexuality (references which John Boswell persuasively argues may refer more to male prostitution than to homosexuality per se), struggled mightily to rescue Christianity from a narrow religious moralism (witness his attack on religious superstitions surrounding circumcision), and to place it on the foundations of community and love for the neighbor.

Republican Rome, like Golden Age Greece, tolerated homosexual practices. Until the late Middle Ages, the secular authorities largely ignored homosexuality, leaving the regulation of this behavior to the Church. As persecution began to build, Aquinas seems to have condemned homosexuality and other sexual deviations less on theological grounds than as a concession to changing political values. But by the sixteenth century in England, Henry VIII (in part because of his quarrel with Rome) made sodomy or "buggery" matters of the criminal law, to reduce the authority of the Church. The American colonists incorporated the English statutes, making homosexuality a capital offense. Apparently, in the years before the American Revolution, only one person was put to death under this law.[11] Nineteenth-century England was another story. According to one authority, "[M]en were regularly hanged for homosexual relations in nineteenth-century England—sixty in the first three decades of the century and 'another score under naval regulations.'"[12]

In our times, the trend has been to remove the ancient prejudices and superstitions preserved in the antisodomy statutes in the states—twenty–six states have done so. And some locales have passed gay civil rights ordinances to protect against discrimination. Recently in Georgia, a homosexual male entered federal court arguing that charges of sodomy brought against him for acts committed with a consenting partner in his own home were unconstitutional.[13] While the federal district court ruled against him, the federal circuit court reversed, arguing that these cases demanded a more strict scrutiny if they were to pass the constitutional test. In other words, the state had to demonstrate that it had a compelling interest in legislating against homosexuality, and that this legislation was the most limited means available to achieve its purpose.

The Supreme Court, for the time being, has rejected this view.[14] By a 5 to 4 vote in Bowers v. Hardwick, the Court upheld the right of the majority to legislate against homosexual acts, committed even in private, on the grounds that repugnance for homosexuality is an ancient and deeply rooted community sentiment. In an earlier decision, the future Chief Justice compared these laws to public health legislation to prevent the spread of communicable diseases. Justice Rehnquist, in 1978, said that laws controlling homosexuals are constitutionally akin to "whether those suffering from measles have a constitutional right, in violation of quarantine regulations, to associate together with others who do not presently have measles."[15] Rehnquist echoes James F. Stephen in the nineteenth century when he said, "Vice is as infectious as disease, and happily virtue is infectious, though health is not. Both vice and virtue are transmittable, and, to a considerable extent, hereditary."[16]

The decision of the Supreme Court is a threat to the entire advance of the privacy decisions of the past two decades. The work of the Court in trying to untangle the claims of moralism, and the claims of public health, by forging a new equality that combines the common good and the right to be left alone in new ways, has been left dangling. If the Court's ruling is to be reversed, the thesis that legal moralism threatens the public health as well as the rights of all citizens, including gays, must be pressed even more vigorously.

Sexual Practices and Paternalism

A sound public health policy depends on both loosening and tightening the bonds of community. Rejecting moralism does not mean that society can have nothing to say about sexual practices. Sex per se, and that includes homosexual sex, is not the business of community. But sexual practices that threaten the common health are.

Sexual practices can have many consequences for the public health. Private conduct, even sexual conduct, which threatens compelling community interests like health and safety, is not beyond the reach of regulation, even if the individuals involved are consenting adults. Of course, there are overwhelming practical limits to this principle, but affirming it is important nonetheless.

Human sexuality is an imperative drive like hunger or safety, and sexual practices, at least in private, are likely very resistant to legal prohibition or regulation. Nevertheless, the public health official cannot ignore sexual practices that are unsafe, dangerous, and a threat to all. Public health information campaigns must not flinch from promoting a standard of sexual conduct that is safe and prudent from everyone's standpoint.

The sexual practices of male homosexuals have become a central controversy in the AIDS debate. According to investigators, many AIDS patients report 1,000 sexual partners over a single lifetime,[17] a notorious statistic overshadowing discussion of AIDS prevalence. It is not surprising that those most widely exposed to the risk of infection should become the first AIDS cases.

An authoritative survey of gay sexual practices reveals that this kind of strenuous sexual activity remains confined to a minority; nevertheless, one third of all male homosexuals surveyed nationally reported that they had more than 50 to 70 sexual partners in the previous year.[18] Gay men report that they participate in sexual contact with persons unknown to each other "very frequently" or "fairly frequently." Favorite cruising places for casual sex have included parks and public restrooms, as well as the back rooms of bars where the owners permit such liaisons. Another site for casual sex is the bathhouse, which many gay men prefer because so little effort is required to make contacts.

Another index to the sexual practices of male homosexuals is sexually transmitted diseases. Individuals who are exclusively homosexuals for a considerable part of their lives constitute 5 to 10 percent of the adult male population, according to Kinsey's estimate. If the statistics are reliable, this group accounts for a third of all cases of infectious syphilis, a high rate of gonorrhea, and an increasing rate of hepatitis A and B. Gay males are also at much greater risk for bacterial and enteric diseases like amebiasis and giardiasis. The risk of herpes and other dermatologic disorders is also much greater among gay males.[19]

In 1977, in New York City, 55 percent of all reported cases of syphilis occurred in homosexual males, even though syphilis, among heterosexuals nationwide, has been declining at a remarkable rate. Homosexual men are reported to be ten times more likely to contract syphilis than heterosexuals.

The epidemic of sexually transmitted diseases among homosexual males is in significant part a result of sexual liberation. Gay liberation meant far more than sexual liberation, but a heavy price has been paid for some of the forms sexual liberation has taken in the gay community. The freedom to have multiple sexual contacts with strangers in one evening, and to continue this practice over a period of years, has exposed hundreds of thousands, perhaps one to two million individuals, to a deadly virus. If recent reports are borne out, exposure to the virus may bring the full-blown AIDS disease to as many as 25 to 40 percent of those infected, a much higher risk than originally thought. The spectre of as many as 250,000 to 400,000 cases (the current level of deaths is 15,000), will dramatically increase societal pressures to blame the victim.

As the toll of the disease among homosexuals mounts, the deadly risks associated with homosexual sex are likely to have the greatest impact in reshaping homosexual life. Words like "promiscuity" are regarded by gays with deep suspicion as covert attacks on homosexuality itself. To minimize suspicion we should observe the distinction between restrictions for sexual standards protecting the common life and restrictions promoting an official sexual morality. Frequent sexual activity is of no interest to the law and the community unless it escalates the risk of serious disease. When the disease is AIDS, the community interest becomes paramount, and official educational campaigns should discourage high-risk sex with strangers. Even if such practices as oral and anal sex are presently beyond the law, informed self-interest should help work to bring sharp declines in free-wheeling sex with strangers.

Should public officials go beyond education? Should, for instance, police monitor gay "cruising" for sexual liaisons where there is a high likelihood of contacts between strangers and where the risk of spreading infection is very high? Here the potential for abuse by the police is very great, and the boundaries between controlling homosexuality per se, versus protecting health and safety, are extremely blurred. The likely outcome will be only to make heterosexuals feel (falsely) reassured and the gay community discriminated against.

The major debate has concerned closing or regulating public places such as bathhouses where dangerous sex is practiced. San Francisco took such steps, but the New York City health authorities took a different position. While the state health officials ultimately overruled them, New York City officials argued that the impact of such closings would be minuscule in terms of the overall threat. Still, the public health official is not required to demonstrate that the closings or regulation will result in containing the epidemic. But at the same time, officials should take steps to assure all concerned that the aim is to regulate the public health, not homosexuality, tipping the scales toward regulation versus outright closing. It may well be that regulation, and in the worst cases outright closings, could be a potent symbol for community action.

On the other hand, some argue that these commercial establishments ought to be used to promote safer sex. This tactic has a familiar ring, something like getting the liquor industry to promote "responsible drinking." An industry that has an interest in promoting casual sex—whether bathhouses or bars—is unlikely to be seriously interested in a health education campaign. Realism should guide our regulatory policy. The goal is to restrict commercial establishments that have an interest in unsafe sex—places where sex between strangers is promoted as a commodity. The fact that some hotels, incidental to their doing business, have couples among their guests practicing high-risk sex, is not an adequate argument against closing bathhouses or bars where casual sex is a main feature.

The lead in any public discourse about gay sexual practices must come from the gay community itself. Such a change can only come from a full and extensive dialogue, which should be open, frank, and based on as much careful and dispassionate research as is possible. At all times the participants should remind themselves that the discussion is about public health, not moralism.

Gay people who object that the majority community ought not control the private behavior of consenting adults forget that membership in the community—which is the ground of public health protections against AIDS—carries obligations as well as benefits. Paternalism to defend the common life protects the health and safety of sexual partners and helps solidify the norms of the shared community. At the present time, frequent sexual activity among strangers promotes spread of a deadly disease. Until this disease is controlled we all share a common interest in a more conservative and restrictive standard for sexual morality.

For their side, homosexuals need to take the leadership and to call for self-imposed restrictions. This is already happening. Also, health statistics in San Francisco and New York City suggest that thousands of gays are altering their lifestyles. Many gay leaders have begun publicly to repudiate the fast-lane life. Political prudence suggests that if gay people want gains against discrimination in housing, employment, medical care, and insurance, then their leaders should speak out against dangerous sexual practices within their community.

I have devoted very little attention to intravenous drug users, a high-risk group that will likely grow more important in the AIDS epidemic. There are many parallels between the problems of preventing AIDS among drug users and homosexuals, not the least of which is that many drug users are homosexual. It is unclear which activity—unsafe sex or contaminated needles—is the primary mode of transmitting AIDS for many individuals. Both activities are illegal, at least in many places, and both groups are the target of deep societal fears and prejudices. The biggest difference is that drug use itself presents a strong health risk for the addict whereas homosexuality per se does not.

Society will certainly have to reevaluate the restrictions in many states on availability to addicts of sterile needles and syringes. Also, as the disease spreads through heroin users, we may have to reopen the controversial question of whether heroin addicts should be registered and furnished safe supplies of heroin by physicians as the most practical way to control the spread of AIDS in the population.

Above all else, for both these groups we should keep our eyes on the central issue—the many ways in which centuries of religious and social superstitions and prejudice stand in the way of improving the public health. Modern public health rests on a complex equality that replaces traditional restrictions with limits rooted in protection against actual harms. Equating the public health with simplistic restrictions on homosexuality per se will only result in fruitless debates over matters like quarantine and isolation, public health strategies that have little role in this epidemic. Hoping for a technological shortcut in the form of a vaccine is not realistic and can cost tens of thousands of lives, especially if this hope keeps us from facing the task of public education and reform of our laws against homosexuality. These reforms can help prepare the way for altering sexual lifestyles among the gay community. The public health community should take the lead and, state by state, demand the repeal of harmful statutes and restrictions on gay life. The health of the body politic depends on rejecting the communal disease of sexual prejudice.

NOTES

1. For a good discussion of "moralism," see Hugo Adam Bedau's discussion in Edwin M. Schur and Hugo Adam Bedau, *Victimless Crimes* (Englewood Cliffs, NJ: Prentice-Hall, 1974). See also Joel Feinberg, *Social Philosophy* (Englewood Cliffs, NJ: Prentice-Hall, 1973) and H.L.A. Hart, *Law, Liberty, and Morality* (New York: Vintage Books, 1963); Ronald Dworkin, *Taking Rights Seriously* (Cambridge: Harvard University Press, 1977), Chapter 11; and A.D. Woozley, "Law and the Legislation of Morality," in *Ethics in Hard Times*, Daniel Callahan and Arthur Caplan, eds. (New York: Plenum, 1981).

2. James Fitzjames Stephen, *Liberty, Equality, Fraternity*, R.J. White, ed. (Cambridge: Cambridge University Press, 1967).

3. John Stuart Mill, "On Liberty," in M. Cohen, ed., *The Philosophy of John Stuart Mill* (New York: Modern Library, 1961), pp. 155–319.

4. Bedau, p. 90.

5. Lord Patrick Devlin, *The Enforcement of Morals* (Oxford: Oxford University Press, 1959).

6. See H.L.A. Hart, "Social Solidarity and the Enforcement of Morality," *The University of Chicago Law Review* 35 (1967), 1-13, for one of the best critiques of the thesis that society is held together by a specific moral practice.

7. "Prevention of Acquired Immunodeficiency Syndrome (AIDS): Report of Interagency Recommendations," *Morbidity and Mortality Weekly Report* 32:101–103, March 4, 1983.

8. See Barry Adkins, "GMHC Accepts Grant from CDC for Sex Education Research," *The New York Native*, February 10–16, 1986, p. 8. For a good discussion of the potential for an anti-AIDS campaign to serve as a cover for a campaign to control homosexuality, see "AIDS—A New Reason to Regulate Homosexuality?" *Journal of Contemporary Law* 11 (1984), 315–43.

9. *Roe* v. *Wade*, 410 U.S. 113 (1973).

10. The source of his history of Roman and Christian attitudes toward homosexuality is John Boswell's *Christianity, Social Tolerance, and Homosexuality* (Chicago: The University of Chicago Press, 1980).

11. See Robert Oaks, "Perceptions of Homosexuality by Justices of the Peace in Colonial Virginia," in *Homosexuality and the Law.* (A Special Double Issue of *The Journal of Homosexuality*) 5 (1979/80), 35–42.

12. These data are found in Bernard Knox's book review, "Subversive Activities," *The New York Review of Books*, December 19, 1985, p. 3. Knox was reviewing Louis Crompton's *Byron and Greek Love, Homophobia in Nineteenth-Century England* (Berkeley: University of California Press, 1985).

13. Kenneth R. Wing, "Constitutional Protection of Sexual Privacy in the 1980s: What *Is* Big Brother Doing in the Bedroom?" *American Journal of Public Health* 76 (February 1986), 201–04. The Georgia case is *Bowers v. Hardwick* 760 F2d 1123 (11th Circ. 1985).

14. *Bowers v. Hardwick*, 478 U.S.—, 92 LEd2d 140 (1986).

15. See David A.J. Richards, "Homosexual Acts and the Constitutional Right to Privacy," and "Public Manifestations of Personal Morality: Limitations on the Use of Solicitation Statutes to Control Homosexual Cruising," in *Homosexuality and the Law.* (A Special Double Issue of *The Journal of Homosexuality*), 5 (1979/80), 43–66. The 1978 case is *Ratchford v. Gay Lib*, 424 U.S. 1080, 1082, reh'g denied, 435 U.S. 981 (1978).

16. Stephen, p. 146.

17. See Mary E. Guinan, et al., "Heterosexual and Homosexual Patients with the Acquired Immunodeficiency Syndrome: A Comparison of Surveillance, Interview, and Laboratory Data." *Annals of Internal Medicine* 100 (1984), 213–18; and H.W. Jaffe, K. Choi, and P.A. Thomas, et al., "National Case-control Study of Kaposi's Sarcoma and *Pneumocystis Carinii* Pneumonia in Homosexual Men: Part 1. Epidemiological Results," *Annals of Internal Medicine* 99 (1983), 145–51.

18. Karla Jay and Allen Young, *The Gay Report* (New York: Summit Books, 1977).

19. Terry Alan Sandholzer, "Factors Affecting the Incidence and Management of Sexually Transmitted Diseases in Homosexual Men," in *Sexually Transmitted Diseases in Homosexual Men: Diagnosis, Treatment, and Research.* Ed. David G. Ostrow, Terry Alan Sandholzer, and Yehudi M. Felman (New York: Plenum, Medicae Book Co., 1983), pp. 3–12. The estimates of the numbers of gay males in the adult population is from *Sexual Behavior in the Human Male* by Alfred C. Kinsey, Wardell B. Pomeroy, and Clyde E. Martin (Philadelphia: W.B. Saunders Co, 1948) (The Kinsey Report).

Medical Confidentiality:
An Intransigent and
Absolute Obligation

Michael H. Kottow

Author's Abstract

Clinicians' work depends on sincere and complete disclosures from their patients; they honour this candidness by confidentially safeguarding the information received. Breaching confidentiality causes harms that are not commensurable with the possible benefits gained. Limitations or exceptions put on confidentiality would destroy it, for the confider would become untrustworthy and the whole climate of the clinical encounter would suffer irreversible erosion. Excusing breaches of confidence on grounds of superior moral values introduces arbitrariness and ethical unreliability into the medical context. Physicians who breach the agreement of confidentiality are being unfair, thus opening the way for, and becoming vulnerable to, the morally obtuse conduct of others.

Confidentiality should not be seen as the cozy but dispensable atmosphere of clinical settings; rather, it constitutes a guarantee of fairness in medical actions. Possible perils that might accrue to society are no greater than those accepted when granting inviolable custody of information to priests, lawyers and bankers. To jeopardize the integrity of confidential medical relationships is too high a price to pay for the hypothetical benefits this might bring to the prevailing social order.

Michael H. Kottow, "Medical Confidentiality: An Intransigent and Absolute Obligation," *Journal of Medical Ethics* 12 (1986): Reprinted by Permission of the Author and the *Journal of Medical Ethics*.

The contemporary expansion of ethics in general and medical ethics in particular harbours the danger of increasing scholasticism to the point where not even pressing practical problems are being offered workable solutions. People involved in health care may end up by distrusting the discipline of ethics, thus increasing the improbability of agreement between pragmatists and analysts.[1] Even traditionally straightforward practices, such as confidentiality, have been subject to extensive review and analysis which have proved incapable of offering committed stances or unequivocal guidelines for action.[2,3] In an effort to illustrate that more stringency is desirable and possible, the status of confidentiality as an exceptionless or absolute commitment is here defended. It should be stated at the outset that I share general skepticism about absolute ethical propositions,[4] and that confidentiality is here not defended as an inviolable moral value—a position that would be self-defeating—but as an interpersonal communications strategy that ceases to function unless strictly adhered to. Confidentiality is a brittle arrangement that disintegrates if misdirected in pursuance of other goals and, since it is a necessary component of medical practice, care should be taken to safeguard its integrity.

Defining Confidentiality

The following definition of confidentiality is used: A situation is confidential when information revealing that harmful acts have been or possibly will be performed is consciously or voluntarily passed from one rationally competent person (confider) to another (confidant) in the understanding that this information shall not be further disclosed without the confider's explicit consent. The harm alluded to may be physical, but moral damage alone may also be the subject matter of a confidential exchange. When this sort of communication occurs in a medical setting it constitutes medical confidentiality.

What Is at Issue in Confidentiality Conflicts?

The main ethical controversy around confidentiality concerns the assessment of whether more harm is done by occasionally breaching confidentiality or by always respecting it regardless of the consequences. As long as the physician gathers private information, that is information that only concerns the confider and harbors no element of past or potential harm, confidentiality will concern exclusively the patient and any disclosure would be nothing but a malicious or at the very least gratuitous act of the physician, of little or no moral significance. It seems redundant to discuss other instances of confidentiality than those involving either the possibility of impending harm or testimonial of past injury, for these are the fundamental cases where dilemmas arise and a breach of confidence must seek justification.

Breaching is defended on the ground that the harm announced in the confidence is severe and can possibly only be averted by the confidant's disclosure.[5,6,7] Exceptionless confidentiality, on the other hand, is upheld by the idea that breaching will relentlessly harm the confider, subjecting her or him to precautionary investigations and constraints of some sort, perhaps even with unavoidable defamatory consequences. The harm purportedly averted is merely potential and all the less likely to occur, the more exorbitant and preposterous the threatener's claims are. After all, excessively vicious menaces may well be uttered by psychotics who are rationally incompetent and therefore not protected by a pledge to confidentiality they can neither honour nor demand. Furthermore, the practice of confidentiality is in itself damaged by breaching because its trustworthiness is disqualified. Ultimately, degrees and probability of harm are so difficult to assess[8] that they will hardly deliver an intersubjectively acceptable argument for or against confidentiality, except for one: Breaching confidentiality can not be a significant and enduring contribution against harmful actions, for these are no more than potential, whereas the damages caused to the confidant, to the practice of confidentiality and to the honesty of clinical relationships are unavoidable.

Perhaps less elusive is the conflict of rights—and their correlative obligations—which ensue in confidential situations. Confidentiality is an agreement bound by the principle of fairness,[9] it gives the confider the right to expect discretion whereas the confidant has the right to hear the truth, but also the obligation to ensure guardianship of the information received. It could be argued against this right that past victims might be vindicated or potential ones helped by divulging confidential information that seems critical, and that these victims also have a right, namely to vindication or protection. In order for the victim's right to prevail, the confider must involuntarily forfeit her or his right to secrecy, which the confidant will forcefully violate by divulging information against the confider's will. This forfeiture of the confider's right can only occur subsequent to the confidence, for it is triggered by the contents of the confider's disclosure. To avoid the risk of losing the right to secrecy, confiders would have to confide falsely or not at all, a strategy that would erode their legitimate and initially granted right to be impunibly outspoken, distort or reduce confidentiality to lies and irrelevancies, and destroy both the confidant's right to hear the truth and the institution of confidentiality.

Medical Confidentiality

Physicians would appear to be under the *prima facie* obligation to respect the right to secrecy, but also to abide by the right of potential victims to be protected. In cases involving moral conflict they must necessarily override one of these rights. Infringing certain rights for the sake of other rights may be justifiable, but it leaves a sediment of negative feelings of regret, shame or guilt.[10,11] It is an unhealthy and paralyzing notion to know that the relationship one enters into with patients may unexpectedly turn into a situation of conflict, infringement of rights, and guilt. This guilt may be compounded by the awareness that breaching relates to a family of dubious practices that misuse information obtained by resorting to deception or even duress. Of course, confidentiality is enacted in the unfettered environment of medical encounters, but its breaching infringes the rights of the confiders, harms them, and abrades confidentiality as an institution, all this in the name of elusive values and hard-to-specify protective and vindicative functions.

In the case where a physician believes the patient's exorbitant threats and alerts the police, a morally questionable principle becomes involved. The patient has sought the clinical encounter and proffered information on the understanding that this is necessary for an efficient therapy and also that the relationship with the physician is protected by a mantle of confidentiality. Confidence is offered and accepted in medical acts, and known to be an indispensable component of the clinical encounter, thus enticing the patient to deliver unbiased, unfiltered, uncensored and sincerely presented information.[12]

Consequently, it appears contradictory and perverse first to offer confidentiality as an enticement to sincerity, only subsequently to breach it because the information elicited is so terrible it cannot remain unpublicized. Confidence is understood as an unconditional offer, otherwise it would not be accepted, and it appears profoundly unfair to disown the initial conditions once the act of confiding has occurred.

Should one decide to introduce exception clauses, it would only be fair to promulgate them beforehand, allowing every potential confider to know what to expect. But officially sanctioned exceptions would have the undesirable side effect of creating a second-class kind of medicine for those cases where the patient considers it too risky to assume confidentiality. The communication between patient and physician would in these cases be hampered and would thus render the patient's medical care less than optimal.

Gathering Confidential Material

The covenant of confidentiality only obtains if information is voluntarily and consciously given. No question of confidence arises unless the relationship involves rational, conscious and free individuals. But subtleties arise in the medical context when incriminating information reaches the physician unintentionally. Does this information fall within the confidence pact in virtue of being part of the clinical encounter? Or does it obey independent rules because it occurred marginally to the intended doctor/patient relationship?

During the clinical encounter a perspicacious physician may find tell-tale signs of matters the patient did not intend to disclose (skin blemishes perhaps caused by alcohol excess, suspiciously pinpoint pupils, injection marks). This involuntary information transfer might not seem at first to fall under any confidentiality agreement according to the above presented definition. Nevertheless, it is the product of a conscious interaction between patient and physician. In consulting a doctor, a person implicitly accepts the risk of surrendering more information than intended but at the same time understands herself or himself to be under the protection of confidentiality. Information fortuitously gained within the freely chosen association of the clinical encounter is to be considered confidential and treated in the same way as information voluntarily disclosed by the patient. Everything that happens in the interpersonal relationship of a clinical encounter is confidential.

Are There Exceptions to Confidentiality?

Exceptions to unrelenting confidentiality[6] have been invoked for the sake of the confider (paternalistic breaching in general and medical consultations as a special case thereof), in the name of potentially endangered innocent others, in the name of institutional or public interests, and less explicitly, in cases where the confidant is potentially in danger.

Confidentiality Throughout Time

Confidants may consider the potential harm of divulging information they have had in custody eventually to diffuse after the confider's death, so that a posthumous revelation will not be injurious. The contrary position that harm after death is possible is too weak to support obligations to the dead.[13] A more convincing approach suggests that posthumous disclosures may be harmful to surviving persons. If the death of a famous politician should prompt a physician to uncover his knowledge about the deceased's homosexual inclination, still-living patients of the same physician might register with distaste and fear the possibility that private information about them could eventually be disclosed after they died. This suspicion may well be unsettling and therefore harmful to them, especially if they happen to believe in some form of "after-life," the quality of which would be polluted by indiscretions occurring after their biological death. Also to be considered are the negative effects a disparaging disclosure might have upon surviving family members as well as groups of individuals with whom the deceased had a commonality of interests. Death does not cancel the obligation of confidentiality, which remains of import to all survivors within the radius of interests of the deceased.

Paternalistic Breaching

A commonly suggested exemption to confidentiality is that some patients' interests might be better served by physicians' indiscretion.[14] Harming confiders for their own purported good is like forcing therapeutic decisions on patients for the sake of their health care. Such stern paternalism has nothing to recommend it, for it is generally agreed that autonomous individuals are not to be compelled into undergoing medical procedures they have explicitly rejected. If rationally competent patients refuse a medical procedure that would do them good, the physician is not authorized to insist, let alone proceed. Rationally competent individuals are allowed to take decisions against their own interests and this does not make them irrational, as some have misleadingly suggested.[15] Why, then, should confidentiality function differently? If patients wish certain knowledge to be kept confidential even if this course of action injures their own interests, they are entitled to do so and no one, not even the physician, has the right to breach confidentiality in the name of patients' welfare.

Medical Consultations

Multi-professional care seems to offer plausible alibis to breach confidentiality for the sake of the confider.[16] It has been argued that patients negotiate confidentiality with their primary care physician and that if additional professionals are involved in the patient's care they are to report to the confidant physician. This position is discarded by those who believe that patients, in as much as their autonomy is respected, are to renegotiate—or count upon—confidentiality with every physician involved. Such a line of thought has much to recommend it since every physician/patient encounter may unveil unedited information which the patient is willing to discuss in a certain setting but is reluctant to have brought to the attention of the primary-care physician. Consultations and other expansions of a medical care programme do not serve as an excuse to exchange information about patients against their will. If they did, they would be supporting double morality and possibly double-quality medicine, where primary health care would have a paternalistic format embedded in trust and confidence whilst secondary and tertiary services would operate in a contractual setting. This would not be acceptable, it being preferable that each act of confidence be equally and nontransmittably entrenched in all medical encounters.

Harm to Innocent Others

Another major exception invoked against absolute confidentiality concerns the aversion of damage to uninvolved and innocent third parties. These are the oft-quoted cases of the doctor telling the bride that her fiancé is homosexual, or calling the wife because he is treating the husband for venereal disease. Escalating examples include informing authorities about a confider's intention to kill someone, as well as encounters with terrorists at large.

This postulated exemption to confidentiality is self-defeating. Firstly, if physicians become known as confidence-violators, problem-ridden patients will try to lie, accommodate facts to their advantage or, if this does not work, avoid physicians altogether.[17] Physicians would then be unable to give optimal advice or treatment to the detriment of both the reluctant patients and their threatened environment. It is better to treat and advise the syphilitic husband without informing the wife than not have him come at all for fear of undesired revelations.

Physicians who believe themselves in possession of information that must be disclosed in order to safeguard public interests are contemplating preventive action against the putative malefactor. Like all preventive policies, breaching confidentiality is difficult to analyze in terms of costs/benefits: Is the danger real, potential or fictitious? What preventive measure will appear justified? How much harm may these measures cause before they lose justification? Since physicians will rarely be instrumental in deciding or carrying out preventive actions, they have no way of knowing in advance whether taking the risk of honoring confidentiality will eventually prove more or less harmful than breaching it.

If physicians play it safe and commit frequent breaches of confidentiality they will unleash overreacting preventive programs, at the same time progressively losing credibility as reliable informers. On the other hand, should they remain critical and carefully decide each case on its own merits, they will be equally suspect and unreliable informers, for their conscientiousness and judgment might well deviate from what other authorities, notably the police, consider adequate.

In apparently more delicate cases it could be argued that physicians might subject their cooperation with the authorities to some conditions in order to defuse the dramatic moment. They may suggest that violence be refrained from, that their own intervention be kept secret, that the preventive action be discreet. But certainly, if physicians accept that their confidential relationship with patients is conditional, they must consequently expect authorities to handle their own role as informants in a similarly unpredictable and contingent way. Physicians who breach confidentiality cannot expect to be protected by it just because they have exchanged the confidant for the confider role. Physicians who are known to take confidentiality as a prima facie value cannot demand that the authorities they are serving by disclosing information should honor their request for discretion. For similar reasons they must expect some patients to become increasingly inconsiderate or even vicious. By breaking confidentiality, physicians are helping sustain a language of dishonesty and they cannot expect violence-prone patients to refrain from blackmailing, threatening, or otherwise molesting them. As a physician, I would be most unsettled if it became a matter of policy that my colleagues violated confidentiality for the public good, for it would leave me defenceless when confronted with a public offender. No amount of promising would help, since physicians would already have a reputation as unpredictable violators of agreements.

Who should control the policy of confidentiality in medicine anyhow? If public interest demands a catalogue of situations where the physician would be under obligation to inform, medicine becomes subaltern to political design and starts down a treacherous path. Should one prefer to leave the management of confidentiality to the physician's conscience and moral judgement, public interest would not be relying on a consistent and trustworthy source of information. Fear of either political misuse or personal arbitrariness should make us wary of opening the doors of confidentiality for the sake of public interest.

What about possible conflicts between the frailties of public figures and the purported interests of society? National leaders from time to time suffer from disabilities due to old age and the question is raised whether the attending medical team are under an obligation to publish full-fledged clinical reports. It must again be brought to mind that the medical team have been commissioned not to safeguard the public interest but to care for the health of this individual who happens to be influential. Consequently, the medical team's duties remain in the clinical realm, not in the political arena. Furthermore, if the leader in question were in such a precarious situation as to constitute a public danger, his political mismanagement would become obvious to other individuals more qualified to take public decisions and would not require the physicians to play the role of enlightening figures. Observers of the political scene have preferred to suggest constitutional amendments and political measures to cope with this problem, being aware that cajoling physicians out of their commitment to confidentiality is no solution.[18]

Competing Claims to Confidential Material

This issue refers to conflicts arising from individual interests colliding with those of groups or institutions. It differs from those previously discussed in that here physicians do not necessarily engage in active disclosure but restrict themselves to a one-sided cooperation. The emphasis here is not so much on harm being prevented—

although this also plays a major role—but on conflicting parties claiming the physician's loyalty.

Company doctors doing routine examinations of employees are under obligation to report even disparaging findings, for their duty is to the commissioning company. By failing to report an epileptic bus driver or a hypertensive pilot, the doctor is deceiving the company and hindering its efforts to secure safe transportation. If, on the contrary, the same bus driver or pilot goes to the private office of a doctor unconnected with his employer, there would be no excuse for unauthorizedly reporting any finding to the company, for the physician is now being commissioned by the individual, not by the institution, to perform a medical act under the mantle of confidentiality. If this results in the bus driver continuing to work under precarious conditions it means that the company has not established an efficient medical service to check its drivers and is negligent. Physicians are to declare themselves explicitly and unmistakably loyal to those who engage their services for, again, the legitimate claim to confidentiality lies in the act of entering an agreement, not in the contents of the confided material.

Not even these competing claims of loyalty can be settled unless a robust and relentless position in favor of exceptionless confidentiality is upheld. If a physician owes loyalty to an institution, he has no right to misuse the confidence of his employer in order to honour any personal desire for confidentiality. Conversely, when physicians are committed to the confidential situations that arise in their consulting rooms, they lack the right to infringe this agreement to the benefit of other interests.

Does Risk to the Confidant Justify Breaching?

The situation could arise where the patient's revelations contain threats of harm or disclosure of damage already done directly to the confidant physician, his or her family members, or their interests. Can the physician disclaim the obligation to confidentiality in the name of self-defense? If physicians were morally allowed to breach confidentiality in defense of their own interests it would mean accepting the principle that one can inflict harm upon others for self-interested reasons. It has already been stated that in disclosing confidential information there is no adequate way of comparing amounts of harm inflicted with harm prevented, so it might well occur that a person brought about severe harm to others in an effort to avert a fairly trivial or improbable harm to her or his own interests, comparable to killing a burglar who is running away with some property—perhaps no more than a loaf of bread. Since an unbiased view can hardly be expected from someone who believes his interests to be in jeopardy, legal systems do not tolerate self-administered justice and condemn, albeit with leniency, injuring others in the face of putative menace to self-interests. Physicians may not safeguard their own interests by mishandling patients, so why should they be allowed to cause harm by breaching confidentiality only because they believe or fear their interests to be imperilled?

Although imaginary situations can be concocted that make it awkward to insist on not breaching, the basic attitude should still be to respect confidentiality to the utmost. Admittedly, if the patient's disclosure implies impending harm to the confidant, the moral obligation to the confidential relationship is weakened in its core, but this admission requires a double qualification: First, such situations are highly improbable and therefore of little paradigmatic interest; second, even if they should obtain, breaching confidentiality should be used as a last, certainly not first, resort to resolve the conflict, precisely because there is no suasive justification for employing confidentiality as a weapon to avert harm.

Concluding Remarks

Confidentiality is a widely recognized implicit warranty of fairness in clinical situations and thus constitutes a technically and morally essential element of efficient medical care. If breaches of confidentiality occur, they do so necessarily after the communication and therefore retroactively introduce unfairness into the clinical encounter. A situation that is potentially, even if only occasionally, unfair can no longer be described as fair, especially if breaching occurs unpredictably. All possible exceptions to an attitude of unrelenting confidentiality lead to morally untenable situations where harm avoided versus harm inflicted is incommensurable, and rights preserved are less convincing than rights eroded. Confidentiality collapses unless strictly adhered to, for even occasional, exceptional or otherwise limited leaks are sufficient to discredit confidentiality into inefficiency.

The clinical encounter is consistently described as a confidential relationship. If this statement is adhered to, there can be no room for violation without making the initial statement untrue. Nor can the description be qualified—"usually confidential"—or made into a conditional—"confidential unless"—statement, for these half-hearted commitments are, from the confider's point of a view, as worthless as no guarantee of confidentiality at all. Confidentiality cannot but be, factually and morally, an all or none proposition. It might perhaps be easier to present a plausible defense of conditional confidentiality, but the ethical atmosphere of the clinical encounter, the autonomy of patients, and the sovereignty of the medical profession are all better served by making confidentiality an unexceptional element of medicine.

NOTES

1. MacIntyre A. Moral philosophy: what next? In: Hauerwas S, MacIntyre A, eds. *Revisions: Changing Perspectives in Moral Philosophy.* Notre Dame/London: University of Notre Dame Press, 1983: 1–15.

2. Thompson I E. The nature of confidentiality. *Journal of Medical Ethics* 1979; 5: 57–64.

3. Pheby D F H. Changing practice on confidentiality: a cause for concern. *Journal of Medical Ethics* 1982; 8: 12–18.

4. Anscombe G E M. Modern moral philosophy. In: Anscombe G E M. *Ethics, Religion and Politics.* Oxford: Blackwell, 1981: 26–42.

5. Walters L. Confidentiality. In: Beauchamp T L, Walters L, eds. *Contemporary Issues in Bioethics.* Encino/Belmont: Dickenson, 1978: 169–175.

6. *Handbook of Medical Ethics.* London: British Medical Association 1981.

7. Anonymous. Medical confidentiality [editorial]. *Journal of Medical Ethics* 1984; 10:3–4.

8. Carli T. Confidentiality and privileged communication: a psychiatrist's perspective. In: Basson M D, ed. *Ethics, Humanism, and Medicine.* New York: Liss, 1980: 245–251.

9. Rawls J. *A Theory of Justice.* Cambridge, Mass: Belknap Press, 1971: 342–350.

10. Melden A. I. *Rights and Persons.* Oxford: Blackwell, 1977: 47–48.

11. Morris H. The status of rights. *Ethics* 1981; 92: 40–56.

12. Veatch R. M. *A Theory of Medical Ethics.* New York: Basic Books, 1981: 184–189.

13. Levenbook B B. Harming someone after his death. *Ethics* 1984; 94: 407–419.

14. Veatch R M. *Case Studies in Medical Ethics.* Cambridge/London: Harvard University Press, 1977: 131–135.

15. Culver C M, Gert B. *Philosophy in Medicine.* New York: Oxford, 1983: 26–28.

16. Siegler M. Medical consultations in the context of the physician-patient relationship. In: Agich G J, ed. *Responsibility in Health Care.* Dordrecht: Reidel, 1982: 141–162.

17. Harvard J. Medical confidence. *Journal of Medical Ethics* 1985; 11: 8–11.

18. Robins R S, Rothschild H. Hidden health disabilities and the presidency: medical management and political consideration. *Perspectives in Biology and Medicine* 1981; 24: 240–253.

Invisible Minorities, Civic Rights, Democracy: Three Arguments for Gay Rights

Richard D. Mohr

FOR ROBERT W. SWITZER

IN WHAT FOLLOWS, I give three related arguments for the inclusion of sexual orientation in such legislation as the U.S. 1964 Civil Rights Act as a characteristic for which a person may not be discriminated against in employment, housing and public services.[1] I will be arguing that such protections from discrimination are necessary enabling conditions for gays having reasonably guaranteed access to an array of fundamental rights—both civic and political—which almost everyone would agree are supposed to pertain equally to all persons. For gays, these rights are eclipsed, I will argue, in consequence of the *indirect* results which widespread discrimination has when it affects members of invisible minorities.[2]

The arguments here are not, then, general arguments for civil rights legislation based on the *direct* or immediate deleterious effects which discrimination in employment, housing, and public services would have on *any* person or even on society as a whole and which might on their own be sufficiently grave to justify a government ban on all but good faith discriminations in these areas—a ban which *per accidens* would catch gays within its broad protective reach. Such direct deleterious effects might include affronts to personal dignity, self-reliance, general prosperity, and individual flourishing.[3]

Richard Mohr, Ph.D., "Invisible Minorities, Civic Rights, Democracy," *Philosophical Forum*, 13, no. 1 (Fall 1985): 1–24. Reprinted by Permission of the Author and the *Philosophical Forum*.

Libertarians and other political minimalists tend to dismiss as irrelevant or inflated assessments of the nature and gravity of these possible direct effects and so have generally been unmoved by such arguments for civil rights legislation and its coercive intrusions into the private sector. I shall be arguing that even if the direct effects of such discrimination are not sufficient on their own to warrant the state's deployment of its monopoly of preemptive coercive forces (and this I here leave an open question), nevertheless if social realities are such that discrimination (actual or prospective) indirectly but determinately has the effect of denying access to certain universally recognized rights—the denial of which draws into doubt the very rule of law, then this effect does warrant state action on almost any account of what constitutes legitimate state action.[4]

The arguments would apply equally well to other invisible minorities whose members are subject to widespread discrimination merely on the basis of their minority status rather than on the basis of their capacities, talents, or needs. By invisible minority I mean a minority whose members can only be identified through an act of will on someone's part rather than merely through the observation of a person's day-to-day actions in the public domain. Thus, severely physically and mentally challenged people would rank along with racial classes, gender classes, and some religious and ethnic groups as visible minorities, whereas diabetics, assimulated Jews, atheists, and released prisoners would rank along with gays as invisible minorities.

The arguments only presuppose the acceptability of a governmental system which is a constitutionally regulated representative democracy with a developed body of civic law. Such in broad outline is the government of the United States and its various states. The arguments, then, hold that gay civil rights are a necessary precondition for the proper functioning of this system. Specifically, they hold: (1) that gay rights are necessary for gays having reasonably guaranteed access to judicial or civic rights; (2) that gay rights are necessary for gays having reasonably guaranteed access to the political rights of the sort found in the First Amendment of the U.S. Constitution; and (3) that gay rights are necessary if democracy is consistently and coherently to be given a preference-utilitarian rationale.

I

I wish to argue that civil rights for gays can be ethically grounded as being necessary preconditions for gays having equitable access to civic rights. By civic rights I mean rights to the impartial administration of civil and criminal law in defense of property and person. In the absence of such rights there is no rule of law. An invisible minority historically subjected to widespread social discrimination has reasonably guaranteed access to these rights only when the minority is guaranteed nondiscrimination in employment, housing, and public services.

For an invisible minority, possessing civil rights has the same ethical justification as everyone's having the right when on criminal trial to have a lawyer at government expense. A lawyer through his special knowledge and skills provides his client with *access* to the substantive and procedural rights of the courts—rights to which a layman left to his own devices would not have reasonably guaranteed access. Without the guarantee of a lawyer, judicial rights are not equal rights but are rights of the well-to-do.

All would agree that judicial rights are rights which everyone is to have, and moreover, as in the case of having a lawyer at state expense, is to have in that strong sense of rights by which an individual can make demand claims based on them. All individuals must be assured the right to demand from government access to judicial procedures. Judicial rights ought not to be debased to the level where judicial access can only not be prohibited by government, but need not be guaranteed by government. This debasement would give judicial access the same status that abortion now has in the U.S.; it cannot be prohibited, but is not guaranteed for those who want or even (in most cases) need it. Civic rights ought not to be mere immunities and they ought not to be restricted only to certain classes.

Imagine the following scenario. Steven, who teaches math in a suburban high school and coaches the swim team, on a weekend night heads to the city to try his luck at Up and Coming, a popular gay cruise bar. There he meets Tom, a self-employed contractor, who in his former life sired two sons by a woman who now hates him, but who is ignorant of his new life. Tom and Steve decide to walk to Tom's nearby flat, which he rents from a bigot who bemoans the fact that the community is going gay and refuses to rent to people he supposes to be gay; Tom's weekend visitations from his sons are his cover.

Meanwhile, at a nearby Children's Aid Home for teenagers, the leader of the Anglo gang is taunting Tony, the leader of the Latino gang, with the accusation of being a faggot. After much protestation to the contrary, Tony claims he will prove to the Anglos once and for all that he is not a faggot and hits the streets with his gang members, who tote with them the blunt and not so blunt instruments of the queer-basher's trade. They descend on Tom and Steve, downing their victims in a blizzard of strokes and blows. Local residents coming home from parties and others walking their dogs witness the whole event.

Imagine that two miracles occur. One, a squad car happens by, and two, the police actually do their job. Tony and another of the fleeing queer-bashers are caught and arrested on the felony charges of aggravated assault and battery, and attempted murder. Other squad cars arrive and while witnesses' reports are gathered, Steve and Tom are taken to the nearest emergency room. Once Steve and Tom are in wards the police arrive to take statements of complaint from them, complaints which will engage the wheels of justice in what appears to be an open and shut case. But Steve knows the exposure of a trial will terminate his employment. And Tom knows the exposure of a trial would give his ex-wife the legal excuse she desires to deny his visitation rights, and he knows he will eventually lose his apartment. So neither man can reasonably risk pressing charges. Tony is, therefore, released, and within twelve hours of attempting murder, he returns to the Children's Aid Home hailed by all as a conquering hero. Gay rights are a necessary material condition for judicial access.

Any reader of gay urban tabloids, like Chicago's *GayLife*, San Francisco's *Bay Area Reporter*, Boston's *Gay Community News*, Toronto's *The Body Politic*, Washington's *The Blade*, knows that the events which I have sketched—miracles excepted—are typical of daily occurrences. Every day gays are in effect blackmailed by our judicial system. Our judicial system's threat of exposure prevents gay access to its protections. The example I have given of latter-day lynch law falls within the sphere of criminal justice; even more obviously the same judicial blackmail occurs in civil cases. Nor are the offending parties always outsiders to the community whose civic access is thus limited:

Similarly, lesbians can be sexually harassed by other lesbians. Some lesbians may foist sexual attentions upon other lesbians who already have lovers, for example. To a large extent lesbians who are victims of nondiscriminatory [i.e., peer-on-peer] sexual harassment will be on their own. A lesbian will tend to reject any suggestion that she initiate a civil suit against her female harasser. Fearing that she will be laughed out of court, or *doubting the wisdom of publicly proclaiming her sexual preference*, the lesbian is apt to handle her problem in informal ways.[5]

These "informal ways," though, are bound to be unsatisfactory. For insofar as they try to circumvent the law and yet require for their warranted success the sort of justified coercion which is the exclusive preserve of the state's police powers, they will at a minimum result in violation of the law,[6] and more likely end in attempted usurpation of the law.[7]

It is unreasonable to expect anyone to give up that by which he lives, his employment, his shelter, his access to goods and services and to loved ones in order for judicial procedures to be carried out equitably, in order to demand legal protections. Even if one were tempted to follow the libertarian and say that these are in fact reasonable expenses to pay for making the choice of living an open lifestyle, that a person always makes trade-offs among his necessarily limited options, and that this condition does not warrant the state coercing *others* on his behalf—even if one believed all that, one would not, I think, go on and say that these costs are a reasonable price to pay to see one's assailants dealt justice or to enter a court of equity.

Now what is bitterly paradoxical about this blackmail is that it is a necessary concomitant of two major virtues of the fair administration of justice. The first is that trials are not star chamber affairs, but are open to scrutiny by public and press. The second is that defendants must be able to confront the witnesses against them and have compulsory process for obtaining witnesses in their favor, while conversely prosecutors must have the tools with which to press cases on behalf of victims; in consequence, determinations of guilt and innocence must be based on a full examination of the facts. The result of these two virtues is that trials cast the private into the public realm.

The Supreme Court itself has recognized that public exposure of the private realm necessarily attends the workings of justice:

> [A]ll the values to which we accord deference for the privacy of all citizens ... must yield ... to our [nation's] commitment to the rule of law. This is nowhere more profoundly manifest than in our view that "the twofold aim [of criminal justice] is that guilt shall not escape or innocence suffer." We have elected to employ an adversary system of criminal justice in which the parties contest all issues before a court of law ... The very integrity of the judicial system and public confidence in the system depend on full disclosure of all the facts.... (Burger, C. J. for a unanimous court in *United States v. Nixon*, 418 U.S. 683, 708, 713, 709 [1974]).

That trials cast the private into the public realm gives the lie to those condescending (would-be) liberals who claim that what gays do in private is no one else's business and should not be anyone else's business, so that they neither need rights nor deserve rights—lest they make themselves public.[8] If the judicial system is to be open and fair, it is necessary that gays be granted civil rights. Otherwise judicial access becomes a right only for the dominant culture.[9]

In being de facto cast beyond the pale of civic procedures, gays, when faced with assaults on property and person, are left with only the equally unjust alternatives of the resignation of the impotent or the rage of man in a state of nature. Societies may remain orderly even when some of their members are denied civic procedures. Many tyrannies do. But such societies cannot be said to be civil societies which respect the rule of law.[10]

In October 1984, the governor of California signed a bill making actionable as civil suits assaults on gays which are motivated by an animus against gays.[11] In March of the same year, he had vetoed a civil rights bill which would have protected gays from private employment discrimination. Given the experience of gays, the former legislation will prove virtually pointless in the absence of the latter.

II

In the same 1938 case in which the Supreme Court programmatically withdrew its attention from the field of economic legislation, it set forth an agenda for itself in the area we now call civil liberties. The Court recognized *inter alia* that "legislation which restricts those political processes which can ordinarily be expected to bring about repeal of undesirable legislation" might need "to be subjected to more exacting judicial scrutiny under the general prohibitions of the Fourteenth Amendment than are most other types of legislation" (*United States v. Carolene Products Co.*, 304 U.S. 144, 152n4). Even more perceptively the Court recognized that social, as opposed to legal, forces also might have the result for some groups of effectively excluding their participation in the political life of the nation: "Prejudice against discrete and insular minorities may be a special condition, which tends seriously to curtail the operation of those political processes ordinarily to be relied upon to protect minorities" (ibid.).[12]

I will argue that widespread social prejudice against gays has for them this very effect about which the Court, at the level of principle, so perceptively worried—the virtual eclipse of political rights. I will argue that in the absence of gay civil rights legislation, gays are—over the range of issues which most centrally affect their minority status—effectively denied access to the political rights of the First Amendment, that is, freedom of speech, freedom of press, freedom of assembly, and freedom to petition for the redress of grievances. Further, gays are especially denied the emergent Constitutional right of association—an amalgam of the freedoms of speech and assembly—which establishes the right to join and be identified with other persons for common (political) goals.[13]

This eclipse of political access is most evident if we look at gays severally. Put concretely, does a gay man who has to laugh at and manufacture fag jokes in workplace elevators and around workplace coffee urns, in order to deflect suspicion from himself in an office which routinely fires gay employees, have freedom to express his views on gay issues? Is it likely that such a person could reasonably risk appearing in public at a gay rights rally? Would such a person be able to participate in a march celebrating the Stonewall Riots and the start of gay activism? Would such a man be able to sign, let alone circulate, a petition protesting the firing of a gay worker? Would such a man likely try to persuade workmates to vote for a gay-positive city-councilman? Would such a man sign a letter to the editor protesting abusive reportage of gay issues and events, or advocating the discussion of gay issues in high schools? Such a man is usually so transfixed by fear that it is highly unlikely that he could even be persuaded to write out a check to a gay rights organization.[14]

In the absence of 1964 Civil Rights Act protections, the vast majority of gays is effectively denied the ability to participate equally in First Amendment rights, which are supposed to pertain equally to every citizen *qua* individual. First Amendment rights, like other such rights, apply directly to citizens or persons as individuals. They do not apply directly to groups and only derivatively to individuals.[15] It will not do then to suggest that even if some, or even most, gays cannot reasonably participate in politics, this is unproblematic on the alleged ground that other gays—those who are open about their minority status—may voice the interests of those who are not. This position simply confuses individual rights, like First Amendment rights, with group "rights." The position further naively assumes that gays uniformly have the same interests and espouse the same views on any given gay issue, so that one simply needs to know one sociological fact—percent of gays in the general population—to know the extent to which some publicly espoused gay interest is held.[16]

If further, for a moment, gays are viewed collectively as a potential political force, it should be clear that for a group that—fanciful contagion and recruitment theories of causation aside—is a permanent minority, it is hardly fair to be further encumbered by having the majority of its members absent through social coercion from the public workings of the political process.

If First Amendment rights are not to be demoted to privileges, to which only the dominant culture has access, then invisible minorities that are subject to widespread social discrimination will have to be guaranteed protection from those forces which maintain them in their position of invisibility. Civil rights protections are a very long step in that direction.

Now, it might be argued that First Amendment rights are to be construed as mere immunities, that they merely prevent the government from interfering with certain types of actions, so that as long as the government and its agents do not, say, refuse parade permits to gays, smash up the gay press, deny the formation of gay student groups on state university campuses, and the like, then in fact gays do have First Amendment rights just like everyone else.[17] In these circumstances, it would be reasonable to say that gays are *free from* active government interference in their political designs. Nevertheless, gays would still remain effectively denied the *freedom to act* politically.

Whatever else First Amendment rights might be, they have as one of their chief rationales and purposes not merely *not making impossible* the procedures of democracy, but also actually promoting, enhancing, and making likely the proper working of democratic processes. To this end, then, First Amendment rights need somehow to be construed not merely as immunities, as the mere absences of government interference, but as somewhat stronger rights. Indeed, they need to be realized as powers which place the government under a certain liability.

Democratic government should operate under the liability not only of removing its own possible interference with the dissemination of political views, but also of removing those forces in society in general which block the *potentially effective* dissemination of political views.

At a minimum, potentially effective political activity requires that the political position espoused is widely and pointedly disseminated. Only with the widespread and lively dissemination of political ideas is it possible for a minority political position on social policy to have a chance of becoming government policy and law. If the majority never has the opportunity to change its opinions to those of the minority, political rights would be otiose. It would seem incumbent upon government, then, to militate against those social conditions and mechanisms by which majority opinion perpetuates itself *simply by the elimination* of the hearing of alternative possible policies, or what is as good, *the reduction* of alternatives to the mere slogans of strawmen.

Now it is not a requirement for democratic process that minority opinions must at some point carry the day and become the majority opinion, as a sign that the system is working correctly. All that is required is that minority opinions have their day in the court of the body politic, that majority opinion should not be allowed constantly to win out *by default*.

To this end, government must prohibit nongovernment agents from interfering with the political activities of individuals and groups. Thus, for instance, because we consider the freedom of assembly to be a power rather than merely an immunity, we insist not only that political rallies, say, should be immune from government interference but also we deem it a major obligation of government and its police actions to make actual as a power the right of people to hold rallies by prohibiting goon squads and hecklers from disrupting political rallies. The goon performs an act considerably worse than simple assault when he strikes a speaker; the assassin an act worse than murder. A special need for police action against the goon and assassin arises over and above normal police activities of protecting civic rights.[18] Analogously, bigoted employers are the goon squads and hecklers who, when unrestrained by law, deny gays access to political rights. Civil rights legislation for gays would be considered an essential part of the police activities of the state.

Only when the government protects gays against discrimination in housing, employment, and public accommodation will they have First Amendment rights as powers. For all potentially effective political strategies involve *public* actions. More specifically, all the actions protected by the First Amendment are public actions (speaking, publishing, petitioning, assembling, associating). Now, a person who is a member of an invisible minority and who must remain invisible, hidden, and secreted in respect to his minority status as a condition for maintaining his livelihood, this person is not free to be public about his minority status or to incur suspicion by publicly associating with others who are open about their similar status. And so he is effectively denied all political power—except the right to vote. But, voting aside, he will be denied the freedom to express his views in a public forum and to unite with or organize other like-minded individuals in an attempt to elect persons who will support the policies advocated by his group. He is denied all effective use of legally available means of influencing public opinion prior to voting and all effective means of lobbying after elections are held.

Such denials to minorities of First Amendment rights as powers differ in kind depending upon the minority affected; and remedies vary accordingly. Blacks, for instance, though constituting a visible minority, nevertheless, as the result of being in general poorer than whites, are effectively denied First Amendment rights as powers, since blacks are, for financial reasons, effectively denied the political use of such expensive mass media tools as purchasing television time and newspaper space.[19]

For gays, it is not poverty *per se* which effectively denies gays First Amendment rights. Indeed gays are, as Kinsey showed, dispersed nearly homogeneously throughout all social and economic classes. Rather it is the recriminations that descend upon gays who are publicly gay that effectively deny them First Amendment rights and might even more effectively deny to them these rights than poverty denies them to blacks, since the poor but visible at least have available to them such inexpensive but limited methods of public communication as sit-ins, marches, and demonstrations. Gays—as long as job discrimination is widespread—are effectively denied even these limited modes of public access.

On the one hand, the closeted condition of most gays has meant that nothing remotely approaching the widespread dissemination of views on gay issues necessary for any potentially effective political strategy has occurred in this country or any other. The condition has caused gay political organizations to be small, weak, inbred, ill-financed, impermanent, and subterranean. It greatly curtails any outreach to the nongay world, leaving such organizations largely "to preach to the converted." Membership tends to stand in inverse proportion to an organization's public profile; thus memberships in gay religious and other largely hermetic social organizations far outstrip those in gay political organizations.

In consequence, any widespread portrayal of gays and gay issues has been left entirely to the mercies of the mass media, which, however much they may preempt political discussion and activity, are no substitute for them. The general media have their own agenda, which includes politics largely to the extent that politics is entertaining. Regarding gays, the mass media have been able to see little beyond the titillation of fear and death. Such titillation after all is largely what keeps the mass media massive. It would be fanciful to say that hidden amongst the columns devoted to AIDS, congressional scandals, and serial murderers, we see something like a robust national debate of gay issues.[20] The most that can be said of the media (especially and ironically the antigay polemics of the New Right) is that they have begun to break down the taboo that has previously surrounded even the mere mention of homosexuality.[21]

On the other hand, local dissemination of views is also impeded. Indeed, the closeted condition of gays blocks the most effective sort of political communication in which gays in particular might engage with others—personal conversation. Social reality is such that many people do not know or think they do not know any gay people firsthand. Such widespread ignorance is a breeding ground for vicious stereotypes. Problems compound when misunderstanding is added to ignorance. Many people *sort of* think they know that someone, say, a workmate is gay. But given the way the workmate acts, especially in avoiding certain topics, in being selectively "absent" from social intercourse or in confusingly broadcasting mixed messages, others think the gay person is embarrassed about his status and so do not initiate any discussion of it, and so further they are left with the impression that there is something wrong with gays because gays themselves seem to act as though there is. The nongay person oddly fails to realize that the gay person may have or—what comes to the same—may *suppose* he has solid prudential reasons for his skittish behavior.

When this widespread ignorance and misunderstanding combine with gut reactions to gays of fear and loathing or even just queasiness and discomfort, mere reportage (even accurate reportage) about gays or mere abstract discussion (even insightful discussion) of gay issues has little chance of success in changing the attitudes by which people conduct their lives. When people's attitudes are informed by deeply held emotional responses—ones perhaps central to their conceptions of themselves—reason's hope is slight. The most effective way of changing nongays' views about gays is for nongays to interact personally with some openly gay people.[22]

Such interaction is almost the only way to cut through stereotypes and fears, which when left unchecked tend mutually to aggravate one another into dangerous frenzy.[23] At a minimum, personal contact generally reveals as sheer paranoia much of the fear some people have of gays. And yet such personal outreach of gays to the nongay person is not likely to occur, however willing the nongay person, as long as a gay person has to put his job and other major interests on the line to make the contact. It is after all at the job site and in certain public accommodations that people tend to have the sorts of contacts with others, initially strangers, which might lead to personal conversations. And yet it is exactly in these locations that a gay person is most likely to encounter discrimination if he is open about his status. And so the most effective avenue of communication for gays about the issues of importance to them as gays is effectively blocked in the absence of civil rights protections.

The California Supreme Court has taken cognizance of the adverse impact that employment discrimination has on political participation by gays. Prior to 1979, Pacific Telephone and Telegraph had an explicit company policy of firing gay employees. No systematic measures were taken by the company to find out who its gay employees were, but "manifest homosexuals," that is, gays who said they were gay or "made an issue of" being gay, were regularly fired. In a groundbreaking case, *Gay Law Students Assn. v. PT&T Co.*,[24] the court ruled that such firings of "manifest" gays violated the plantiffs' political freedoms in violation of the sections of the California Labor Code which forbid employers from preventing employees from engaging or participating in politics (sections 1101, 1102). The court recognized, for the first time in U.S. legal history, the special political plight of gays as an invisible minority. It acknowledged that if they are to have political rights, gays must be free to be open about who they are. After holding that the struggle for gay rights is political activity covered by the Code, the decision reads, in relevant part:

> A principal barrier to homosexual equality is the common feeling that homosexuality is an affliction which the homosexual worker must conceal from his employer and his fellow workers. Consequently, one important aspect of the struggle for equal rights is to induce homosexual individuals to "come out of the closet," acknowledge their sexual preferences and to associate with others in working for equal rights. In light of this factor in the movement for homosexual rights, the allegations of the plaintiffs' complaint assumes a special significance (24 Cal. 3d 458, 488).

Here the court recognizes that the ability to be openly gay is a necessary prerequisite for gays, *qua* gays, having any effective political rights. The California Labor Code, in its political dimension, stands to the First Amendment as the 1871 Civil Rights Act, with its remedies for procedural abuses to equal protection, stands to the Fourteenth Amendment. These very general legislative acts turn the immunities of the Amendments into effective powers.

Now I do not think that in the absence of such legislation the courts themselves should take the step of construing Constitutional guarantees as powers rather than as mere immunities,[25] by ruling, say, that First Amendment rights entail rights to welfare and education as necessary enabling conditions for the equitable realization of First Amendment rights. As long as the courts merely say in what ways the government *may not deploy* its monopoly of coercive forces against individuals and systematically avoid mandating (except as compensation for violations of Constitutional immunities) that the government *must deploy* its monopoly of coercion in some way, then the courts, while retaining the legitimate capacity to construe Constitutional rights broadly, avoid the conservative's common charge that in dilating Constitutional guarantees the courts mistakenly act like Platonic Guardians and usurp the proper power and function of legislatures.[26] But the very last thing that Platonic Guardians do is to dispense to individuals immunities from state coercion. Their core activity, *like that of legislatures*, is essentially to deploy coercive force against individuals by either prohibiting or compelling acts in the private sector. If courts avoid coercing the private sector, they systematically avoid intruding into the essential activity of legislatures.

If, however, civil rights protections are to remain creatures of legislatures rather than the courts, the problem arises that the majority is left as the judge of its own fairness to minorities. Those most in need of such protections seem the least likely on their own to acquire them. Here the California case is instructive to political strategists. The labor code covers gays without explicitly mentioning gays. Yet the omission is neither a ruse nor an oversight. Rather, the labor code appeals to general principle and general social realities, and in doing so, is broad enough in scope that many people will find it attractive legislation, for many can imagine themselves as potential beneficiaries of it. And so the likelihood of enacting such legislation is greatly enhanced.

That nonlegal social forces hinder robust political life to an even greater extent than does government coercion has been eloquently stated by J. S. Mill:

It is [social] stigma which is really effective [in stopping] the profession of opinions which are under the ban of society.... In respect to all persons but those whose pecuniary circumstances make them independent of the good will of other people, opinion ... is as efficacious as law; men might as well be imprisoned as excluded from the means of earning their bread. Our merely social intolerance roots out no opinions, but induces men to disguise them or to abstain from any active effort for their diffusion.[27]

Mill probably underestimated the effects of social intolerance in rooting out or even inverting opinions. He shows virtually no awareness of the possibility that a member of a despised group may so thoroughly absorb the values of his culture regarding his group that he becomes an unwitting participant in his own oppression. Gays seem particularly prone to this mangling of their beliefs about themselves.[28] However, Mill is certainly correct in his general assessment of the effects of social ostracism and job discrimination in blocking the diffusion of unpopular beliefs and forcing their holders into lives of disguise. And though Mill never mentions homosexuals here or elsewhere in *On Liberty*, he could not have picked a clearer illustration for his general thesis.

The meager energies and monies of the gay rights movement have been directed almost exclusively at trying to get 1964 Civil Rights Act protections for gays.[29] Without these legislated rights, which would begin to bring them into the procedures of democracy, gays have not even been able to begin thinking about the substantive issues on which gays reasonably would want to exert influence in democratic policy making, issues, for instance, concerning sex and solicitation law, licensing, zoning, immigration policy, judicial and prison reform, military and police policy, tax law, education, medical and aging policy, affirmative action, law governing living associations and the transfer of property, and "family" law. By being effectively denied the public procedures of democracy, gays are incapable of defending their own interests on substantial issues of vital concern.

It is important to remember that the 1964 Civil Rights Act and similar legislation reasonably enough contain exemption provisions that allow for employment discrimination on the basis of an otherwise protected characteristic, *if* a business can show that the discrimination is reasonably necessary to the operation of the business, that is, that the discrimination is a discrimination in good faith. So, for example, it is reasonable for a bank to discriminate in its hiring practices against the invisible minority that consists of repeatedly convicted embezzlers, even though this minority may be organizing politically to try to reform embezzlement laws. However, given exemption provisions for discriminations based on *bona fide* occupational qualifications, ex-convicts, as an invisible minority subject to widespread discrimination, should be, as they are in a few jurisdictions, included within the reach of civil rights protections on the basis of the arguments advanced here. It is also important to note that the arguments for the inclusion of gays as an invisible minority within the reach of the 1964 Civil Rights Act hold good independently of whether gay sexual acts are legal in any given jurisdiction.[30] Whether the moral or legal status of a person's gay-related activities ever raises to the level of a *bona fide* occupational qualification, I leave here an open question.[31]

III

I have suggested that the absence of civil rights protections for gays casts doubt on the fairness of current political *procedures* surrounding democratic voting. I now wish to suggest that the same absence also casts doubt on the adequacy of certain *justifications* for democracy.

Perhaps the strongest argument for democracy is that democracy is justified on utilitarian grounds. Those who try to justify democracy deontologically as the institution which most directly gives expression to individual dignity simply overestimate the significance of political activity and voting in people's lives. The *consequences* of a democratically enacted statute may be great for an individual, but for the vast majority of people, an individual's *contribution* to the democratic system—unless he is political by profession—is slight in his overall pattern of life. Campaigning and voting are sporadic activities. They are neither activities by which individuals sustain their day-to-day lives nor those in which everyday activities culminate. At least one never hears anyone say "I work that I might vote" or "I live that I might vote." And so politics and voting are not integrative principles nor even integral parts of day-to-day life. They are not activities in terms of which any but a few do or should define their lives. The childless curmudgeon who religiously votes against school levies is no more dignified than the social worker who, caught up in a flurry of commitments, fails to vote. The resident alien is not deprived of essential dignity by his inability to participate fully in the mechanisms of democracy.[32]

This is not to deny that many, even most, of the things that individuals do in their day-to-day lives have political overtones. As nearly all of everyday discourse is devoted to persuading people of this or that, or asserting to others the value of this or that, an individual's day-to-day activities will tend to shape other people's views in ways that may well register at the ballot box, but this registration is usually an entirely incidental and unconscious spinoff effect of day-to-day activities and not what motivates them or gives them importance in individuals' lives.

To make democratic politics the paradigmatically human activity is also to place it uncomfortably at odds with soundly held beliefs that voting should be restricted in what it may achieve. If one views voting as the paramount human value and if voting is not to be made a hollow activity, a mere formal ritual, in virtue of having its effects voided, then one will be committed to a pure, direct democracy operating without substantive Constitutional restraints and holding out the prospect that law can be the mere amassing of prejudice—a position virtually everyone would reject.

Further, voting is not even to be viewed as a value on a par with Constitutional rights. Now, the Court has persistently claimed for a century that voting if not *the* fundamental right at least *a* "fundamental right" on the ground that voting is "preservative of all rights" *(Wick Yo v. Hopkins*, 118 U.S. 356, 370 [1886]) or, put somewhat more modestly, because voting is "preservative of other basic civil and political rights" *(Reynolds v. Sims*, 377 U.S. 533, 562 [1964]); cf. *Harper v. Virginia Bd. of Elections*, 383 U.S. 663, 667 [1966]). The Court, however, in these cases simply is conceptually confused. For democratic voting and its deployment of the state's coercive poers by majority rule are how fundamental Constitutional rights, including "political" rights like speaking and assembling, are impinged and trampled. At best the right to vote preserves *legally* engendered rights, not Constitutional rights. The mere expansion of the franchise to include some minority does not guarantee the minority equal protection of the laws. Therefore, voting is a fundamental right not as Constitutional rights are fundamental, but in consequence of whatever role democracy properly plays in the constellation of just political institutions.[33]

In sum, democracy is a better registrar of desire than of dignity. And as such, democracy is best justified in utilitarian terms.

It is reasonable to suppose that the policies that represent the wishes of the most people will be the policies which will most likely maximize utility. For given the complexity of *predicting* precise consequences of social policies for large and complex populations, relying on the *preferences* of the people in general rather than on the *predictions* of social engineers as likely indicators of future utility seems eminently reasonable.[34] It is precisely in the area of economics and other areas which are productive on a large scale of the public objects of desire (e.g., automobiles, clean air) that democracy is going to be the most accurate guide for social policy and least justifiably accused of irrationally burdening liberty.

However, if preferences pure and simple were the whole rationale for establishing social policy, social policies could be determined simply by direct democracy, as manifest in referenda and plebiscites.

For democracy coherently to have a preference-utilitarian justification, though, requires that a distinction be drawn between an individual's internal and external preferences. His internal preferences are preferences for goods and services *for himself.* His external preferences are preferences that he has for things *for persons other than himself.* To be *coherent*, preference-justified democracy must discount and disregard a person's external preferences. For the man who has external preferences and who would have society act upon them is assuming for himself the role of social engineer—a role discredited by the very premises of the argument justifying democracy in terms of preferences.[35] Further, if democracy is to be an *accurate* gauge of likely utility maximization, it must for this reason discount external preferences. For in general it is unlikely that anyone other than a person himself will know what is best for himself; hardly anyone will hold another's interest in the same regard that he holds his own (see Mill, pp. 74-75). Those individuals whose interests one might plausibly put on a par with one's own will be those with whom one has intimate or familial relations, which in the main ought to be covered by privacy rights and so fall outside the purview of democratically engendered law.

If, in consequence, external preferences are to be disregarded in the calculus of preferences, then direct democracy can not be the instrument for this measurement. For referenda and plebiscites give equal weight to internal and external preferences; they give equal weight to the views of bigots and nonbigots. The remedy—where the distribution of powers rather than immunities is concerned—is a form of representative democracy in which the elected official, it is hoped, is rational enough and impartial enough to rise above popular prejudices taking into account only the internal preferences of his constituents. A legislator who discounts external preferences is not to suffer the accusation of moral elitism, for he is acting in accordance with sound democratic principles.[36]

Now, there are two sorts of external preferences, which the rational legislator must discount. He must, on the one hand, discount the crass egoist's preferences for disutilities to be distributed to others and discount the possible attendant sadistic pleasures which the egoist might take in seeing other people's plans defeated.[37] On the other hand, the legislator must disregard the preferences of the altruist, who wishes to see the utilities of others promoted, and discount the possible masochistic pleasures which the altruist might take in seeing the plans of others succeed.[38]

The rational legislator will sift through his mail, public debates, editorials, letter columns, and all the other modes of public discussion of social policies and will winnow out external preferences. The legislator in this scheme is as justified in disregarding the altruistic opinions of the well-intended heterosexual (or would-be heterosexual) do-gooder who writes him supporting gay-positive legislation, as he is in disregarding the opinion of the religious zealot who desires state persecution of gays.

If this system of justification for democratic procedures is to work, it presupposes that people can present publicly their opinions on social policy as desires for things for themselves. They must be able to present themselves publicly as members of classes of which they in fact are members, so that they can promote legislation which benefits them as members of their classes. ·

For preference-utilitarianism to be a coherent rationale for democracy, everyone must be permitted to present himself in public debate as what he is. For preference democracy to be coherent, gays must be free to present themselves publicly as gays; and gays are effectively precluded this option, if the means by which they live can be removed from them at whim for being publicly gay. Civil rights protections for invisible minorities are a necessary prerequisite for coherent democratic processes.

Further, aside from this procedural justification for gay rights, once the distinction between internal and external preferences is drawn, it should be obvious that gay rights legislation has a strong independent utilitarian justification. For, with external preferences dropped from the calculus of preferences, the only conflict of internal preferences which remains—assuming permissible discrimination-in-good-faith exemptions in hiring—is a conflict between, on the one hand, the preferences of some employers to be whimsical, arbitrary and so, irrational in their hiring practices and, on the other hand, preferences of gays to avoid the deep and continuous anxiety that attends leading an existence of systematic disguise.

IV

Current society puts gays in the queer position of not being able to fight for gay rights unless gays are already "out" and gays cannot be "out" unless gays already have gay rights. Paradoxically, gays can not get gay rights, unless they already have them. This "particularly vicious circle" was noted over thirty years ago by an author himself closeted. Little has changed:

On the one hand ... the social punishment of acknowledgment [of one's homosexuality is] so great that pretense is almost

universal; on the other hand, only a leadership that would acknowledge [its homosexuality] would be able to break down the
barriers ... of discrimination. Until the world is able to accept us
on an equal basis as human beings entitled to the full rights of life,
we are unlikely to have any great numbers willing to become
martyrs ... But until we are willing to speak out openly and
frankly in defense of our activities and to identify ourselves with
the millions pursuing these activities, we are unlikely to find the
attitudes of the world undergoing any significant change.[39]

The author perhaps overestimates the potential effectiveness of
martyrs,[40] but his main point is sound. As an invisible minority, gays
cannot fight for the right to be open about being gay, unless gays
are already open about it, and gays cannot reasonably be open
about being gay, until gays have the right to be openly gay. One
would hope that once society was made aware of this paradox, if
society had any sense of decency and fair play, it would on its own
move to establish civil rights for gays.

NOTES

1. An earlier version of this paper was presented to the American Philosophical Association's Eastern Division meetings for 1981. An abstract of it
appears in *Journal of Philosophy*, 78 (1981), 608–609.

2. For discussion of the extent of employment discrimination against homosexuals, see Martin P. Levine and Robin Leonard, "Discrimination against
Lesbians in the Work Force," *Signs*, 9:4 *(The Lesbian Issue)* (1984), 700–
710, and Martin P. Levine, "Employment Discrimination against Gay Men,"
International Review of Modern Sociology, 9:5–7 (July-December 1979),
151–163.

3. Elsewhere I have sketched arguments to suggest that such direct effects
do sufficiently motivate civil rights legislation and sometimes even justify
with special force such legislation for gays: "Gays and the Civil Rights Act,"
QQ: *Report from the Center for Philosophy and Public Policy*, 4:2 (1984),
12a–13a, and "How to Argue for Gay Rights," *Christopher Street*, (#84,
June 1984), 46a–48a. If one is independently convinced by these arguments
from direct effects, the additional arguments of this paper should cause one
to elevate the ranking of gay political work from simply being worthwhile
to being important or even compelling in the hierarchy of one's political
commitments.

4. For libertarian argument against the 1964 Civil Rights Act generally, but
for some government involvement in assuring access to courts and political

processes, see for example Anne Wortham, "Individualism versus Racism" in *The Libertarian Alternative*, ed. Tibor R. Machan (Chicago: Nelson-Hall, 1974) pp. 403–407.

5. Rosemarie Tong, "Lesbian Perspectives" in *Women, Sex, and the Law* (Towtowa, NJ: Rowman & Allenheld, 1984) p. 187; italics added to suggest euphemism or understatement.

6. Example: in December 1982, the only two women's bars in NYC—unwilling, not without reason, to rely on police protections—initiated a "women only" door policy to protect patrons from persistent harassment from nongay males. This action, of course, violated state liquor codes (among others) which bar sex discrimination. The result: Both establishments lost their licenses and were closed by the state (Tong, p. 186). I leave here as open questions whether such a door policy could be justified as a private sector affirmative action program or whether, given the historically central role of bars in the development and maintenance of gay and lesbian communities, the license revocations should be subject to successful challenge as violations of the Constitutional right to (political) association. On this role, see John D'Emilio, *Sexual Politics, Sexual Communities: The Making of a Homosexual Minority in the United States, 1940–1970* (Chicago: Univ. Chicago Press, 1983) pp. 30–33, 49–51, especially 97–99, 107, 186. *Caveat emptor:* Usually, though not always, such Constitutional challenges to civil rights ordinances have worked against rather than in favor of gay and lesbian interests, especially when religious rights have been invoked. See, for example, *Gay Rights Coalition of Georgetown University Law Center v. Georgetown University* (#CA5863-80 D.C. Superior Court, October 14, 1983) (municipal civil rights ordinance with sexual orientation protections cannot force a church-affiliated university to recognize a gay student group) or *Walker v. First Presbyterian Church*, 22 F.E.P. Cases 762 (Cal. Super. Ct., 1980) (Free Exercise Clause voids application of municipal gay employment protections to gay church organist).

7. For a grisly example of such vigilantism—a case of revenge over an alleged violation of personal rights in which the avenger is in no position to seek recourse in the law—see Tong, p. 189; for further examples and analysis, see "Lesbian Battering," *Gay Community News*, 11:25, January 14, 1984, 8, 13–17.

8. For portraits of such liberal condescension to gays and the general inability of non-gays to understand gay life, see David Leavitt, "Territory" and "Dedicated" in *Family Dancing* (New York: Alfred A. Knopf, 1984).

9. Inequitable procedures and results tend to characterize those criminal cases with gay victims which do go to trial. In this regard, gay experience parallels that of blacks. The life and liberty of gays and blacks simply count for less than the life and liberty of members of the dominant culture. This devaluation of gays and blacks registers in the sentencing of their assailants to punishments which are disproportionally weak when compared to similar cases with nongay and white victims.

Frequently queer-bashers as "just All-American Boys" by judges who hand them suspended sentences. See for example, "2 St. John's Students Given Probation in Assault on Gay," *The Washington Post*, May 15, 1984, I describing a case in which the permanently injured victim had been stalked, beaten up, stripped at knife point, slashed, kicked, threatened with castration and pissed on. (cf. Editorial, *The Washington Post*, May, 22, 1984, 14). This judicial devaluation of gays also registers in the disproportionately frequent success in gay victim cases of extreme procedural measures which benefit the accused by effectively gutting or voiding sentences. For instance, youths who, in virtue of the extreme violence of their alleged crime, could be and would be expected to be tried as adults are tried rather as children. For example and analysis, see Richard Steinman, "Looking Back at Bangor," *Gay Community News*, 12:18, November 17, 1984, 5, a case in which the victim was hurled from a bridge and drowned. On this case, see also *The New York Times*, July 16, 1984, 17; July 18, 16; July 29, 18; August 1, 19; August 22, 12; October 2, 27; and especially September 17, IV, 14, and October 6, 6.

Alternatively, juries in gay victim cases will readily accept insanity and other "diminished capacity" defenses once it becomes clear that the facts of a case themselves point inevitably to a verdict of guilt. In 1981 a former NYC Transit Authority policeman, claiming to be doing the work of God, machine-gunned down nine victims, killing two, in two Greenwich Village gay bars. His jury found him innocent due to mental illness (*The New York Times*, July 25, 1981, 27, and July 26, 1981, 25). The best known example of a successful "diminished capacity" defense is Dan White's voluntary manslaughter conviction for the 1978 assassinations of Harvey Milk and George Moscone, respectively gay supervisor and liberal mayor of San Francisco. For analysis of what has became known as the "Hostess Twinkie defense," see Randy Shilts, *The Mayor of Castro Street: The Life and Times of Harvey Milk* (New York: St. Martin's, 1982), pp. 308–325; see also Robert Epstein and Richard Schmeichen's Academcy Award winning documentary *The Times of Harvey Milk*, A TC Films International Release (1984).

Or again, juries will typically find a homicide to be "justified," if the killer claims his act was merely a panicked response to a sexual overture. Assaults on gay men are also typically construed by police and juries as self-defense. See for examples and discussion, Pat Califia, " 'Justifiable' Homicide?". *The Advocate*, #367, May 12, 1983, 12.

Or again, juries will simply discount testimony from gay witnesses. D'Emilio writes of the trial of seven police officers caught in a gay bar shakedown racket: "The defense lawyer cast aspersions on the credibility of the prosecution witnesses ... and deplored a legal system in which 'the most notorious homosexual may testify against a policeman.' Persuaded by this line of argument, the jury acquitted all of the defendants" (p. 183).

10. In this section, I have not intended to address a complementary problem of criminal justice for gays: whether, when gays stand accused of crime or pursue civil litigation, they get fair treatment from police, bench, and

jury. For some eye-opening examples of patently prejudicial and abusive treatment of gays from the bench, see Rhonda R. Rivera's magisterial "Our Straight-Laced Judges: The Legal Position of Homosexual Persons in the U.S.," *30 Hastings Law Review* (1979), 799–955, and for a history of police abuses of criminal procedures against gays, see D'Emilio, pp. 14–15, 30, 49–51, 70, 110–111, 120–121, 157, 182–184, 187–188, 193–194, 200–201, 202, 206–207.

To the extent that civil rights legislation for a group tends to legitimate that group in the eyes of society as a whole, gay civil rights legislation would in fact increase the likelihood of gays getting fair trials. The issue is complex, but I doubt that this benefit outweighs the general inappropriateness of government throwing its weight behind one or another lifestyle or class, *even when* this weight is viewed as a matter of compensatory justice to classes; so correctly Justice Stewart:

> The Legislative Branch of government is not a court of equity. It has neither the dispassionate objectivity nor the flexibility that are needed to mold a race-conscious remedy around the single objective of eliminating the effects of past or present discrimination (dissenting opinion, *Fullilove v. Klutznick*, 448 U.S. 448, 527 [1980]).

I am inclined to agree with neo-conservatives that gay civil rights legislation is not warranted *if* its main purpose and effect are simply a symbolic legitimizing of gays. See Jean Bethke Elshtain, "Homosexual Politics: The Paradox of Gay Liberation," *Salmagundi*, 58–59 (1982-3), 255.

11. While I think that all assaults (or at least highly aggravated ones, as queer-bashings almost always are) should *qua* assaults be actionable as civil suits, I do not think that they should be actionable (especially with punitive damages) *simply in virtue* of some political dimension of the assault, such that the only distinguishing feature between actionable and non-actionable assaults is simply the assailant's social or political beliefs and attitudes. Indeed to the extent that a law draws a distinction based solely on the political dimension of some violent act, the law should be declared unconstitutional on First Amendment grounds.

12. In this circumstance, laws affecting discrete and insular minorities "may call for correspondingly more searching judicial inquiry" (ibid.). To date, race, alienage, and, to a lesser degree, gender require special judicial protections from the political process. Gays also ought to be considered a discrete and insular minority *on the very ground* that the Court gives in establishing the classification, namely, that prejudice tends to push the minority group out of the political process. See John Hart Ely, *Democracy and Distrust* (Cambridge: Harvard Univ. Press, 1980), pp. 162–64. See also Justice Brennan's dissent from denial of certiorari *Rowland v. Mad River Local School District*, (53 U.S.L.W. 3614/U.S. February 25, 1985).

If given the status of a "suspect" class with attendant Constitutional protections under the Fourteenth Amendment, gays would be largely spared legislation that is targeted specifically against them. They would be guaranteed rights as *immunities* or certain negative freedoms, but this protection alone is nowhere near a sufficient guarantee of gay social justice. For as long as gays, even with immunity rights, still remain outside the political system, they will not be able to register their *interests*, however well protected their (immunity) *rights* may be. At a minimum, gays require for social justice that public policy take their interests into account. Beyond that, though, remains, of course, the problem of what the just weighting and realization of those interests should be.

13. See Lawrence Wilson and Raphael Shannon, "Homosexual Organizations and the Right of Association," *Hastings Law Journal*, 30 (1979), 1029–1074, and Donald Solomon, "The Emergence of Associational Rights for Homosexual Persons," *Journal of Homosexuality*, 5 (1979-80) 147–155.

14. Some organizations, like National Gay Rights Advocates, desperately aware of this last problem's magnitude, set up fundraising account "fronts" with innocuous sounding names, like "Legal Foundation for Personal Liberties," in an attempt to ease money, if not persons, out of the closet. Many organizations simply dissimulate, lying by omission or vagueness in assuming for themselves closeted names; thus the national gay political action committee baptizes itself "The Human Rights Campaign Fund."

15. "It is true that in *Griswold* the right to privacy in question adhered in the marital relationship. Yet the marital couple is not an independent entity with a mind and heart of its own, but an association of two individuals each with a separate intellectual and emotional makeup. If the right to privacy means anything, it is the right of the *individual*, married or single, to be free from unwarranted governmental intrusion into matters so fundamentally affecting a person as the decision whether to bear or beget a child," *Eisenstadt v. Baird*, 405 U.S. 438, 453, emphasis in original.

16. The "letters" column of gay tabloids are regularly littered with frequently vituperative but always anonymous contributions of those who claim that open gays do not represent their interests, indeed positively destroy their interests. These authors though are in a pretty hopeless position politically; the column is their only outlet, an incredibly narrow one at that, and readers reasonably enough are going to doubt the convictions and the courage of conviction of those who resort to anonymity. Such doubt is the reason most mainstream tabloids decline publication of anonymously submitted letters.

More generally, as D'Emilio, writing of the years bridging 1980, claims: "the [gay] movement itself shows no unanimity as to the social rearrangements that equality would require" (p. 247).

17. For the *status quaestionis* of gays and the First Amendment, see José Gómez, "The Public Expression of Lesbian/Gay Personhood as Protected Speech," *Journal of Law and Inequality*, 1 (1983), 121–153. See also *National Gay Task Force v. Oklahoma City Board of Education*, 729 F. 2d

1270 (10th Circuit, 1984) (law permitting the dismissal of a teacher for advocating or encouraging homosexuality ruled unconstitutional on its face); aff'd Oklahoma City Board of Education v. National Gay Task Force, (53 U.S.L.W. 4408/U.S. March 26, 1985).

18. Meting out greater penalties to the goon and assassin than to a typical assailant or murderer does not punish the criminal simply on the basis of his political views, as it does in the case of the queer-basher (see note 11 supra). Rather the criminal here is given a greater punishment because the result of his action is a greater offense—the disruption of legitimate government. It is true that but for his political views he probably would not have committed the greater offense, but that is irrelevant.

19. For a general defense of First Amendment rights as powers and for an application of the view to blacks, see Alan Gewirth, Human Rights (Chicago: Univ. Chicago Press, 1982), pp. 310–328.

20. Little in this regard has changed in the last thirty years: "When articles did find their way into the press or periodicals, they tended to focus on scandal, tragedy, or stereotypical images of homosexual and lesbian life. Gay women and men rarely enjoyed the opportunity to express in print their own views about their lives," D'Emilio, p. 109, writing of the period 1956–1960.

Can the liberal press serve as a proxy for gays in the discussion of gay issues? In December 1984, the Berkeley City Council passed domestic partner legislation which gives gay couples the same city employment benefits as married couples. This was the first successful piece of domestic partner legislation in the country and so a major gay news story. Yet The New York Times thought this beacon worthy of but twenty-three words and failed even to mention that the law applied to and was designed for gays, choosing rather to focus its three inch article on Eldridge Cleaver's presence at the council meeting ("Berkeley Council Backs Friendship Benefits," December 7, 1984, 12). Subsequently, Cleaver's presence was made a feature in the Times's Sunday "Ideas and Trends" column, where however no mention at all was made of the domestic partner legislation ("The Trials of Cleaver," December 9, 1984, IV, 7). See also n. 40 infra.

21. On this important role of antigay polemics, see D'Emilio, p. 52. The January 1985 issue of Moral Majority Report (7:1) contains three articles on gay issues, the March issue four, covering AIDS, First Amendment issues, privacy rights, C.I.A. employment, gay parents and domestic partner legislation. The cover of the February issue features a photograph of two gay men in affectionate embrace. In context such reportage is but editorial fodder; even so, to an extent, it defeats itself. For what is intended to shock the reader and elicit an immediate sense of revulsion also, as a side effect, informs and desensitizes the reader. He who sees men kissing in an image accompanying a conservative funding solicitation will be less surprised when he sees the original on the street. The more conservatives discuss gay issues, the less they can rely on automatic social responses which are fueled by fear of the unknown.

Conservative attention to gay issues runs another risk as well. For many people the traditional taboo on even discussing gay issues may be one of the chief mechanisms by which homosexual desire is kept from waxing into consciousness and act. See Michael Slote's "Inapplicable Concepts and Sexual Perversion" in *Philosophy and Sex*, ed. Robert Baker and Frederick Elliston, 1st ed. (Buffalo: Prometheus, 1975), pp. 261–267. See also Renaud Camus' forward to *Tricks: 25 Encounters* (New York: St. Martin's, 1981) p. *xi*: "Still other [homosexuals], and doubtless they are even today the majority, are unaware of such tastes because they live in such circumstances, in such circles, that their desires are not only for themselves inadmissible, but inconceivable, unspeakable. They possess no discourse of accommodation with which [they might] assume such desires and could change lives only by changing words."

22. The State of Oregon conducted a study of gay employment discrimination and found that positive attitudes toward gays in the workplace index closely to the degree of workers' firsthand acquaintance with gays (State of Oregon, Department of Human Resources, *Final Report of the Task Force on Sexual Preference*, Portland: State of Oregon, Department of Human Resources, 1978, pp. 73–87). For a review of the empirical literature on stereotyping of gays, see Alan Taylor, "Conceptions of Masculinity and Femininity as a Basis for Stereotypes of Male and Female Homosexuals," *Journal of Homosexuality* 9:1 (1983), 37–53, especially 37–44.

23. I do not wish to be taken as naively suggesting that personal contacts will explode stereotypes with the efficacy with which a pin will do in a balloon. For stereotypes are not simply mistaken inductions from a skewed sample of particular experiences; rather to a large extent stereotypes are the product of ideology and are sustained by cultural rather than personal transmission. Particular experience, then, can only begin to blunt their force and undo their damage. I do, though, wish to suggest that little else can.

24. *Gay Law Students Assn. v. Pacific Telephone and Telegraph Co.*, 24 Cal.3d 458, 595 P.2d 592, 156 Cal. Rptr. 14 (1979).

25. Exceptions are those few rights in the Constitution that explicitly are powers, namely, the right to compulsory process for producing witnesses on one's behalf and Thirteenth Amendment rights against slavery and involuntary servitude.

26. See for example Chief Justice Burger's dissent in *Plyler v. Doe*, 457 U.S. 202 (1982): "The Constitution does not constitute us as 'Platonic Guardians' nor does it vest in this Court the authority to strike down laws because they do not meet our standards of desirable social policy.... The Court employs, and in my opinion abuses, the Fourteenth Amendment in an effort to become an omnipotent and omniscient problem solver" (at 242–243), quoted in Justice O'Connor's dissent in *Akron v. Akron Center for Reproductive Health, Inc.*, 462 U.S. 416, 453 (1983). This view simply confuses immunities and powers.

27. J.S. Mill, *On Liberty*, ed. Elizabeth Rapaport (Indianapolis: Hackett, 1978), pp. 30–31, cf. *xv*.

28. See Andrew Hodges and David Hutter, *With Downcast Gays: Aspects of Homosexual Self-Oppression* 2nd ed. (1974, Toronto: Pink Triangle Press, 1979) and Barry Adam, *The Survival of Domination: Inferiorization and Everyday Life* (New York: Elsevier, 1978), especially chapter 4.

29. Success has been slight. Only some forty to fifty municipalities have such legislation and only Wisconsin among the states has such legislation. Municipal protections are generally limited in scope, tend to have weak enforcement provisions, have frequently been voided by popular referendum and have been successfully challenged as unconstitutional violations of state charter provisions which grant powers to cities.

30. As of September 1985, gay sexual acts remain criminal offenses in twenty-five states and the District of Columbia.

31. For the beginnings of an analytic for assessing claims of good faith discrimination against gays, see Richard Mohr, "Gay Rights," *Social Theory and Practice*, 8 (1982), 31–41; reprinted in *Moral Issues*, ed. by Jan Narveson (Toronto: Oxford University Press, 1983), pp. 347–355 and in *Philosophical Issues in Human Rights*, ed. Patricia Werhane (New York: Random House, 1985).

32. For a critique of the view that politics represents the central medium for dignity and human value, see Gerald Doppelt, "Rawls' System of Justice: A Critique from the Left" *Nous*, 15 (1981), 259–307.

33. The Court is vaguely aware of this contingent status of what is fundamental about voting, even though the awareness stands at odds with the Court's "preservative of rights" analysis. Thus the Court correctly holds that "the right of suffrage is a fundamental matter *in a free and democratic society*" (emphasis added, *Reynolds v. Sims*, at 561–562) and more fully, that "though not regarded strictly as a natural right, but as a privilege merely conceded by society according to its will, under certain conditions, nevertheless [voting] is regarded as a fundamental political right" (*Wick Yo v. Hopkins*, at 370).

The value of the role which democracy plays in any system of just institutions will more than sufficiently warrant bars to most democratically generated restrictions and regulations of the franchise—even if voting is not given the same rank of importance as Constitutional rights. *Reynolds v. Sims* reaches the right result.

34. For a related argument to this end, see Ronald Dworkin, *Taking Rights Seriously* (Cambridge, MA: Harvard Univ. Press, 1977), p. 233.

35. This argument is similar to an argument that Dworkin makes only in passing to the effect that in many cases counting a person's external political preferences (say, for some group not to get some scarce resource,

when the person does not want or need the resource for himself) will simply be self-defeating from a utilitarian standpoint (p. 235 middle). I do not wish to commit my argument to Dworkin's assumptions that the right to treatment as an equal is the most fundamental of rights (p. 273) and that taking external preferences into account in social policy is wrong as violating that right (pp. 234–235, 275–276).

Even the necessary proviso in any utilitarian justification for democracy that each person's preferences are to count for one can be justified in purely utilitarian terms without appeals to general principles of equality. For, given the presumption that we are only considering conscious homo sapiens as voters and are not including in the franchise, say, comatose individuals or especially sensitive creatures from space, and given that people are more equal than unequal in their sensitivity and in the volume of their desires, then it seems likely that assigning one non-weighted vote to each will be a more accurate gauge in general of overall preference than if we try to establish some (unimaginable) mechanism to weight votes for small variations in either sensitivities or intensities of preferences.

36. So correctly Dworkin, p. 255, but contrast p. 276 (bottom), where it is claimed that the mechanisms of democracy are incapable of winnowing internal and external preferences. In the latter passage, though, Dworkin simply runs together the mechanisms of direct democracy and representational democracy. The numerous cases in which city councils have passed gay civil rights legislation only to have it overturned by vast margins in referenda would suggest that legislators can on occasion raise above the prejudices of their constituents. The solution to the problem is not to abandon all hope that legislatures might effect a refined utilitarianism, opting instead for a democratic system awash in prejudices and checked only by Constitutional immunities. The solution is for the Court to resurrect the Guarantee Clause of the Constitution (Art. IV, sect 4) from the deadletter status to which it was assigned in *Baker v. Carr*, 369 U.S. 186, 224 (1962) and to void most referenda procedures.

37. I disagree with Dworkin that external preferences are no "less a source of pleasure when satisfied and displeasure when ignored, than purely personal preferences" (p. 276). The pleasure of external preferences satisfied is illusory in intensity. For such pleasures are parasitic upon a mere perceived *contrast* of one's situation to that of another's—and are not consequences of anything one has done or experienced on one's own. Such pleasures have a similar status to the mere absences or cessations of pains. We can discount such pleasures *even on a utilitarian account*. Again, we need not resort to a theory of rights to rid the utilitarian calculus of external preferences; see n. 35 *supra*.

38. See Dworkin, pp. 235, 277 top. Whatever the moral worth of the altruist's acts and their masochistic pleasures, the intensity of the pleasures is again illusory based not upon anything that one's self has accomplished or experienced directly.

39. Donald Webster Cory [pseud.], *The Homosexual in America* (New York: Greenberg, 1951), p. 14. For the strange history of "Donald Webster Cory," subsequently the antigay polemicist Edward Sagarin, see D'Emilio, pp. 33, 57, 98, 139, 167–169.

40. Thus during the 1985 nationally televised Academy Awards, a seemingly ingenuous presenter could describe a documentary on the assassination of an activist gay elected-official (see n. 9 *supra*) merely as "a film about American values in conflict," *GayLife*, 10:39, March 28, 1985, X, p. 1. Had the film not won the award, no one in the audience of millions not already in the know would have learned that the film even had a gay content. As it was, the award recepients made mention only of their subject's pride, not his death, while those in the know were left with the suspicion that the Academy supposes that killing gays is an "American value."

AIDS Discrimination: Its Nature, Meaning, and Function

David I. Schulman

AIDS IS LIKE A stain on a microscopic slide, highlighting preexisting chronic social problems the way a stain brings into sharp relief the characteristics of certain organisms. For those resistant to confronting such problems—drug abuse or inequitable health care delivery, for example—there is a temptation to attribute them to AIDS, as if our resolution of these issues had been effective until AIDS destroyed our social stability.

AIDS discrimination laws prohibit people from treating AIDS as an exception to all social norms, as the cause of social ills it merely exacerbates. The policy crises surrounding AIDS may force society to adjust those norms. But AIDS discrimination laws require that society adjust all like behavior equally, not merely single AIDS out for exception.

Epidemics threaten the ties that bind communities together, driving societies to victimize some to bind back together the rest. Yet law can help overcome this ancient human impulse to fracture in times of crisis. This article examines several ways to do just that regarding AIDS.

It first discusses the nature of AIDS discrimination and draws lessons from the work of those first charged with enforcing AIDS discrimination laws. It then briefly examines two emerging AIDS

David I. Schulman, Supervising Attorney, AIDS/HIV Discrimination Unit, Los Angeles City Attorney's Office, "AIDS Discrimination: Its Nature, Meaning, and Function," *Nova Law Review*, 12 (1988): 1113–1140. Reprinted by Permission of the Author and the *Nova Law Review*.

legal issues, the special problems posed by recalcitrant HIV-infected individuals who knowingly place others at unreasonable risk of infection, and the problems presented by those who are both infected with HIV and mentally ill. The article then comments upon the role of law in fashioning effective AIDs education programs.

This article concludes, in the section entitled "The Threat of AIDS Euthanasia," with an analysis of the potential impact of AIDS upon health care delivery. It examines the depersonalizing nature of institutionally based chronic care and proposes a new public-private partnership to combat its effects, a partnership designed to deinstitutionalize chronic care.

Throughout the article, the underlying theme is the importance of looking clearly and in new ways at the challenges which lie before us in responding fully and humanly to AIDS.

I. The Nature of AIDS Discrimination[1]

AIDS discrimination is like other forms of discrimination familiar to Americans insofar as it is the unfair treatment of individuals based upon irrational fears and prejudices about groups. However, since AIDS discrimination varies in unique respects from other types of discrimination, its character must be carefully examined and new efforts created to overcome its particular divisive and destructive effects.

American society has learned that deeply embedded prejudices against race, for example, are difficult to alter by education alone; they usually require new, positive life experiences, as well before such attitudes change. But, Los Angeles's, New York's, and San Francisco's AIDS discrimination units have discovered that prejudices against people with AIDS can be dramatically reversed with education about the medical facts of AIDS. However, the staff of these units have also learned about the immense fears about AIDS which block comprehension of the basic medical facts. They have learned that fears about AIDS as a disease and AIDS as the harbinger of social disorder must be addressed before the fight against AIDS discrimination can be truly successful.

A. Fear of the Disease

The fear of AIDS as a disease is fivefold. Each express a powerful social taboo which, by its very nature, must be overcome since taboos protect individuals from deep-seated fears.[2]

The first fear concerns human sexuality. American society's difficulty in public discussion about sexual matters is signaled by the continued lack of consensus about the content of sexual education in the public schools despite thirty years' debate. It is, of course, also signaled by the deep divisions in the nation over gay rights. Yet learning the medical facts necessary to halt HIV's spread requires frank public discussion about sexual activities.

The second fear involves stigma.[3] It is one of the cruelest ironies of the epidemic that its impact is greatest among those already stigmatized: gay men and intravenous drug abusers (many of whom are black or brown).[4] Labeling some groups dangerous, unclean, or aberrant functions to externalize what is feared by the normative group.

Projecting what is feared outside the normative social group strengthens its social bonds during times of social crisis, such as epidemics, when those bonds are threatened. It does so, however, at the expense of the nonnormative groups. In a democratic society, where equal rights are guaranteed for all, this primal impulse to stigmatize presents a tremendous challenge, for neither stigmatizing nor the wholesale isolation of others halted the spread of bubonic plague, leprosy, or syphilis, and there is no reason to believe that it would halt the spread of AIDS.[5]

Worse, stigmatizing others obstructs the social cooperation necessary to control the epidemic's further spread; infected people identified as "them" and treated punitively naturally become less willing to contribute voluntarily to the social efforts needed for control.[6] The majority group's disapproval of stigmatized groups' characteristics and habits also obstructs the delivery of education necessary to halt the spread of the virus among these groups. People of color, for instance, have complained that AIDS education efforts are often ineffective because, by ignoring crucial cultural differences, they impede those at risk from effectively comprehending and utilizing the information.

For example, too many efforts have relied heavily on written material despite the high illiteracy rates among blacks and Hispanics. Too little material has been available in Spanish. Material directed at gays cannot educate about stopping HIV's spread if it is predicated on the assumption that gays should not be gays. Fear of stigmatized groups, then, intensifies the epidemic through its divisiveness at a time when social cooperation is essential.

The third fear is the fear of being helpless. Despite government entitlement programs, many continue to presume that people should take care of themselves and that families and communities should take care of their own. Yet despite the persistent nature of this presumption,[7] society's sense of community has eroded, so that when people do need each other when they become sick, truly human caring is difficult to arrange. Yet AIDS demands that society create new ways to mobilize communities' capacity to provide care, comfort, and medical treatment,[8] especially since the emerging AIDS treatment modalities like AZT will prolong the lives of those who are ill but, tragically, exacerbate the epidemic's growing numbers.

The fourth fear concerns mental illness. Society has never resolved its ambivalence and fears about the mentally ill. Yet AIDS potentially will create vast numbers of HIV-demented individuals requiring care from mental health care systems, exacerbated, as well, by the accomplishments of medical treatment modalities.[9]

The fifth fear—death—has always, of course, been the most overwhelming. Yet death has uniquely modern overlays which make it even more difficult to think or talk about today. Death was once part of everyday life, a family and communal event regularly witnessed by everyone. With modern medicine's advances, however, it has been removed to specialized institutions. Experts care for the dying. Experts bury the dead. Most Americans never see a corpse except in carefully cosmeticized viewings before burial.

Whereas death used to occur rapidly from illness, accident, old age, or assault, today's medical prowess prolongs life until death occurs slowly, in increasingly debilitating stages. Since infections can now be fought off with antibiotics, it is slow, lingering death, isolated from community and family, ministered by technically competent professionals, which Americans dread. As society's response to death becomes increasingly phobic, so, too, is the response to those infected with an incurable, invariably fatal disease. They force, after all, an unwelcome recognition of one's own mortality, with its anticipation of a comfortless death.

B. Fear of Social Disorder

The fear of social disorder can be as primal as the fear of death, for it is the fear of chaos. Epidemics can obstruct or even halt the normal functioning of society. Afflicted people drop out of work force, removing their economic contributions from society. At the same time, they strain societal resources for they need medical care, food, shelter and companionship.

As more and more places fall empty in the social structure, panicked people place their individual survival needs over the social obligation to cooperate with others: social relationships collapse, people abandon relatives, there is mass hysteria and mob looting.[10]

In all times past, when disorder and panic threatened the ties that bind, law and force were used to blame, isolate, and scapegoat the stigmatized to bind together the normative group. Focusing social panic onto already stigmatized groups is an ancient and primary response. America's national character reflected this shameful impulse as recently as World War II when the United States Supreme Court upheld the scapegoating and isolating of Japanese-Americans as a means of dealing with our fear of war.[11]

Civil rights thinking, however, has evolved since the Second World War. That development is not the product of "special interests" intent upon fracturing the whole, as some suggest. Rather, America's maturing understanding of civil rights is a remarkable bulwark today against the ancient impulse to victimize others; these recent advancements are as remarkable and critical for enabling America to withstand the impact of AIDS as are recent advancements in science.

Civil rights will not provide easy answers to the agonizing policy questions presented by AIDS. But civil rights cannot "give way" to the "demands" of public health, as some insist, for both civil rights and public health laws seek to ensure the vitality of the body politic.

Since the great racial struggles began thirty-five years ago, civil rights law has become a process which teaches Americans how to be civil, even when they are frightened, indeed, especially when they are frightened. Events such as AIDS remind people of epidemics past, of battles of each against all for scarce resources, of how, as Camus observed, "officialdom can never cope with something really catastrophic."[12]

But today, for the first time, civil rights reminds American society of something else.[13] An archaic form of the word "remember" is "re-member," to bring all members back into the whole. Civil rights enable American citizens to re-member those who are unpopular, those who are disenfranchised, even those who are frightening, remember that in a democratic society all are members of the whole.

II. AIDS Discrimination Laws

A. *Introduction*

Randy Shilts, in his landmark study of the early years of AIDS in America, marked the end of the epidemic's first great cultural wave with Rock Hudson's announcement that he had the disease in July 1985.[14] One month later, Los Angeles City Councilmember Joel Wachs successfully led a drive to enact the nation's first AIDS discrimination measure, undoubtedly aided by the favorable climate created by the movie star's announcement. Los Angeles' new law,[15] passed unanimously by the City Council, began AIDS' second great cultural wave, that of policy-based responses to the epidemic.[16]

The national impact of the council's action was immediate and widespread. Network news programs covered the event and *The New York Times* endorsed the measure.[17] The Los Angeles City Attorney's Office, given enforcement powers under the ordinance, was flooded with complaints under the new law and complaints about the new law. Letters to the editor appeared in the local press reflecting elation at the enlightened action of the council and terror at the prospect that the new law would force thousands to be exposed unwillingly to the disease.[18]

Los Angeles's law was the first statute to provide clear and unambiguous discrimination protection for people infected with the AIDS virus (HIV). Many attorneys had already anticipated that the analytical concepts of physical handicap rights law applied well to the dilemmas presented by HIV. In fact, litigation was already underway to determine whether people with AIDS were to be included within California's housing and physical handicap rights protections at the time of the council's action.[19]

Los Angeles's action provided critical leadership at a time when no other legislative or executive body was prepared to enact into law what scientists had known for some time, that HIV could not be casually transmitted.

Normally, legal measures regarding epidemics emanate from the federal government, reflecting the widespread nature of an epidemic. It is emblematic of the madness of the social phenomenon surrounding AIDS, however, that the process was reversed— a municipal government first incorporated scientific knowledge into social policy.[20]

B. Structure[21]

Los Angeles officials wisely fashioned their ordinance upon familiar principles of physical handicap law, for this enabled attorneys unfamiliar with the arcana of HIV to share a familiar vocabulary—*reasonable accommodation, otherwise qualified, bona fide occupational qualification*—no small comfort when first confronting the tidal wave impact of AIDS upon law. It also enabled citizens to recognize the council's action within a familiar social framework.

In the months that followed Los Angeles's action, four California cities followed suit.[22] Since then, many states have re-interpreted their physical handicap protections to include people with AIDS and a number of additional cities in California and elsewhere have passed AIDS-specific statutes. Most importantly, a series of federal court rulings have held AIDS to be a protected handicap under federal law.[23]

AIDS discrimination laws, whether AIDS-specific or part of a general physical handicap scheme, are similarly structured. Besides people infected with HIV, they usually protect people wrongly thought to be infected with HIV, since handicapped rights protections are intended to prohibit the irrational injury of any individual because of prejudice about physical disabilities. The classic example involves people recovered from cancer. Such people fortunately are no longer handicapped. However, irrational employers frightened of cancer might still wish to discriminate against them were they not entitled to handicapped rights protections.

So too, AIDS discrimination laws protect people who might be associated with irrational fears about AIDS, people like family members, care-givers, and gay men. The widow of a man who died of AIDS only agreed to appear on television to discuss the prejudice she and her husband had faced when the producers of the program arranged for her to be filmed in shadow and allowed her to use a pseudonym.[24] This widow, although uninfected, is entitled to the full range of protections afforded by laws such as Los Angeles's should she continue to suffer further discrimination.

The forerunners of Los Angeles's law was the physical handicap civil rights protections of the Federal Rehabilitation Act of 1973, enacted by Congress at the end of the activist civil rights era, after the racial struggles and the beginnings of the women's movement. Most states soon followed Congress's action with similar statutes regarding private employment, housing, public accommodations,[25] and state government activity.[26] Los Angeles's AIDS discrimination law, and all other AIDS-specific statutes and executive orders which followed, drew directly upon the constitutional framework of these earlier physical handicap projections.

That framework established the fundamental assumption that society wished to treat people in decisions about jobs and services as free individuals, unimpaired by others' irrational beliefs and attitudes. Physical handicap laws and their sub-set, AIDS discrimination laws, require that decisions must be based upon sound medical evidence applied in a fair and equal manner. Professors Larry Gostin and William Curran, Harvard School of Public Health, have recently considered the level of scrutiny courts should apply in weighing and balancing the rights these laws create and the duties public health measures entail.[27]

Gostin and Curran argue that scientific and constitutional understandings have sharpened considerably since the early part of the century (when most current public health statutes and rulings were formulated). Originally, only a rational basis was necessary for a public health statute to pass constitutional muster, for the power to regulate public health was understood to emanate from the police powers of the state to ensure safety and security. Even by the turn of the century, however, courts had already begun to scrutinize much more closely both the scientific basis for the statute and the appropriateness of the methods to be used to achieve its end. The case of Jew Ho v. Williamson[28] is illustrative.

Plague broke out in the Chinatown area of San Francisco. The authorities imposed a quarantine around the region, a rational measure to control the epidemic's spread. However, the exact boundaries drawn by San Francisco's public health officials were gerrymandered to include the homes of Chinese residents living outside the area of outbreak and to exclude the homes of Caucasians living within the area. The health authorities argued that this action was rational, given the likely associational patterns involved in transmission. The Jew Ho court held, however, that this argument was insufficient to justify the level of government intrusion imposed by quarantine.

Gostin and Curran argue that courts today should impose a heightened level of scrutiny to determine the constitutionality of public health measures which affect constitutional or statutorily defined rights. Such measures must not be justified merely by the importance of achieving a public health end. Because public health measures interfere with fundamental rights—such as the right to associate freely and to maintain privacy, measures which also ensure a healthy body politic—such measures today need to have ends and means that fit tightly.

No one would argue, however, that civil rights protections should sanction unsafe situations; such laws must never give one the right to place others at unreasonable risk to their health.[29] What is critical, however, is the rationality of the analysis. When the burden on others to protect themselves from infection is minimal—as in the case of blood-borne infectious agents such as HIV—then one should not refuse to take those precautions and insist, instead, upon imposing more onerous burdens on those infected.[30]

When the burden on others to protect themselves from infection is unreasonable—as in the case of airborne agents, which would require that everyone wear masks all the time to avoid exposure— then one may burden those infected, even to the extent of restricting their freedoms. Los Angeles demonstrated this commitment to balancing when it amended its law in June 1986[31] to incorporate the workplace guidelines,[32] issued by the federal government's Centers for Disease Control three months after the law's enactment, to provide guidelines for risk prevention in the workplace.

AIDS discrimination laws hold that if people infected with HIV merely present health threats others can reasonably avoid, then the burden is on others to take those precautions, rather than violate infected people's fundamental rights. If HIV-infected individuals are otherwise physically capable of continuing to perform their jobs, they have a right to keep working.

The test for continued suitability of employment, as in all physical handicap rights contexts, is whether the person with HIV is *otherwise qualified* to perform the task. For example, an individual in a wheelchair who can still type and answer phones has a right to continue working as a secretary. Employers or service providers must *reasonably accommodate* the special needs created by the handicap. They cannot say, "You are fired because your chair won't fit behind the desk"; they have the duty to move the desk away from the wall. However, musical directors need not cancel their tap dance numbers. Being able to tap dance is a *bona fide occupational qualification* of that particular job; people in wheelchairs are not *otherwise qualified* to tap dance.

If HIV-infected people begin to perform their jobs poorly, they are to be judged by the standards we use to judge others who begin to perform their jobs poorly. Perhaps they should be transferred to less demanding positions. Perhaps they should be retrained. Perhaps they should be warned about poor performance, with review rights and appeals. But it is important to remember that we already have guidelines and standards for dealing with people whose job performance deteriorates. Individuals divorce, abuse alcohol or drugs, suffer from Alzheimer's and other diseases. Discrimination laws insist that we treat HIV-infected people similarly to others in similar positions. If HIV-infected individuals require reasonable accommodation, then we must accord them the same rights and privileges we accord others who require reasonable accommodation such as permission to work at home or flexible hours to accommodate changes in energy level.

The inclination, however, is to treat AIDS as a special case, an exception to the rule. A nursing director at a medical center said she allowed pregnant nurses to opt out of treating HIV patients. "This was not discriminatory, however, HIV-infected patients are at high risk for cytomegalovirus (CMV). Pregnant nurses should avoid exposure to CMV. Therefore, it is rational to let them opt out of HIV care." She was asked "Do they have the same right to opt out of pediatrics care? Isn't it true that there is an equally high prevalence of CMV among children?" The nurses did not have a similar right. The seemingly rational basis of CMV risk masked the irrational fear of providing care for people with HIV. It might be reasonable to argue that pregnant nurses should not work with either HIV-infected people or sick children. But it is not reasonable to have a policy which excuses them from one population and not the other.

C. Remedies and Enforcement

AIDS discrimination laws provide for traditional discrimination remedies. Injunctive court orders can be sought by city attorneys and by private attorneys to halt discriminatory practices.[33] Private attorneys can seek damages for their clients to recompense for injury, but city attorneys cannot.[34]

Early in the Los Angeles City Attorney's experience with the new law, the need to develop nontraditional methods of enforcement was soon recognized.[35] Initially, four deputy city attorneys with full-time assignments elsewhere handled inquiries and complaints on their overtime. They reviewed over fifty discrimination complaints and began to forge a philosophy of early intervention and mediation. One case demonstrated the importance of prohibiting discrimination even against people who are not infected. A local health club attempted to refund the membership fee of a skinny gay member (who it turned out, was not infected) because of pressure from other club members. They were concerned that since he was skinny and gay, he must have "it." Through early intervention and education, the City Attorney's Office was able to resolve the case without litigation.

These volunteer attorneys eventually determined, however, that they did not have the time to develop the technical expertise necessary to address the myriad questions being posed, particularly the core questions about virus transmission. In December 1985, the City Attorney successfully sought the creation of a full-time deputy city attorney position to enforce the new law.

During my first six months, I reviewed fifty-three complaints, held three hearings, responded to fifty-eight community and professional inquiries and twenty-three media contacts, attended thirty-six professional or community meetings, and spoke to nineteen groups, including the Los Angeles County Medical Association, the Gay and Lesbian Chapter of the ACLU of Southern California, the Screen Actors Guild, and to community and professional representatives of the Hispanic community. Our office assisted the California Continuing Education of the Bar Institute to create two-day AIDS and law conferences for lawyers. During my first full year, I reviewed ninety-three complaints, held five hearings, handled one hundred and twenty community and professional inquiries, responded to forty-eight media contacts, attended seventy-five meetings, and spoke to forty different groups.

During the first five months of my second year, the number of complaints fell by almost half to twenty-four and I held only one hearing, but the number of community and professional inquiries more than doubled to one hundred and five. The number of media contacts (twenty-six) remained about the same, the number of meetings dropped (twenty-five), and the number of speaking engagements increased to twenty-nine. Hopefully, the reason for the drop in complaints was directly attributable to the outreach efforts.[36] I also coordinated the creation of a model AIDS education project to be required as a condition of probation for anyone convicted of a misdemeanor drug or sex crime, assisted the Los Angeles County Bar Association in the creation of a volunteer lawyer referral service for people with HIV, and participated in a City Attorney Crimes of Hate Task Force to deal with the rise in incidence of attacks on gay men.

In response to complaints that dentists were not accepting AIDS patients, I held a hearing that brought together leaders from the local dental professional associations, professors from the dental schools at UCLA and USC, and AIDS medical experts. We hammered out a concensus which led to the local professional associations creating a coalition committed to teaching dentists proper infection control techniques, combating AIDS fears among dentists, and raising money for a local AIDS dental clinic.

Another case involved a man who worked in an accounting unit of a large Los Angeles medical center. A twelve-year employee, he had recently returned from an AIDS-related medical leave of absence to face rumors flying about his work center regarding his condition. Nasty notes were left on his desk, telephones were sprayed with disinfectant, and he was shunned. I contacted the corporate counsel for the medical center and discovered that an AIDS education program had been initiated in the company but had not yet reached the accounting unit. Counsel agreed to schedule a session for this unit immediately and, the following week, the man reported that the atmosphere had been transformed. I later discovered that this man had been deeply involved in setting up a job fair for his local church parish and died the week before the fair began. However, he had finished all the organizing details and the fair was dedicated to his memory. A friend of his reported that without a doubt the extra few months of peace at work had enabled him to make this one last gesture of giving to others.

Comparing cases and strategies, my colleagues in New York and San Francisco and I agree upon several common themes. We had each observed how useful our laws[37] were in stimulating interest in the community in learning about AIDS among many previously unaware,[38] if for no other good reason than the fear of breaking the law. We had also learned the critical importance of emphasizing early intervention and medication of complaints.

AIDS discrimination complaints are particularly ill-suited to the adversarial process. The stress of litigation is unhealthy for everyone, but particularly for those infected with HIV, whose major lifestyle change must include a reduction in stress. Furthermore, people with AIDS often will not survive the time protracted litigation can take, even with expedited court procedures.[39]

The negotiating posture of AIDS discrimination cases is also different from other discrimination cases. AIDS discrimination complainants in the typical employment-related case are often prepared to settle if their health coverage is guaranteed, whereas others are prepared to wait until a full cash settlement for all damages is reached, for most HIV-infected people will become too sick to support themselves until a full settlement is reached and may not survive at all. Furthermore, HIV-infected people often cannot risk the further stigma and discrimination to which litigation threatens to expose them, even with the confidentiality safeguards available to litigants.[40]

AIDS discrimination suits also risk creating adverse public reactions, since they involve issues which are anxiety-provoking. For example, there was a great deal of backlash, confusion, and polarization of opinion following the Justice Department memorandum issued in June 1986[41] holding that discriminatory actions based upon irrational fears of contagion were not prohibited by the Federal Rehabilitation Act of 1973. That opinion was issued in response to a Department of Health and Human Services request for guidance on the applicability of federal law in that regard. Similarly, the *Markowski* blood-selling case[42] and the *Jasperson* nail salon case[43] raised a great deal of consternation, even as both suits sought to establish important rights.

Moreover, the employment protection provision of California's municipal ordinances are extremely vulnerable to challenges asserting that they are preempted by state law.[44] Plaintiffs' attorneys proceeding under these provisions face the risk that a procedural ruling sustaining a preemption challenge would be misinterpreted by the public as a substantive ruling on the merits of such protections, further compounding the public's confusion and mistrust of public authorities regarding AIDS (a confusion and mistrust regularly manipulated by some who claim concern about AIDS).[45]

Finally, the opportunity for litigation is further curtailed for government offices, since their enforcement powers are limited to filing injunctive relief actions.[46] Such actions not only require a higher burden of proof than an action for damages, they also require a fact situation suitable to an order for injunctive relief, an order often made unnecessary through negotiation, and in the case of personal services, thought by some[47] to be insupportable as a matter of law.

These problems are no secret to defense attorneys in AIDS discrimination cases. They are, however, the other major reasons, aside from the success of early intervention and mediation, why AIDS discrimination cases rarely go to court.

But defense attorneys, fully taking the range of tactical truths about AIDS cases into account, can integrate competent representation with compassionate understanding. For example, a twenty-seven-year-old woman with a degenerative neurological condition could no longer live on her own despite regular visits from a social worker and a home health aide. The intermediate care facility which had accepted her for placement refused to admit her when it learned she was HIV-infected. The bruise on the woman's head from a fall she had suffered attested to the need for a rapid resolution to her problem.

When she filed a complaint with the City Attorney's Office, I quickly investigated the matter and contacted the facility's attorney. This attorney was thoroughly familiar with AIDS legal issues and could have advised his client to contest the matter as a defense tactic so that the woman could have won the legal battle and lost her war to find a safe environment quickly. Instead, this practitioner aggressively educated his client about the legal duties involved, the practical measures to be taken to implement HIV-related procedures, and arranged placement for the woman in a matter of days.

D. Conclusions and Recommendations

1. Policymakers must take into account the unique strategic aspects of AIDS discrimination cases, and fashion appropriate remedies emphasizing alternative dispute resolution. For example, hospitals should offer binding arbitration to HIV-infected patients to resolve promptly breaches in confidentiality which might quickly mushroom into a discrimination case.

2. AIDS discrimination laws with effective enforcement mechanisms are vital at all three levels of government—federal, state and local. It is an extremely useful negotiating tool for local government attorneys to have powerful state and federal investigative agencies backing them up, particularly when they can indicate in good faith that these agencies are prepared to accept locally negotiated settlements as settlements in full of potential state and federal claims. But sometimes, only highly flexible, locally based government units can intervene quickly and draw on local relationships of mutual trust and respect to ensure successful rapid resolution of AIDS discrimination cases.

3. AIDS discrimination legislation at the state and federal level must contain language which ensures that local laws are not voided on pre-emption grounds. Otherwise, courts may hold that state or federal regulations so thoroughly occupy the field of AIDS discrimination that local jurisdictions may not also regulate the area.

4. Government AIDS discrimination units must firmly commit to community outreach education programs which can prevent AIDS discrimination cases from occurring in the first place.

5. Local government attorneys must draw on local trust relationships to carry AIDS education programs to segments of the community otherwise resistant to such information.

6. Impact litigation is essential in strategically appropriate cases to establish needed case law and send a message to those in the community who would not otherwise comply with applicable legal standards.

III. Recalcitrant Individuals

It is beyond the scope of this article to examine thoroughly the issue of "recalcitrants," those HIV-infected individuals who put others at an unreasonable risk of infection. However, a brief examination of the dynamics surrounding a highly publicized case in California illumines the complexities of this issue.

In June 1987, Joseph Markowski was arrested while attempting to sell his HIV-infected blood to a plasma center and was charged with attempted-murder by the District Attorney.[48] Ironically, several months before, AIDS activists had brought intense pressure to bear on the California Association of Local Health Officers when they learned that the organization was reviewing draft guidelines regarding recalcitrants.

California law, as well as many other jurisdictions, assigns virtual absolute authority to public health officers regarding control of recalcitrants. However, these statutes had rarely been used since the nineteen twenties, and the California association wanted to develop internal guidelines to ensure a uniform response throughout the state. The activists opposed this process on the basis that it was immoral to devote resources to a negligible factor in the spread of AIDS at a time when many more effective public health educational measures had yet to be implemented.

Markowski changed the position of many of the activists in a hurry. Upon seeing the frightened public response to the case, they soon argued that such matters should be handled confidentially by public health officials rather than prosecutors. Prior to Markowski, these activists had failed to recognize that the government's duty to act varies radically, depending on whether people are merely sick or present a threat to others.

One of government's most fundamental functions is the preservation of public order. Definition of that order is open to debate. But the vision of a man, no matter how helpless and desperate, selling AIDS-infected blood to a plasma center, no matter what the heat-processing procedures of the center might be, carried the sort of primal sense of threat which must be accounted for in any AIDS analysis.

Andrew Moss, an epidemiologist at the University of California, San Francisco, acknowledged the need for this accounting at a conference on AIDS cosponsored by UCSF and the Society for Health and Human Values.[49] Dr. Moss stated that the San Francisco Public Health Officer's delay in making his decision about San Francisco's bathhouses damaged the public's trust in the willingness of officials to act. Moss theorized that government inaction had created in the public's mind a perception of a leadership vacuum, a perception creating intolerable conditions of fear for the public.

Yet the criminal justice system is a poor place for dealing with public health matters. It is adversarial and, in matters of HIV transmission, requires evidence-gathering intrusions into intimate matters. The issues involved in charging someone criminally with recalcitrant behavior regarding the virus's spread sets us apart, one against another, concerning a social crisis which requires communal responses. In dealing with recalcitrants, society must, amidst the other demands of the epidemic, find ways to do so which address the legitimate need for a sense of safety without furthering polarizing the community.

IV. HIV, Mental Disabilities and Civil Liberties

Our ambivalences and fears about the mentally ill have never been resolved. Yet HIV-demented people will vastly swell the ranks of the mentally ill. The vision of mentally ill people infectious for a deadly disease could lead to a deterioration in public attitudes toward all people with mental illness. This is particularly likely if hysteria explodes because the public first learns of the overwhelming implications of HIV neurological destruction from sensationalistic mass media coverage rather than from responsible public officials.[50]

The numbers of HIV individuals requiring mental health care will rise in part because immunological treatment modalities are quite likely to improve, enabling individuals to live longer but in the process raising the likelihood of eventual mental impairment. This rise in numbers will also result from the likelihood that some number of those HIV-infected who are immunologically resistant will eventually go on to develop neurological difficulties. These rising numbers will further burden already straining mental health and chronic care facilities and raise vast problems in law regarding competency and intent.

The challenge this aspect of the epidemic poses can only be dimly perceived. One likelihood is the restigmatization of all who are mentally ill once the public comes to associate some mentally disabled with infectiousness for a deadly disease. A second is the likelihood of the creation of separate and unequal institutional care facilities for those whose handicaps are non-HIV-based and those who are demented or neurologically disabled and HIV-infectious. A third is an acceleration of the crisis in institutionally based chronic care as more come to perceive the structural inadequacies of such institutions.[51]

HIV-demented individuals involuntarily committed to custodial facilities raise a chilling set of constitutional rights problems. Has the institution the right to test for presence of the virus without consent? How will others involuntarily committed into the same setting protect themselves from infection? What level of due process rights should be available to employees of these institutions as well as to those committed? How does the presence in these institutions of those committed because of recalcitrant behavior regarding spread of the virus affect these questions?[52] And how can our answers to these questions abide by our fundamental constitutional commitment not to create separate and unequal facilities?[53]

V. Fashioning an Education Program to Combat Discrimination[54]

Teaching about the duties that we learn from the law can make learning the medical facts about AIDS easier. When we understand our duties to others regarding confidentiality and discrimination, we learn behavior which reinforces clear medical messages about AIDS. Our experience in Los Angeles helping to implement the City of Los Angeles' AIDS education program for its 33,000 employees has confirmed this.

Unlike most other AIDS education programs, ours has two goals. All programs seek to teach about preventing further spread of HIV. But the program mandated by the Los Angeles City Council on October 13, 1987, gained Surgeon General C. Everett Koop's praise because it also requires education about AIDS legal issues: how to ensure confidentiality in the workplace, prevent discrimination, and protect against liability.

The program began with special briefing sessions for elected officials and department heads to make sure there would be knowledgeable leadership. AIDS task forces are being created within each department to coordinate workplace education and problem-solving efforts. Each department has been ordered by the Council to accomplish three objectives: educate its employees; review and revise all policies and procedures in light of AIDS medical and legal information; and adapt daily department interactions with the community to further public education about AIDS. An illustration from the Department of Transportation provides a good example of the program's potential impact.

Drivers in city programs to transport the disabled learned in training sessions that it is illegal to refuse to transport people with HIV. Instead of merely being told that, however, with the resentment and misunderstanding that can create, everyone was taught why. No precautions are necessary to prevent the spread of AIDS in the normal course of transportation, since transmission requires infected blood or semen to have direct contact with another individual's blood system. Should a passenger bleed or vomit (which might contain blood), drivers were taught to clean up the mess or assist the passenger only after donning gloves to create a barrier against the virus entering through possible cuts or abrasions on the hands—and *always* to don the gloves.

The drivers learned what everyone must—that they need not know who has AIDS and who does not since their lawful and medically safe action should be the same in either case: Use gloves to clean up all blood or vomit. Passengers who question the use of gloves learn accurate medical information about HIV transmission from the drivers. Gay men or intravenous drug users who might otherwise feel singled out will not since everyone receives similar treatment. The likelihood of HIV transmission in such a setting is tiny. But gloves are a reasonable response to just that tiny theoretical possibility some have urged as justification for more tyrannical measures against people with HIV. Everyone learns that protection of an individual's rights and the public's health adds up to the same thing—reason and fairness.

VI. The Threat of AIDS Euthanasia[55]

A. *Introduction*

Perhaps the greatest form of discrimination is to feel dismembered, cut off from all hope. The impersonal nature of institutionally based chronic care has already raised immense dilemmas in this regard for American society. Rather than feeling remembered as respected members of the human family, many individuals, often in concert with personal physicians, are quietly choosing to curtail treatments and end their lives rather than endure further pain and hardship from chronic illness and disease. Such decisions may be rational when viewed from the perspective of the individual. When viewed from a policy perspective, however, the conditions leading to such decisions warrant reexamination. When the mounting toll of the AIDS epidemic threatens to increase the numbers of such individuals manyfold, a continued unwillingness to consider altering the underlying conditions of such a problem amounts to a de facto policy of euthanasia.

Since the Quinlan[56] case first brought to the nation's attention in 1976 the profound issue of when we "pull the plug," remarkable changes have occurred in our attitudes toward death and in the balance of power between individuals and health care institutions. The holding in the 1986 Bouvia[57] case would have been unimaginable before *Quinlan*—that competent adults may refuse medical care even if doing so ends life. Yet the standard enunciated in Bouvia is emerging as a basic doctrine regarding the right to medical treatment.

Hospice has evolved since Quinlan as an alternative care philosophy for the terminally ill, offering humane care in the home made possible through the coordinated effort of interdisciplinary professional teams, family, friends and trained support volunteers. During this time, too, new legal devices like living wills and durable powers of attorney have also emerged, strengthening one's capacity to choose the kind of care desired.

While emerging legal standards, hospice, and durable powers of attorney strengthen one's autonomy and control over the depersonalizing aspects of institutionally based chronic care, other developments since *Quinlan* are altering the power relationships between individuals and institutions in ways that are not so benign. DRG's (diagnostically related groups), a new reimbursement scheme, assign lump sum payments based on the category of ailment rather than upon actual services rendered, creating incentives for physicians to mass produce medical care rather than tailor it to individuals' unique needs. Such new systems of health care delivery as pre-paid plans and health maintenance organizations also create institutional pressures upon physicians regarding individual care decisions.

B. The Problem of Chronic Care

The problem of chronic care has its root in the tremendous increase in acute care effectiveness in the twentieth century. That success has been marked by a phenomenal rise in the power and scope of medicine's capacity to overcome medical trauma. This power has emerged from the efficiency of institutionalized professional care, coordinated with sophisticated technological advancements. This rise in the power and scope of medicine, however, has altered the rate of morbidity. A century ago, and forever before, most individuals died rapidly of trauma or infection. The late twentieth century is the first era in which most will survive to die slowly from a new host of repressive causes brought forth because of the survival rate from acute disease made possible by medicine's power.

It is not surprising, then, to discover that America's early attempts to deal with the new issues of chronic care would be modeled upon the decisions made regarding care of the elderly, choosing institutionalized professionally dominated modes. Yet chronic care is not amenable to the institutionally based combination of technique and management so successful in acute care settings. Chronic care requires a fundamentally different response, one grounded in the meaning and solidarity of community, family and friends.

One's broken leg needs to be set expertly and fast, and the patient may not suffer overmuch from brusque orthodpedic surgeons and nurses forcing him or her to take one's temperature every three hours.

However, the dynamics of care for the chronically ill are far different. Altering senses of self, particularly of loss, must be addressed. In chronic illness, especially degenerative illness, mental, physical, and emotional health interact in complex interweavings relating to senses of control, autonomy, dependence, involvement, and the fear of abandonment.

C. The Dying Process, AIDS, and Euthanasia

For those suffering irreversible, degenerative illness, all rationalizations about future benefit and present discomfort come to naught, means and ends come resoundingly together. It is not surprising, then, that the logical inconsistency of the acute care model and the chronic care condition should be felt most acutely by the dying. Institutional care, predicated necessarily upon the needs of institutions for procedures and rules, conflicts fundamentally with the needs of dying individuals for meaning now. This conflict when combined with AIDS creates the frightening preconditions for a policy of de facto euthanasia.

The HIV-infected are presenting massive new demands for medical and neurological chronic care. Those needing this care will be primarily gays and minority groups. The combination of the depersonalizing nature of institutionally based chronic care, the right to refuse such care, the increasing scarcity for all of institutionally based care resources because of the demands of the epidemic, and the socially unpopular nature of those creating the intense new demands upon such resources can scarcely not result in hostilities.

It is reasonable, in such an atmosphere, to consider that the HIV-infected will come to understand that it would be wise to exercise the right to refuse care. It need not be mandated. No legislation need even articulate such an unthinkable policy. But euthanasia can become a social reality, first for the HIV-infected, then for others who are institutionally bound, through a social unwillingness to develop other forms of health care services, ones which do not trample upon one's sense of personhood.

D. A Proposal for Home-Basing Chronic Health Care Services

Implementing home-based chronic-care treatment programs requires both reorienting presently existing health care institutions and altering the role of family, friends and volunteers in the process of care. Most health care institutions recognize the inherent dangers of the AIDS epidemic upon their fiscal and institutional stability. They fear the overwhelming numbers HIV threatens. They fear the impact upon residency programs, and staff morale. They should welcome carefully coordinated efforts, then, to develop new methods of home care such as those being developed by San Francisco's gay community.

These efforts, to be properly stewarded, require the creation of a new national Commission on the Deinstitutionalization of Chronic Care. While it could be modeled after the commission on the abuse and neglect of children, its mandate should be broad, like the Marshall Plan or the Works Project Administration, for it must be capable of rationalizing the flow of federal dollars and the application of federal, state and local regulatory standards.

Incentives should be attached to federal dollars to require hospitals and out-patient facilities to combine home-based care with functions they continue to be suited best to deliver. Federal dollars allocated to home health agencies must mandate home health education as a central function of such agencies, enabling family and friends to learn the skills necessary to make possible extensive home care. Government must also encourage churches, synagogues, and other communities of faith to draw on the teachings of their traditions and help finance the mobilization and training of congregational and community volunteers to provide the routine yet vital support services necessary to enable family and friends to care for their own at home.

This approach on a massive scale does potentially change weekly patterns of life. Yet a new ethos of caretaking that redefined the nature of one's weekly chores—an hour or two as a home care volunteer, folding laundry or running errands, along with work, shopping, and aerobic classes—could help regenerate the care and communal values so badly needed today.

Such home care programs, however, must be coordinated through multi-focal, community-based facilities whenever possible. Since HIV has a disproportionate impact upon the inner-city poor, such programs would have a powerful effect. Inner-city-based facilities coordinating home care programs which require as an essential component the education and involvement of family, friends, and neighbors would powerfully reorient relationships by altering the oftentimes destructive nature of institutionally based services upon the poor.

For members of inner-city areas, the self-help and professional support created by such programs would transform their perceptions of the helping role of the professions. For care professionals, the paternalism inherent in institutionally based care models which burdens professionals' self-esteem would be lessened. For middle-class volunteers assisting inner-city efforts, such programs offer the basis for strengthening religious and civic values.

This vision of care, however, cannot be only for those infected with HIV. Justice mandates that successful aspects of such programs be applied appropriately to issues of care regarding the frail elderly, those with Alzheimer's, the neurologically impaired, any who require chronic care. This would address a great secret in the health care world regarding AIDS, the fear that AIDS will overwhelm other health care programs, for good-hearted, long-committed workers in other health areas fight unseemly feelings of resentment and anger about the front-page status of AIDS.

E. Conclusion

Most American religious institutions are centrally committed to relieving human suffering, yet many people feel dismembered from a religious sense of self. With AIDS as a catalyst, a new ethos of caring in our religious institutions could be constructed. That ethos would have to include all who were concerned, not merely the religiously involved. But it makes sense to begin with religious institutions because of their ideological commitments to human service, their preexisting networks of potential volunteer labor and their low-overhead administrative structures. These factors make them a promising choice for an organizing base, coordinating with other community organizations and supported by government dollars, to slightly alter the nature of daily American life.

If society fails to consider these issues of care, then it risks creating for everyone, not merely those infected with HIV, de facto conditions of widespread euthanasia without even having to call it by its name. Enough is already known about the despair that sets in from the necessarily depersonalizing effects of intimate care from hired hands rather than from those who love us for ourselves. The choice to continue business as usual in planning to deliver HIV-related health care in institutional settings rather than at home will drive many, many people to choose to refuse care earlier than they might otherwise. We need not utter the word "euthanasia" in the legislature. We need not confess our underlying discomforts about most people infected with HIV, that they are gay, or drug users who are black or Hispanic. We need not say that we wish them dead. We need merely ignore what we already know.

In California, a proposed November 1988 ballot initiative would legalize active euthanasia—the assented to killing of one person by another—for the first time in the United States. The proposal is hedged in by numerous safeguards. The organizers of the initiative originally told members of the Bioethics Committee of the Los Angeles County Bar Association that they expected the effort to enact their measure to take five years. That was eighteen months ago, in the fall of 1986.

The Euthanasia Initiative speaks to people's unprecedented despair about the end of life. It is immoral in the same fashion that society's failure to confront the issue of chronic care is immoral—by seeming to leave individuals with no alternative to the indignities of their final days but to end them quickly. The challenge of AIDS is, ultimately, the challenge to find alternatives which do not permit that despair to transform all people from "us" to "them."

NOTES

1. I owe a great deal to Professor St. Clair Drake for my insights into the general nature of prejudice. Professor Drake is the co-author (with Horace Cayton) of the landmark study of black urban life, BLACK METROPOLIS: A STUDY OF NEGRO LIFE IN A NORTHERN CITY.

2. *See generally*, M. DOUGLAS, PURITY AND DANGER: AN ANALYSIS OF CONCEPTS OF POLLUTION AND TABOO (1966); V. TURNER, THE RITUAL PROCESS: STRUCTURE AND ANTI-STRUCTURE (1969); and R. Alder, *Tum'ah and Taharah: Ends and Beginnings*, THE JEWISH WOMAN (1976).

3. For the classic work on the subject of stigma, *see*, E. GOFFMAN, STIGMA: NOTES ON THE MANAGEMENT OF SPOILED IDENTITY (1963). For a survey of racial minority issues, *see* AIDS Discrimination Unit, New York City Commission on Human Rights, AIDS and People of Color: The Discriminatory Impact (Nov. 13, 1986); N. Nickens, Nat'l Minority AIDS Council Report on AIDS and Ethnic Minorities (available from M. Nickens, 744 Fell St., San Francisco, CA 94117); and Martinez, *AIDS: The Crisis in Latino L.A.*, L. A. WEEKLY, October 30-November 5, 1987, at 10. For a provocative and disturbing account of gay issues of stigma, *see* Mohr, *AIDS, Gay Life, State Coercion*, 6 RARITAN (1986). For a discussion of AIDS, stigma and euthanasia, *see infra*, section VI.

4. It is useful in this regard to consider how our response to AIDS might have been different had the epidemic broken out among white, middle-class, happily married midwestern businessmen or examine our response to the small outbreak of Legionnaires' disease.

5. For an authoritative discussion of past public health measures and their appropriateness for the AIDS epidemic, *see* Brandt, *AIDS: From Social History to Public Policy*, 14 LAW, MED & HEALTH CARE 5-6 (1986) at 231.

6. *See infra*, section III.

7. For a discussion of the nature of the American character, *see* R. BELLAH, R. MADSEN, W. SULLIVAN & A. TIPTON, HABITS OF THE HEART: INDIVIDUALISM AND COMMITMENT IN AMERICAN LIFE (1985). For a discussion of the importance of character in culture, *see* A. MACINTYRE, AFTER VIRTUE: A STUDY IN MORAL THEORY (2d ed. 1984).

8. *See infra*, section VI. D.

9. *See infra*, section IV.

10. *See* W. MCNEILL, PLAGUES AND PEOPLE (1976).

11. Korematsu v. U.S., 319 U.S. 432; 87 L.Ed. 1497; 63 S.C. 1124 (1943).

12. A. CAMUS, THE PLAGUE 117–118 (1972).

13. The recent Bork hearings demonstrated how thoroughly embedded into the fabric of society the civil rights transformation has become. Southern Democratic senators explained their "no" votes by declaring that their constituents would not tolerate a constitutional reexamination of the new values forged in the civil rights struggles.

14. RANDY SHILTS, AND THE BAND PLAYED ON: POLITICS, PEOPLE AND THE AIDS EPIDEMIC (1987), p. 585.

15. L.A. MUN. CODE section 45.80 *et. seq.*

16. For example, the first bi-weekly newsletter devoted solely to these matters, AIDS, POLICY & LAW, began six months later. *See* Oliver, *AIDS: An Uncharted Legal Field*, LOS ANGELES TIMES, April 3, 1986, part 1, p. 1.

17. Editorial, *The Only Weapon Against AIDS*, NEW YORK TIMES, August 18, 1985, section 4, p.18.

18. *Letters to the Times*, LOS ANGELES TIMES, August 26, 1985, part 2, p. 4.

19. California Department of Fair Employment and Housing v. Raytheon Company (*Real Party Interest* John Chadbourne), FEHC Dec. No. 87–04.

20. *Cf.*, M. FOUCAULT, MADNESS AND CIVILIZATION: A HISTORY OF INSANITY IN THE AGE OF REASON (1965).

21. For an excellent general introduction, *see Law, Social Policy and Contagious Disease: A Symposium on Acquired Immune Deficiency Syndrome (AIDS)*, 14 Hofstra L. Rev. 1 (1985), especially Leonard, *AIDS and Employment Law Revisted, id.* at 11, and Dolgin, *AIDS: Social Meanings and Legal Ramifications, id.* at 193.

22. West Hollywood, Berkeley, Oakland and San Francisco.

23. *School Board of Nassau County v. Arline*, 107 S.Ct. 1913 (1987) (holding that persons with contagious diseases are protected by the physical handicap civil rights provisions of the Federal Rehabilitation Act of 1973); Chalk v. U.S. District Court (Orange County Dept. of Education, *real party in interest*), 840 F.2d 701 (9th Cir. 1988) (holding that *Arline* protects people with AIDS); and Thomas v. Atascadero Unified School District, 662 F. Supp. 376 (C.D. Cal. 1987).

24. *Hour Magazine* (FOX TELEVISION broadcast Sept 18, 1987).

25. Contrary to the apparent common meaning of the term, "public accommodations" in a legal context is a term of art used to describe the broad ambit of civil life—retail establishments, restaurants, medical and dental services, motels and hotels, theaters, parks, etc.

26. *See* Leonard, *supra* at note 21.

27. W. J. CURRAN, L. GOSTIN AND M. CLARK, ACQUIRED IMMUNE DEFICIENCY SYNDROME: LEGAL AND REGULATORY POLICY (1986); Gostin and Curran, *Public Health and the Law*, 77 AMERICAN JOURNAL OF PUBLIC HEALTH 2 at 214 (1987). For an excellent review of Curran and Gostin's book, *see* Rosoff, *The AIDS Crisis: Constitutional Turning Point?*, 15 LAW, MED & HEALTH CARE 1-2 (1987) at 80.

28. 103 F. 10 (C.C. N.D. Cal. 1900).

29. *Cf.* L.A. MUN. CODE section 45.93(B). In *Arline, supra*, note 23, the matter was referred back to the trial court for a determination of the risk Mrs. Arline's infectious tuberculosis presented to others (having held in its decision only that she was entitled to the due process provisions of the Federal Rehabilitation Act).

30. For a further discussion of reasonable precautions to prevent HIV transmission in workplace, *see infra*, section V.

31. L.A. MUN. CODE section 45.93(B)(2).

32. 34 MORBIDITY & MORTALITY WEEKLY REPORT (1985) at 681.

33. In New York and San Francisco, the human rights commissions investigate and mediate, and request city attorney action on appropriate cases. In Los Angeles, the City Attorney's Office fulfills all three functions.

34. This exclusion is based upon the general principle that it is inappropriate to use taxpayer money to assist private citizens to recover money damages. It is thought that contingent fees in damage cases create sufficient incentive for private attorneys to take such cases. It is thought appropriate, however, for government attorneys to seek court orders to halt discriminatory behavior because such actions create a healthier climate for everyone and may not include the monetary award necessary to make it economically feasible for private attorneys to seek them.

35. *See supra*, section I.

36. A similar analysis regarding San Francisco's drop in cases was offered by the San Francisco Human Rights Commission. *See* 3 AIDS, POLICY & LAW (February 24, 1988) at 8.

37. Which, in the case of New York City, was a municipal ordinance prohibiting physical handicap discrimination interpreted to include AIDS, rather than an AIDS-specific statute.

38. And with that point in mind, entitled the paper was presented at the Third International Conference on AIDS in Washington, D.C. *Municipal AIDS Discrimination Laws as Public Health Education Tools for Preventing HIV Transmission.*

39. For example, John Chadbourne, the real party in interest in the landmark California employment case of *DFEH v. Raytheon, supra*, note 19, died in January 1985, twenty-five months before the Commission issued its ruling that AIDS was a covered handicap under California law. While this dramatically demonstrates the general incompatibility of the litigation process with the needs of people with AIDS, impact litigation—litigation which clarifies disputed points of law—is nonetheless essential in the battle against AIDS discrimination. Recent cases such as *Chadbourne, id., Chalk and Thomas, supra* at note 23, have been critical in strengthening the negotiating posture of AIDS discrimination plaintiffs. Furthermore, Mr. Chadbourne knew full well that he might not live to see his case resolved, but believed that his fight to establish the legal rights of people with AIDS added meaning and value to his life. But most cases are not impact litigation cases, and plaintiffs must face the harsh realities of protracted litigation. For an excellent discussion of alternative strategies for resolving AIDS, disputes, *see* Stein, *Strategies for Dealing with AIDS Dispute in the Workplace*, THE ARBITRATION JOURNAL (September 1987) at 21.

40. Marjorie Rushforth, lead attorney in *Chalk supra* at note 23, revealed at the AIDS and law panel discussed *infra* at note 53, that within two hours after she filed John Doe papers in the case, an *Orange County Register* reporter had determined the name of her client by an analysis of facts which had to be alleged in the complaint. It was not too difficult to find out *which* male special education teacher in the Orange County school district had just returned from a medical leave of absence.

41. Office of Legal Counsel, U.S. Department of Justice, Memorandum for Ronald E. Robertson, General Counsel, Department of Health and Human Services, Re: Application of Section 504 of the Rehabilitation Act to Persons with AIDS, AIDS-Related Complex, or Infection with the AIDS Virus. The position of the Department was generally repudiated by the U.S. Supreme Court the following March in the *Arline case, supra* at note 23.

42. *See infra*, section III.

43. Jasperson v. Jessica's, No. WEC 10966 (Sup. Ct., L.A. Cnty. filed Mar. 23, 1988) (order denying permanent injunction).

44. *See, e.g.*, Los Angeles City Attorney Report No. R-85-0711 at 1, 2 (Aug. 13, 1985); Letter from Legislative Counsel of California to Assembly member Art Agnos (Nov. 7, 1985); and Letter from the Attorney General's Office, California Dept. of Justice to State Senator Bill Locker (May 2, 1986).

45. *Cf., e.g.*, ANTONIO, THE AIDS COVER-UP? (1986) and Scott, *Playing Politics with Death: Radical Homosexuals and the AIDS Epidemic*, PASSPORT MAGAZINE at 2 (June 1985) (published by Calvary Chapel of West China, CA).

46. *Cf., e.g.*, Los Angeles Municipal Code section 45.90(B)(2).

47. For example, the court in *Jasperson, supra* at note 43, wherein Judge Waddington denied the plaintiff's request for an injunction prohibiting the defendant from refusing him service, in part, because the court refused to "[C]ommand defendant to administer a pedicure, and, if she refused, subject her to incarceration until she complied," *id.* at 8.

48. On December 1, 1987, the attempted murder charges against Markowski were dismissed by Los Angeles Superior Court Judge Ron Coen, who held that the prosecutors had failed to show that he had intended to kill anyone when he sold his plasma. Instead, Coen said, "The defendant's ... intent was ... to make enough money to support himself." Harris, *Charges Dropped Against Donor of AIDS-tainted Blood*, UPI (Dec. 2, 1987 at 1) (NEXIS). On March 2, 1988, a jury acquitted Markowski of the remaining charges of attempted poisoning.

49. "AIDS and the Medical Humanities," April 10–11, 1986.

50. For instance, immediately after TIME and the ATLANTIC MONTHLY carried cover stories on AIDS and heterosexuals in February 1987, the waiting

period at Los Angeles County's alternate test site mushroomed from ten days to eight weeks. For a thoughtful discussion about the role of the media in the epidemic, *see* Check, *Public Education on AIDS: Not Only the Media's Responsibility*, 15 HASTINGS CENTER REPORT 4 (Dec. 1985) (special supplement at 27).

51. *See infra* at section VI.

52. *See supra* at section III.

53. For a thoughtful analysis of these emerging problems, *see* panel discussion transcript, *AIDS and Civil Rights*, Whittier College School of Law Symposium, (March 4, 1988). (Transcript available from Whittier College School of Law, 5353 West Third Street, Los Angeles, CA 90020.)

54. Taken from Schulman, *AIDS and Public Policy: Using Law Against Fear to Re-member Society*, (opinion piece, LOS ANGELES TIMES, March 13, 1988, part 5, p. 3.

55. *See also*, Schulman, *Stopping AIDS Euthanasia*, 2 TIKKUN 3 at 14 (July/August 1987) and Vrolyk, *AIDS and Euthanasia: Is There a Morally Dubious Connection?*, BIOETHICS INSTITUTE NEWSLETTER (April 1988), Northridge (CA) Hospital Medical Center.

56. In the Matter of Karen Quinlan, 70 N.J. 10; 335 A.2d 647 (1976).

57. Elizabeth Bouvia v. Superior Court of Los Angeles County, 179 Cal App. 3d 1127; 225 Cal. Rptr. 297 (1986).

HIV AND THE ROLE OF COMMUNITY

Introduction

FOR THOSE OF US who see in the AIDS battle a struggle for a renewed American way of life and a way of health care provision that is entirely more humane and responsive than it has been for decades, the concept of community is very important. Community holds a promise of the full recovery of people who have been shut out of power. Community can restore the dignity of life and the ability to steer one's life in consort with others. If health is ever to mean more than access to health care, it can do so only if people can present their needs not only *to* institutions of care but to each other and find responsiveness. Part of health is the power to direct one's life and the individual context of one's life. And part of healthy power—power that is not adversarial and competitive—is *shared* power: power that involves others in a circuit of interdependence.

Community has always been a fact of life. In a country of ethnic groups, it is not hard to see how pervasive the phenomenon of community must be. But in a country explicitly devoted to "singleness," to competitive community (sports), to geographic isolation (the "car culture"), to the ideologies of the "private" and of the "individual," it is easy to see how hard community must be to maintain.

"Community" has always meant a group of people linked by their identification with a culture. In the United States the notion of culture has been expanded beyond the notion of an ethnic, geographic, or economic culture to also include a culture of need, a culture of struggle, a culture of sexual preference, a culture of fate. "Community" means essentially that one can be identified through others and share a life view and a fate that is ever, as in any relationship, being revised and renewed.

What has occurred in the HIV epidemic is that groups of people have found a way not only to press for the services they needed from a meager and depleted health, employment, and educational official-dom. More important, they have identified with each other and have invented structures that offered an array of emotional, psychological, philosophical, religious, and economic support. One must say that the "AIDS community" has offered HIV-infected people and those close to them a way to establish relationships with familial strangers who provide the support and ways of going on with living.

The articles in this chapter offer a number of ways in which to think about the issue of community. The first three articles treat the issue of community in light of the needs of specific groups of people affected by the epidemic. The first article by Peter Arno, addresses the service model of medical provision as it works and must increasingly work in community-based organizations.

Public health crises or general health issues are regarded mono-lithically by public health experts and the health establishment only so long as the definitions of health needs remain the province of experts. As soon as communities are empowered enough to have a say in their own health needs, the understanding of health needs changes and reflects the needs that exist in the lives of the affected. HIV policy is increasingly informed by the differences in community needs. Besides the obvious epistemological issue here of disease and health, the service issue looms large for Americans who lack primary care—care that is the basic relationship that can establish the agenda of needs that an individual has that they cannot meet for themselves. The Arno article shows how important services in the community are for the assessment of health needs, the coordination and continuity of their provision, and the accessibility of their placement for people who are largely at the mercy of a devastating and debilitating illness.

Nancy Stoller Shaw shows how important community organizing is for HIV prevention. HIV prevention's most crucial element is education and the means or ability to protect oneself. Education cannot occur through posters and public health announcements. Education must occur through a process of enlightenment and empowerment. This is what Stoller calls for. However, as is the case with women, education and its consequent empowerment must also change the dynamics of relationships built upon disenfran-chisement and fear. Women, traditionally disempowered in a society stratified by racism, class, heterosexism, and, finally, pervasive sexism, must not only address themselves to preventive health behavior but must do so in a context where new empowering and preventive behaviors will be threatening and are likely to meet consistent resistance.

Education and new behavior will be meaningless unless women are able to get help and services. Women confront the epidemic differently from men as a result of the multiple burdens and social habits (and strengths) of their everyday lives. Shaw outlines the role that political engagement has in helping women confront the epidemic. It is an important and altogether pervasive look at the obstacles to health and freedom that confront women in America.

Like the Shaw article, the article by Ronald Braithwaite and Ngina Lythcott points to the necessity of community organizing in the black community and Latino populations. Echoing Shaw's concern for women of color, this article seeks to find the link between past organizing efforts when groups have been almost completely politically (and therefore at all other levels) disenfranchised and the present emergency that AIDS offers those already politically vulnerable.

The drug-using community is a disenfranchised population direly in need of services and health care access and almost singularly unable to organize toward that end. "Against All Odds: Grass-roots Minority Groups Fight AIDS," taken from a 1988 *Health/PAC Bulletin* article, attempts to answer the question of what would be useful in securing this desperately needed help.

Surprisingly little has been written about the successful alternative health care system developed by gay communities across America. HIV infection, like mental illness, drug addiction, disability, and cancer, requires an exquisite coordination of services if those affected are to get on with their lives. The American health care system is a highly fragmented one and its public sector, as well as the public entitlement programs that fund it, are in great disarray. The need for coordination is even more pronounced today than it has been in the past due to the disappearance of basic care centered in the family physician or internist in solo or group practice.

Organized care—care that is coordinated—is health care that can identify patient needs as patients move through the trajectory of sickness. It focuses upon different stages of illness that urgently require various medical, mental health, and social services. Ideally, it is community-based, accessible geographically and culturally, since "needs" depend not only upon levels of morbidity and disability but also upon the strengths of social, familial, and community networks, as well as upon the commitment of caretakers and health institutions. The Gay Men's Health Crisis (GMHC) is an organization that seeks to provide basic, coordinated care to people with AIDS and it does so through an elaborate use of paid and volunteer staff. The description contained in this chapter of the philosophy and practice of GMHC could serve as a model for other community-based centers. The world owes the Gay Men's Health Crisis and other organizations like it—the Shanti Project in San Francisco (see "A Week on Ward 5A" included in this chapter), BEBISHI in Philadelphia, the Minority Task Force on AIDS of New York—a large debt for their leadership, advocacy, organizational skill, and incredible innovation in providing a complex of services to thousands upon thousands of PWAs as well as for providing educational and caretaking models for the world of HIV.

Cities can be communities, too, if enough people in them identify with each other. San Francisco, the city with the highest rate of HIV infection in the United States, committed itself very early to helping those affected by HIV disease. The coordination of services that San Francisco has provided for the last ten years to its citizens and the unique blend of public, private and volunteer services is known and applauded worldwide. It is called the "San Francisco Model of Health Care Delivery." But as "A City Responds" shows, the San Francisco model is crumbling. It is no longer possible for the community alone to continue almost exclusively to respond to its own needs without sizable state and federal help. This article shows what even a community as large as the city of San Francisco can do in providing responsive, humane care to the sick. But it also shows the limits of voluntarism. San Francisco has operated in crisis for ten years. Services are worn out, donations are dwindling, and there is pervasive burnout in the entire array of service providers. It is possible for communities to be the center of health care, but this cannot be done in an economic vacuum.

"Bearing Witness" is an eloquent essay on the human cost of AIDS by George Whitmore, a writer with AIDS. He describes the PWAs he met and worked with, a foster grandparent and a homeless child with AIDS "residing" in a South Bronx hospital among them. Whitmore candidly describes both his own struggle and theirs. "Bearing Witness" brings home for the reader the painful experience of HIV and the right we all have to autonomy, identification, and respect. At the end of his story, George Whitmore describes visiting Frederico, the child with AIDS, and seeing him as the tiny embodiment of his own fate and wanting desperately for Frederico what he wanted for himself—to live.

George Whitmore did not live. He died in April 1989. But he did bear witness to a time, an anonymity, a struggle that is both entirely private and ineluctably communal.

An Expanded Role for Community-Based Organizations

Peter Arno, Ph.D.

IN THE EARLY DAYS of the AIDS epidemic, there was an enormous and unanticipated need for medical, public health, social, and educational resources. Local governments were unwilling or unable to provide this broad range of human and social services and in New York and New Jersey, as elsewhere in the country, an array of community-based organizations (CBOs) arose to fill the gap. CBOs—generally defined as nonprofit, grass-roots agencies that emerge to serve a particular and well-defined constituency—have served persons with AIDS and their families in a number of vital ways, including:

- Public health education
- Psychosocial counseling
- Practical support, particularly help with day-to-day activities such as cooking, cleaning, laundry, shopping, and transportation
- Home health care services
- Housing
- Government benefits advocacy
- Legal protection, such as fighting employment and housing discrimination
- Access to health care, including providing referrals, and access to clinical trials and experimental drugs

Peter Arno, Ph.D., "An Expanded Role for Community-Based Organizations," *The Crisis in AIDS Care: A Call to Action*, Working Group of the Citizens Commission on AIDS, March 1989, pp. 33–46. Reprinted by Permission of the Citizens Commission on AIDS of New York City and Northern New Jersey.

By providing a broad array of social services, CBOs play a pivotal role in promoting continuity of care and case management for large numbers of AIDS patients. The availability of community-based services allows many patients to remain outside hospitals or reduce their length of stay when medically appropriate. In addition, these services facilitate the care of patients at home by friends, family members, and health care personnel. The economic contributions of CBOs, as well as their impact on service provision, are thus critically important to patients, local health care systems and municipal governments. AIDS service organizations have relied heavily on volunteer labor since the inception of the epidemic. This approach has thus far worked relatively well in the gay community, although there are concerns about burnout, availability of volunteers, and long-term viability. In poor, minority neighborhoods, however, the use of volunteer labor in community-based organizations is significantly more problematic. Those CBOs which do provide services in these neighborhoods must rely primarily on paid staff, supplemented by a limited number of volunteers.

As AIDS spreads increasingly into poor communities, it will be important either to expand the funding of CBOs so that paid staff can be hired or to develop new models of care. In this section, we review the potential of community-based organizations as a means of delivering services in both the gay and the minority communities and probe the limitations of voluntarism.

The Role of Community-Based Initiatives

With the recognition that AIDS was disproportionately affecting gay men, the gay community galvanizes its resources to create self-help voluntary organizations such as the Gay Men's Health Crisis in New York and the Hyacinth Foundation in New Jersey. Building upon human rights movements of the 1960s and 1970s, gay men were able to organize politically and financially in a way that less cohesive groups at risk, such as intravenous drug users (IVDUs), were not.

The need for and success of these voluntary organizations have been demonstrated repeatedly. In San Francisco, for example, the extensive development of outpatient services, which rely on volunteer-supported CBOs, has helped reduce unnecessary use of the hospital by AIDS patients.[1,2,3] The gay communities of New York City and northern New Jersey have helped build effective educational, advocacy, and service organizations that annually provide hundreds of thousands of hours of direct services to persons with AIDS.[4]

However, the organization and administration of large volunteer networks require substantial financial support from public and private sources and significant commitments from a pool of volunteers, neither of which is assured in the future. It remains unclear whether current levels of voluntarism in the gay community can be maintained. Emotional burnout among paid and unpaid staff is an important operational issue in any volunteer organization, but it is intensified among AIDS groups, whose staff members continually bear witness to the suffering and death of their colleagues and the people they serve.

Also threatening future provision of services is the fact that many of the first AIDS-specific organizations have functioned successfully only within their constituent group, which is mainly white, middle-class, gay men. With a few notable exceptions, they have not been able to meet the needs of patients in minority communities. In 1987, for example, the Gay Men's Health Crisis added to its caseload an estimated 47 percent, 15 percent and 17 percent of New York City's newly diagnosed AIDS cases among white, blacks, and Hispanics, respectively.[5]

As the epidemic shifts increasingly toward poor, inner-city communities, the demand for health and social services mounts. In neighborhoods already suffering from a host of other debilitating social problems, including poverty, unemployment, racism, lack of adequate housing, educational opportunities, substance abuse and teenage pregnancy, AIDS does not always receive priority. The increasing numbers of women, children and IVDUs diagnosed with AIDS is creating complex new pressures on fragile family support systems, such as child care and foster care, which will intensify during the next few years. (For more information on this topic, see Section Two: "The Special Needs of Women, Children, and Adolescents.")

Housing is the most critical non-medical need of people with AIDS or HIV illness. The most common reason for inappropriate hospitalization of AIDS patients is the lack of adequate housing where outpatient care can be delivered. The extent of homelessness or precarious living arrangements is estimated to affect between 2,000 and 5,000 persons in New York City alone.[6] A recent study of 174 hospitalized AIDS patients who are also IVDUs indicated that 40 percent are either homeless or precariously housed at the time of diagnosis and hospitalization.[7] As more IVDUs become ill over the next few years, this will translate into thousands of individuals in need of housing. (For more information on this topic, see Section Two: "Housing, Homelessness, and the Impact of HIV Disease.")

Poverty and unemployment place severe restraints on the development of new community-based organizations or the expansion of existing CBOs in many minority neighborhoods. Volunteers in inner-city neighborhoods have traditionally donated their services mainly through their churches or political organizations; efforts to combat teenage pregnancy and juvenile crack use have recently received the greatest attention.

A few community-based groups, relying primarily on volunteer labor, have emerged to deal with AIDS in poor communities but the level of organizational development among these groups has not been on a scale necessary to meet the rising service needs. Self-help efforts among IVDUs and their sexual partners have also been slow to emerge. In addition to the health and social problems stemming from drug addiction, a number of other obstacles to internal mobilization exist. There is no tradition of collective self-organization and the very behaviors around which people might organize are illegal. Moreover, there is internal competition and conflict within the drug subculture.[8,9]

One positive sign of change is that City, State, Federal and private dollars are increasingly available for AIDS, enabling a number of established organizations to broaden their programs to include AIDS-related services. Emmaus House, which works with minority home-less, and Covenant House, which helps adolescents, are two notable examples; other well-established social service agencies, including Lighthouse for the Blind and Cancer Care, now include individuals with AIDS or HIV-disease among their constituents and have begun to plan for the services they need. Human Service Agency Executives Concerned about AIDS, a coalition of mainstream and AIDS-specific groups, is facilitating this process.

Until the political and church leadership of the minority communities speak out forcefully on AIDS, however, the work of both established and fledgling CBOs is likely to be hampered. Political leaders have been fearful—with some justification—that representing AIDS as a minority issue will diminish the current level of public support for all AIDS programs. The stigma of homosexuality among blacks and Hispanics and the conservative values that permeate many of the churches in minority communities has also stifled indigenous support for AIDS work by CBOs.[10]

Although many black and Hispanic churches are active in the community, providing foster care programs, adult education, food, and shelter to impoverished individuals and their families, the leadership has failed to respond collectively to the AIDS crisis. According to Reverend John Vaughn, executive director of East Harlem Interfaith, "In Spanish Harlem we are at a point where the gay community was five years ago."[11] Although there is a growing willingness in Spanish Harlem to talk about homosexuality, cultural and theological traditions foster resistance, fear, and denial within the community as a whole. The refusal of many pastors to take an active role can often be directly linked to their fear of accusations that they are advocates for gay or gay themselves. Reverend Lee Wesley, executive director of the Minority Task Force on AIDS, has suggested that "homophobia" is the principal reason most church leaders are reluctant to take a more active stance in the AIDS crisis.[12] In addition, churches face an overwhelming number of other social problems on a daily basis and their modest resources are already stretched to meet the myriad other needs of their congregations.

The willingness of many churches to foster the work of AIDS-focused CBOs is thus contingent upon individual pastors and their particular theological and ideological beliefs. Some activists *have* played important roles in helping to build community-based AIDS initiatives and there are already some vital church-sponsored programs in place. Of particular note are the Lunch for Life Program at the Yorkville Pantry, the Upper Room AIDS Ministry, God's Love We Deliver, AIDS Interfaith, St. Peter's Momentum Outreach and Project Brave.

St. Peter's Momentum Outreach Program, serving approximately 400 persons with AIDS and their families, is the largest of these church-sponsored programs. It is primarily maintained by volunteers from St. Peter's Lutheran Church. With private sector support, mainly from the Robert Wood Johnson Foundation, this model program is being replicated at seven sites throughout the New York metropolitan area to provide food and supportive services to people with AIDS.[13,14] Another church-sponsored CBO, God's Love We Deliver, has grown significantly since it was founded in the summer of 1985; currently it delivers free gourmet meals daily to approximately 130 homebound persons with AIDS.[15]

Unmet Needs

One rough gauge of the need for additional AIDS-related health and social services was recently demonstrated by the national request for proposals issued by the Robert Wood Johnson (RWJ) Foundation's AIDS Prevention and Service Projects Initiative.[16] In the largest response in the Foundation's history, 1,026 grant proposals totalling $537 million were received in July 1988. More than half the proposals were from CBOs. According to Dr. Leighton E. Cluff, RWJ Foundation president: "The response reveals what is, in effect, a national assessment of community needs in the fight against AIDS. We were not surprised by this enormous response but we are sobered by it. The proposals represent the voice of people who are actually fighting this epidemic."[17]

Nationally, 54 projects were selected by the Foundation and $16.7 million dollars in awards were recently announced. New York and New Jersey alone submitted 140 and 48 proposals totalling $87.5 million and $22.3 million dollars, respectively. These figures far exceed the level of state-only expenditures for AIDS (exclusive of Medicaid) for fiscal year 1988, which are estimated at $39.9 million in New York and $7.9 million in New Jersey.[18]

Two other calls for substantial increases in funding AIDS-related health care and social service needs have recently been issued in New York, one focused on city agencies,[19] the other on state programs.[20] The Committee for AIDS Funding, a diverse coalition of 22 community-based AIDS service providers in New York City, recommended an additional budget allocation of $41,321,713 for New York City alone. The New York AIDS Coalition, comprised of more than 70 individuals representing different communities affected by AIDS around the state, has called for $139,707,785 in additional state funding. These funding requests are for the coming fiscal year, focus on non-mandated spending, and are geared mainly toward improving community-based ambulatory care services and programs.

Community-based AIDS organizations were surveyed in New York City and northern New Jersey by the Citizens Commission on AIDS in the Spring of 1988. The following problems, ranked in order of importance, were identified. In New York: (1) lack of funding; (2) staff shortages; (3) discrimination against gays and minorities; (4) lack of adequate housing; and (5) insufficient drug treatment slots. In New Jersey; (1) lack of funding; (2) lack of public education; (3) lack of adequate housing; (4) lack of psychosocial support for patients and their families; and (5) lack of adequate home health care. CBOs from both states serving primarily ethnic minorities were more likely to identify inadequate funding as a major problem than CBOs serving other groups.

Conclusion

Community-based organizations have played a crucial role in responding to the needs of the AIDS epidemic but their potential is far from being realized. Although there has been much discussion of the value of CBOs in promoting the continuity of care and case management of large numbers of AIDS patients, there has been no systematic planning with public agencies or the private sector.

Beyond the issue of unrealized potential lies the reality that voluntarism has inherent limitations. Efforts to impose on minority communities models that have worked so effectively among gay groups are unlikely to succeed. Thus, it is imperative that the model of CBOs using paid labor be expanded and that other innovative approaches be adequately supported. One promising development is that recent government contracting and funding from the private sector are beginning to push established community groups toward incorporating AIDS services in their mission. But greater efforts to foster a more proactive role in response to AIDS must be made by black and Hispanic church and political leaders and by the private sector if the common needs of minority communities are to be met.

NOTES

1. R. T. Chen, et al. "Use of hospitals by patients with AIDS in San Francisco," *New England Journal of Medicine* 319 (1988): 1671–2.

2. P. S. Arno and R. G. Hughes, "Local policy responses to the AIDS epidemic: New York and San Francisco," *New York State Journal of Medicine* 87 (1987): 264–72.

3. P. S. Arno, "The nonprofit sector's response to the AIDS epidemic: community-based services in San Francisco," *American Journal of Public Health* 76 (1986): 1325–30.

4. P. S. Arno, "The future of voluntarism and the AIDS epidemic," in D. E. Rogers and E. Ginzberg, eds., *The AIDS Patient: An Action Agenda* (Boulder and London: Westview Press, 1988), 56–70.

5. Ibid.

6. P. Smith. Testimony before the President of the New York City Council, City Hall, New York. 1 November, 1988.

7. E. Drucker et al., "IV drug users with AIDS in New York City: A study of dependent children, housing and drug addiction treatment," (Unpublished paper: July 1988).

8. S. R. Friedman et al., "AIDS and self-organization among intravenous drug users." *The International Journal of Addiction* 22 (1987): 201–19.

9. D. C. Des Jarlais et al., "AIDS among intravenous drug users: a sociocultural perspective," in D. Felman and T. Johnson, eds., *The Social Dimensions of AIDS* (New York: Praeger, 1986).

10. E. Hammonds, "Race, Sex, AIDS: The construction of other," *Radical America* 20 (1987): 28–36.

11. Interview by Nelson Fernandez from the Citizens Commission on AIDS with John Vaughn, Executive Director of East Harlem Interfaith, a religious-based community organization whose goals include the development of a network of religious and secular organizations which work together to create structural social change. 28 October, 1988.

12. Interview by Peter Arno from the Citizens Commission on AIDS with Reverend Lee Wesley, Executive Director of the Minority Task Force on AIDS, 25 April 1988. The Task Force advocates for more effective AIDS prevention and treatment modalities in minority communities and provides limited services to minority persons with AIDS and their families, including a telephone information and referral service, a volunteer "buddy" program and free weekly meals.

13. L. E. Cluff, "Grants awarded under the Robert Wood Johnson Foundation's AIDS prevention and service projects initiative," (Special memorandum to members of Congress, governors, selected federal officials, foundation executives and corporate executives: 12 December, 1988).

14. Interview by Nelson Fernandez from the Citizens Commission on AIDS with Peter Avitable, founder and executive director, St. Peter's Momentum Outreach Program, 27 December, 1988.

15. Interview by Nelson Fernandez from the Citizens Commission on AIDS with James Kirkpatrick, Business Manager, God's Love We Deliver, 28 December, 1988.

16. L. E. Cluff, "Grants awarded under the Robert Wood Johnson Foundation's AIDS prevention and service projects initiative," (Special memorandum to members of Congress, governors, selected federal officials, foundation executives and corporate executives: 12 December, 1988).

17. L. E. Cluff, cited in *AIDS/HIV Record* (August 1988).

18. M. J. Rowe and C. C. Ryan, "Comparing State-only expenditures for AIDS," *American Journal of Public Health* 78 (1988): 424–9.

19. Committee for AIDS Funding, *Funding agenda for community-based HIV/AIDS service programs in New York City FY 1989–1900* (December 1988).

20. New York AIDS Coalition, *Funding agenda for community-based AIDS programs and services in New York State* (November 1988).

Preventing AIDS Among Women: The Role of Community Organizing

Nancy Stoller Shaw

WITHIN THE UNITED STATES, the AIDS epidemic is highly structured by race, class, sexuality, and gender. This structure has developed because its cause, the Human Immunodeficiency Virus (HIV), is transmitted primarily through intimate social or sexual contact in a society composed of many cultures and communities which are subject to varying degrees of separation, segregation, and boundary-crossing. Although HIV disease, including its most severe manifestations, Acquired Immunodeficiency Syndrome (AIDS) and AIDS-Related Complex (ARC), has struck every segment of American society, it is especially and increasingly an illness of the poor and of ethnic and sexual minorities. As we move into the 1990s, this will be more the case than ever.

There are three current and important tasks for American society in responding to the epidemic: prevention, care, and cure. Although current research indicates that the progress of HIV disease can be

Research for this article was partially supported by faculty research funds from the University of California, Santa Cruz. An earlier version was presented at the National Institutes of Health's Conference, "Women and AIDS: Promoting Healthy Behaviors," In September, 1987. Melia Franklin and Gilda Zwerman provided welcome editing assistance.

Nancy Stoller Shaw, "Preventing AIDS Among Women: The Role of Community Organizing," *Socialist Review* 100 (Fall 1988): 77–92. Reprinted by Permission of the *Socialist Review*.

slowed, cure is not yet a possibility. Prevention and care are two avenues which *can* be pursued. Because AIDS is a socially transmitted and socially preventable disease, the best way to contain it is probably *not* through health department flyers, television messages by celebrities, or doctors' entreaties, but through changing the patterns of interaction within communities. Changing community behavior also requires changing attitudes, values, and power structures. An effective route to these changes is community organizing. In fact, until there is a vaccine, this may be the most promising way to halt the epidemic. To explore this argument, I will focus on the challenge of preventing AIDS among women.

Women with AIDS: A Profile

As of June 13, 1985, 5,136 adolescent and adult women in the United States and Puerto Rico had been diagnosed with AIDS.[1] The majority are intravenous drug users (52 percent).[2] The second most common risk category is heterosexual contact (26 percent), which rose from 21 percent over the last year alone.[3] The infected male sexual contacts of these women were IV drug users (67 percent), bisexual men (16 percent), hemophiliacs (1 percent), or men with other or undetermined sources of infection.[4] Nationally, 11 percent of women with AIDS contracted HIV from blood transfusions. In a small number of cases (8 percent), the source of transmission is unknown; most of these cases are believed to be heterosexual transmission in situations where the woman did not know that her partner might be infected. A few are cases where the woman died before she could be interviewed. AIDS among lesbians can generally be traced to the same source of infection as for heterosexual women. Only one case of woman-to-woman transmission has been documented in the United States: that transmission was most probably through blood-to-blood contact.[5]

Although these women are linked by similarities of biology and diagnosis, they are divided by the multiplicity of cultures and classes to which they belong. Both before and after diagnosis, some of their challenges may be similar: poverty, living in a sexist society, negotiating sexual encounters in an environment in which HIV infection is a possibility. But the forms of these challenges, the contexts in which they occur, and the access to family and/or peer support vary considerably. One set of AIDS prevention techniques or models of care would be grossly insufficient to serve all of them. If we examine their diversity, we will see why AIDS prevention and community service strategies which recognize and respond to community variety are especially crucial for women.

Nationally, women constitute approximately 8 percent of all AIDS cases since 1981, a figure which increased from 7 percent in early 1987. Women with AIDS are concentrated in four states: New York, New Jersey, Florida and California. In five states (New Jersey, Connecticut, Florida, Rhode Island and New York) as well as Puerto Rico, they constitute 10 percent or more of all reported AIDS cases.[6] These six locations are also marked by high rates of infection among IV drug users and by greater than average incidence of heterosexual transmission of HIV. Within these areas, the majority of women with AIDS are black (51 percent), while white women comprise 28 percent of the total and Latinas 20 percent.[*]

Not surprisingly, most women with HIV disease are also poor and uneducated. In a pattern similar to that of intravenous drug-using women, they have backgrounds of early family loss and emotionally or physically absent parents.[7] Many left home in their early teens and turned to drugs or prostitution for survival. More than half have children under 18, and caring for these children is often the primary emotional focus of their lives. Women diagnosed with AIDS are predominantly between 13 and 39 (79 percent), which makes them significantly younger than men with AIDS, and indicates that more were infected in their teens than is the case with men.[8] It is common for them to express low self-esteem, place their children and their male partners ahead of themselves in terms of importance, and to deny their own needs to meet the needs of others.

These women and others with similar backgrounds are individually isolated and unable to present an agenda of needs. Their futures are currently linked to those of the ethnic, geographic, social, and economic communities to which they belong. If we are to prevent HIV transmission to and from women such as these, in the various communities that comprise our nation, we will need innovative programs which can reach them in comprehensible, locally available forms.

Unfortunately, many of the AIDS prevention programs for heterosexuals and IV drug users are directed by and/or for men. While these programs do and will have some impact on the female members of the community, prevention programs which are designed to assist in women's survival (and the survival of their children) must go beyond the needs of men.

[*]National rates of HIV infection and illness are much higher among black women and Latinas than among whites.

If each woman's chance of survival remains primarily in the control of her sexual partner(s) or in self-management of a drug addiction for which woman-appropriate treatment programs do not exist, then many lives—both male and female—will be inevitably lost. Community-based programs will need to address both women's specific educational needs and their relative powerlessness. Education without the power to implement it will only produce despair.

Individual and Social Change

Outreach alone cannot prevent AIDS. Local and national policies and cultural practices must also be transformed. Many local governments as well as the US federal government do not view AIDS as a health emergency. Racism, disinterest in the poor, and contempt for gay men have created an atmosphere in which most Americans are willing to passively accept the idea that over 100,000 people in racially or sexually stigmatized groups will die from a completely preventable disease. The same public evinces little interest in AIDS prevention in these "high risk" communities unless there is some fear that the epidemic might "spill over"—for example, through blood transfusions, male bisexuality, or female prostitution—into the "wider community," to the "rest of us." One consequence of these attitudes is an emphasis on education and personal behavior change by "groups" at risk (backed up with threats of quarantine), without new social policies which are needed if education is to be effective and if behavior changes in large segments of the population are going to occur.

For example, physicians have been instructed by health departments to advise patients to use condoms,[9] but community norms for both men and women are not supportive of condom us and most physicians teach neither technique nor negotiation skills.[10] Consequently, little change of the sort that can prevent transmission of HIV has occurred in sexual behavior. Condoms are expensive, available only in limited locations, and they are provided to the public without adequate education for safe and effective use. Added to those problems is the relative powerlessness of women when confronted with male sexual demands.

Effective use of condoms by women and men will require three components: greater availability of free or very low-cost condoms, understandable information on how to use them properly, and the power to use them. All three components require community intervention. In other words, AIDS prevention for those at risk of HIV infection through sexual contact can only be accomplished through basic changes both in community sexual norms and in the economics of preventive health programs.

For those whose risk of AIDS is through dirty needles, social changes ultimately require a revision of the relative power of the drug economy in American ghettos, barrios and other poor communities. Such change has been a goal of these communities for a number of years, but poor neighborhoods, which are highly dependent on government services, have been unable on their own to end the drug trade which weakens them. Their attempts have not been supported by local, state, or federal agencies and they have not had the power to force that support.

In fact, in some cases government drug policies have run counter to strategies known to help prevent HIV infection. For one, the Reagan administration has gutted federal support for the already inadequate number of drug rehabilitation programs, despite its antidrug posturing. Further, it was not until this year—a full six years after the connection between sharing needles and AIDS transmission became clear—that the National Institute on Drug Abuse began to fund its first experimental needle exchange program. This delay did not occur because there was no evidence that such programs can be useful: evidence to the contrary had already been accumulated in parts of Britain with exchange programs. The United States forbade needle exchange primarily for moral reasons—the same justification that was given to block the provision of condoms in both prisons and high schools, despite their obvious value in these locations.

It is this widespread, federally sanctioned complacency that has helped lead me to the conclusion that local community organizing efforts, based in the communities with the most serious risks of infection, are the most immediate route to saving lives and creating networks of compassion. In preventing AIDS, the second half of the slogan, "Think globally, act locally," may well be the most important.

Community Change, Community Power

In order to study community change and AIDS prevention, it is necessary to have a clear definition of community. For the purposes of this article, a community is defined as a group of people who identify themselves as linked by culture, social organization, language, common experience or fate. When I discuss community change I am referring to changes within the group as well as to changes between the group and the external social or political structure in which it exists.

The degree of control or management of the changes process vested in the local community can vary from 0 to 100 percent. Hypothetically, at one end of the continuum a community would have no control over the process, and local or national government would attempt to rigorously regulate sexuality and drug use through law and the criminal justice system. Quarantines of people infected with AIDS represent an extreme form of this approach. At the other extreme, a local community would have a network with economic and political resources and the opportunity and ability to define and pursue health priorities and goals. This latter scenario has been the case in some gay communities and in scattered ethnic communities. These organizing projects generally survive on donations from within the communities in which they are located, with minor support from foundations or government agencies.

Somewhere in the middle of the empowerment continuum are community-oriented primary health care programs, such as those which work on a block-by-block basis to help neighborhoods define and address health concerns with the support of a medical center or health department.[11] Although this is also a promising approach, there are still few AIDS prevention projects of this type.[12] Community-based AIDS prevention projects which are connected to health departments can be seen as somewhat reflecting this model.[13]

It is now commonly accepted among public health officials that AIDS-prevention programs should be tailored to the communities in which they are located. This awareness has led to the provision of materials and events that are culturally appropriate (in terms of language, graphics, and other content), often distributed by community members or leaders. Such distribution and education programs may be considered "community based" in the sense that they operate from a community location or use community culture or structure.

Programs which are described as "community controlled" do not necessarily reflect the needs and interests of all members of the community. Women—and especially women with HIV—are often excluded from planning and managing these prevention and service programs. This is partly because women comprise a small proportion of those known to the HIV-infected in the U.S. It is also partly because some HIV-infected women are active drug users and/or seriously ill with AIDS-related infections, and such women are incapable of major sustained involvement in AIDS prevention or care. But the primary reason for women's exclusion is neither lack of numbers, illness, nor apathy: it is the institutionalized sexism and racism which relegate black women and Latinas to subordinate— and sometimes invisible—positions in organizations ranging from health departments and government administrations to substance abuse programs, AIDS programs, and ethnic advocacy groups. In short, women are neither seen nor heard.

A consequence of this exclusion is that women's needs take a back seat. Health educators write brochures asking women to protect their men and children. Saving their own lives is mentioned last. Further, while men are told to use condoms, women may hear that they should "consider discussing" their use. AIDS residences, food banks, drug programs, and support groups focus on the individual and his or her support network. Provisions to help a mother with her children are often tacked on or delayed as afterthoughts.

Organizing Models

Communities vary in degree and type of organization. A small migrant labor camp in central Florida may have only rudimentary social institutions, while an East Harlem Puerto Rican neighborhood may be filled with a variety of schools, churches, associations, and familial networks. A neighborhood in San Francisco may have black residents from the American South, Panama, Ethiopia, the Caribbean, as well as third-generation Californians. All three locations (Florida, East Harlem, San Francisco) could have high rates of HIV infection. Community mobilization designed to reach women and to combat the spread of HIV would vary considerably from one location to the other. For example, at the labor camp in Florida, one might work through a health clinic or a prenatal care program, while in San Francisco, one might target churches and cultural associations with high rates of participation by women.

Many groups have attempted to change daily life in community settings by organizing the members of the community so that they can have greater control over the basic institutions which determine their lives. The settings for such work range from traditional neighborhood organizing and unions to movements for ethnic liberation, peace, and women's rights. Some of the best known of the neighborhood organizing work in the United States has been done by Saul Alinsky or others utilizing his techniques.[14] The essence of the Alinsky approach is the identification of community values, traditions, interests, leaders, and factions, followed by the organization of people who are spread among the factions but are essentially powerless because they have been divided and unorganized. Alinsky believed that community power was a value in itself. He was less concerned with the specific issues around which the community was organized and more concerned with the development of a powerful organization which could leverage material goals from the local or state government. The value of the Alinsky model to those working in AIDS prevention is its flexibility, and the wealth of knowledge concerning its application in a variety of situations. One limitation of the approach is that many local phenomena are controlled by larger forces (such as national economic policy and consequent health priorities and funding) and are therefore not amenable to control by strictly local organizations.[15]

Attempts at community organizing in the 1960s and 1970s built on the techniques of the Alinsky model, but more often followed a strategy of linkage with similar organizations within a region, or in some cases, nationally. These organizations, such as the Student Non-violent Coordinating Committee (SNCC), Student for a Democratic Society (SDS), and later, the Association of Community Organizations for Reform Now (ACORN), combined local community empowerment with national structures. As national organizations, they attempted to develop unified strategies that would produce national social policies in accord with their goals.

Other relevant models of organizing from which lessons can be drawn for AIDS prevention include: (1) union organizing, especially within large-scale settings and where health issues are involved; (2) the welfare rights movement of the late 1960s, in particular the experience of the National Welfare Rights Organization, which mobilized thousands of welfare recipients to disrupt welfare offices and insist on more services;[16] (3) community-based disease prevention projects, such as the Community Heart Disease Prevention Trials[17] and the National Cancer Institute Community Intervention Trial for Smoking Cessation;[18] and (4) national public health intervention and mobilization models, such as those in China, Cuba, and Nicaragua.

Community Organizing and AIDS

If community organizing is to reach women at highest risk for HIV infection and disease, it will need to be located in communities with significant populations of blacks and Latinos. In 1987, the National AIDS Network surveyed 250 AIDS organizations concerning their participation in AIDS prevention work in minority communities, where the majority of women at risk for HIV infection can be found. Very few organizations served areas with significant minority populations, nor were minorities a significant component of their caseload. This was true for both educational and service organizations.[19]

On the other hand, considerable grass-roots community organizing focused on the AIDS epidemic has been done within gay communities. When gay male communities were first denied public resources for AIDS prevention in the early 1980s, they organized themselves to raise private money and to apply political pressure to public agencies. In San Francisco, where the gay community had already established itself economically and politically, this two-pronged approach was effective in reducing viral transmission rates and in providing generally compassionate care.

In 1983, with small grants from the city health department, gay community organizations in San Francisco began major AIDS prevention campaigns. At that time the opinion was publicly expressed around the country—and even within some segments of the gay community—that gay men infected with HIV or at risk of infection were "sex addicts" who had such low self-esteem that they believed that they deserved AIDS and were incapable of changing their sexual behavior.[20] However, as a result of the community organizing and education campaigns, the San Francisco HIV transmission rate associated with gay sexual contact had dropped from 12 percent to 2 percent by 1985, and the following year it dropped even further. Additionally, the city developed a pattern of medical and social services which have been cited as national models of both humane and economic care.[21]

A crucial component in the development of the "San Francisco experience," as it has been called, has been the active role of the gay and lesbian community, not only in the provision of services, but also in the exercise of political power. Grass-roots organizing of the gay community in the 1970s, especially in the Castro district, resulted in large gay Democratic clubs and the inclusion of both open and closeted gay and lesbian staff throughout the city bureaucracy. When gay community leaders responded to the AIDS epidemic, they utilized the political power of the clubs, combined with the community's growing power in the bureaucracy to force a response from the city's health department. When the response was deemed inadequate, but no more could be forced at the time, the economic power and the local organizing skills were turned to the development of community-based alternatives to public services.

For example, when the San Francisco Department of Public Health refused to print sexually explicit educational material, the Harvey Milk Democratic Club, and later, the San Francisco AIDS Foundation, printed explicit brochures and posters from their own funds.

Gay community activists, joined by others with concerns about AIDS, raised funds, lobbied, campaigned, and built new organizations. In some cases, they went around the law. Illegal activities included the provision of unapproved medicines, civil disobedience, and individual assistance to those seeking a final escape from pain. These activities were overwhelmingly supported by the gay community, in which there was a widespread belief that the community must make its own priorities, rules, and responses to survive the epidemic.

Most ethnic minority communities cannot draw on the financial resources that are available to the (predominantly white) gay community. They have also been unable to force a public (governmental) response sufficient to provide the AIDS prevention and medical care services needed in their communities.[22] At the same time, they suffer from pervasive poverty, inadequate health services, poor health, a drug use epidemic, and a rapidly growing rate of HIV infection and disease.

It is sometimes stated that community organizing to prevent the spread of AIDS in minority communities is unrealistic. Some believe that key elements in the communities at risk are either unable or unwilling to change. Alternatives most commonly suggested are mass media approaches, working with individuals or small groups, or more traditional social control strategies. A brief glance at two high-risk groups, previously written off as intractable, indicates that such assumptions can be wrong.

Drug users, a group that comprises a significant proportion of people of color with AIDS, are often described as "unable to change." However, a New Jersey Health Department study conducted in 1986 of addicts who were provided with vouchers for treatment indicated that the overwhelming majority of intravenous drug users will seek care and rehabilitation in a therapeutic environment if it is available.[23] In fact, even President Reagan's AIDS Commission found that the most important obstacle to preventing AIDS among drug users is the lack of adequate treatment programs, and lengthy waiting lists for those in existence. Furthermore, research on women who are drug-dependent indicates that a major impediment to their survival and to their ability to change is the lack of women-appropriate treatment.[24]

Another group which is often scapegoated as unscrupulous HIV infectors of innocent populations are female prostitutes. However, research conducted by the Centers for Disease Control found no differences in HIV infection rates between prostitutes and other women, despite the fact that prostitutes average many more sexual encounters, including higher rates of intercourse.[25] Those prostitutes who are either infected through sexual contact (sometimes by their steady partners) or through drug use often continue to use condoms with customers. Also, prostitutes in both the United States and Europe are currently educating themselves about AIDS and are developing risk-reduction programs which include condom use, drug abuse prevention and safety, education of customers, and legal protection against the scapegoating process. The prostitutes most involved in this work are those who were already organized locally, nationally and internationally prior to the AIDS epidemic through organizations such as COYOTE in the United States and the Red Thread in the Netherlands and elsewhere in Europe.[26]

An important contradiction in the attitude of the state toward prostitutes and AIDS is seen in the fact that some prostitute education programs are being partially state funded, as in California and the Netherlands, at the same time that repressive legislation is being passed against prostitutes under the auspices of preventing the spread of the virus. For example in 1988, the California legislature (by an overwhelming majority) enacted legislation which allows mandatory HIV testing of anyone convicted of prostitution charges. Previously a misdemeanor, prostitution became a felony if engaged in by an HIV-positive person, regardless of the type of sex act involved. This legislation will have its greatest impact on poor black women, who make up the majority of women infected with HIV and the majority of prostitution arrests. They can be forced to undergo non-confidential antibody testing, the results of which will be placed in governmental files. They will also face prison time for the "crime" of having been infected with HIV.

Direct Action and Self-Help

By 1988, "direct action" AIDS focused organizing projects had spread to over twenty American cities. The best known, Act-UP of New York City, staged die-ins, demonstrations on Wall Street and at City Hall, and helped to sponsor civil disobedience at the U.S. Supreme Court after the National Gay and Lesbian Rights March in October, 1987. A national network of such organizations now exists. The organizations in the network and the network itself are primarily based in the gay community and have a special focus on the needs of people who are already infected with HIV. Consequently, their primary concern has been treatment, including research and access problems. Matters such as prevention, and agreement on a political analysis or a strategy to combat racism, poverty, or sexism in services, have had a lower priority for these groups.[27] Concerns over access to treatment, however, have moved many members of the network in the direction of support for greater state funding of health care. The most loudly cheered demands at some rallies are those for national health care and/or health insurance. It is to be expected that if the composition of the network changes, the focus of the action will also change.

The large numbers of people with AIDS in these direct action groups give their demonstrations the feel of a mass movement. However, until the movement is more firmly linked to women's issues and to black, Latino and other minority communities, the AIDS direct action movement will probably have limited utility for the women who are most affected by the epidemic.

In addition to the direct action tradition, political activity focused on AIDS could incorporate lessons from the women's health movement of the 1960s and 1970s. The women's "self-help" movement produced some important changes in health care and the analysis of health issues that are relevant to any organizing concerning AIDS and women. The institutional changes include an important increase in the number of women physicians, a somewhat greater role for women in setting health policy, the increased recognition of the right of women to control their own bodies, and the establishment of women's clinics and other women-focused services in both the private and public sector. Coincident with these changes has been the development of feminist analyses which utilize gender-sensitive socioeconomic models to understand women's health. The self-help movement, epitomized by self-examination and the rise of feminist and collectively run clinics, combined forces with the feminist pressure for changes in the medical establishment to produce the new and reorganized services for women.[28]

In some cities these services are now providing the base for services and advocacy for women with AIDS. The Women's AIDS Network of the San Francisco Bay Area (founded in 1983) and the Women and AIDS Project in New York State (begun in 1986) are two examples of broad-based feminist advocacy networks whose members are also predominantly involved in direct health services to women. The political focus of these and similar organizations throughout the US is on policies which predominantly affect women of color. Nevertheless, many of the most active women in the networks are white. The discrepancy is partially due to the tendency of ethnically identified health activists, including women, to work in ethnically identified organizations. Women's AIDS advocacy work through the networks has generally been sensitive to issues of race and class. However, the AIDS epidemic presents feminist AIDS activists with a challenge that reflects—and could potentially ameliorate—some of the color and class contradictions of its leadership and members.

Investing Resources

In 1988, the Robert Wood Johnson Foundation, one of the largest funders in the area of health policy, announced its intention to begin funding innovative, community-based AIDS projects. Health departments, state and federal agencies are also moving slowly in this direction. But the question still remains: which communities will be targeted for these resources and how will they be selected?

From an ethical standpoint, the most appropriate communities for organizing projects are those in which the members have a high risk or rates of infection. Communities which meet this criterion include urban black, Latino, and Native American communities; prison populations and the families of prisoners; and gay male communities. Population groups at high risk within their communities (which may be formed into subcultures or subcommunities) include: teenagers (because of high rates of sexual activity without protection); IV drug users, their partners and families; and sex partners of infected members of a community.

It is important to remember, however, that risk is a relative term: compared to the residents of Boise, Idaho, San Franciscans are at high risk, while residents of Boise are at higher risk than people in Stanley, Idaho, which is a much smaller town. But any drug user who has shared needles in the last ten years is at higher risk than anyone else in the categories just mentioned. Even within certain states there are factors that can cloud the determination of who is most at risk for HIV infection. For example, although California is in the top four states nationally in absolute numbers of cases of AIDS among women, women constitute only 2 percent statewide of those diagnosed. This is because there are so many gay men in California with AIDS. Risk factors for California women with AIDS are divided almost equally among IV drug use (25 percent), heterosexual contact (31 percent), and transfusions (30 percent).[29] Transfusions, and consequent transfusion-related HIV infections,* are more common among whites and Asians than among blacks and Latinos, which also affects the racial distribution of HIV infection in the state. However, within the state, blacks still have the highest rates of infections from intravenous drug use, heterosexual intercourse, and "undetermined sources." And the gay/bisexual risk for black men is close to that for whites.[30] The cumulative meaning of these statistics is that although there may be more white women and men with AIDS in California, the current risk of HIV infection is far greater for a black woman than for her white counterpart.

A second factor one might consider in initiating a community organizing project is the power of the community members individually or collectively to marshall resources to protect themselves from HIV. Variables such as access to wealth, political power, education, and community organization affect this ability. In the United States, the AIDS epidemic has struck individuals and communities which vary widely in their ability to control key resources such as medical care, prevention campaigns, civil liberties protections, and public and private social services. If AIDS prevention is going to work for women, one goal of organizing should be to increase their control of these resources.

Most women at risk of HIV infection and/or AIDS lack the economic and social power to protect themselves from the epidemic. Community organizing is a method of mobilizing and involving women in a process of social change that results in heightened ability of the community to control key aspects of its destiny. Community organization is not sufficient to prevent AIDS in every individual. But it is a necessary step to develop the resources, norms, rewards, and sanctions needed within the community to sustain any individual behavior change. New economic resources, housing, drug treatment centers, battered women's shelters, accessible health services and childcare, as well as legal resources, are probably necessary for women in specific communities to stay off IV drugs and be safe in their sexual relationships.

We do not yet know how effective community organizing will be for AIDS prevention. The San Francisco gay experience gives us a clue and we can speculate from the histories of other organizing projects. But more research is needed in other communities. Com-

---

*Since the introduction of HIV antibody testing in 1985, transfusions no longer represent a significant risk of infection.

munity organization projects are complex and their study requires appropriate methodology. One goal of AIDS prevention research in this area should be comparison of the effectiveness of different organizing strategies in controlling the AIDS epidemic. Research could be done in several black and Latino communities within one large metropolitan area or state (in order to control for epidemiological and/or political factors). Several organizing techniques could be studied. Interventions could include not only the community organizing *per se*, but a variety of AIDS-prevention techniques, such as support groups, media messages, behavior modification, counseling, and so on.

Data concerning the organizing processes and their impact on the community's institutions and social relations, including individual behavior, would be collected over time. The natural complexity of human social relationships and social change would require the collection and analysis of qualitative as well as quantitative data. And because we know that intervention of any sort is better than nothing in preventing AIDS, it would not be ethical to have a "control" community with no intervention as part of the sample under study, although one could examine epidemiological data from similar communities which did not have intervention and/or research projects.

Without a diverse approach, which community organizing and community control implies, we are condemning not only these women, but their communities, to long slow deaths. If we opt for life, let us opt for the conditions which make it possible.

NOTES

1. CDC, "AIDS Weekly Surveillance Report," June 13, 1988.

2. Guinan, Mary and Ann Hardy, "Epidemiology of AIDS in women in the United States: 1981 through 1986," *JAMA*, vol. 257, no. 15 (April 17, 1987), pp. 2039–2042.

3. *Ibid.*

4. *Ibid.*

5. M. Marmor, L.R. Weiss, et al., "Possible Female-to-Female transmission of Human Immunodeficiency Virus," (letter), *Annals of Internal Medicine*, vol. 105 (December, 1986).

6. Guinan and Hardy, "Epidemiology of AIDS in Women ..."

7. Catherine Maler, "Women with AIDS and ARC in San Francisco," in *Women and AIDS Clinical Resource Guide*, Nancy Shaw, ed (San Fran-

cisco AIDS Foundation, 1987); Carolyn McCall, Jan Casteel, and Nancy Shaw, *Pregnancy in Prison: A Needs Assessment of Perinatal Outcome in Three California Penal Institutions* (State of California Department of Health Services, 1985).

8. Guinan and Hardy, "Epidemiology of AIDS in Women ..."

9. C. Horsburgh, et al., "Preventive Strategies for Sexually Transmitted Diseases for the Primary Care Physician," *JAMA*, vol. 258, no. 6 (August 14, 1987), pp. 815–821.

10. M. Solomon and W. DeJong, "Recent Sexually Transmitted Disease Prevention Efforts and Their Implications for AIDS Health Education," *Health Education Quarterly*, vol. 13, no. 4 (Winter, 1986), pp. 301–316.

11. See the following for some examples of this type of community-oriented primary health care: D. Werner and B. Bower, *Helping Health Workers Learn* (Palo Alto, CA: Hesperian Foundation, 1982); and Richard Couto, *Streams of Idealism and Health Care Innovation* (New York: Teachers College Press, 1982).

12. National AIDS Network," AIDS Education and Support Services to Minorities: A Survey of Community-Based AIDS Service Providers" (Washington, DC: 1987).

13. See P. Harder, et al., *Evaluation of California's AIDS Community Education Program* (Sacramento: Office of AIDS, California Department of Health Services, 1987).

14. S. Alinsky, *Reveille for Radicals* (New York: Vintage, 1969).

15. See Robert Fisher and Joseph M. Kling's "Leading the People," In *Radical America*, vol. 21, no. 1, February 1988, for a comparison of Alinsky's strategy with that of the American Communist Party, which emphasized overt ideological leadership in local activism.

16. Frances Fox Piven and Richard A. Cloward, *Poor People's Movements* (New York: Vintage, 1979).

17. J. Farquhar, et al., "The Stanford Five-City Project; An Overview," In *Behavioral Health: A Handbook of Health Enhancement and Disease Prevention* (New York: J. Wiley & Sons, 1984) and J. Farquhar, et al., "Community Education for Cardiovascular Health," *Lancet*, no. 1 (1977), pp. 1192–1195.

18. A. McAlister, "Community Studies of Smoking Cessation and Preventions," in *Health Consequences of Smoking for Chronic Obstructive Lung Disease: A Report of the Surgeon General* (Washington, DC: Public Health Service, 1984).

19. National AIDS Network, "AIDS Education and Support Services to Minorities ..."

20. See P. Harder, et al., *Evaluation of California's AIDS Community Education Program* (Sacramento, 1987), p. 129.

21. W. Winkelstein, et al., "The San Francisco Men's Health Study: Reduction in Human Immunodeficiency Virus Among Homosexual/Bisexual Men, 1982–84," *American Journal of Public Health* (June, 1987).

22. AIDS Discrimination Unit, "AIDS and People of Color: The Discriminatory Impact" (New York: New York City Commission on Human Rights, Nov. 13, 1986, xerox); "Access of Hispanics to Health Care and Cuts in Services: A State-of-the-Art Overview," *American Journal of Public Health* (May–June, 1986).

23. J. Jackson and L. Rotkiewicz, "A Coupon Program: AIDS Education and Drug Treatment," Paper presented at the Third International Conference on AIDS (Washington, DC: June, 1987).

24. J. Mondanaro, "Strategies of AIDS Prevention: Motivating Health Behavior in Drug Dependent Women," *Journal of Psychoactive Drugs*, vol. 19, no. 2 (April–June, 1987).

25. "Antibody to Human Immunodeficiency Virus in Female Prostitutes," *JAMA*, vol. 257, no. 15 (April 17, 1987).

26. Interviews, Gail Pfetersen (Red Thread), December, 1987; Gloria Lockett, Priscilla Alexander (COYOTE), June, 1988.

27. Interview, Vito Russo, Act-UP, June, 1988.

28. For a review of these changes, see E. Lewin and V. Olesen, eds., *Women, Health, and Healing: Toward a New Perspective* (New York: Tavistock, 1985).

29. California Department of Health Services, "California AIDS Update," June, 1988.

30. California Department of Health Services, "February Surveillance Report," March 2, 1988.

Community Empowerment as a Strategy for Health Promotion for Black and Other Minority Populations

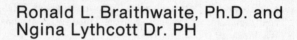

Ronald L. Braithwaite, Ph.D. and Ngina Lythcott Dr. PH

Today's despair is a poor chisel to carve out tomorrow's justice.[1]

Rev. Dr. Martin Luther King, Jr.

THE HEALTH STATUS OF blacks, other minorities, and the poor remains unconscionably low when contrasted with that of white Americans. This disparity is not new but is an historical trend that can be seen across all categories of the leading causes of death and disease. In August 1985, the *Report of the Secretary's Task Force on Black and Minority Health*[2] noted that minorities experienced approximately 60,000 "excess deaths" annually. Margaret Heckler, who was then the secretary of the U.S. Department of Health and Human Services, emphasized that the disparity is "an affront both to our ideals and to the ongoing genius of American Medicine." The six major contributors to the disparity between black and white death rates are cancer, cardiovascular disease and stroke, diabetes, chemical dependency, homicide and accidents, and infant mortality. Since the 1985 report, blacks and Latinos, in particular, also have evidenced a disproportionately high rate of Acquired Immunodeficiency Syndrome-related deaths.[3]

Ronald Braithwaite and Ngina Lythcott, "Community Empowerment as a Strategy for Health Promotion for Black and Other Minority Populations," *Journal of the American Medical Association* 261, no. 2 (January 13, 1989): pp. 282–283. Reprinted by Permission of the Authors and the *Journal of the American Medical Association*.

Congressman Louis Stokes recently reported that the health care system in America is by and large two-tiered: the affluent, who occupy one tier, receive adequate health care and the poor, who occupy the other, do not.[4] At a time when our nation is making remarkable breakthroughs in medical care, this state of affairs is inexcusable. It is not difficult to postulate what Dr. Martin Luther King, Jr., would have to say about this serious disparity; and Jesse Jackson's words serve as inspiration when he says that "it's about the politics of inclusion, not exclusion."

Poverty and powerlessness create circumstances in people's lives that predispose them to the highest indexes of social dysfunction, the highest indexes of morbidity and mortality, the lowest access to primary care, and little or no access to primary preventive programs. Poverty of the spirit and of resources remains *the* antecedent risk factor of preventable disease. Dr. King[1] said, "When people came to see that in spite of progress their conditions were still unsufferable, when they looked out and saw more poverty ... despair began to set in. Unfortunately, when hope diminishes, the hate is often turned most bitterly toward those who originally built up the hope."

Powerlessness is a structural problem that is embedded in and reinforced by the fabric of our social institutions. Community empowerment and self-reliance are valuable strategies that need to be promoted on a large scale for poor communities. Jesse Jackson speaks of American society as a quilt with many different patches, many cultures and perspectives. Yet we find most black Americans, Latinos, and other economically disadvantaged groups immersed in poverty and in the quagmire of premature death and disability. Thus, America's quilt is tattered, if complete.

Freire's work with communitywide illiteracy in Brazil involved concepts that might prove useful to the American medical community.[5] In his view, the individual becomes powerless in assuming the role of "object," acted on by the environment, rather than "subject," acting in and on the world. The individual, thus, is alienated from genuine participation in the construct of social reality. Powerlessness, for Freire, results from the passive acceptance of oppressive cultures. In summary, the sense of powerlessness is viewed as a construct of continuous interaction between the person and his/her environment. It combines an attitude of self-blame, a sense of generalized distrust, a feeling of alienation from resources of social influence, an experience of disenfranchisement and economic vulnerability, and a sense of hopelessness in the sociopolitical struggle. Fuchs[6] raises the question, "Who shall live?" Certainly one scenario could observe the poor and disenfranchised rising up and saying, "We will not submit to this neglect any longer."

Several approaches to community empowerment have emerged from the early community organizing efforts of Alinsky[7] and Kahn.[8] Community empowerment is a process of increasing control by groups over consequences that are important to their members and to others in the broader community.[9] Research by McKnight[10] on health and empowerment suggests that it is impossible to produce health among the powerless but that it is possible to allow health by transferring tools, authority, budgets, and income to those with the malady of powerlessness. Dr. King[1] said, "However much we may try to romanticize the slogan [Black Power], there is no separate Black path to power and fulfillment that does not intersect White paths, and there is no separate White path to power and fulfillment short of social disaster that does not share that power with Black aspirations for freedom and human dignity. We are bound together in a single garment of destiny."

During the 1960s, the concept of community empowerment grew from its roots in social action ideology. In this context, low-income people were encouraged to become genuinely involved in making decisions and addressing policy issues that affected the quality of life in their respective communities. The self-help perspectives of the 1970s and the health promotion movement of the 1980s offer hope for the 30 to 40 million Americans who lack private or public health insurance coverage.

Victor Fuchs, author of *The Health Economy*[11] and *Who Shall Live?*[4] addresses the pitfalls of the U.S. health care system from an economic perspective. Among the remedies he suggests, health education and health promotion are the options likely to yield the greatest benefits. Fuchs's hypothesis has become a tenable one because now there is less disagreement in the health field regarding the impact of cholesterol, lack of exercise, cigarette smoking, and other aspects of lifestyle or morbidity and mortality. Access to structured health promotion programs through employer benefit programs and/or private health clubs is available primarily to the middle and upper classes due to the high cost of the programs and the limited resources of others in our country. Primary prevention must become available to the black, brown, and other minority communities if the tide of systemic neglect of these groups is to be addressed.

Following the assassination of Dr. King, many inner-city communities did rise up in anger and frustration. The U.S. congressional response was the War on Poverty. This legislated public reaction had its successes and failures; the key question is why we require national tragedy and bloodshed to evoke a public response. Could we not have an equally active response to reasoned, peaceful expressions of concern? Is violence the only way the cries of the poor and disenfranchised of our society can be heard?

The legislative response to the 1985 *Report of the Task Force on Black and Minority Health* was to create an Office of Minority Health. This office was appropriated only a $3 million budget to address the health promotion and disease prevention concerns within the black, Latino, Native American, and Asian-American communities. Needless to say, this amount was woefully inadequate. It is time to do away with incrementalism and other bandages. The health community needs to develop comprehensive and culturally sensitive approaches to address the complex and multifaceted issues of minority health and wellness.

The Henry J. Kaiser Family Foundation, based in Menlo Park, Calif, has assumed a leadership role with its ten-year initiative for health promotion. The foundation has begun a national effort to reduce preventable morbidity and mortality due to cancer, cardiovascular disease, adolescent pregnancy, substance abuse, violence, and accidents through a grant-funding mechanism. The foundation has funded the Health Promotion Resource Center at Morehouse School of Medicine, Atlanta, to provide technical assistance in community-based health promotion for minority and poor communities. The Carnegie Corporation also is providing support for this effort.

The approach of the Health Promotion Resource Center uses community development as the vehicle and community-based health promotion intervention as the change model. An important aspect of this approach facilitates the development of a decision-making community coalition board to identify its health promotion priorities, to inventory its resources, and to build coalitions with the public and private sectors to access other resources and to address policy and manage resources in support of health interventions. This approach also develops community leadership for health promotion and advocates community health promotion. The expectation is that community organization and development for health promotion is a model that will improve the community's ability to address other important quality-of-life issues as well as to improve the health status of its members.

Because health behaviors are culture-bound, primary prevention efforts that address preventable disease and illness must emerge from a knowledge of and a respect for the culture of the target community to ensure that both the community organization and development effort and any interventions that emerge are culturally sensitive and linguistically appropriate. For the poor, such an empowerment approach to health promotion is like a sleeping giant— when it rises up, all will know that the historically disenfranchised will be more self-reliant and healthier.

NOTES

1. King ML: Black power, in Baker RK (ed): *Afro-American Readings*. New York, Van Nostrand Reinhold Co. 1970.

2. *Report of the Secretary's Task Force on Black and Minority Health*. US Dept of Health and Human Services, 1985.

3. Minorities and AIDS: Knowledge, attitudes and misconception among black and Latino adolescents. *Am J Public Health* 1988; 78:55–57.

4. Stokes L: The health of black America. *Health Aims* 1988:6 3–4.

5. Freire P: *Education for Critical Consciousness*. New York, Seabury Press, 1973.

6. Fuchs VR: *Who Shall Live?* New York, Basic Publishers, 1983.

7. Alinsky SD: *Reveille For Radical*. New York, Vintage Books, 1969.

8. Kahn S: *How People Get Power*. New York, McGraw-Hill International Book Co., 1970.

9. Fawcett SB, Seekins T, Whang PW, et al: Involving consumers in decision-making. *Social Policy* 1982:13: 36–41.

10. McKnight JL: Health and empowerment. *Can J Public Health* 1985:76:37–38.

11. Fuchs VR: *The Health Economy*. Cambridge, Mass., Harvard University Press, 1986.

A Week on Ward 5A

Ed Wolf, Shanti Staff Counselor, Ward 5A

(All client names have been changed to maintain confidentiality.)

SEVEN DAYS A WEEK, every day of the year, there are Shanti counselors on Ward 5A to offer support to all who come here—patient, visitor and staff alike. We are counselor, advocate, educator, handholder, masseur, facilitator, and mediator all rolled into one.

There are currently seven of us, offering our services throughout the hospital. Together we are gay and straight, male and female, HIV-positive and HIV-negative, black, brown, and white. As a team we speak Spanish, French, Greek, and English. Some of us are raising kids, one is a grandparent, some take dance classes, some go kayaking and camping. Some have their own private practice, some are planning to go back to school. We keep journals, we cook, and some of us do volunteer work for other organizations.

Together we work as a team. Two, three, or four of us on the ward at any one time. We know we can lean on each other, learn from each other, and rely on each other. The days here can be very intense, and we use each other to unload, to enliven, to comfort.

Ed Wolf, "A Week on Ward 5A," *Eclipse*, the Shanti Project, Spring 1989. Reprinted by permission of the Shanti Project.

Sunday

Ann spoke to me this evening about her brother, who is dying of AIDS. Ken was able to speak to her several days ago, but is now incoherent. Ann is from out of town and is filled with feelings of grief and loss. The doctors told her last week that Ken wouldn't live past Friday, and now, two days later, he's still alive. We spoke about the dying process and why it might be taking him so long to die. Is he ready yet? Has he said his goodbyes? Has she said hers?

She spoke tenderly, of how her brother's impending death has reopened for her an old wound, the death of her infant daughter several years ago.

We discussed together her ability to deal, and to cope, and to find ways to carry the immeasurable sadness she is experiencing.

Earlier this evening I spoke with a young man who had recently been diagnosed with pneumocystis. He described how his "journey" with AIDS was progressing, of his KS diagnosis last year, of the day he was first told he was HIV-positive. He asked me if I had taken the HIV-antibody test. I told him that I had, and that I had tested negative. I told him one of my first reactions had been "why me?" He told me he had the same reaction to his tests results. Together we explored the randomness of things and the importance of separating judgment from the events that come into our lives. Before I left his room, he said he had recently stopped asking "why me?" "Nowadays," he said, "I ask 'what's next' "?

Monday

This morning, as I get ready to go to work, I wonder if Ken and his sister will still be at the hospital. Has he died during the night?

As Shanti counselors at San Francisco General Hospital, we are privileged to come into people's lives while they are experiencing extraordinary circumstances. We may become involved with a patient and his or her loved ones for several days or several weeks; often there's only enough time for a single visit. We are constantly opening up to new people and letting go of familiar faces. During my two days off-duty this past week, half of the ward was discharged and an equal number of patients were admitted. We often have feelings of incompleteness, of unfinishedness, with the rapid comings and goings of the patients and the visitors with whom we work. I am always reminded that life on the ward magnifies the larger picture—how we are all constantly walking in and out of each other's lives.

Every morning at 11 o'clock the Shanti counselors, social workers, and the charge nurse come together for report. Together we go over every patient with AIDS or ARC in the hospital and assess their varying needs. These patients are going home today; someone's being transferred to 5A from the Intensive Care unit. Someone's mom has come to see him for the first time since his diagnosis—can one of the Shanti counselors be sure to check in on them later today? Ken is still alive; his sister needs help finding a chaplain.

There are three Shanti counselors on duty today and we divide and prioritize the patients to be seen. I will follow up on Ken and his sister, but first there's someone a nurse wants me to talk with.

He's not a patient here. He's sitting in a chair in the corridor, a young black man who has just recently arrived in San Francisco. Jim tells me he has little money and needs a place to stay, says that he is HIV-positive, feels weak and tired all the time, and is having trouble keeping his food down. He has not been diagnosed with either AIDS or ARC—can I help him?

I explain how without an actual AIDS/ARC diagnosis he cannot receive the services he's requesting through Shanti. I suggest some of the emergency shelters in San Francisco, some of the food lines, where to go for food stamps and general assistance. I encourage him to make an appointment at Ward 86, the outpatient clinic here at SFGH. Jim tells me the horrific story of his past year, of his enlistment in the military, of the standard blood tests they now require, and the shock he felt when he was rejected by the local board because he was HIV-positive.

Shunned by family and friends, he has come to San Francisco because "I heard how they help people here." As we part in the hallway, I am filled with a sense of helplessness and concern.

As I go in to see Ken, I am struck by the sound of his breathing. It is loud and labored, and the oxygen coming from the wall fills the room with a harsh hissing. He lies on his side; he cannot speak. His sister is not in the room, but his lover, Bill, is at his bedside, looking very tired and very sad. We talk about the death of his father and the similarity of the pain of losing a dad and a lover, the pain of losing anyone we love, of being left behind. I gently touch Ken's arm as Bill tells me a little about their seven years together; a special trip one summer, a mountain they had climbed. He has been wondering if Ken can still hear. As we talk he decides he probably can, and that these bittersweet sharings of their life together are like a memorial service. We wonder what it would be like to hear one's own memorial service, and decide it would be okay to know that you are missed, that you had left many loving memories behind. The sadness in the room swells up and as Bill cries, I gently move my hand and place it on the heart of the man in the bed.

As the day draws to a close, I check in with one of my coworkers. He listens as I describe the sadness that I felt in Ken's room, and how difficult it was for me to let the young HIV-positive man walk away down the hall, unable to do more for him. He tells me of an especially good connection he made with one of the patients, and how happy he is that another went home today.

Tuesday

As I enter through the main lobby of the hospital this morning, I find myself wondering if Ken is still alive.

The day begins in a rush as I encounter Ken's sister in the hallway. Ann has already extended her stay here in San Francisco for two days—she must get to the bus station and return home to her children and other responsibilities. But Ken is still alive. How can she leave him? We move into an empty room on 5A and sit together. Her eyes are swollen from all the crying she has done in the last few days. She says to me, "I must go and I can't go."

At first I am struck with the seeming impossibility of this dilemma. I experience a growing sense of my own inadequacies in trying to help in some way. I also know that this woman has her own answers and that she doesn't need me to tell her what to do. She sought me out to be a supportive presence, to be a sounding board perhaps, to discuss and explore her own options. As she tells me of her situation at home, it becomes increasingly clear that she must return to her children as soon as possible.

I ask her if she can tell Ken what she is telling me, how much it hurts to be leaving him now. We begin to talk about permission and the startling similarities between her need for permission to go home and Ken's need for permission to die in his own time, on his own terms.

She decides that she can do this. I ask her if she'd like me to come with her to Ken's room, and she softly says, "Thank you, no." As we return to the hallway, I give her a parting hug and know that I will not be seeing her again.

The tone of this interaction seems to reverberate through the rest of the day. I have lunch in the hospital cafeteria with one of the chaplains, and as he tells me about a recent weekend retreat he attended, I know that several floors above us Ken and his sister are gently parting.

Later in the day I meet with Alfredo, who is here visiting his brother Ramon. Ramon has pneumocystis, is from Mexico, and is far from his family. I listen as Alfredo speaks of life in Mexico City and the AIDS epidemic there, and for just a moment I see Ann looking out a bus window, heading home.

Wednesday

The first half of every Wednesday is devoted to getting together with the other counselors. We alternate, from week to week, between support group and case presentations. This morning one of the counselors discussed an especially difficult series of interactions he had with a patient who was having problems with the nursing staff. We then had a business meeting and a short support group. Through these first four hours of the day, I repeatedly thought of Ken.

Wednesday is also discharge planning day, when many outside AIDS service agencies come together with the in-house staff to discuss the discharge plans for all PWAs and PWARCs currently in the hospital. It is here that I find out that Ken is still alive. The medical team reports that his "deep pain reflex" is gone and he is now comatose.

When the meeting ends, I go to see Ken. There is no one visiting. The room is filled with balloons, flowers, and get-well cards. Someone has placed a small teddy bear on the pillow near his head. Ken seems peaceful. His breaths are very short and far between as I place my hand on his chest and breathe with him for a while. I tell of some of my interactions with his sister and his lover, and that they have told me they will be all right. I tell him it's okay to let go. I become aware of my own wish that his suffering will end soon, today, now. I am aware then of the necessity of my having to let go, of respecting the mystery of how and when any of us die.

The day is quickly coming to a close as I leave Ken's room and go to see one more patient. He was here a year ago and I remember him well. I have pulled our old chart on him and read through some of the previous conversations we had.

As I enter his room, I perceive how much Marvin has changed since we last met. His body is extremely thin; he is too weak to stand on his own. But the biggest change is in his mental status. He has been diagnosed with HIV dementia and is here awaiting placement.

Five of the sixteen patients on 5A this week are here because of dementia and the placement problems it creates. Because of the level of difficulty experienced in trying to connect with someone who is demented and the anguish it can cause the visitor, demented patients often spend a lot of time alone.

Today as I sit with Marvin, I find myself working hard to connect in any possible way. I ask about the television show he is watching; the lunch he has just been fed. I read all his get-well cards out loud and ask him about each of the senders.

Because his responses are minimal, I feel I have not connected. As I begin to leave his vacant eyes follow me and he asks, "You're not leaving yet, are you?"

I sit down and tell him I can stay a little longer. I am touched and moved by his question. I sit with him in silence now as he gazes blankly at the television, and I hold his hand. I assumed that my presence had not been felt and, in doing so, had almost missed the connection we were so clearly sharing.

Thursday

Today is my last day on the ward before a three-day weekend, my birthday weekend as a matter of fact, and I have made plans to go to the mountains. After 2-½ years on 5A, I have found it very important to take care of myself, especially on my days off. As I get ready for work, I think of the full week I've already had.

When I get to the hospital I see that Ken is still alive.

Morning report runs longer than usual because the census is very large.

All 16 beds on 5A are full and another 16 patients are on other wards. There are 14 patients with penumocystis, many newly diagnosed. There will be a lot for the weekend counselors to do.

I go and say good-bye to Ken. A friend is visiting, and so is Ken's Shanti volunteer. Ken's breathing seems very faint, too delicate and weak to be keeping him alive. As I leave, I know I will not see him again.

I check in with Alfredo. His brother is doing better physically, but not as well emotionally. He wants to bring their mother up from Mexico City, but there are financial as well as visa problems. The social worker is doing what she can, but nothing is definite. Alfredo seems very tearful today and when I ask him if he's cried since his brother's diagnosis, he says, "Yes, but alone, so no one sees. It is important for me to be strong for my brother."

I am glad to learn that the man with pneumocystis whom I had seen earlier in the week continues to do well. He is no longer using oxygen and most of his energy is spent dealing with the side effects of the medications he is on. He looks forward to going home soon.

As I am charting the many interactions of the day for the counselors who will be following me, a nurse tells me there is a man in the patient lounge looking for me. Before I can finish what I am doing, Bernard comes into the office and sits down. He is someone with whom I have worked before, another man suffering with dementia. It has been several weeks since his discharge. He had been upstairs on a locked unit for several months and was visited many times by myself and the other counselors. He is extremely agitated and out of control, has been drinking, and is suicidal. I see immediately that he needs to go to Psych Emergency and be admitted. As we talk, I keep him focused on where he is and who he is with, that he is in crisis and with someone who cares about him. With the help of the social worker, I find out that he can only be admitted by his doctor who is over on Ward 86, a ten-minute trip from 5A.

We walk together across the hospital grounds, my arm across his shoulders. He tells me of some of the good times and bad times he's been through since we last saw each other. As I leave him with the team on Ward 86, I am aware of the special relationship I have with him. No matter how many times he may be discharged and readmitted, I or one of the other counselors will be here for him in whatever capacity he needs.

When I return to 5A and finish up my charting, I see a note on the blackboard. It tells of a patient who was recently discharged from 5A and who has died at home.

I go to a shelf and pull out a thick red scrapbook, the 5A book of keepsakes; of names and faces and poems and thank yous. In the front are page after page of lined entries, divided into years, the names of men and women who were patients on 5B/5A and the date of their death. I enter the last name and the date, and know that sometime over the next few days, someone will come behind me and enter Ken's name.

My work week is over.

I put on my jacket, ride down the elevator, and go through the main entrance of the hospital, out into the night air. I think of Ken's sister, Ann, and how she is surely at home by now. I think of several patients who will be going home from 5A during the days I will be off. And I think of Ken, who is going home too. I feel the sadness that this week has touched in me and then, looking expectantly toward the coming weekend, head off for home myself.

Against All Odds: Grass-roots Minority Groups Fight AIDS

William Deresiewicz, Health/PAC Bulletin

1988

ONE DAY THREE YEARS ago, Curtis Wadlington learned that a close friend had AIDS. The friend was in a hospital, and his family didn't want him home.

"His family was dysfunctional," Wadlington says. "A lot of IV drug use. So I brought him home with me and took care of him for the last ten months that he lived." Remembering that time now, Wadlington speaks softly, almost monotonously, his face impassive, his eyes burning.

"I ended up leaving my work—taking care of him was a full-time job," he says. His friend was in and out of the hospital until he died. "The nurses weren't doing what they should be doing. The workers wouldn't clean his room. A lot of days it was just me and him."

So for ten months Curtis Wadlington took the place, for his dying friend, of the entire social welfare system of their city, Philadelphia, of much of the public health system, and even of the AIDS service network, since the Philadelphia AIDS Task Force, the city's local private AIDS organization, all but refused to help him.

Wadlington's experience as a social worker taught him how to get what he needed—"who to holler at"—but, he thought, what about

"Against All Odds: Grass-roots Minority Groups Fight AIDS," *Health/PAC Bulletin*, Spring 1988. *This article is based on reporting by* Bulletin *editors William Deresiewicz and Joe Gordon, and was written by Deresiewicz. Health/PAC board members Robert Cohen, Arthur Levin, Ann Umemoto and Richard Younge provided research assistance.* Reprinted by Permission of *Health/PAC Bulletin*.

all the people who were going through the same thing and didn't know the system?

Curtis Wadlington's friend was black, a part of the "other" AIDS epidemic—the one that gets scant notice in the media, the one that has found virtually no place in the nation's consciousness, the one that receives the smallest crumbs from the crust that the federal government throws to AIDS education and counseling. Forty percent of the 52,000 people with AIDS (as defined by the Centers for Disease Control) are black, Hispanic, Asian, or Native American; among women and children, the proportion is twice as high. In large cities, over half the people with AIDS are members of minority communities. In some of New York City's largest black and Hispanic neighborhoods, more than 2 percent of all infants are born with AIDS-infected blood.

By the end of 1981, the first year of the epidemic, the AIDS surveillance reports published by the CDC showed that 20 to 25 percent of those with the disease were black or Hispanic. Epidemiologists saw by the following year that those numbers would steadily grow, that, like hepatitis, another disease that passes through blood and semen, AIDS would invade the black and Hispanic communities through the sharing of needles among intravenous drug users, through intercourse among homosexual and bisexual men, and through sex between women and drug-using and bisexual men. Their prognosis was correct: The proportion of AIDS cases found among blacks and Hispanics has grown steadily, and everything now known indicates that those two groups will bear ever-greater shares of the epidemic.

The federal response to the crisis of AIDS in minority communities has been criminally slow. The CDC held its first conference on minority AIDS in August 1987, and established a minority section of its National AIDS Information and Education Program last December. Not until February did the President's AIDS Commission release a draft report acknowledging the severity of the epidemic among blacks and Hispanics. Federal money earmarked for minority AIDS is only now being released; none has yet reached its target.

Minority communities were left to combat AIDS on their own, without the wealthy donors and sensitivity to sexual issues that allowed the white gay community to organize in the face of prejudice and neglect. Within the last three years, dozens of minority AIDS groups have come into being, all relying overwhelmingly or exclusively on the volunteer efforts of poor and working-class people.

This is the story of such groups, and of one in particular: BEBASHI of Philadelphia—Blacks Educating Blacks About Sexual Health

Issues—the organization Curtis Wadlington joined in order to help other blacks avoid the pain and frustration he went through for his dying friend.

BEBASHI was organized three years ago by Rashida Hassan, an infection-control nurse and longtime activist within the city's black community. At the time, 98 black Philadelphians had been diagnosed with the disease. Hassan's first task was to convince people that AIDS is actually a black problem. Resistance came from two sources: white gay men and blacks themselves.

"Although the gay community was saying it's not a gay white disease," Hassan recalled during a conversation earlier this year, "AIDS brought about a tremendous gay community empowerment. They said, 'No, we don't want AIDS to be classified as a gay disease, but on the other hand it's given us an opportunity to speak out in ways we haven't been able to before.'"

In fact, Hassan worked at the Philadelphia AIDS Task Force until frustration with the group's lack of response to black concerns led her to organize BEBASHI. "I came into a climate," she recalled, "where I had to say: 'Like everything else in our society, people of color are disproportionately affected, and I'm not going to let my community be the last one to be dealt with again.'" Hassan spoke with the patience of a teacher and the understated irony of someone who's had to put up with a lot of idiocy.

That same perception of AIDS as a gay white disease thwarted Hassan's efforts to mobilize black leaders. "The last thing they wanted to know was that there was some kind of deadly disease, primarily associated with gay men, affecting their community," she said. "As many leaders told me: "We've got enough stigma, we don't need to add AIDS to it.""

But Hassan wasn't daunted. "I knew about the incubation period," she said, "and I thought if we start now, we might have a chance to beat the numbers." She gathered several of her colleagues in health care—nurses, health educators, social workers—to form BEBASHI. At first the group operated out of the living room of one of its members, but BEBASHI's contacts within health care led to an informal arrangement with District 1199C, the Philadelphia local of the National Union of Hospital and Health Care Employees. Since 1986, the union has provided BEBASHI with free office space and covered its operational expenses. The group, with a staff of 4 and 30 regular volunteers, works out of a single room crowded with pamphlets and festooned with public-health posters; the door is always open and the phones ring constantly.

While BEBASHI seeks to educate all members of the black community, it focuses on gay men, IV drug users, and young people. Targeting programs to the first group has proved difficult. Unlike gay white men, gay blacks don't have a network of political and self-help organizations, because to identify with one another in this way would expose them to double discrimination from white heterosexuals. Nor do gay blacks live in separate neighborhoods. As Hassan said, "People in the black community are not ostracized because of sexual orientation. They live next door, because where else are you going to live?"

BEBASHI distributes condoms and literature in the city's few black gay bars and organizes "home parties"—safer-sex Tupperware parties. "We talk about basic AIDS transmission," Hassan said. "We have a visual aid that we use to show you how to use a condom. We talk about erotic behavior, that sex isn't dead because you have to use a condom."

Like other cities, Philadelphia faces a critical shortage of drug-treatment programs, so protective measures for IV drug users must be implemented within the context of addiction. "IV drug users will tell you that they're very careful who they share their needles with," Hassan said. "That means that at least they're thinking about it." Other AIDS workers have found many addicts to be hostile to AIDS education, resentful of being told, essentially, that they should modify their sexual or drug behavior for the sake of a society that has abandoned them.

Curtis Wadlington talked about his work as coordinator of BEBASHI's youth programs. Sitting across from Hassan at his cluttered desk in the back of the office, he explained that educating young people about AIDS means counseling them about life. "When you start to talk about AIDS," he said, "you end up talking about relationships, school, stress, being yourself, physical and mental health, caring about other people."

Hassan also stressed work with youth: "The younger your audience is," she said, "the more likely you are to reach someone who hasn't had sexual activity. We tell them that part of being an adult is accepting responsibility. We talk to them about self-empowerment, getting them to see that there is actually a reason to save themselves."

Much of BEBASHI's work addresses the black community at large. The group believes the best way of educating people to reduce their risk of contracting AIDS is by talking with them directly. Last year, BEBASHI gave over 750 presentations at schools, community centers, and churches, and sent volunteers out five days a week to talk to people and distribute condoms in gay bars, drug-treatment centers, and the city's commercial sex district. Forty percent of Philadelphia's blacks are illiterate; what brochures BEBASHI does publish present information as briefly as possible, and are understandable to people with second-grade reading levels. The group also appears regularly on Philadelphia's two black radio stations, its best source of publicity, and runs workshops for health professionals, workers in social welfare organizations, and black journalists.

It is often said that AIDS is a magnifying glass for our society, revealing the worst and best in ourselves and our nation. The worst is well-known: homophobia, racism, extreme poverty. BEBASHI is part of what's best, as are dozens of other organizations working in black, Hispanic, Asian, and Native American communities around the country. These include the New York Minority AIDS Task Force, the Hispanic AIDS Forum of New York, the San Francisco Black Coalition on AIDS, the Minority AIDS Project of Los Angeles, the Kupona Network of Chicago (the name means "to get well" in Swahili), HERO (Health Education Resource Organization) of Baltimore, Portland's People of Color United Against AIDS, and the National Native American Prevention Center on AIDS, based in Oakland.

While the history and activities of these groups have been shaped by the politics of their cities and the needs of the particular communities they serve, they have much in common. Many have expanded their activities beyond providing education and information on AIDS to include programs in support of those who have contracted the disease. The New York Minority AIDS Task Force runs group counseling for people with AIDS, people with AIDS-related complex, and families of infected individuals, and has set up an AIDS buddy program. HERO provides legal services and housing, albeit in small numbers, for people with AIDS who have lost their homes. Ron Rowell of the National Native American Prevention Center says he devotes a great deal of time to educating nurses and other health professionals about AIDS within his community.

The Kupona Network, which also provides housing, and recently opened a drop-in center for people with AIDS, has been unusual in receiving support from local Chicago officials. "The city health department recognized the importance of what we wanted to do," says its director, Tim Offut. "They encouraged us to form and are doing whatever they can to assist us."

The younger groups—those in cities where AIDS emerged relatively recently—are learning from the older ones. Portland's People of Color United Against AIDS has developed a systematic strategy for disseminating information, first developing a cadre of educators, then going out into the community at large. Amani Jabari, the group's director, has also learned to discuss AIDS infection not in terms of risk groups, but of risk behaviors, to make clear that being gay or taking drugs intravenously does not in itself make one more vulnerable to contracting the disease or pass a death sentence. Talking to gay men, IV drug users, and others about what they can do to reduce their risk lessens their feelings of helplessness and avoids stigmatizing them.

Organizers of nearly all these groups have had to overcome resistance and even hostility from white AIDS organizations, who, they say, resented minorities asking for a piece of the small pie the gay groups had fought so hard to win. Minority-run organizations were disdained as "Johnny-come-latelies," and were told they would have to refight the same battles white organizations were already beginning to win. "There are people within white male communities," says Amanda Houston-Hamilton, a physician with the San Francisco Black Coalition on AIDS, "who, no matter what their sexuality, are racist."

Even when white AIDS organizations conceded the need for education and counseling among blacks and Hispanics, they insisted on remaining in charge, on "owning AIDS," as several activists put it. Suki Ports, former director of the New York Minority AIDS Task Force, says that organizations like the Gay Men's Health Crisis were loath to surrender their reputation as the experts on AIDS even though the programs they had developed for mostly middle-class white men were inappropriate for people of different status, educational level, and ethnicity.

Nor have minority AIDS organizations received much encouragement from existing institutions within their communities. The most influential and all-pervading institution in black and Hispanic communities is the church, and most churches have been very slow in confronting the epidemic. Never before having dealt with issues of sexuality in any but the most dogmatic way, they have neither the framework nor the appetite for discussions of homosexuality, adolescent sexuality, or safer sex. But there are ways for churches to help even without confronting these issues—by counseling families of people with AIDS, running programs for drug users, and stressing the importance of AIDS prevention for the preservation of the family. A growing number of churches have begun such programs, often in response to pressure from minority AIDS groups.

While the churches' reluctance to confront the epidemic stems from religious taboos, it also reflects the stigma that many in minority communities attach to homosexuality. Many blacks and

Hispanics with AIDS, Suki Ports says, find that revealing their condition cuts them off from friends, family, and community.

In addition to this, Hassan and other grass-roots organizers point out that the major national black organizations—the NAACP, the Southern Christian Leadership Conference, the Urban League—have so far done very little in the fight against AIDS.

Yet the obstacles white AIDS groups and the black and Hispanic leadership have placed in the way of minority AIDS organizations are like pebbles compared to the monumental public health problems in whose shadow these communities have lived for generations; inadequate health services, medical indigency, malnutrition, unemployment, a dearth of decent housing. "People walk in with AIDS, but they also walk in with poverty," says the Reverend Carl Bean of the Minority AIDS Project in Los Angeles, a group he founded in 1985 upon discovering that no one in his city was addressing the problems of black people with AIDS. "We're dealing with mothers who have to grease the crib legs and place them in cans of oil to keep the rats off the crib, kids who still hunt down soda bottles to buy potato chips for a meal."

"People of color with AIDS," Hassan says, "come with all the social problems that you can think of: they're unemployed, they're probably going to be homeless if they're not already, they don't have health insurance." They are thrown at the mercy of overburdened social welfare systems that often do everything in their power to deny them help. AIDS, she explains, has become an excuse to deny public housing, health care, and psychiatric services to people in need.

What resources do minority AIDS organization have to educate their vast communities about AIDS prevention and offer help and comfort to the thousands who have contracted the disease? Private contributions and volunteers—"peanuts and love," as one activist put it. This may resemble the situation white AIDS groups faced until several years ago, but, black organizations pointed out, it's even worse. Minority communities can't draw on the kind of wealth that can generate a million dollars in a single evening; Rashida Hassan tells of collecting 5 and 10 dollars at a time from neighbors. And volunteers, as Suki Ports explains, are much harder to recruit in places where people need every minute for survival.

Yet even today the most well-funded groups run primarily on volunteer effort. And, as Curtis Wadlington says, "When we say 'volunteer' we should say 'crazy people,' because they volunteer an eight-hour day." BEBASHI, like other groups, has been able to stay afloat with small city service contracts, enough to pay for Hassan's salary, at least. The group was recently awarded a $100,000 grant from the City of Philadelphia, which brings its total operating budget to a quarter of a million dollars, about a tenth of what Curtis Wadlington estimates is needed to educate Philadelphia's 600,000 blacks effectively. Still, that's way ahead of the $100,000 budget of the New York Minority AIDS Task Force, one of the major minority AIDS service organization in a city of over three million blacks and Hispanics.

Only tax dollars can provide the sums needed to turn the rising tide of AIDS in minority communities. Yet as of this writing, Congress has allotted only $10 million for AIDS education and information programs in minority communities. Of that total, $7 million went first to states, which then issued requests for proposals (RFPs)—invitations to community-based groups to apply for grants for specific projects. The states are evaluating the responses they have received.

There are several problems with RFPs. Each embodies certain values, which, according to Paul Moore, head of the AIDS Initiative of New York City's Health and Hospitals Corporation, tend to be those of the white middle class. Advances in our understanding of AIDS tend to be long in reaching the bureaucrats who draft them. "San Francisco to this day is writing RFPs that say that AIDS is a gay white disease," Amanda Houston-Hamilton says.

The RFP system, as Amani Jabari points out, is based on the idea that organizations should fight with one another for funds. The name of his group, in fact—People of Color United Against AIDS—reflects the attempt of minority AIDS groups in Portland to cooperate with each other despite the efforts of the state health department to force them into competition. The biggest problem with applying the RFP system to AIDS funding is the time it takes. The $7 million allocated to states will not reach the streets until June, more than nine months after it was appropriated.

An additional $3 million has been appropriated for national minority AIDS organizations like the National Minority AIDS Council. This money, too, will go through a system of RFPs, and will finally be dispensed in September. The $10 million total, taken out of the roughly $100 million Congress has appropriated to AIDS education and information overall, comes in the eighth year of an epidemic that from its very beginning had at least a 20 percent minority component.

Paula Van Ness, head of the CDC's Office of AIDS Education and Information, points out that much of the money already allocated to fight the epidemic has gone to services—programs for children, for

IV drug users—that, while not specifically targeted to minority communities, serve members of those groups. She also maintains that decisions about AIDS funding are made by Congress, not by the CDC. "If I had my way," she says, "I'd be spending a billion dollars on education alone. But no one cares what I want."

AIDS has been and is still perceived as a disease that has yet to affect the "general population." Large segments of the public and the media continue to see it as a disease confined to certain outgroups who brought it on themselves. Rather than leading the country toward an acknowledgment of the scope of the epidemic, Congress has pandered to popular prejudice and distrust. "We're in an election year," Van Ness says. "Some people think AIDS has been overplayed." Every day that's wasted means more lives lost; the federal and state response to AIDS so far amounts to negligent homicide on a vast scale.

When will AIDS get the money it needs? "It won't be until case numbers nationally reach a million," Rashida Hassan says. "People will literally be dying in the streets."

Until then, the Rashida Hassans and Curtis Wadlingtons will continue to fight for the survival of their communities. Wadlington learned a long time ago that no one else will fight for them, and that ordinary commitment isn't enough. "We tell people in training," he says, "that it's down to the real stuff now—either we sink or swim. Because a lot of people are going to die in the next five years, and we're going to need that mentality just to save the few."

Supporting People with AIDS: The GMHC Model

Lewis Katoff, Ph.D. and
Susan Ince, M.S.
and the staff of the
GMHC Client Services Department

It started with love. And courage. And a terrifying realization that there was no other choice.

In 1981, confirmed and rumored cases of "gay-related immune deficiency" numbered in the dozens—and the traditional helping professions had no response to the fears and needs of those whose lives were touched by the new, mysterious, and deadly illness.

Six concerned men founded the Gay Men's Health Crisis to provide information and to raise money for research. They used their first donations to establish a hotline.

The calls poured in. With questions. With fears. And with stories more heartbreaking than they had ever imagined. True-life dramas of neglect, of abandonment, of bewilderment and abuse.

The volunteers of GMHC responded to the emergency, rapidly organizing a wide range of support services for friends and strangers whose medical conditions would later be called AIDS and ARC.

The help they offered was different from traditional medical or social services—more like the help that a family or close-knit community would offer someone in need. Like the help that lesbians and gay men offer the informal family networks they create.

Lewis Katoff, Ph.D., Susan Ince, M.S., and the staff of the GMHC Client Services Department, "Supporting People with AIDS: The GMHC Model," Reprinted by Permission of the Authors and the Gay Men's Health Crisis.

> "The needs were pressing, obvious,
> and overwhelming—it didn't take a genius
> in organizational development
> to understand the suffering."
> —Rodger McFarlane
> Former Director, GMHC

Over the years, organization became a survival issue for GMHC and other community-based groups who struggled to respond to the growing and changing nature of the epidemic. Eventually, GMHC's client services program expanded to involve more than 5000 volunteers and to serve more than 6000 clients. From the beginning, GMHC served as a prototype for others who wanted to provide emotional and practical support to people with AIDS.

This manual offers an organizational look at GMHC's client services. It is intended to provide community organizations and service providers with a detailed introduction to how the services work and how the systems evolved. Each section will describe the rationale behind organizational decisions, look ahead to upcoming challenges, and answer common practical questions from groups as they identify and address unmet needs in their local communities.

Today, the AIDS epidemic and the world are very different than when GMHC was founded. The number of cases has skyrocketed beyond the most dire predictions. And society has developed some capacity to respond.

This manual is not intended to be a step-by-step formula for organizations or a full description of the compassionate and creative work of GMHC volunteers. It is a description of one organizational model, offered so that service providers can take whatever they find valid and adapt it for the needs in their community.

Client Services Overview

> "All of GMHC's client services
> begin with the assumption
> that a diagnosis of AIDS or ARC
> is catastrophic—the threatened or actual
> disruption of all parts of a person's life."
> —Lewis Katoff
> Director of Client Services

Before very recently, most people who received the AIDS or ARC diagnosis felt that life was over. That there would be no more opportunities. No more career, no more chance for love. Many felt as if they were already dead, emotionally if not physically.

With that as the premise, client services are meant to be a lifeline—the means for a person to reestablish the ability to live life fully, within the limitations of the illness. To reconcile with families. Regain a sense of control. Reconnect with other people. Reestablish activities that are personally meaningful.

When most people think of client services, they think of crisis intervention workers and buddies. But today, three out of four GMHC clients do not receive these services. They make use of a variety of other GMHC tools and services which are available to PWAs as they make the enormous adjustments the disease may require.

GMHC's client services include:

1. Intake and referral—the client's initial assessment and ongoing guide to services
2. Crisis intervention services—the buddies, crisis intervention workers, and crisis management partners who are there when clients need caring one-on-one support in order to deal with the social, behavioral, practical, and emotional consequences of their illness
3. Group services—professionally led support groups for PWAs and their care partners
4. Recreation—opportunities for socializing and reactivating life
5. PWA telephone team—peers who stay in touch when a client is homebound or hospitalized
6. Financial services—information and advocacy so clients get the benefits they have earned
7. Legal services—aids in planning and bringing back control, as well as fighting discrimination

Intake Department

Greeting and Guiding

The intake department is the central nervous system of client services. It receives signals from inside and outside GMHC, rapidly analyzes needs, and sets in motion a coordinated response from GMHC's many branches.

When GMHC started, the function of intake could most closely be likened to that of emergency medical triage in an isolated hospital—rapid determination of the severity of needs and routing the client into the organization's available services.

Now, GMHC is no longer the only agency prepared to provide support services for PWAs, and many people are referred to outside services. The intake interview now entails a fuller assessment, and it is followed by ongoing referral and monitoring.

The intake department has four major components—registration, intake interview, referral planning, and monitoring.

I. Registration

Not everyone who contracts GMHC client services is automatically registered with the agency. Preregistration screening, which is usually done during the initial telephone call to an intake staffperson, redirects three callers for every one who is registered and scheduled for an intake interview.

Preregistration screening focuses on several questions:

• Is the potential client making the contact?

Potential clients must register directly, for considerations of confidentiality and informed consent.

Exceptions are made if a person is severely ill, does not speak English (and no translator is available), or has no access to a telephone. In these cases, the intake clinician will speak to a relative, social worker, or very close friend to determine whether registration with GMHC is appropriate. Pediatric cases are registered by the child's legal guardian.

• Is the person eligible for GMHC services?

There are two requirements for eligibility.

Diagnosis. GMHC clients must have a diagnosis of AIDS or ARC. For potential clients whose diagnosis is in doubt, the intake person will help them phrase the necessary questions in order to elicit a clear diagnosis from their physician.

Residence. GMHC serves residents of the five boroughs of New York City, and may also assist nonresidents undergoing an extended hospital stay in the city.

• Does the person want services available to nonclients?

A person can contact GMHC's legal department or ombudsman's office without becoming a GMHC client. For example, someone may just want an answer to a specific financial question. However, in order to be eligible for the complete range of services, people must go through the intake process.

• Is the person willing to participate in the intake evaluation?

All potential clients are informed that the intake involves meeting with someone for at least two hours and talking frankly about what's going on in their lives.

• Could the person be better served elsewhere?

Certain services, such as housing assistance and pastoral counseling, are outside the scope of GMHC, and the caller is referred elsewhere.

When a client is registered, preliminary information is recorded (basic demographics, diagnosis, contact information) on a registration card, and an intake staffperson assigns an intake clinician.

II. The Intake Interview

> "It's a teaching session,
> a welcome wagon, a resource directory,
> and maybe the only time that
> a client sits down to discuss
> some important life issues."
> —Daniel Korte
> Director, Intake Department

About 150 new intake assessments are performed each month. These wide-ranging, one-on-one interviews last from ninety minutes to four hours. They may be done at the GMHC office or in hospitals spread throughout the city; however, most intake sessions are scheduled at the client's home to ensure psychological comfort and to allow a more realistic needs assessment.

The intake volunteer has considerable freedom in structuring the interview, establishing rapport, pacing the interview, phrasing questions, giving information, and assessing the need for immediate advocacy or intervention.

The interview covers client needs for physical and emotional support, along with family background, sexuality, medical, psychiatric, and mental health history, drug and alcohol use, employment and financial status, and leisure-time interests.

In addition to its role as an information-gathering procedure, the intake session is an important intervention in its own right. Some key functions of intake are as a:

• Focusing session.

The intake session helps clients focus on and understand their situation better—to think about where they are with their illness and the resources that are available to them.

It helps clients assess their current circumstances and also look toward the future and their own choices. What could financial planning mean for themselves and loved ones? What would they like to get out of supportive counseling?

• Space to discuss sensitive issues.

The few hours with a GMHC volunteer may be the first time that clients have ever been encouraged to reflect on and speak openly about a variety of sensitive topics—with the security of knowing that they will not be burdening or frightening a family member or friend, and that they will not be medically labelled for their thoughts.

Sexuality, suicidal thoughts, family relationships and disclosures about money may all be highly charged areas, and it may be the first time the person has been able to talk in a comfortable situation.

• Teaching session.

Clients often see the intake clinician as the AIDS expert. Intake volunteers are free to answer questions from their knowledge and experience. However, intake clinicians do not give medical advice, even if they are medical professionals. Intake clinicians can help clients figure out how to ask their own doctor for the information they need, or may help them identify a more appropriate person to ask.

• Welcome wagon.

The full range of GMHC services is described, whether or not the clinician anticipates that a given service will be needed or appropriate for that particular client. The intake clinician and client discuss and decide together which referrals to GMHC services should be made.

Intake reports may contain impressions and observations, but no "diagnosis" of a client's problems. Diagnostic categories are not as useful to lay volunteers as are careful word-pictures of a client.

III. Referral Planning

> "People's needs often change,
> due to the nature of the illness, the moods,
> the roller-coaster effect. At one intake, my
> client was very sick, allergic to his medicine,
> and all he could think about was getting help
> paying his bills. Within two weeks of our talk
> he realized that peer support
> is great to have, and asked for a
> crisis intervention worker."

All referrals for clients following intake are made under the direct supervision of the intake staff and with the assistance of office volunteers specifically assigned to intake.

After the complete intake report is reviewed, a one-page summary is prepared and copied for each service receiving a referral.

Among the policies for GMHC client services referral are the following:

- Volunteers cannot make referrals without client consent. If the intake volunteer feels strongly that a client would benefit from a service he/she doesn't want, that may be noted, with explanation, in the intake report. A staffperson may then recontact the client to reintroduce the possibility of that service and answer any questions before the treatment plan is finalized.
- No clinician can refuse to make a referral requested by a client, even if the clinician feels the service would not be appropriate. During the intake, the volunteer helps a client anticipate how a particular service might be used, by describing its purpose and limitations.

For example, a client who has heard about crisis intervention workers (CIWs) may specifically request this service. When asked how he/she intends to use the service, the client may only anticipate calling the CIW occasionally to get emotional support. The intake volunteer can explain the crisis aspect of the CIW role, can reassure the client that if a crisis emerges a CIW can be assigned later, and can offer other avenues for gaining emotional support (e.g., recreation, group services, occasional calls to the hotline).

IV. Ongoing Monitoring

The intake department remains involved throughout a client's relationship with GMHC.

1. New Requests for Referral

Whenever a current client needs referral to a new department, the client contacts the intake department and his or her treatment plan is reasssessed and updated.

2. Follow-up on Inactive Clients

Client files are kept within the intake department. A sticker on the outside of the files indicates the month of the last client contact. (The person filing a note from a buddy or showing attendance at a recreation activity in June will place a June sticker on the chart.)

If three months go by without contact, a volunteer calls to check up on the client. This helps monitor referrals, identifies unmet needs, updates client files, and helps assess client satisfaction.

Volunteers make the contact phone call from the GMHC office, under the supervision of a staff member. The format is a brief structured interview with questions about changes in health and emotional status, satisfaction, and unmet needs.

After the call, a client's chart may be refiled as deceased, inactive, or in need of treatment-plan reassessment.

3. Follow-up on Active Clients

To evaluate services more realistically and assess unmet needs, GMHC is beginning to contact a random sample of active clients to obtain their evaluation and reaction to service provision.

Volunteer Intake Clinicians

Intake clinicians must be able to perform an informal, yet complete, psychosocial assessment, and to communicate what they have learned in a way that is meaningful to lay volunteers, stripped of medicalese or psycho-jargon.

Thirty-five percent of these volunteers are mental health professionals; 40 percent are in other people-oriented professions such as nursing, education, or guidance counseling; and 25 percent are persons who have gained experience through their volunteer work with GMHC.

Group supervision meetings are held monthly. In addition, each intake report and treatment plan is reviewed by staffpeople who make the formal referrals, thereby providing ongoing review and supervision concerning the thoroughness and appropriateness of the interview, write-ups, and planning for services.

Four mandatory in-service trainings are offered per year. Recent and upcoming topics for the full-day sessions include:

- Neurological manifestations of AIDS
- Suicide
- Family therapy and family systems
- Cultural diversity: issues for volunteers working with clients from dissimilar backgrounds

In addition, optional in-service seminars are offered for intake clinicians to increase their familiarity with the workings of other GMHC services.

Crisis Intervention Services

Smoothing the Rough Edges

Crisis intervention services offers one-on-one volunteer assistance to PWAs. Volunteers perform a range of services as unique as the individuals involved: holding a hand; rehearsing what to say to Mom; carrying laundry; confronting a doctor; planning a daughter's funeral; listening to gripes and dreams for the future.

A volunteer may be there until the client dies, or may celebrate as the client regains equilibrium after a crisis and returns to work, or even becomes a GMHC volunteer.

Types of Crisis Intervention Workers

I. Crisis Intervention Workers

> "Over fifty, no family no friends,
> and trying to stay away from alcohol.
> I was desperate and panicked
> when they assigned my CIW."

Crisis intervention workers (CIWs) provide emotional support to PWAs, actively and carefully listening and responding as needed during a time of crisis. They maintain close contact (usually four to eight hours a week) while striving to strengthen the client's natural support systems. CIWs help clients organize the information and resources that they need. With the client's direction, they serve as a liaison to the social service/medical bureaucracy.

CIWs are not therapists or best friends.

2. Buddies

> "Someone who would go into the homes
> of people who were ill
> and do their shopping, walk the dog,
> clean up a little bit.
> Buddies were people who would act, toward strangers,
> as ethically they would act toward friends."
> —Dan Bailey
> GMHC Boardmember

Buddies assist PWAs (either at home or in the hospital) with daily living activities. A client may need someone to go to the bank, to help get to the doctor, or to cook a meal on the days the home attendant is gone.

Buddies are not nurses, maids, or substitutes for adequate discharge planning and home care services. They are caring peers who, during a crisis, are willing to lend a hand with daily tasks in order to free clients to put their limited energy into more healing, life-affirming activities. A client may be capable of shopping, but if it is so exhausting that it means missing group therapy or dinner with a friend, then shopping is an important use of the buddy.

Although they are not primarily assigned as peer counselors, their emotional support may be what the client values most.

While a CIW's work can sometimes be done over the phone, buddies usually visit a client several times a week. To facilitate frequent contact, buddies are assigned to clients in their own neighborhoods.

3. Crisis Management Partners

Crisis management partners (CMPs) are prepared to provide both CIW- and buddy-type services.

Always blurry, the distinction between CIWs and buddies is increasingly difficult to delineate. Clients requiring crisis intervention services usually have an array of needs, which include advocacy and physical and emotional support. The exact needs may change quickly and dramatically over the weeks and months.

GMHC hopes to train increasing numbers of CMPs, and fewer CIWs, in the future. An all-CMP volunteer program may be the only practical model for communities that are geographically dispersed or have a limited volunteer pool.

4. Pediatric Volunteers

In 1985, GMHC started a special program to reach children with AIDS. Pediatric volunteers provide emotional and practical support to children within both the hospital and family setting.

In addition to being a primary source of affection and social contact for children with AIDS, pediatric volunteers frequently serve as an advocate for the child and the family as housing and schooling decisions are made.

Because of the demanding nature of most children's cases, as well as the importance of consistency, two volunteers are routinely assigned to each pediatric case. These volunteers are organized into a separate team and receive more intensive supervision and guidance from staff clinicians.

How It Works

More than six hundred volunteers, members of thirty-seven volunteer teams, work for crisis intervention services.

Referrals for CIW, buddy, or CMP service are received by a coordinator on the GMHC staff, who contacts the leader of a team which has indicated it can accept another client.

The coordinator calls the team leader and describes the case. If the team leader has a volunteer who might be a good match, he/she provisionally accepts the case and contacts the volunteer.

The volunteer reads the intake report and arranges to meet with the client. After that, the amount and type of support offered is determined between them, with the volunteer getting supervision from the group leader during weekly telephone contact and monthly team meetings. Each volunteer only has access to the chart for his or her own client.

CIS volunteers try to keep a treatment plan, including short-term goals and the means they will use to achieve them. They keep records of all direct and indirect contacts with the client, and submit their notes and time records monthly.

Support and Supervision
"Volunteers are terribly afraid
they might do something wrong

and it will have disastrous, possibly fatal,
consequences for the client.
And 99.98 percent of the time, that's a groundless fear."
—Richard Dunne
Executive Director

Adequate support and supervision for volunteers are crucial.

Initially, GMHC tried to provide support for buddies via general meetings every few weeks. It didn't work. A consistent, small percentage of the volunteers attended the meetings, but many volunteers dropped out. Much more support was needed.

Now, GMHC uses a group model for support and supervision at all levels. Volunteers have monthly team meetings led by a team leader who is also a volunteer. Team leaders, in turn, have supervision meetings led by a staffperson.

"I'm not a group person,
but for this the group model works."

Each volunteer is assigned to a team of about a dozen volunteers doing similar work (CIW, buddy, or CMP). Volunteers are required to attend monthly team meetings held at a regularly scheduled day and time.

At team meetings, volunteers are responsible for:

• Briefly presenting what is happening with their case, which may include types of contact, progress in achieving certain goals, feelings about the interaction and support given.

"Teammates could recognize the value of
what someone else did
more than they could recognize the value
of what they did. So reporting
in a team meeting worked very well."
—Judd Mattes
Former buddy captain

• Offering and receiving emotional support and supervision. As one volunteer expressed it, "It's OK to feel angry or bored. It's like a new romance or anything else. For a while it's the greatest, and then it settles into a routine."
• Submitting notes for review and inclusion in the client's chart.

The team meeting may also include announcements from GMHC and information on new and changing services throughout the community; participation by a staffperson; or an outside speaker on a specific topic of concern to team members (such as dealing with clients' anger, handling bereavement).

There is no GMHC budget for the operation of teams. Team meetings are held outside the agency environment, usually rotating between the apartments of conveniently located team members who have sufficient space.

Each team develops its own personality and way of sustaining its members. Some are quite social—gathering outside regular team meetings for picnics, parties, and outings. Other teams feel that their members have very full business and social lives outside of GMHC, and a more businesslike atmosphere is maintained.

Backup for CIS Volunteers

For CIS volunteers to perform this demanding work on an ongoing basis, it is vital that backup support is available:

- When you can't be there.

CIS volunteers make a commitment to their client, but it is critical that they have adequate backup if there is an emergency in the client's (or their own) life.

> "We have to appreciate
> what a volunteer goes through when a client
> needs them urgently and they can't leave work."
> —CIW team leader

Most teams are organized in clusters to provide this support. In a 2 x 2 cluster, two volunteers are assigned to two clients. Each meets with the client and has access to the client's chart. Day-to-day support needs may be divided as arranged with the client, or one person may serve as backup to the primary volunteer. Sometimes a single complex case is best handled by two volunteers working together.

If backup is not available within the cluster, team leaders can always be called.

- When a client has psychiatric problems.

The Coordinator of Crisis Intervention helps with treatment planning, and consults and supervises all cases involving psychiatric or neuropsychiatric disorders.

- When a client dies.

After a client dies, the volunteer can turn to members of the team for understanding and support. Volunteers can take the time they need to grieve before accepting a new client, knowing that they are still a member of the team and are welcome at team meetings.

If a volunteer has lost three clients, a break from CIS work is encouraged—perhaps a shift to the speaker's bureau or another department involved in less direct service.

- When you don't know the answer.

Many teams have a team nurse or team financial specialist. They may never have their own client, but are available to answer questions and help volunteers determine whether a problem requires immediate attention or referral to another service.

It is fine for CIS volunteers to tell a client they don't know the answer to something—and to help the client find out by calling on GMHC volunteers and staff for direction.

- When the client just wants to talk.

Sometimes "just talking" is important therapy, and volunteers appreciate its value. As an example, one client was a woman living with her father, who didn't know her diagnosis. She was poorly informed and needed someone to talk to and ask questions of as they came up.

> "When your client gets a check in the mail,
> you're a hero.
> When your client needs a sounding board,
> it's hard to feel that you're doing
> a good job, that you're doing enough."

A distinction is made between peer support and friendly socializing. If a volunteer is primarily meeting a client to talk and go to the movies, it may be time to reassess with the client what the current needs really are. It may be time for the client to graduate to an "inactive" status, knowing that a volunteer can be reassigned at a later date if needed.

- When a client doesn't need you anymore.

The goal is to help clients reenter their own social network and develop new relationships. Team members can help a volunteer recognize, and appreciate, when it is time for a client to graduate from crisis intervention services.

"A CIW helped me figure out
what to tell my boss
and how to keep my health insurance.
After that, I was most interested
in talking to other PWAs
and people who knew about experimental treatments."

Supervision of Team Leaders

Team leaders are usually volunteers with significant on-the-job training. Each group has two co-leaders, so the leaders can divide backup and paperwork duties and lend each other support.

Team leaders are required to attend monthly supervision meeting. In addition, new team leaders receive additional supervision for at least six months.

Group Services

Talking It Out

Isolation, confusion, depression, anxiety. The emotions surrounding an AIDS or ARC diagnosis can be overwhelming, and are particularly difficult to deal with in the face of an uncertain physical prognosis, shifting social supports, and economic and political barriers.

Although all client services at GMHC are aimed at providing psychosocial support, group services is the department which formally addresses the psychological and mental health needs of clients. GMHC believes that therapy groups are an effective and efficient way to help clients adjust.

Therapy groups offer PWAs the opportunity to deal directly with social, emotional, and behavioral consequences of AIDS, to foster a network of mutual support and problem-solving, and to observe role models among other persons who are coping with the stress associated with the disease. Groups also provide clients with the chance to socialize in a relaxed and relatively informal atmosphere, thereby reducing social isolation and withdrawal.

Thirty percent of GMHC clients request group services, and over forty different groups meet weekly. Clients are referred to group services through the intake department, either as a result of their initial evaluation or in a later request.

In addition to the therapy groups for people with AIDS, groups are also available for relatives or friends who are the care partners of PWAs, and for parents, couples, and the bereaved. Rather than a full intake, these people undergo an abbreviated registration process in the intake department.

Intake clinicians and peer counselors may encourage participation in groups for clients who are feeling depressed, anxious, or out of balance; who want to talk to other PWAs; or who have questions about a new diagnosis.

All groups are led by mental health professionals on a volunteer basis.

Types of Groups Offered

1. Ongoing AIDS Therapy Groups

Therapy groups meet weekly. Most meet at one of the GMHC offices, but therapists may also use their own office space.

> "I've had a regular therapist for two years,
> but the groups at GMHC offered
> something quite different,
> a support I really needed."

People feel more than they can say individually; it helps to hear another person say it. The underlying goal of all talk-therapy groups is to help people verbalize, rather than internalize, their emotions. For PWAs such therapy helps remove one source of stress that can lead to further physical deterioration.

Specific goals for a group are as individual as the groups themselves. Even though all groups are structured as professionally led talk-therapy, the actual content and benefits may encompass:

- Strengthening social support. PWAs often need support to deal with the indignity and frustration of being a patient within the U.S. health care system. In the group setting, PWAs can share experiences, strategize, and bolster their skills at dealing with rigid and unfamiliar bureaucracies.
- Coming out. For many people, telling family and friends of an AIDS or ARC diagnosis means coming out to these people for the first time. Relationships may shift alarmingly or disintegrate during illness. Family, relationship, and intimacy issues are the top priorities among many groups.
- Sharing information. Clients often use groups to ask questions and swap resources about new treatments or available supports.

- Expressing difficult emotions. Significant persons in clients' lives often shrink from discussions of illness, loss, or mortality. Clients are encouraged to express and explore their feelings in therapy groups.

A GMHC client who has been newly referred to group service but is not recently diagnosed as having AIDS or ARC will tentatively be assigned to an existing group. The therapist for that group contacts the client and arranges an introductory interview. Together they make the decision about whether the individual will join the group.

Clients who join an AIDS therapy group area are asked to do four things: (1) to make a twelve-week, renewable commitment to the group; (2) to participate; (3) to be supportive to one another; and (4) to maintain confidentiality.

2. Walk-in AIDS Therapy Groups

> "I was offered a therapy group, but just couldn't
> make the commitment
> while my life was in such chaos.
> Drop-in groups give me
> a place to talk when I can."

Each week there are regularly scheduled drop-in groups for PWAs and PWARCs. There are very few requirements for participation in these groups. There is complete anonymity, no commitment to ongoing therapy, and no pressure to speak or to actively participate.

Walk-in groups are especially helpful for clients who:

- Have erratic work or treatment schedules, or those who travel frequently.
- Have severe problems dealing with intimacy. The disease exacerbates a lot of intimacy issues, calling into question how close, or how distant, a person wants to be from other human beings and how much emotional energy he/she wants to put into relationships. Because self-disclosure and the development of ongoing relationships are not required, walk-in groups are very popular with clients for whom intimacy is a major issue.

3. Short-term Groups for the Newly Diagnosed

People come to group services at varying points in the history of their disease. For newly diagnosed clients, GMHC offers four-session orientation groups, with a new group beginning the first week of every month. GMHC will soon offer short-term groups especially for persons newly diagnosed as having ARC.

The purpose of the short-term groups is to help clients become acclimated to working within GMHC and to become comfortable with group dynamics and open self-expression. For many newly diagnosed people who feel perfectly healthy, there is great fear and anxiety about meeting PWAs who have severe physical manifestations such as visible lesions or severe weight loss.

By dealing with such fears immediately and directly, GMHC has found that clients are better prepared to start group therapy and are less likely to withdraw from a group. It can also be disruptive to the progress of ongoing groups to continually integrate new clients who need answers to many basic informational questions.

After the four weeks, members of the newly diagnosed group (usually about fifteen people) may stay together to form an ongoing group.

4. Care Partners Groups

Ongoing and walk-in groups are available for friends, lovers, or relatives who help care for PWAs.

A care partner can make use of GMHC group services even if the PWA with whom they are involved is *not* a client. In some cases, a PWA's denial of his or her illness and subsequent failure to utilize support services is a source of tremendous stress to the care partner—and the primary reason that he/she seeks group support.

In the next year, GMHC plans to offer separate therapy groups for care partners who are also PWAs.

5. Parents' Groups

A weekly parents' group allows parents of adult PWAs to lend each other support and understanding. Group members seem to benefit tremendously from the peer support. Working with a therapist, they can also explore difficult feelings.

The parents' group is open to parents of nonclients. Not infrequently, the support is sought by the parent of a PWA who lives in another town.

6. Couples Groups

When group services first began, couples affected by AIDS contacted GMHC for answers to questions concerning sexual intimacy. A couples workshop—a fairly structured, four-week group—was developed in response to such questions.

It later became apparent that AIDS had a dramatic impact on the dynamics of a couple's relationship. There were many expressions of anger and fear, withdrawal and distrust. To answer the needs raised by the illness, GMHC offers three couples groups, each with six couples and led by volunteers with experience in couples or family counseling. Groups are ongoing, operating on a twelve-week, renewable cycle. This therapy is increasingly requested.

Couple status is self-defined—GMHC does not make a distinction based on sexual orientation or the nature of the couple's relationship.

GMHC previously offered separate groups for persons with Kaposi's sarcoma and for IV drug users. While GMHC recognizes the diversity of PWAs and their physical challenges, these distinctions are no longer made. Clients come to GMHC already feeling stigmatized and set apart by having AIDS. GMHC did not want to divide and stigmatize people any further by implying that only those with similar lesions, or a similar mode of transmission, could understand their feelings or be a source of support.

Volunteer Group Therapists

Eighty therapists volunteer with the group services department, conducting forty groups per week. Volunteers all have extensive experience as counselors, but come from a variety of clinical backgrounds—social work, clinical psychology, psychiatry, training in psychoanalytic institutes, and psychiatric nursing. About 60 percent of volunteer therapists are gay men, working in private practice or within agencies. The other 40 percent are primarily female therapists.

Each volunteer is individually interviewed and screened for clinical experience, emotional stability, AIDS experience, and feelings about working within a gay-defined agency. Experience in leading groups is *not* a prerequisite because of the scarcity of therapists with specific group training or experience.

Therapists who contact the GMHC volunteer office are told about group services, and usually meet with the department before participating in the three-day general training.

Volunteer group therapists are required to:

- Complete simple paperwork after each weekly session, writing a brief note about each client's participation and significant issues for that week.
- Make a one-year commitment. At the end of the contract, the volunteer meets with the coordinator to evaluate the experience and to make a decision about renewing the contract.

Therapists stay at GMHC an average of two years, with some staying five.
- Attend biweekly supervision groups.

Support and Supervision

Group therapists face many challenges in this volunteer work. Some issues that may be different from their usual practice are:

- Understanding and accepting negative transference. Although therapists may find it perfectly understandable intellectually, it may nonetheless be difficult or even intolerable for them when clients express anger and dislike toward them. As authority figures, group leaders are often the target of PWAs' anger.
- Defining success. People come into groups because they want to stay alive and they want to use psychological means to help them stay well. Therapists would also like to make people well, but if they hold this out as an unrealistic and unacknowledged success measure, it may cause great emotional stress.
- Countering early training to "be nice to sick people." Sometimes being therapeutic and "being nice" are at odds. "If a client with AIDS or ARC is berating a therapist, and that person's response is to treat them nicely, they're creating a very crazy world for that person," observes Richard Wein, Ph.D., who until recently was GMHC group services coordinator.

To assist group leaders and ensure high-quality group services, GMHC has several levels of support and supervision:

1. Co-leaders

Most therapy groups are co-led by two therapists. This is encouraged for two reasons. First, since the content of the groups is very difficult, it is helpful for leaders to have someone to process the content with following each session. Second, group leaders should be able to take a vacation or a break without disrupting the ongoing group.

Groups run fifty-two weeks a year with no break. If there is no co-leader, a substitute therapist acts as facilitator during the therapist's absence (and does not attempt to alter the direction the group is moving in). The necessity for continuity of care has been demonstrated frequently. For example, one therapist took a two-week vacation from a group that had functioned several months. During the break, five of the nine clients were hospitalized.

2. Supervision Groups

Each therapist is required to attend a ninety-minute supervision, group every two weeks. There is usually a mix of therapists with different backgrounds and therapeutic approaches. Supervision groups are led by a staff clinician with extensive experience in group therapy, and serve several purposes:

- Training. Supervision groups are also therapy groups and are designed to serve as a training model.
- Case supervision. Therapists are encouraged to discuss group issues or "difficult" clients during supervision.
- Therapy. All of GMHC's volunteer therapists express feelings of incompetence and helplessness. Therapists expressing "no problems," "no questions," or "no desire for supervision" are likely to be covering over these painful feelings. Such feelings are discussed frequently during supervision.

> "Those best able to do this work—and
> none of us are very good at it—
> are those who are able to contemplate
> their own mortality and the mortality of people
> who they care about and love,
> without invoking some kind of strong defense
> which would be either counterproductive
> or injurious in nature."
> —Richard Wein, Ph.D.

Therapists' own early experiences and personalities may cause them to interact with clients in ways that can either facilitate or hinder the progress of the group. The supervision group is a place to bring out and talk about these issues, both for the personal growth of the volunteer and for the success of the group.

Recreation Department

Reactivating Lives

Recreation services started modestly, with a Friday evening social and a movie. Now, 65 percent of clients—currently, about thirteen hundred people—participate in activities which range from crochet to candlelight dinners, from cooking classes to circus outings.

GMHC's recreation center is open five days a week, with a variety of weekend outings and cultural activities. The center includes a large open space, surrounded by separate office and small classroom spaces. It includes a kitchen, eating area, mini-gym, and small private rooms for massage, counseling, etc.

Goals of Recreation

"I was offered group therapy,
but couldn't see myself sitting in a circle
with a bunch of guys
talking about their feelings."

Recreation services offers clients a place to meet other PWAs outside of formal group therapy. It also provides a means for PWAs to reactivate their social lives at a time when they may have an excess of free time and a lack of money, physical strength, and self-esteem.

Referral

Clients are referred to recreation services through the intake department, either following the initial interview or later.

After referral, a client is invited to a group orientation, held two to four times per month. At this small, social meeting, the range of recreation services is described, along with the rules regarding participation.

This structured group orientation provides the client with an opportunity to see the recreation facility and meet other people coming in for the first time, thereby avoiding the stressful experience of walking into a group of strangers who already seem busy and comfortable with one another.

No formal recreation therapy plan or individual goals are set for clients. Significant aspects of a PWA's life may be dictated by medical therapy, financial limitations, and requirements of government agencies—all of which may result in feelings of dependency and lack of control. Recreation services attempts to offer clients maximal autonomy and input into their personal use of the services and how the services, as a whole, evolve.

Types of Recreation Services

I. Nutrition

A wide spectrum of nutritional problems is associated with AIDS. Some are physical—loss of appetite, nausea, diarrhea, fat intolerance, lactose intolerance, pain on swallowing, increased caloric needs, heightened need for sanitary preparation of food, and debilitating fatigue which may interfere with food preparation. Other nutritional problems are social—a severely reduced food and restaurant budget, cooking and eating alone for the first time, or housing with inadequate cooking and food storage facilities.

> "It can be a vicious cycle.
> An immune-suppressed person
> develops diarrhea. In response, he stops eating,
> loses weight, and becomes more immune-suppressed.
> He needs to know how to eat
> to battle the diarrhea and maintain his caloric intake."
> —Ori Caroleo
> Recreation Services

GMHC's nutrition program has three components:

1. *Nutrition Counseling.* Volunteer professional nutritionists offer individual counseling to GMHC clients. For a week prior to the session, the client is asked to keep a log of all foods consumed. The counseling offers:

- General information about proper food preparation, storage, and nutritional value
- Individualized nutritional and dietary assessment
- Training in how to monitor and assess nutritional needs and food intake
- Suggestions for eating changes to help remedy specific eating problems
- Encouragement to participate in group activities involving food
- Adjustments of client's favorite traditional foods to meet current nutritional needs

To adapt to a growing demand for nutritional counseling, the recreation department is initiating group nutrition counseling. With this format, there is a preliminary group counseling session, including a general discussion and distribution of informational materials.

Individual monitoring and follow-up for specific questions is then made available.

2. *Cooking classes.* GMHC offers six-session cooking groups for clients who want to learn to translate nutritional advice into planning and preparation of simple meals. Cooking groups prepare and eat meals planned with the advice of a volunteer nutrition counselor.

3. *Meals/Socials.* Meals are the most popular recreation service. GMHC offers two lunches and one dinner per week, cooked and served by volunteers. Meals are nutritionally balanced, providing large portions and a sampling of alternative food therapies (vegetarian, yeast-free, etc.).

> "I enjoy eating more
> when I'm with other people—
> and I won't deny that it's
> a big help on my food budget."

II. Stress Management

PWAs are under a tremendous amount of stress, which can further depress an already suppressed immune system. Recreation services offers two types of stress reduction programs for clients.

1. *Stress-reduction class.* For clients who have a limited understanding of stress management, an eight-week class is available to familiarize them with what stress is; sources of stress; and the impact of diet, lifestyle, and recreation.

In the class, clients sample various strategies for reducing stress.

2. *Access to stress-reducing techniques.* For clients who already appreciate the importance of such activities to enjoy and master yoga, t'ai chi, visualization, martial arts, and trager techniques.

III. Leisure Education

> "I was a lawyer."
> "I was a waiter."
> "I was an actor."
> "I was a hair stylist."
> —PWAs asked about what they do

AIDS often strikes people at a stage in their lives when they are largely focused on career activities and advancement. The diagnosis may mean losing the job—and along with it whatever identity and self-esteem were associated with it.

Clients can use the classes and activities of the recreation department to help refocus their identity on what they do in their free time instead of during the work day. A variety of classes and outings enable people to develop their leisure activities with a group and under the guidance of someone enthusiastic and knowledgeable in the specific area.

In addition, there is access to many theater and movie tickets for low-cost socializing, as well as free massage and haircuts.

There is a higher priority placed on offering a variety of activities than on selecting those which will appeal to the largest number of clients. In one case, a discussion group was usually attended by only one client. Since the two volunteer leaders did not object, and it was the only activity that the client was attending, the group continued for several months before other clients joined.

A monthly calendar of recreation activities is distributed, and new classes are announced on posters and given feature treatment in the eight-page monthly recreation newsletter.

IV. Volunteering

"My life had been very crowded
with work, with drugs, and with people.
Now, none of those things is in my life anymore.
I stay busy as a volunteer, and I like that the others
at the rec center really appreciate what I do."

Clients are encouraged to share their job-related and other skills and energy as GMHC volunteers. One of every four clients becomes a volunteer. They participate in all aspects of the program's operation, including office work, budgeting, cooking, helping maintain supplies and facilities, and leading groups and classes.

Volunteer opportunities are advertised in the classified section of the recreation newsletter.

Volunteers

A wide range of volunteers participates in recreation services. Professional volunteers may provide a service—such as massage, nutrition counseling, or haircutting. Others share their professional skill or hobby with a class.

In fields where it is applicable, volunteers must have obtained their professional license or work under supervision. Volunteers must *not* enter into a fee-generating relationship with GMHC clients.

Recreation volunteers are also active in preparing and cleaning up after meals, in logging attendance and making new clients feel welcome, and in the recreation office.

Each volunteer participates in the three-day general client services training and is then interviewed by the recreation director.

For supervision and support, recreation volunteers work in close communication with the staff and attend monthly supervision meetings.

Financial Advocacy

Claiming the Help That's Been Earned

> "Total financial crisis
> is what first brought me to GMHC."

In the United States, financial hardship and confusion almost always accompany AIDS. The financial advocacy department receives nearly one hundred new referrals per month—and more than 90 percent of GMHC clients use the agency's financial services at least once.

Financial advocacy has five goals:

- To assess the benefit eligibility of all clients
- To educate clients and volunteers in the benefit application process
- To advocate for individual clients with various entitlement agencies
- To provide emergency funds for clients who are unable to provide for food and other necessities
- To identify repeated problems in entitlement programs and advocate for policy and program change

The financial advocacy department has recently been reorganized to meet these goals more efficiently and with greater empowerment of clients. The approach has shifted from application processing to the present approach of client education with step-by-step guidance and individual advocacy on an as-needed basis.

1. Case Management

> "It was worse than a nightmare.
> I used to get
> physically sick every time I had to deal
> with the welfare office."

Almost every PWA, at some point, will come in contact with government entitlement programs—social security, Medicaid, etc.

When financial services started at GMHC, the goal was to remove the client completely from having to deal with bureaucracies and agencies. The intention was that PWAs could put their emotional and physical strength to better use in other aspects of life than in hassling with caseworkers.

The financial advocates attempted to provide management of clients' financial affairs. In one-on-one reviews of the client's financial situation, entitlement programs were introduced and eligibility for various benefits was assessed. The financial advocate completed application forms and kept copies of forms and supporting documents on file at GMHC.

Even when benefits were obtained smoothly and rapidly, this system sometimes created more stress for clients than it reduced. The less clients knew about entitlement agencies, the more frightening the systems became. A phone call from a caseworker, or a missed check, could instill understandable panic in clients who had been shielded from the application process.

2. Step-By-Step Guidance

> "When I got help from the financial service,
> they did everything for you. I appreciated it
> at the time but regretted it later
> when I had to deal directly with the agencies.
> It's important to learn the system."

When the client load became overwhelming, GMHC instituted benefits clinics for the many clients who were neither homebound nor hospitalized. After benefit eligibility was assessed (via a financial services questionnaire and a phone interview with a financial advocate), a group of eight to ten clients was scheduled to meet with one or two volunteers. At the clinic, clients were led, page by page, step by step, through the applications for all pertinent benefits (not unlike some college financial-aid seminars).

The atmosphere at these clinics was intended to be simultaneously relaxed, intimate, and anonymous. Clients gathered around a table and shared problems and experiences between line-by-line instructions. Full names were not exchanged, and the second volunteer was available to take aside anyone with a specific question pertaining to individual financial circumstances.

3. Education with Backup

Financial advocacy now includes education as the initial approach to helping clients gain needed services.

Clients are telephoned by a financial advocate, a GMHC staffperson, who does an initial assessment of the person's current financial situation and benefits eligibility.

Using this information, an individual financial packet is created for the client. It contains:

- All necessary applications
- Detailed fact-sheets for each application, including a description of benefits, instructions for filling out the form, addresses for filing, and when/how to follow up on the application
- Envelopes for mailing
- File folder for records
- Financial records sheet to record all applications and contacts with agencies
- General information and tips on filing
- Contacts and phone numbers at various agencies

Following the initial assessment, each client is offered one of the following options:

- To have the packet mailed so the client can complete and file applications with the written help provided.
- To register for a benefits seminar. Depending on the client's needs, the seminar format may be a question-and-answer session or, like the previous benefits clinics, a step-by-step guide through financial aid applications.
- To attend a question-and-answer forum for clients who are still working and not ready to file for benefits (geared toward preventive financial planning to avoid later problems).
- To be assigned a financial advocate for one-to-one support throughout the application process (for clients who need individual support and guidance).

At any point, a client may decide to register for a benefits seminar, to call financial advocacy with questions or problems, or to be reassessed for a change in benefit eligibility or for an emergency financial grant.

Starting in 1984 with a private donation to GMHC, the financial advocacy department has been able to offer small emergency grants. These grants (up to a total of four hundred dollars) are highly restricted—reserved for persons with a very minimal income who have already exhausted other means of support (such as family and friends) and who are waiting for benefits to start. Emergency grants are most commonly used to pay for prescriptions, rent, or to prevent utilities from being cut off for nonpayment. Occasionally, in cases of extreme emergency, a second grant is given. This must be approved by the financial director, client services director, and executive director.

Advocacy

Financial advocates on staff at GMHC address individual client difficulties and tackle systemic problems. The need may be as straightforward as finding out why a check didn't arrive, or as complex as picking up the pieces when a client has no money, eviction is imminent, and a prescription must be filled.

The financial advocates attempt to establish and maintain good contacts within the various entitlement agencies. Representatives of the agencies helped in the development of the education fact sheets for each entitlement program. They have a lot to gain—GMHC is doing the agencies a favor by helping people submit complete and accurate applications. The city of New York has recognized this service by helping to fund the work of the department.

Volunteers

Financial advocacy uses fewer volunteers than other client services at GMHC. Volunteers work mainly in three capacities:

- Providing office clerical assistance. The clerical support team, currently all GMHC client-volunteers, assists with the mounds of forms, supporting documents, and educational materials by gathering statistics, photocopying and updating information packets.
- Assisting homebound and incapacitated clients. Volunteers visit homebound clients to help fill out forms and to make copies of necessary documents.
- Monitoring financial assistance. About six weeks after the original financial assessment and applications process, a monitor telephones each client to review progress and alert the staff to problems, questions, or possible new service needs.

What the volunteers have in common is patience, attention to details, sensitivity, and good listening skills. Financial volunteers receive a special one-day training in addition to the full crisis intervention training.

The actual advocacy work of the financial department is handled by staffpersons. In working with agencies and bureaucracies, it is important to have consistency in people available for contact during the regular workday.

Volunteers do *not* assess clients' eligibility for benefits. The rules are complex and frequently change, and it has been a relief for most volunteers to know that such a critical responsibility is not on their shoulders.

Legal Services

Restoring Control to the PWA

Upon diagnosis, the PWA suffers an erosion not only of the immune system, but of the social support network, financial status, and legal rights. To provide a sense of empowerment and greater control, GMHC offers an array of legal services through volunteer attorneys. The services are meant to offer concrete solutions to practical legal problems that emerge for many PWAs.

The GMHC legal services department can be likened to a law office which has a general practice, or to a legal services clinic with very few eligibility restrictions. The unique aspect is that all of the work relates to the diagnosis of AIDS.

Who Is Served

The Legal Services Department serves persons with AIDS and ARC, regardless of whether that person is a client of GMHC. Restrictions on service include:

1. Residency. GMHC can only offer legal services to persons in New York City. Persons from upstate New York and neighboring states are referred to attorneys and legal services in their communities.
2. Income. GMHC prepares wills free of charge for people who have less than $5,000 worth of assets OR who make less than $25,000 per year.

This restriction is made in order to put the limited resources of the department to best use, and to better serve the PWA. The department provides valid, basic wills; anyone with substantial assets may benefit from more sophisticated estate planning.

3. Diagnosis. While GMHC is designed to serve persons with AIDS and ARC, within the Legal Services Department there is an important exception. If a person has been discriminated against because they are *perceived* to have AIDS, GMHC legal services will get involved whether or not the perception is correct.
4. Service required. GMHC does not become involved in issues (such as a divorce or a business dispute) not directly related to the client's diagnosis.

Referral

During the intake process, a one-page legal questionnaire is completed. It is designed to assess whether clients need to consult with an attorney regarding common legal problem areas. It also introduces the idea that wills and powers of attorney are prudent planning for most individuals. Through a series of questions, clients are asked whether they:

- Would like a lawyer to draw up or review an existing will
- Would like to designate someone to handle their business or medical affairs should they become incapacitated
- Need assistance with documents related to immigration law
- Are suffering landlord/tenant problems
- Need help dealing with creditors
- Are having insurance problems
- Are being discriminated against in employment, housing, hospitals, or other public accommodations

A decision on whether a legal services referral is desired and appropriate is made during the intake session. Whether or not a legal referral is made, the client receives "Legal Answers About AIDS," a sixteen-page GMHC brochure which provides answers to common legal questions and information about the legal services available at GMHC. Some of the information is general, but other answers refer to specific laws in New York State.

1. Wills and Powers of Attorney

> "Your will is your last laugh.
> It is your ball game, and you can
> do almost anything you like."
> —Mark S. Senak, J.D.

Inheritance laws apply to family members only (spouse and children, followed by parents). Gay couples have no such rights unless they do something affirmative to obtain them. A will is the only way to provide for non-family members.

Ambulatory clients requesting assistance with wills or powers of attorney sign up for a wills clinic, held four evening per week.

One or two volunteer attorneys staff each clinic, with a maximum of three clients per attorney in an evening.

Although called a clinic, the evenings consist of individual consultations between each client and volunteer attorney. The consultations include:

- Providing information and support for legal planning. Clients are told what a will can accomplish and how it works; and the consequences of dying without a will. GMHC information emphasizes the individual empowerment and personal expression of formulating a will.
- Gathering essential information—names and addresses of all close relatives, whether or not they will be named in the will.
- Ascertaining and recording the client's wishes.
- Drafting the will, starting from a basic will draft form provided by GMHC.
- Familiarizing client with other legal tools—a general power of attorney, a medical power of attorney and a living will declaration are explained and made available during the session.
- Encouraging clients to express their wishes regarding funeral arrangements and child custody, although these are not legally binding.

Putting the will into action. The attorney returns completed forms to GMHC for word processing of the final will. The client is then invited to the office for a brief execution ceremony under the supervision of a volunteer attorney (and in strict accordance with New York State law).

At this session, clients are once again acquainted with powers of attorney and a living will, which can be executed at that time if they wish.

Nonambulatory clients are also served by volunteer attorneys who agree to visit their home or hospital room. Although procedures are basically the same, volunteers have greater responsibility in nonambulatory cases. This includes making an assessment of the client's competence and recording any necessary notes for the client's file which will support the contention of the client's lucidity.

2. Insurance

Problems with insurance companies are widespread, often tricky to solve, and not restricted to PWAs. The most common problems with health insurance are:

- Pre-existing condition. The insurance company refuses to pay a claim because the claimant knew or should have known that he had the condition at the time of taking out the policy.
- Misrepresentation. The insurance company refuses to pay a claim, alleging misrepresentation of pertinent information on the insurance application.
- Stalling. The company delays payment indefinitely on sizable claims, waiting for supervisory approval or review.
- Inability to maintain insurance after leaving a job. GMHC advises people on how to make full use of their conversion rights under state and federal laws.

PWAs and non-PWAs increasingly find themselves "risked-out" of life insurance—denied policies because of a suspicious zip code, occupation, medical history, or same-sex beneficiary. In many areas, insurance companies may require that an applicant submit to an HIV-antibody test.

3. Discrimination

Discrimination against a person because of disability, or presumption of disability ("He's thin and gay, he must have AIDS"), is prohibited in New York State. Successful legal remedy has been obtained in instances of discrimination in employment, public accommodation, and housing.

4. Landlord/Tenant

Landlord/tenant problems can be a direct result of AIDS, usually involving housing discrimination, failure to pay rent while awaiting benefits, or harassment by a landlord who has become aware of the tenant's diagnosis.

5. Debtor/Creditor

GMHC lawyers can help to alleviate the stress of being hounded by creditors a PWA has no ability to pay. Although clients frequently ask about the option of bankruptcy, it is rarely a useful or necessary choice.

6. Immigration

An increasing number of GMHC clients are undocumented workers who do not have the citizenship status or on-the-books employment records to qualify for federal assistance programs. GMHC has been successful in obtaining limited recognition and benefits for individuals under the rules of the Voluntary Departure Program.

Volunteers

About two hundred attorneys volunteer with GMHC's legal services. Initially, the attorneys were recruited through word of mouth—largely through members of the Bar Association for Human Rights, a gay and lesbian bar association in the greater NYC area.

When attorneys volunteer, they are invited to a three-hour training session and given GMHC's "Volunteer Attorney Procedure Manual" covering estate planning, insurance, discrimination, landlord/tenant disputes, debtor/creditor disputes, and immigration.

A City Responds

Elizabeth Fernandez

IN THE EARLY 1980s, there was puzzlement and there was grief, but strongest of all was fear, fear distilled with dread.

A modern scourge that had no name was coursing through a benevolent city, a mystery that ravaged robust bodies and sent young men to their graves.

In short order, a virulent virus was identified and the illness given a proper medical name. Gay men and lesbian women, a group with enormous political and economic clout but often fractious as an entity, were galvanized in a unified force. They pioneered a landmark social-service network and spurred government response to the strange sickness.

And San Francisco became, for the world to hail and duplicate, the sterling prototype of a city best coping under the siege of AIDS.

The touted San Francisco AIDS model, a system of home care relying primarily on community volunteers and only secondarily on the medical industry, helped set national public policy. It contributed to the development of AIDS programs in cities from Dallas to Berlin.

But today, at a crossroads in the disease, the model is fatigued to the point of collapse. San Francisco, harder hit per capita by the AIDS epidemic than any other city in the country, is virtually tapped out, financially and emotionally.

Elizabeth Fernandez, "A City Responds," *San Francisco Examiner*, a Special Reprint, 20–24 June 1990. Reprinted by permission of the *San Francisco Examiner*.

SAN FRANCISCO LIVES WITH AIDS

June 1981—First articles appear in San Francisco's Sentinel (a gay newspaper) referring to a mysterious and "unique pneumonia" attacking gay men and causing deaths in Los Angeles.

Summer 1981—UCSF virologist Jay Levy and his colleagues are among the first three groups worldwide who say they've identified the HIV virus. His lab is the first to show that the virus infects not only immune-system cells, but brain and other cells as well.

1981—A 20-month-old Bay Area boy dies of AIDS after receiving contaminated blood provided by San Francisco's Irwin Memorial Blood Bank. His death is one of the first two in the nation linked to a blood transfusion and prompts the development of blood-donor screening tests.

1981—UCSF clinicians begin treating patients whose symptoms are later recognized as those of AIDS. By March of 1983 the clinic is well-established.

1981—Shanti Project, a counseling service for people with life-threatening illness and their families, started in 1974, begins seeing people living with AIDS. It is San Francisco's first support group for people with AIDS, before the disease even had an official name.

1982—The San Francisco AIDS Foundation opens its doors on Castro Street. In 8 years, it has grown from handling a half dozen clients to its current caseload of 2,225 on a budget of $4.5 million.

May 1983—First AIDS Candlelight March, now a nationwide phenomenon, is held in San Francisco and involves simultaneous city marches in New York and Los Angles.

July 1983—Ward 5B, S.F. General Hospital, becomes the first separate ward in the nation for in-patients with AIDS.

1985—An outgrowth of the nationwide "guerrilla clinics" movements. Project Inform begins acting as a clearinghouse that searches out, tests and disperses information on unapproved and experimental drugs. The drugs are made available to people living with AIDS, without FDA approval.

March 1985—Irwin Memorial Blood Bank becomes the first major institution of its kind to implement the HTLV-3 AIDS antibody test in screening donors to protect its blood supplies.

September 1985—Open Hand becomes the first food service in the nation to deliver meals to people living with AIDS in San Francisco.

October 1985—As part of an AIDS protest; placards bearing names of those who've died are placed on the walls of San Francisco's Federal Building. Cleve Jones builds on the idea, and the AIDS memorial quilt is begun.

October 1985—AIDS/ARC Vigil begins at the United Nations Plaza, in which demonstrators chain themselves to the doors of the Federal Building. The vigil is the first act of civil disobedience approved by a city government, in the form of a resolution of support by San Francisco's Board of Supervisors.

December 1985—UCSF dermatologist Marcus Conant and Dr. Jay Levy are the first to establish that latex condoms prevent the transmission of AIDS.

1986—UCSF researchers, under the leadership of Dr. Paul Volberding, are among the first to test AZT on AIDS patients.

April 1987—S.F. Health Dept. kicks off annual Safe Sex/ Condom Giveaway (4000 condoms and information pamphlets are passed out) at the Oasis and Caesar's Latin Palace, as part of its education campaign to inform Latinos about AIDS transmission.

July 1987—First annual AIDS Walk marks one of San Francisco's first broad-based grass-roots involvement in AIDS fund-raising. Moms, dads and kids in strollers walked alongside people with AIDS to raise $667,000. The AIDS Walk now raises $1 million annually.

September 1987—Pope John Paul II speaks to 62 people with AIDS at Mission Dolores Basilica. This is a major public acknowledgment of the Vatican's concern for people with AIDS, including homosexuals, whose lifestyle was called "an intrinsic moral evil" in 1986.

November 1988—Prevention Point begins an underground needle exchange program to check the spread of AIDS among IV drug users using contaminated needles. It trades more than 2,500 needles a week, making it larger than any of the five legal needle exchanges in Seattle; Tacoma, Wash.; Portland, New York City and Boulder, Colo.

January 1989—Protesting members of SANE (Stop AIDS Now or Else), an AIDS activist group, demand more affordable health care and compassion for people with AIDS and close the Golden Gate Bridge for 34 minutes during morning rush hour, creating an hours-long traffic jam; 25 demonstrators are arrested. (The bridge has been closed only 12 times in its history.)

July 1989—San Francisco Health Commission unanimously votes to allow condom distribution in the city jails to prevent further infection among the inmates. It is the first such step taken by a city government in California, where sexual contact between inmates is a felony, and third in the nation.

March 1990—San Francisco's Board of Supervisors unanimously approve legislation allowing city employees to donate the sick leave and vacation time to co-workers with catastrophic illnesses, including AIDS.

"The system is not prepared to deal with the doubling of cases expected in the next 12 to 18 months," says Pat Christen, head of the San Francisco AIDS Foundation. "The San Francisco model will not be able to support the need if there is not a massive infusion of funds."

Pushing the model to the brink, the lethal virus is penetrating broader segments of San Francisco society, striking the poor, minorities and intravenous drug users. These groups are traditionally the least equipped to set up a volunteer network, cornerstone of the gay community's response.

This city, where 100 people die of AIDS a month, has reached "the barrier," in the phrase of Dr. Paul Volberding of UC-San Francisco.

The signs of exhaustion are most vivid on the faces of front-line soldiers who have spent much of the last decade battling the medical enigma:

On the Castro psychologist who no longer allows himself to hope when he hears rumors of an AIDS cure.

"There have been so many mythical cures," says Leon McKusick. "There's five seconds when you start to think, my God, could this be over, but then reality checks back in."

On the community worker fighting to staunch the spread of the deadly virus into the black community.

"The drug epidemic is rampant, unemployment is rampant," says Gerald Lenoir, director of the Black Coalition on AIDS. "There are other priorities. When we come around and say AIDS, people don't want to hear it."

And on the exhausted young man who sadly left his post last month with the Names Project quilt, bombarded by sickness in the office and at home with his partner, Garth Wall.

"We've worked, believing we could make a difference," says Dan Sauro, 36. "But there is a cumulative effect. It's numbing. I almost find it hard to react these days, to feel.... Just yesterday I was at a memorial service for a friend and I felt no emotion. Maybe it's a self-protection kind of thing."

With an average of six people a day now being diagnosed with AIDS, the jagged statistical markings on The City's mortality charts have inexorably risen—5,692 people have died, the highest per-capita rate in the nation. Another 8,700 have been diagnosed and as many as 18,000 to 35,000 residents may also be infected with the virus that destroys the body's immune system, leaving it defenseless against devastating infections.

"We are a grief-struck city," says Dr. Sandra Hernandez, director of the San Francisco AIDS Office. "There has been a tremendous loss of young, vital life. It has set a tone of grief and fatigue and loss. It affects us everywhere, in our social life, in our business life. It has created a whole new demand of health care from a population who normally would be alive and well at the age of 32. It is changing the face of San Francisco."

Three days before Dr. Paul Volberding arrived at San Francisco General Hospital in July 1981, the first patient with the peculiar lesions checked in.

"I walked in and there it was," Volberding says.

Medical textbooks offered little advice. They told the young oncologist that Kaposi's sarcoma was a benign tumor afflicting elderly men. Volberding saw a 22-year-old with an aggressive tumor.

As the months passed, more and more young gays were afflicted with the same symptoms of purple spots and weight loss. In an unusual teamwork effort, local physicians and scientists collaborated with the gay community, holding town hall meetings and pooling limited knowledge.

A hallmark that came to characterize the disease was that it commonly affected the young—young men who were sick, young physicians who tried to help them. To doctors, the toxic new malady represented a singular challenge.

"It was an incredibly exciting period, in a lot of ways more so than it is now. In the early days, no one knew anything," says Volberding, an associate professor of medicine at UCSF and director of the AIDS program at S.F. General.

Holly Smith of the Shanti Project, one of the best-known volunteer groups, remembers the social stigma attached to the "gay disease," the fearsome uncertainties. "We didn't know if it was transmitted by air or by towels. It was this great unknown," says Smith, 36.

Hitting as it did almost exclusively in the gay community in the first years, AIDS became an unprecedented catalyst for community work.

From a hodgepodge of political and social clubs, an army of social-service volunteers was born, creating revolutionary programs to help stricken brethren. Not simply medical, but practical help was given—cooking, cleaning, services to help the sick stay home and out of the hospital.

This corps lobbied for blood testing when it became known that the HIV virus was sexually transmitted, and many fought to close public bathhouses, a symbol of gay liberation but also a dangerous source of contagion. They drafted safe-sex guidelines, and they demanded money from city coffers.

They became a new generation of heroes.

Given such prodding, The City responded to the surging crisis by instituting educational programs and portioning millions from civic revenues to fight the new disease. By many accounts, San Francisco officials mounted the fastest and most efficient municipal response to AIDS in the country.

In a rented second-floor office on Castro Street, with a single phone, a chair and a folding table, the AIDS Foundation was born, becoming a major link on the AIDS lifeline.

"The day the phone was installed, it started ringing and it's never stopped," says Cleve Jones, 35. "A line of men were outside the door that week, all with the same symptoms. There was no place else to go. They are all dead now."

Today Jones, one of the first AIDS activists, smiles as he flings his arm the length of Market Street. "This is my block," he says. It is neither ego nor exaggeration. Several of the buildings on the block belong to Jones-inspired organizations, most prominently the Names Project quilt, a 16-acre patchwork representing at latest count, 13,000 people around the country dead of AIDS.

"This is something all San Francisco should take pride in," Jones says. "Working-class, ordinary people with no special training were able, despite the terror of the situation, to create what was necessary.

"When I walk down Castro Street, I'm accompanied by ghosts, but always very proud. The epidemic proved something to us. We really are a community."

In less than a decade, the lethal virus sparked an explosion of social service in San Francisco, from five AIDS organizations in 1982 to 172 today.

The services run from educational and preventive to those that distribute free clothes, to a Zen hospice group, even to a pet-care program. With so many groups, cost inefficiency was inevitable, forcing a recent move to streamline and consolidate.

"I've never seen two agencies fighting over the same client," says Robert Munk, executive director of AIDS Service Providers Association of the Bay Area. "But it would be more efficient to have fewer agencies. There is duplication of administrative overhead."

Streamlining efforts have one chief purpose: to bolster the cracking San Francisco model. Overwhelmed by volunteer burnout and underfunding, the model paradoxically is also under growing pressure because AIDS patients are living longer, further straining resources.

"In a way we've shot ourselves in the foot," Munk says. "San Francisco has mounted an incredible crisis response, but it's lunacy to think we can continue with it."

To some of the more militant AIDS activists, the model was inadequate from the start for it relied excessively on volunteers and it failed to extend warnings soon enough to intravenous drug users and to ethnic minorities.

"The model is not a great truth in the sky," says Eric Ciasullo, 27, a member of ACT-UP, which next week plans a major demonstration on the "crumbling" model during an International Conference on AIDS here. "It has always been late responding and it has never fully responded. People who come here should see a system that is desperate and near collapse."

Increasingly, in the face of escalating cases, the local AIDS network is competing for smaller slices of city funds.

At the AIDS Foundation, for instance, the number of clients has climbed by 445 percent in five years, from 500 clients to 2,225, but the proportion of its budget from city funds has dropped from a third to a quarter. The organization in the last 18 months was forced to cut its staff from 75 employees to 55.

"The caseload is exploding but support from the government has declined," Christen says.

What will save the teetering San Francisco model is—not surprisingly—money, all sides agree.

"When people say the model is falling apart, I say the model is getting stronger," says Health Director David Werdegar. "There's much more involvement of the minority community. For all our faults, San Francisco represents the way it can be done.... I take the view that if they give us federal dollars, the San Francisco model will remain a shining example."

The overall goal is to bring $154 million next year to San Francisco from public and private sectors. During the last fiscal year, The City spent nearly $25 million in city revenue on AIDS. State and federal allotments to the San Francisco AIDS Office totaled $15.6 million, and total allocations for the upcoming year are only fractionally higher. But in the next four years, local treatment costs could run as high as $100 million a year, experts say.

Earlier this year, Mayor Agnos unveiled an ambitious blueprint to halt the tailspin dive of The City's model. Generating funding from state, federal and private sources, the $310-million plan would expand drug treatment and care programs.

In the meantime, however, valuable AIDS services are in jeopardy. Illustrating the touch-and-go frailty of some AIDS work, AIDS Benefits Counselors exists on $3,500 a month. The City promised funds for August and September, but the till was empty for June and July. The agency planned to close on May 31.

On May 29, two local residents stepped forward with checks.

"It looked like we were going down the tubes. This has been quite a cliff-hanger," says Audrey Doughty, unpaid head of the group. "We'll be able to get through the summer. After that, who knows?"

They are also struggling for volunteers, from a pool increasingly drained. The Shanti Project, to cite one program, has 63 AIDS patients waiting for volunteers.

Glynn Parmley, a 44-year-old San Francisco lawyer, illustrates the price paid by many AIDS workers.

After five years with the AIDS Foundation, after burying 50 friends, after so much stress he suffered a pinched sciatic nerve, Parmley is on a sabbatical relearning how to live.

"I found I was escaping from my grief and sadness by volunteering," says Parmley. "The more I got involved, the less time I had to think.

"You have to balance your life. You have to say this time is for work, this time is for volunteering, this time is for play. No one knew how to handle it. Most people don't have friends die like this."

AIDS, though, is a disease with an amazing capacity to engender commitment. Exhausted as they are, many AIDS workers say the illness is too gripping, too important to put aside.

Since 1984, junior high math teacher Michael Mank has been a volunteer counselor with the Shanti Project. He's had 13 clients; 12 are now dead. He accompanied them as they chose their caskets and he held their hands as they died.

"I can see them all today," says Mank, who does not have AIDS. "I wonder sometimes if I'm blinding myself to what I'm doing to myself. But it's like going through a war. You won't know until it's over what effect it has on you."

Bearing Witness

George Whitmore

> *And we go,*
> *And we drop like the fruits of*
> *the tree,*
> *Even we,*
> *Even so.*
>
> — GEORGE MEREDITH
> "Dirge in Woods"

Three years ago, when I suggested an article to the editors of this magazine on "the human cost of AIDS," most reporting on the epidemic was scientific in nature and people with AIDS were often portrayed as faceless victims. By profiling a man with AIDS and his volunteer counselor from Gay Men's Health Crisis, I proposed to show the devastating impact AIDS was having on a few individual lives. It had certainly had an impact on mine. I suspected that I was carrying the virus and I was terrified.

Plainly, some of my reasons for wanting to write about AIDS were altruistic, others selfish. AIDS was decimating the community around me; there was a need to bear witness. AIDS had turned me and others like me into walking time bombs; there was a need to strike back, not just wait to die. What I didn't fully appreciate then, however, was the extent to which I was trying to bargain with AIDS; if I wrote about it, maybe I wouldn't get it.

George Whitmore, "Bearing Witness," *The New York Times*, January 31, 1988. Reprinted by Permission of New American Library.

My article ran in May 1985. But AIDS didn't keep its part of the bargain. Less than a year later, after discovering a small strawberry-colored spot on my calf, I was diagnosed with Kaposi's sarcoma, a rare skin cancer that is one of the primary indicators of acquired immune deficiency syndrome.

Ironically, I'd just agreed to write a book on AIDS. The prospect suddenly seemed absurd, but "Write it," my doctor urged without hesitation. And on reflection, I had to agree. I don't believe in anything like fate. And yet clearly, along with what looked like a losing hand, I'd just been dealt the assignment of a lifetime.

That I was able to take it on isn't as remarkable as some might think. Kaposi's sarcoma alone, in the absence of the severe opportunistic infections that usually accompany AIDS, can constitute a fortunate diagnosis. Many Kaposi's sarcoma patients have lived five years and beyond. Although my own disease has steadily accelerated, I'm one of the very lucky ones. Although increasingly disabled, I haven't even been hospitalized yet.

I'm also hopeful—though it gives me pause to write that, since I value realism and pragmatism over the ill-defined "positive attitude" I'm often counseled to cultivate. Last summer, I began taking the antiviral drug AZT in an experiment to test how it works in people with Kaposi's sarcoma. Partly because testing has been completed on so few other drugs in this country, AZT or something like it is our best hope for an AIDS treatment and, in spite of possible severe side effects, it has already been shown to benefit other categories of people with AIDS. I have no doubt that, administered in combination with drugs that boost the immune system, antiviral drugs like AZT will eventually prolong the lives of countless people like me.

But I don't want to give the impression that I'm patiently waiting, hands folded, for that day to come.

When I began taking AZT, I bought a pill box with a beeper that reminds me to take the medication every four hours. The beeper has a loud and insistent tone, like the shrill pips you hear when a truck is backing up on the street. Ask anybody who carries one— these devices insidiously change your life. You're always on the alert, anticipating that chirp, scheming to turn off the timer before it can detonate. It's relentless. It's like having AIDS. At regular intervals your body fails to perform in some perhaps subtle, perhaps not new, but always alarming way. The clock is always ticking. Every walk in the park might be your last. Every rent check is a lease on another month's life. The beeper is a reminder that with chronic illness, there is no real peace and quiet and no satisfaction, not without the sure prospect of complete health. Paradoxically, this same sense of urgency and unrest enabled me to write my book.

Needless to say, reporting on the AIDS epidemic from my particular point of view has had its advantages and handicaps. My book includes my original article on Jim Sharp, then 35, a New Yorker with AIDS, and Edward Dunn, 43, his counselor from Gay Men's Health Crisis, both white gay men, like myself. But it also profiles men, women and children, black and brown, in all walks of life, who have been touched profoundly by AIDS, too. We are more alike than not. If I felt a special affinity for Manuella Rocha, a Chicano woman in rural Colorado who defied her family and community to nurse her son at home until his death in 1986, it was in no small part because I recognized in her eyes the same thing I saw in my own mother's eyes the day I gave her the news about myself. If I was scared sitting for hours in an airless room in the South Bronx with a bunch of junkies with AIDS, it wasn't because I was scared of *them*. It was because their confusion and rage were precisely what I was feeling myself. The journalist's vaunted shield of objectivity was of little use at times like those. On the contrary, what often counted most wasn't my ability to function as a disinterested observer, but my ability to identify with my subjects.

Although some reporters might, I didn't need to be told what it feels like to wait a week for biopsy results or to be briefed on the unresponsiveness of governments and institutions. Nor did I need to go out of my way to research issues of AIDS discrimination—not after I was informed at my neighborhood dental clinic, where I'd been treated for years, that they would no longer clean my teeth.

So, there's much to be said for subjective truth. Nevertheless, I worried for a long time about the morality, even the feasibility, of producing a documentary-style piece of reportage like the one I'd contracted for—that is, without literally putting myself into it, in the first person. It wasn't until I found myself alone in a cabin in the woods, poised to write, that I began to confront just who that "first person" had become.

The MacDowell colony in Peterborough, New Hampshire, is a collection of quaint artists' studios, each isolated from the others on 450 acres of dense woodland. Since 1907, the colony has served as a retreat and a safe haven for generations of writers, composers and other artists, and it surely did for me. But it would be a lie to say that people who go there can escape; up there, in the woods, the world is very much with you. Up there, away from my constant lover and loving friends, at a certain remove from the Catherine wheel of death and mourning that my life in New York had become, off the treadmill of interviews and deadlines, I came face to face with everything I'd successfully evaded about AIDS.

Having it, for instance. Before I went to New Hampshire, it was still possible, even necessary, to pretend that in some essential way I didn't have AIDS in order to keep working. As far as I know, no one I interviewed during the course of researching my book knew that I had AIDS. And the telltale marks hadn't spread to my face.

My body. I hadn't looked at it much.

Before I left for New Hampshire, at the Passover seder with my lover Michael's family, we took turns reading the Haggadah in booklets illustrated with line drawings. When we reached the page with the plagues God brought down on the Egyptians, there was a locust, there was a dead fish with X's for eyes, there was the outline of a man with dots all over him, signifying boils. I stared at the cartoon of the man with the boils. I knew Michael, sitting next to me, was thinking the same thing. My body was like that now. I'd had three lesions twelve months before. Now there were three dozen.

One day in New Hampshire, in the shower, I looked at my body. It was as if I'd never seen it before.

A transformation had taken place and it was written on my skin. When I met Jim Sharp three years ago, I have to confess, I could only see a dying man. A chasm had separated me from him and the other men with AIDS I interviewed for The Times. Even though they were gay, even though most of them were my own age, each one of them remained safely at arm's length. But now the chasm was breached and there was no safety.

Grief, despair, terror—these feelings easily come to mind when AIDS does. They threatened to engulf me when I began writing my book. But what about anger?

When you have AIDS, the fear and loathing, the black paranoia, the everlasting, excruciating uncertainty of AIDS colors everything. When you walk down the street with AIDS, everything in your path is an aggravation, an impediment, a threat—for what in your life isn't now? A cab overshoots the crosswalk. Someone at the head of the line is arguing with the bank teller. All the petty frustrations of urban life get magnified to the limit of tolerance. Not even the infirm old man counting out his pennies at the newsstand is exempt from your fury—or perhaps especially not him, for in the prime of life aren't you becoming just that: elderly and infirm?

It wasn't until I returned to the transcripts of my original interviews with Jim that I realized that he—a voluble ad man with a wicked sense of humor, a short fuse, and an iron will to live—had a special gift for anger, and Jim was now speaking for me, too.

Anger, life-affirming anger was the lesson Jim, Manuella Rocha, and that room full of addicts taught me. Without it, I couldn't have written about the ocean of pain and loss that surrounds us without drowning in it.

My article about Jim Sharp and Edward Dunn was a portrait of two strangers united in adversity. In 1984, after his lover died of AIDS, Edward felt compelled to volunteer at Gay Men's Health Crisis. He couldn't, he said, sit passively on the sidelines while the epidemic raged on. Jim's case was the first one assigned to Edward when he finished his training as a crisis counselor. It was Edward's job to help Jim negotiate the labyrinth of problems—medical, financial, legal—that an AIDS diagnosis entails. In time, they became remarkably good friends as well.

An intensely private person, Edward was willing to expose himself in a series of grueling interviews because he was, I think, desperate to make a difference. The sole stipulation he attached to our work together was that his lover be given a pseudonym. Edward wanted to spare "Robert's" family—who had never been able to acknowledge their son's homosexuality, even unto death—any possible hurt.

Soon after the article came out, Edward brought me a gift. It was a little teddy bear—a nice ginger-colored bear with a gingham ribbon tied around its neck—and I didn't know quite what to make of it. But Edward explained to me that he often gave teddy bears to friends, as they represented warmth and gentleness to him. Later, he asked me what I was going to name mine.

"I hadn't thought of naming it . . ."

"Oh, you have to name him," Edward said.

"I don't know, what do you think?"

"I thought you might call him Robert."

That summer, Jim, a transplanted Texan, moved back to Houston from New York. Then, Edward moved to Los Angeles, saying it was time to begin a new life. Perhaps grandiosely, I wondered if our interviews hadn't played a part in Edward's decision to leave the city—that perhaps they'd served as something of a catharsis or a watershed.

Over the next year and a half, Robert the bear sat on the bookshelf in the hall and only came down when the cat knocked him down. Every once in a while, I'd find Robert on the floor, dust him off and put him back on the shelf. I felt vaguely guilty about Robert. I was no longer in touch with Edward.

*   *   *

It has been called "the second wave" of the AIDS epidemic. Its casualties include, in ever-increasing numbers, drug abusers, their wives and lovers, and their babies. I knew one of those babies.

I first saw Frederico—this is not his real name—one gloomy day last March, in the pediatrics ward at Lincoln Hospital in the South Bronx. Room 219, where Frederico was kept out of the way, is down the hall from the nurses' station. Not many people pass by its safety-glass windows. I doubt that I would have known Frederico even existed had I not been told about him by Sister Fran Whelan, a Catholic chaplain at the hospital.

Sister Fran, a petite woman with a neat cap of salt-and-pepper hair, was instrumental in getting me permission to visit Lincoln to observe its "AIDS team." For a few months, I sat in on meetings, went on rounds with its members, interviewed patients and health-care workers, and attended the weekly support group for people with AIDS.

In the early years of the epidemic, when Sister Fran, a member of the Dominican Sisters of the Sick Poor, began working at Lincoln, there were no more than one or two people with AIDS in the hospital at any given time. By last winter, there were always more than two dozen, with dozens more on the outpatient rolls. Virtually all of the AIDS patients at Lincoln, a huge municipal hospital, were heterosexual, virtually all were black or Hispanic. Although blacks and Hispanics account for some 20 percent of the United States population, they now represent, nationwide, 39 percent of those with AIDS. In the Bronx, rates of AIDS infection are believed to be among the highest in the nation. Currently, one out of forty-three newborn babies there carries antibodies to the HIV virus, indicating that their mothers were infected.

When I first saw him, Frederico was 2½ years old and had been living at Lincoln for nine months. His mother, an alcoholic and former drug addict, had apparently transmitted the AIDS virus to him in the womb. The summer before, a few weeks before Frederico's father died from AIDS, his mother had left him in the hospital. Then she died of AIDS, too. From then on, Frederico was a "boarder baby," one of about 300 children living in New York City hospitals last March because accredited foster homes couldn't be found for them. Frederico happened to be disabled—he was born with cerebral palsy in addition to his HIV, or human immunodeficiency virus, infection—but lots of other children who were no longer ill and had no handicaps remained in hospital wards indefinitely.

Frederico's only visitor from the outside was a distant relation, a

Parks Department worker named Alfred Schult who came to the hospital religiously, on Tuesdays and Sundays. Frederico's mother had been, Mr. Schult later told me, "the daughter I never had." When she died, Mr. Schult sent a telegram to her widowed father in Florida. The telegram wasn't returned, but it wasn't answered, either. Frederico's father's mother, who lived in the Bronx, visited him in the hospital once, I was told. She had custody of Frederico's five-year-old brother, whom she'd sent to Puerto Rico to live with relatives. But no one in Frederico's father's family was willing to take Frederico. Nor was Mr. Schult, ailing himself, able to.

At 2½, Frederico couldn't talk. He couldn't sit up or stand. He couldn't hold a bottle. Since he'd never had any of the cancers or opportunistic infections that spell AIDS, his official diagnosis was AIDS-related complex, or ARC. He had not, however, escaped the stigma of AIDS. Sister Marie Barletta, his patient advocate at the hospital, had to argue long and vigorously with authorities and submit reams of paperwork to get Frederico into a rehabilitation day-care program elsewhere. Unfortunately, just when he was about to go to day care, Frederico got a temperature, so day care was postponed.

The hospital personnel and the volunteers who held and fed Frederico did the best they could.

The day Sister Fran took me to see Frederico, he was sleeping. We stood side by side, peering into his crib.

That day, he was wearing mitts made of stretch-knit bandage material knotted at one end and fastened around his wrists with adhesive tape. These were to keep him from scratching himself or pulling out tubes; sometimes Frederico had to be fed formula through a nasal-gastric tube taped to his cheek and nose, and sometimes he had to be given antibiotics intravenously.

The nurses on Frederico's floor noticed that he picked up everything, every little fungus, every little infection.

Stuffed animals were lined up at the head of Frederico's crib. A musical mobile of circus animals in primary colors was fastened to the headboard. A heart-shaped balloon with the words "I Love You" was tethered to the rail. Frederico was propped up in an infant carrier in the crib, facing a blank wall with a bed-lamp on it and a red sign that said No Smoking/No Fumar.

I stood next to Sister Fran, looking at Frederico. I heard a ringing in my ears. I almost bolted out of the room. Somehow, I kept my feet planted where they were on the floor.

I'd seen eyes unblinking from lesions. I'd spoken into deaf ears. I'd held the hand of a dying man. But nothing prepared me for this.

Frederico was beautiful. In his sleep, he expelled little sighs. His eyelids twitched. He was very fair, with light brown curly hair. His skin was translucent. You could see violet veins through the skin of his eyelids.

I wanted to snatch him out of his crib, snatch him up and run away with him. It was all at once horribly, cruelly clear that I wanted for Frederico what I wanted for myself, and I was powerless.

Later, walking down the hall beside Sister Fran, I struggled to retain my composure.

"It's good the nurses saw you with me," Sister Fran was saying. "Now you can come visit him lots, whenever you like, and there'll be no questions." Sister Fran has her ways. She knew I'd come back.

And I did, more than once. I held Frederico in my arms. He smelled like urine and baby powder, and he was quite a handful. He squirmed in my arms. I was a stranger. He didn't know me. He wanted to be put down.

The day I first saw Frederico, when Sister Fran was distracted for a moment, I took Robert the bear out of the plastic bag I was carrying and set him down among the other stuffed animals in the crib. I had felt I shouldn't come empty-handed. I knew Edward would approve. What I didn't know was that Edward had AIDS and would die before the year was out.

Irony of ironies, Jim outlived Edward, the counselor sent to aid him in his affliction.

Today, Jim lives in a modest bungalow house on a tree-lined street in Houston, where I visited him last June. He's something of a celebrity and has served on the board of the local AIDS foundation. He spends lots of time every day on the phone, dispensing comfort and advice to other people with AIDS. Among his other distinctions, Jim is probably the only man with AIDS in Texas who has lived through the mandatory two-year waiting period there to collect Medicare.

As we sat talking in Jim's living room, I noticed, on the mantelpiece, the stuffed piranha Edward once brought back from Brazil and gave to him, joking that, "This is what you look like when you don't get your way."

I remember vividly my reaction to the piranha, when I first interviewed Jim in New York three years ago—with its slimy hide and repulsive grin, it was the perfect image of AIDS to me. Now it seemed strange to see it in a living room in Texas, alongside all the ordinary things people accumulate. Still fearsome, still bristling with malevolence, the piranha had nevertheless somehow grown familiar, almost domesticated, like the gnawing terror Jim and I and thousands like us have had to learn to accommodate. Every time he has to go to the hospital, Jim told me, he takes along the piranha. It's a kind of talisman.

A week after I got back from Texas, Mr. Schult called to tell me Frederico was dead.

Things had been looking up for Frederico. Sister Barletta had finally gotten him into day care. The agency had placed him in a foster home. But on his second night outside the hospital, inexplicably, Frederico turned blue. By the time the ambulance arrived, he was dead. And for some reason, I was told, the emergency medical service didn't even try to revive him.

I went to the funeral parlor. The long, low, dim basement room in East Harlem seemed full to overflowing with grieving women—Sister Barletta, the women from Frederico's daycare center, nurses and volunteers who'd taken care of Frederico in the hospital—all of them asking why.

Frederico's body lay up front in a little coffin lined with swagged white satin. He was dressed in a blue playsuit with speedboats on it.

"You dressed him in a playsuit," I said to Mr. Schult, at my side.

"And now he's at play," Mr. Schult sobbed. "He's romping in heaven now with Jesus like he never was able to down here."

I held Mr. Schult's arm tightly until the sobbing passed. I couldn't help but notice, the coffin was too small for the top of the catafalque. You could see gouges and scrapes and scars in the wood in the parts the coffin didn't cover. I looked down into the coffin, at the body beyond help. I agreed aloud with Mr. Schult that Frederico was in heaven now, because it seemed to make him feel a little better.

I don't know why, but I always thought Frederico would live.

Contributors

Nancy F. McKenzie, Ph.D., is Executive Director, the Health Policy Advisory Center, New York City.

Anthony S. Fauci, M.D., is Director of the National Institute of Allergy and Infectious Diseases, National Institutes of Health, Bethesda, Maryland.

Peter H. Duesberg, Ph.D., is Professor of Molecular Biology in the Department of Molecular Biology, University of California, Berkeley, California.

Stephen Jay Gould, Ph.D., is Professor of Biology at Harvard University.

Larry Kramer, the co-founder of Gay Men's Health Crisis, is the author of *The Normal Heart*, a play about the HIV epidemic, and an AIDS activist.

Harlon L. Dalton is Associate Professor of Law at Yale Law School and a member of the National Commission on AIDS.

The Working Group on Care and Service Needs of the Citizens Commission on AIDS consists of Peter Arno, Ph.D., and Jesse Green, Ph.D., Co-Chairs; Peter Drucker, Ph.D., Montefiore Medical Center; John Griggs, United Hospital Fund; John Jacobi, Office of the Public Advocate, State of New Jersey; Margaret Nichols, Community-Based Organizations Consultant, New Jersey; Gerald Oppenheimer, Brooklyn College. The final report, *The Crisis in Care* was also prepared by Gary Stein, Carol Levine, and Harold Fernandez of the commission.

Ernest Drucker, Ph.D., is Director of the Division of Community Health, Department of Epidemiology and Social Medicine, Montefiore Medical Center/Albert Einstein College of Medicine, New York City.

Peter Arno, Ph.D., is Assistant Professor, Department of Epidemiology and Social Medicine, Montefiore Medical Center/Albert Einstein College of Medicine, New York City.

Kathryn Anastos, M.D., is Director of the AIDS Clinic at Bronx Lebanon Hospital in New York City.

Carola Marte, M.D., is a physician with the Community Health Project in New York City.

Carol Levine, M.A., is Executive Director of the Citizens Commission on AIDS for New York City and northern New Jersey.

Karen Davis, Ph.D., is Professor and Chairman of the Department of Health Policy and Management at Johns Hopkins University, School of Hygiene and Public Health, Baltimore.

Diane Rowland, Ph.D., is Professor in the Department of Health Policy and Management at Johns Hopkins University, School of Hygiene and Public Health; and Senior Staff Associate, Subcommittee on Health and the Environment, U.S. Congress.

The Clearinghouse Review is published monthly by the National Health Law Program, Los Angeles, California, and Washington, D.C. NHeLP is an advocacy law project serving the poor, minorities, and the aged in their quest for equity and non-discrimination in federal, state, local, and private health care programs.

Jesse Green, Ph.D., is Assistant Professor in the Department of Health Policy Research, New York University Medical Center.

David Barr is an attorney with the Gay Men's Health Crisis in New York City.

Allan M. Brandt, Ph.D., is Associate Professor of the History of Medicine and Science, Department of Social Medicine and Health Policy, Harvard Medical School, Boston.

Ronald Bayer, Ph.D., is Associate Professor and A. Sheldon Andelson AmFar Scholar, School of Public Health, Columbia University, New York City.

Susan M. Wolf, J.D., is Associate for Law, Hastings Center, Briarcliff Manor, New York.

June E. Osborn, M.D., is Dean of the School of Public Health, the University of Michigan, Ann Arbor, Michigan and a Member of the National Commission on AIDS.

Dan Beauchamp, Ph.D., is Professor of Health Policy and Administration, School of Pubic Health; and Professor of Social and Administrative Medicine, School of Medicine, University of North Carolina, Chapel Hill.

Michael H. Kottow, M.D., is Associate Professor of Ophthalmology, University of Chile, Santiago.

Richard Mohr, Ph.D., is Professor in the Department of Philosophy, University of Illinois, Champaign/Urbana.

David I. Schulman was the first full-time government AIDS discimination attorney, is Supervising Attorney for the AIDS/HIV Discrimination Unit, Los Angeles City Attorney's Office, Los Angeles, California, and a member of the National Committee on AIDS of the Union of American Hebrew Congregations.

Nancy Stoller Shaw, Ph.D., teaches Community Studies at the University of California, Santa Cruz. From 1984 to 1987 she was the coordinator of programs for women at the San Francisco AIDS Foundation.

Ronald L. Braithwaite, Ph.D., is Associate Professor, Department of Community Health/Preventive Medicine and Director, Community Health Intervention, Morehouse School of Medicine, Atlanta.

Ngina Lythcott, Dr. PH, is Senior Associate Dean, Dartmouth College, New Hampshire.

Ed Wolf is a Shanti Staff Counselor, the Shanti Project, San Francisco General Hospital.

William Deresiewicz is on the editorial board of *Health/PAC Bulletin*.

Lewis Katoff, Ph.D., is Director of Client Services, Gay Men's Health Crisis, New York City.

Susan Ince is a medical writer in New York City.

Elizabeth Fernandez is a staff reporter for the *San Francisco Examiner*.

George Whitmore died April 1989. He was the author of *Someone Was Here*, a book on the HIV epidemic.

MODERN TIMES ... MODERN ISSUES